Botulinum Neurotoxins and Nervous System

Botulinum Neurotoxins and Nervous System: Future Challenges for Novel Indications

Editor

Siro Luvisetto

MDPI • Basel • Beijing • Wuhan • Barcelona • Belgrade • Manchester • Tokyo • Cluj • Tianjin

Editor
Siro Luvisetto
Institute of Biochemistry and Cell Biology (IBBC)
National Research Council (CNR) of Italy
Italy

Editorial Office
MDPI
St. Alban-Anlage 66
4052 Basel, Switzerland

This is a reprint of articles from the Special Issue published online in the open access journal *Toxins* (ISSN 2072-6651) (available at: https://www.mdpi.com/journal/toxins/special_issues/Botulinum_Neurotoxins).

For citation purposes, cite each article independently as indicated on the article page online and as indicated below:

LastName, A.A.; LastName, B.B.; LastName, C.C. Article Title. *Journal Name* **Year**, *Article Number*, Page Range.

ISBN 978-3-03943-456-5 (Hbk)
ISBN 978-3-03943-457-2 (PDF)

Contents

About the Editor ix

Siro Luvisetto
Introduction to the Toxins Special Issue on Botulinum Neurotoxins in the Nervous System: Future Challenges for Novel Indications
Reprinted from: *Toxins* **2020**, *12*, 601, doi:10.3390/toxins12090601 1

Elina Zakin and David Simpson
Botulinum Toxin in Management of Limb Tremor
Reprinted from: *Toxins* **2017**, *9*, 365, doi:10.3390/toxins9110365 7

Nicki Niemann and Joseph Jankovic
Botulinum Toxin for the Treatment of Hand Tremor
Reprinted from: *Toxins* **2018**, *10*, 299, doi:10.3390/toxins10070299 13

Olivia Samotus, Jack Lee and Mandar Jog
Transitioning from Unilateral to Bilateral Upper Limb Tremor Therapy for Parkinson's Disease and Essential Tremor Using Botulinum Toxin: Case Series
Reprinted from: *Toxins* **2018**, *10*, 394, doi:10.3390/toxins10100394 23

Raymond L Rosales, Jovita Balcaitiene, Hugues Berard, Pascal Maisonobe, Khean Jin Goh, Witsanu Kumthornthip, Mazlina Mazlan, Lydia Abdul Latif, Mary Mildred D. Delos Santos, Chayaporn Chotiyarnwong, Phakamas Tanvijit, Odessa Nuez and Keng He Kong
Early AbobotulinumtoxinA (Dysport®) in Post-Stroke Adult Upper Limb Spasticity: ONTIME Pilot Study
Reprinted from: *Toxins* **2018**, *10*, 253, doi:10.3390/toxins10070253 33

Jong-Min Lee, Jean-Michel Gracies, Si-Bog Park, Kyu Hoon Lee, Ji Yeong Lee and Joon-Ho Shin
Botulinum Toxin Injections and Electrical Stimulation for Spastic Paresis Improve Active Hand Function Following Stroke
Reprinted from: *Toxins* **2018**, *10*, 426, doi:10.3390/toxins10110426 45

Giancarlo Ianieri, Riccardo Marvulli, Giulia Alessia Gallo, Pietro Fiore and Marisa Megna
"Appropriate Treatment" and Therapeutic Window in Spasticity Treatment with IncobotulinumtoxinA: From 100 to 1000 Units
Reprinted from: *Toxins* **2018**, *10*, 140, doi:10.3390/toxins10040140 57

Yoon Seob Kim, Eun Sun Hong and Hei Sung Kim
Botulinum Toxin in the Field of Dermatology: Novel Indications
Reprinted from: *Toxins* **2017**, *9*, 403, doi:10.3390/toxins9120403 69

Parisa Gazerani
Antipruritic Effects of Botulinum Neurotoxins
Reprinted from: *Toxins* **2018**, *10*, 143, doi:10.3390/toxins10040143 87

Roshni Ramachandran, Marc J. Marino, Snighdha Paul, Zhenping Wang, Nicholas L. Mascarenhas, Sabine Pellett, Eric A. Johnson, Anna DiNardo and Tony L. Yaksh
A Study and Review of Effects of Botulinum Toxins on Mast Cell Dependent and Independent Pruritus
Reprinted from: *Toxins* **2018**, *10*, 134, doi:10.3390/toxins10040134 105

Ioana Ion, Dimitri Renard, Anne Le Floch, Marie De Verdal, Stephane Bouly, Anne Wacongne, Alessandro Lozza and Giovanni Castelnovo
Monocentric Prospective Study into the Sustained Effect of Incobotulinumtoxin A (XEOMIN®) Botulinum Toxin in Chronic Refractory Migraine
Reprinted from: *Toxins* **2018**, *10*, 221, doi:10.3390/toxins10060221 . . . . **119**

Elena Fonfria, Jacquie Maignel, Stephane Lezmi, Vincent Martin, Andrew Splevins, Saif Shubber, Mikhail Kalinichev, Keith Foster, Philippe Picaut and Johannes Krupp
The Expanding Therapeutic Utility of Botulinum Neurotoxins
Reprinted from: *Toxins* **2018**, *10*, 208, doi:10.3390/toxins10050208 . . . . **127**

Josephine Sandahl Michelsen, Gitte Normann and Christian Wong
Analgesic Effects of Botulinum Toxin in Children with CP
Reprinted from: *Toxins* **2018**, *10*, 162, doi:10.3390/toxins10040162 . . . . **155**

Yongki Lee, Chul Joong Lee, Eunjoo Choi, Pyung Bok Lee, Ho-Jin Lee and Francis Sahngun Nahm
Lumbar Sympathetic Block with Botulinum Toxin Type A and Type B for the Complex Regional Pain Syndrome
Reprinted from: *Toxins* **2018**, *10*, 164, doi:10.3390/toxins10040164 . . . . **167**

Jihye Park and Myung Eun Chung
Botulinum Toxin for Central Neuropathic Pain
Reprinted from: *Toxins* **2018**, *10*, 224, doi:10.3390/toxins10060224 . . . . **175**

Alba Finocchiaro, Sara Marinelli, Federica De Angelis, Valentina Vacca, Siro Luvisetto and Flaminia Pavone
Botulinum Toxin B Affects Neuropathic Pain but Not Functional Recovery after Peripheral Nerve Injury in a Mouse Model
Reprinted from: *Toxins* **2018**, *10*, 128, doi:10.3390/toxins10030128 . . . . **189**

Ewelina Rojewska, Anna Piotrowska, Katarzyna Popiolek-Barczyk and Joanna Mika
Botulinum Toxin Type A—A Modulator of Spinal Neuron–Glia Interactions under Neuropathic Pain Conditions
Reprinted from: *Toxins* **2018**, *10*, 145, doi:10.3390/toxins10040145 . . . . **207**

Ya-Fang Wang, Fu Liu, Jing Lan, Juan Bai and Xia-Qing Li
The Effect of Botulinum Neurotoxin Serotype a Heavy Chain on the Growth Related Proteins and Neurite Outgrowth after Spinal Cord Injury in Rats
Reprinted from: *Toxins* **2018**, *10*, 66, doi:10.3390/toxins10020066 . . . . **219**

Hyun Seok and Seong-Gon Kim
Correction of Malocclusion by Botulinum Neurotoxin Injection into Masticatory Muscles
Reprinted from: *Toxins* **2018**, *10*, 27, doi:10.3390/toxins10010027 . . . . **233**

Kazuya Yoshida
Botulinum Neurotoxin Injection for the Treatment of Recurrent Temporomandibular Joint Dislocation with and without Neurogenic Muscular Hyperactivity
Reprinted from: *Toxins* **2018**, *10*, 174, doi:10.3390/toxins10050174 . . . . **247**

Domenico A. Restivo, Mariangela Panebianco, Antonino Casabona, Sara Lanza, Rosario Marchese-Ragona, Francesco Patti, Stefano Masiero, Antonio Biondi and Angelo Quartarone
Botulinum Toxin A for Sialorrhoea Associated with Neurological Disorders: Evaluation of the Relationship between Effect of Treatment and the Number of Glands Treated
Reprinted from: *Toxins* **2018**, *10*, 55, doi:10.3390/toxins10020055 . . . . **261**

Marius Alexandru Moga, Oana Gabriela Dimienescu, Andreea Bălan, Ioan Scârneciu, Barna Barabaș and Liana Pleș
Therapeutic Approaches of Botulinum Toxin in Gynecology
Reprinted from: *Toxins* **2018**, *10*, 169, doi:10.3390/toxins10040169 . . . . **271**

Jia-Fong Jhang and Hann-Chorng Kuo
Novel Applications of OnabotulinumtoxinA in Lower Urinary Tract Dysfunction
Reprinted from: *Toxins* **2018**, *10*, 260, doi:10.3390/toxins10070260 . . . . **301**

Matteo Caleo and Laura Restani
Exploiting Botulinum Neurotoxins for the Study of Brain Physiology and Pathology
Reprinted from: *Toxins* **2018**, *10*, 175, doi:10.3390/toxins10050175 . . . . **313**

Veronica Antipova, Andreas Wree, Carsten Holzmann, Teresa Mann, Nicola Palomero-Gallagher, Karl Zilles, Oliver Schmitt and Alexander Hawlitschka
Unilateral Botulinum Neurotoxin-A Injection into the Striatum of C57BL/6 Mice Leads to a Different Motor Behavior Compared with Rats
Reprinted from: *Toxins* **2018**, *10*, 295, doi:10.3390/toxins10070295 . . . . **325**

Luca Bano, Elena Tonon, Ilenia Drigo, Marco Pirazzini, Angela Guolo, Giovanni Farina, Fabrizio Agnoletti and Cesare Montecucco
Detection of *Clostridium tetani* Neurotoxins Inhibited In Vivo by Botulinum Antitoxin B: Potential for Misleading Mouse Test Results in Food Controls
Reprinted from: *Toxins* **2018**, *10*, 248, doi:10.3390/toxins10060248 . . . . **347**

About the Editor

Siro Luvisetto obtained his degree in Chemistry at the University of Padova (Italy). After graduating in 1984, he started his scientific career at the Institute of General Pathology (University of Padova, Italy), where studied mitochondrial physiology with an emphasis on energy conversion during mitochondrial oxidative phosphorylation. In 1987, he was a Visiting Scientist at the Department of Membrane Research of the Weizmann Institute of Science (Rehovot, Israel). In 1988, he obtained a permanent position as a researcher at the National Research Council of Italy (CNR) at the Center for the Study of Mitochondrial Physiology (Padua, Italy). In 1997, he joined the CNR Centre for Biomembranes Study where he changed his research interest toward the biophysics characterization of high-voltage-activated neuronal calcium channels responsible for the familial hemiplegic migraine. In 2001, he moved to Rome where he worked at the CNR Institute of Neuroscience after, then at CNR Institute of Cell Biology and Neurobiology, and, presently, at the CNR Institute of Biochemistry and Cell Biology where he is studying the pharmacology of pain modulation and peripheral nerve regeneration after peripheral nerve injury in animal models. Specifically, his main interest is in the effects of botulinum neurotoxins, serotype A and B, in peripheral regeneration after peripheral nerve injury. Dr. Luvisetto has authored and co-authored more than 90 peer-reviewed journal articles, including reviews and book chapters. He has been an invited speaker at several international and national conferences and meetings. He is an active member of some national and international professional associations. He has served as a reviewer for many scientific journals.

toxins

MDPI

Editorial

Introduction to the Toxins Special Issue on Botulinum Neurotoxins in the Nervous System: Future Challenges for Novel Indications

Siro Luvisetto

National Research Council of Italy-CNR, Institute of Biochemistry and Cell Biology (IBBC), via Ercole Ramarini 32, Monterotondo Scalo, 00015 Roma, Italy; siro.luvisetto@cnr.it

Received: 14 September 2020; Accepted: 14 September 2020; Published: 17 September 2020

Botulinum toxins (BoNTs) are a true wonder of nature. Like Dr. Jekyll and Mr. Hyde, they have a double "personality", making them unique among the toxins of bacterial origin. As Dr. Jekyll, BoNTs are drugs approved for a variety of clinical conditions while, as Mr. Hyde, they are one of the most dangerous toxins, causing botulism. In the past, many studies have extensively investigated the mechanism of action of BoNTs, showing a variety of apparently different mechanisms which have in common the block of the cholinergic transmission, mainly at the neuromuscular junction. These discoveries gave an extraordinary consensus to therapeutical use of BoNTs in human pathologies characterized by excessive muscle contractions, i.e., hypercholinergic dysfunctions including torticollis, blepharospasms, dystonia, and so on. Recently, the list of human disorders in which treatments with BoNTs have produced, or are expected to produce, beneficial effects is long and continuously growing. The ambitious goal of this Special Issue of *Toxins* was to provide an up-to-date picture on the state of studies for the development of new therapeutic treatments with BoNTs, mainly with serotypes A (BoNT/A) or B (BoNT/B). This Editorial is an introduction to the 25 contributions (14 research and 11 review papers) collected in this Special Issue of *Toxins*, which I strongly invite you to read in their original versions.

The first three papers focus on the treatment with BoNT/A of limb essential tremors (ETs), a neurology condition characterized by persistent postural, or kinetic, tremor due to involuntary rhythmic muscle activity of the upper or lower limbs, neck, and trunk. In detail, Zakin and Simpson [1] contributed with an overview on the techniques for BoNT/A injection, together with muscle targeting techniques, in the treatment of ETs. Niemann and Jankovic [2] reported the results of a retrospective study performed on a large database of patients treated with BoNT/A for hand tremor of different origins, mainly ETs but also dystonic, Parkinsonian, and cerebellar. Finally, Samotu et al. [3] analyzed the efficacy of BoNT/A in one open-label trial, with participants affected by Parkinson's disease (PD) and ETs.

Three clinical studies investigated the effects of BoNT/A in post-stroke spasticity (PSS), a common impairment arising from involuntary activation of muscles that often appears after stroke. Rosales et al. [4] performed a clinical trial (ONTIME) in post-stroke patients with spastic paresis, and analyzed the impact of BoNT/A on symptomatic spasticity progression. ONTIME provided evidence that an early BoNT/A injection improved muscle tone, delayed time to appearance of PSS symptoms, and significantly increased time until re-injection. Shin et al. [5] reported results from an open-label pilot study demonstrating that BoNT/A injection into finger and wrist flexors, followed by electrical stimulation of the finger extensor, improved active hand function in chronic stroke patients. Ianieri et al. [6] recalled the importance of performing an accurate evaluation of spasticity to determine how invalidating the symptoms are in order to personalize, for each patient, the optimal doses of BoNT/A, muscles, and injection time.

Another series of papers focuses on new dermatological uses of BoNTs. Kim et al. [7] contributed with a review for the use of BoNT/A in several off-label dermatological indications, including regenerative treatments of hypertrophic scarring and keloids, postoperative scar prevention, rosacea and facial flushing, and post-herpetic neuralgia, all conditions associated with hyperhidrosis, oily skin, psoriasis, and itching.

Itching constitutes another dermatological condition where application of BoNT/A may exert beneficial effects, especially in the treatment of neuropathic itching, a debilitating symptom appearing secondary to several skin, systemic, metabolic, and psychiatric disorders. The action of BoNT/A as an antipruritic agent is exhaustively reviewed by Gazerani [8] who summarizes all the evidence in favor both in animal models and in healthy human volunteers, and in many clinical conditions. The mechanism originating the antipruritic effects of BoNTs is discussed by Gazerani and also by Ramachandran et al. [9], who also give a possible explanation. The authors, analyzing the antipruritic effects of both BoNT/A and B in murine models, showed that both BoNT/A and B exert antipruritic effects in a mast cell/histamine-dependent and -independent manner.

Pain is another condition where the use of BoNTs is very promising. Different approaches have been adopted to treat chronic pain and, among others, the use of BOTOX® (commercial preparation of BoNT/A from Allergan, Inc., Irvine, CA, USA) has been recently authorized as a novel pharmacological indication for the prophylaxis of chronic migraine. In this context, Ion et al. [10] reported the results from a prospective study on the effect of a new BoNT/A formulation, namely XEOMIN® (commercial preparation of BoNT/A from Merz Pharmaceuticals, Inc., Frankfurt am Main, Germany), injected in patients with refractory chronic migraine. Unlike the other commercial preparationd of BoNT/A, XEOMIN® benefits from the absence of binding albumin protein, minimizing allergic reactions. The authors proved that XEOMIN® can be a prophylactic treatment in chronic migraine, effectively reducing the number of attack days, the number of migraine episodes per day, and the drug intake. Expanding the therapeutic uses of BoNTs, not only in pain, but also for overactive bladder, neurogenic detrusor overactivity, osteoarthritis, and wound healing, is exhaustively reviewed by Fonfria et al. [11]. The authors not only reviewed the effects of BoNTs, remote from injection sites, but also the effects of novel formulations, including modified and recombinant toxins, and of novel delivery methods, including transdermal, transurothelial, and transepithelial methods. Another potential analgesic effect of BoNTs is reviewed by Sandahl Michelsen et al. [12], who analyzed the results from a series of studies examining the effect of BoNT/A in alleviating pain in children with cerebral palsy (CP). The authors emphasize the difficulty concerning the treatment of pain in children with cerebral palsy (CP), a physical disability that affects the development of movement and posture in children and a neurological disorder in childhood caused by damage to either the fetal or the infant brain.

Continuing on the topic dedicated to the pain, Lee et al. [13] tested the efficacy of a lumbar sympathetic block with BoNT/A and B as pain therapy for complex regional pain syndrome (CRPS), a neuropathic pain syndrome causing spontaneous pain and allodynia. They found that the lumbar sympathetic block, with both BoNTs serotypes, constitutes a safe method to treat CRPS and, more surprisingly, BoNT/B is more effective and longer lasting than BoNT/A. The effects of BoNTs on CRPS as well as other neuropathic pain are also reviewed by Park et al. [14]. In addition to CRPS, this review also reports a complete overview of clinical studies of BoNT effects for central neuropathic pain, such as neuropathic pain after spinal cord injury, post-stroke shoulder pain, and central pain associated with multiple sclerosis.

In a basic science study, Finocchiaro et al. [15] compared the effect of BoNT/A and B in counteracting neuropathic pain in a murine model of sciatic nerve injury. The results confirmed that BoNT/A reduces neuropathic pain over a long period of time and, in parallel, it induces an acceleration of the regenerative processes of injured nerves, improving the functional recovery of the injured limb. BoNT/B can also reduce neuropathic pain over a long period of time, but, compared to BoNT/A, this reduction is not accompanied by an improvement in functional recovery. Finally, in an interesting review, Rojewska et al. [16] discussed whether and how BoNT/A reduces the development of neuropathic pain, with particular emphasis on spinal neuron–glia interactions and on the role of glial cells in BoNT/A-induced analgesia.

Another experimental study presented by Wang et al. [17] reported the nerve regeneration effects of BoNT/A on injured spinal cords in rats. What renders this paper unusual is the use of the BoNT/A heavy chain (BoNT/A-HC) as a catalytic subunit. This is completely in disagreement with the canonical view that BoNT/A-HC is the subunit necessary to bind to the vesicle presynaptic membrane and to translocate, inside the vesicle, the BoNT/A light chain (BoNT/A-LC), which constitutes the catalytic subunit which, by cleaving the SNARE proteins, blocks the neuronal transmission. The authors found that local application of BoNT/A-HC to the site of spinal cord injury significantly induced an increased expression of growth-associated protein, together with a stimulation of neurite outgrowths. The mechanism by which BoNT/A-HC favors the relief of spinal motor dysfunction after nervous injury remains unknown.

As for novel indications of BoNTs, we should not forget that BoNTs have been considered as agents for inducing controlled paralysis in different muscles of the oral, maxillofacial, and temporomandibular joint region, with the aim to treat dysfunction and dislocation in clinical orthodontics and maxillofacial surgery. Clinical applications of BoNTs in treatment for the correction of severe malocclusion-associated problems, including occlusion after orthognathic surgery and mandible fracture, are reviewed by Seok and Kim [18]. This particular application of BoNTs is based on the principle that the induction of controlled paralysis of masticatory muscles reduces the tensional force to the mandible and prevents relapse, and affects maxillofacial bone growth and dental occlusion. Yoshida [19] performed a study comparing the treatment outcome after intramuscular injection of BoNTs in patients with recurrent temporomandibular joint dislocation (TMD). Restivo et al. [20] reported an interesting effect of BoNT/A in reducing hypersalivation in patients with neurological diseases of different etiologies, including Parkinson's, amyotrophic lateral sclerosis, brain injury, and cerebral palsy.

Two reviews focus on new therapeutic approaches of BoNTs in gynecology and urinary tract dysfunctions. In the first, Moga et al. [21] made a literature review regarding the efficiency of BoNT/A in the treatment of chronic pelvic pain, vaginismus, vulvodynia, and overactive bladder or urinary incontinence. In the second, Jhang and Kuo [22] did a literature review regarding treatment of neurogenic lower urinary tract dysfunction, such as overactive bladder, neurogenic detrusor overactivity, interstitial cystitis, urethral sphincter dyssynergia, dysfunctional voiding, benign prostate hyperplasia, and chronic prostatitis.

Moving on to completely different topics, Caleo and Restani [23] contributed with a review describing the experimental use of BoNTs as a tool to block synaptic function in specific brain areas, with central delivery of BoNTs used to treat pathological brain conditions such as epilepsy, cerebral ischemia, Parkinson's, and prion disease. For obvious reasons, primarily toxicity and toxin diffusion, these studies are still limited to animals. An example of this unusual utilization of BoNT/A is also reported by Antipova et al. [24], who injected toxin directly into the striatum of mice and compared the motor behavior. The authors speculate that locally applied BoNTs could be useful for treating brain dysfunctions that require the deactivation of local brain circuitry.

The last paper was contributed by Bano et al. [25]. This paper reports a relevant observation on the fact that a tetanus neurotoxin (TeNT), a relative of BoNT/B produced by a *Clostridia tetani* strain, is neutralized by antisera raised against BoNT/B. This finding implicates that, although TeNT is not considered a food-borne pathogen, it can be present in foodstuffs and interfere with the detection of *Clostridia botulinum* by the mouse test, giving rise to misleading results. It is interesting to recall that humans are not usually vaccinated against type B botulism but citizens in many countries are regularly vaccinated for tetanus. It might be interesting to investigate whether the human vaccine for type B botulism also protects from certain isoforms of TeNTs.

In conclusion, the papers included in this Special Issue of *Toxins* contributed to the advancement of the state of the art in the novel therapeutic uses of BoNTs. Furthermore, many of the published studies focused on emerging or less investigated applications of BoNTs, in particular for pathologies, thus providing the scientific community with new data supporting better knowledge of the contributions given by BoNTs to improve the health of humanity.

Funding: This research received no external funding.

Acknowledgments: As Guest Editor, I wish to thank all authors and colleagues who contributed to the success of this Special Issue of *Toxins*, and the expert peer reviewers, who performed careful and rigorous evaluations. The valuable contribution and editorial support of the MDPI management team and editorial staff are also acknowledged.

Conflicts of Interest: The author declares no conflict of interest.

References

1. Zakin, E.; Simpson, D. Botulinum toxin in management of limb tremor. *Toxins* **2017**, *9*, 365. [CrossRef]
2. Niemann, N.; Jankovic, J. Botulinum toxin for treatment of hand tremor. *Toxins* **2018**, *10*, 299. [CrossRef] [PubMed]
3. Samotu, O.; Lee, J.; Jog, M. Transitioning from unilateral to bilateral upper limit tremor therapy for Parkinson's disease and essential tremor using botulinum toxin: Case series. *Toxins* **2018**, *10*, 394. [CrossRef] [PubMed]
4. Rosales, R.L.; Balcaitiene, J.; Berard, H.; Maisonobe, P.; Goh, K.J.; Kumthornthip, W.; Mazlan, M.; Latif, L.A.; Delos Santos, M.M.D.; Chotyarnwong, C.; et al. Early AbobotulinumtoxinA (DYSPORT®) in post-stroke adult upper limb spasticity: ONTIME pilot study. *Toxins* **2018**, *10*, 253. [CrossRef] [PubMed]
5. Shin, J.-H.; Lee, J.-M.; Park, S.-B.; Lee, K.H.; Lee, J.Y. Botulinum toxin injection and electrical stimulation for spastic paresis improves active hand function following stroke. *Toxins* **2018**, *10*, 426.
6. Ianieri, G.; Marvulli, R.; Gallo, G.A.; Fiore, P.; Megna, M. "Appropriate treatment" and therapeutic window in spasticity treatment with Incobotulinumtoxin A: From 100 to 1000 units. *Toxins* **2018**, *10*, 140. [CrossRef]
7. Kim, Y.S.; Hong, E.S.; Kim, H.S. Botulinum toxin in the field of dermatology: Novel indications. *Toxins* **2017**, *9*, 403.
8. Gazerani, P. Antipruritic effects of botulinum neurotoxins. *Toxins* **2018**, *10*, 143. [CrossRef]
9. Ramachandran, R.; Marino, M.J.; Paul, S.; Wang, Z.; Mascarenas, N.L.; Pellett, S.; DiNardo, A.; Yaksh, T.L. A study and review of effects of botulinum toxins on mast cell dependent and independent pruritus. *Toxins* **2018**, *10*, 134. [CrossRef]
10. Ion, I.; Renard, D.; Le Floch, A.; De Verdal, M.; Bouly, S.; Wacongne, A.; Lozza, A.; Castelnovo, G. Monocentric prospective study into the sustained effect of Incobotulinumtoxin A (XEOMIN®) botulinum toxin in chronic refractory migraine. *Toxins* **2018**, *10*, 221. [CrossRef]
11. Fonfria, E.; Maignel, J.; Lezmi, S.; Martin, V.; Splevins, A.; Shubber, S.; Kalinichev, M.; Foster, K.; Picaut, P.; Krupp, J. The expanding therapeutic utility of botulinum neurotoxins. *Toxins* **2018**, *10*, 208. [CrossRef] [PubMed]
12. Sandahl Michelsen, J.; Normann, G.; Wong, C. Analgesic effects of botulinum toxin in children with CP. *Toxins* **2018**, *10*, 162. [CrossRef] [PubMed]
13. Lee, Y.; Lee, C.J.; Choi, E.; Lee, P.B.; Lee, H.-J.; Nahm, F.S. Lumbar sympathetic block with botulinum toxin type A and type B for the complex regional pain syndrome. *Toxins* **2018**, *10*, 164. [CrossRef] [PubMed]
14. Park, J.; Chung, M.E. Botulinum toxin for central neuropathic pain. *Toxins* **2018**, *10*, 224. [CrossRef] [PubMed]
15. Finocchiaro, A.; Marinelli, S.; De Angelis, F.; Vacca, V.; Luvisetto, S.; Pavone, F. Botulinum toxin B affects neuropathic pain but not functional recovery after peripheral nerve injury in a mouse model. *Toxins* **2018**, *10*, 128. [CrossRef]
16. Rojewcka, E.; Piotrowska, A.; Popiolek-Barczyk, K.; Mika, J. Botulinum type A—A modulator of spinal neuron-glia interactions under neuropathic pain conditions. *Toxins* **2018**, *10*, 145. [CrossRef]
17. Wang, Y.-F.; Liu, F.; Lan, J.; Bai, J.; Li, X.-Q. The effect of botulinum neurotoxin serotype A heavy chain on the growth-related proteins and neurite outgrowth after spinal cord injury in rats. *Toxins* **2018**, *10*, 66. [CrossRef]
18. Seok, H.; Kim, S.-G. Correction of malocclusion by botulinum neurotoxin injection into masticatory muscles. *Toxins* **2018**, *10*, 27. [CrossRef]
19. Kazuya, Y. Botulinum neurotoxin injection for the treatment of recurrent temporomandibular joint dislocation with and without neurogenic muscular hyperactivity. *Toxins* **2018**, *10*, 174.
20. Restivo, D.A.; Panebianco, M.; Casabona, A.; Lanza, S.; Marchese-Ragona, R.; Patti, F.; Masiero, S.; Biondi, A.; Quartarone, A. Botulinum toxin A for sialorrhoea associated with neurological disorders: Evaluation of the relationship between effect of treatment and the number of glands treated. *Toxins* **2018**, *10*, 55. [CrossRef]
21. Moga, M.A.; Diminiescu, O.G.; Balan, A.; Scirneciu, I.; Baraba, B.; Liana, P. Therapeutic approaches of botulinum toxin in gynecology. *Toxins* **2018**, *10*, 169. [CrossRef] [PubMed]

22. Jhang, J.-F.; Kuo, H.-C. Novel application of OnabotulinumtoxinA in lower urinary tract dysfunction. *Toxins* **2018**, *10*, 260. [CrossRef] [PubMed]
23. Caleo, M.; Restani, L. Exploiting botulinum neurotoxins for the study of brain physiology and pathology. *Toxins* **2018**, *10*, 175. [CrossRef] [PubMed]
24. Antipova, V.; Wree, A.; Holzmann, C.; Mann, T.; Palomero-Gallagher, N.; Zilles, K.; Schmitt, O.; Hawlitschka, A. Unilateral botulinum neurotoxin-A injection into the striatum of C57BL/6 mice leads to a different motor behavior compared to rats. *Toxins* **2018**, *10*, 295. [CrossRef]
25. Bano, L.; Tonon, E.; Drigo, I.; Pirazzini, M.; Guolo, A.; Farina, G.; Agnoletti, F.; Montecucco, C. Detection of *Clostridium tetani* neurotoxins inhibited in vivo by botulinum antitoxin B: Potential for misleading mouse test results in food controls. *Toxins* **2018**, *10*, 248. [CrossRef]

toxins

MDPI

Review

Botulinum Toxin in Management of Limb Tremor

Elina Zakin * and David Simpson

Department of Neuromuscular Medicine, Icahn School of Medicine at Mount Sinai, New York City, NY 10029, USA; david.simpson@mssm.edu

* Correspondence: elina.zakin@mountsinai.org; Tel.: +19-212-241-6983

Academic Editor: Siro Luvisetto

Received: 24 October 2017; Accepted: 8 November 2017; Published: 10 November 2017

Abstract: Essential tremor is characterized by persistent, usually bilateral and symmetric, postural or kinetic activation of agonist and antagonist muscles involving either the distal or proximal upper extremity. Quality of life is often affected and one's ability to perform daily tasks becomes impaired. Oral therapies, including propranolol and primidone, can be effective in the management of essential tremor, although adverse effects can limit their use and about 50% of individuals lack response to oral pharmacotherapy. Locally administered botulinum toxin injection has become increasingly useful in the management of essential tremor. Targeting of select muscles with botulinum toxin is an area of active research, and muscle selection has important implications for toxin dosing and functional outcomes. The use of anatomical landmarks with palpation, EMG guidance, electrical stimulation, and ultrasound has been studied as a technique for muscle localization in toxin injection. Earlier studies implemented a standard protocol for the injection of (predominantly) wrist flexors and extensors using palpation and EMG guidance. Targeting of muscles by selection of specific activators of tremor (tailored to each patient) using kinematic analysis might allow for improvement in efficacy, including functional outcomes. It is this individualized muscle selection and toxin dosing (requiring injection within various sites of a single muscle) that has allowed for success in the management of tremors.

Keywords: botulinum toxin; limb tremors; muscle selection

1. Introduction

Essential tremor (ET) affects approximately 4–6% of individuals over the age of 65 [1]. Patients present with tremor characterized by persistent, bilateral, usually symmetric, postural, or kinetic tremor involving muscles of either the distal or proximal upper extremity. ET may also affect other body regions and functions including the voice, neck, lower limbs, and trunk. Over time, the severity of the tremor may worsen, and typically will affect daily tasks, including dressing, self-care, and feeding. Patients often present for evaluation and treatment once the tremor has begun to affect their quality of life. Oral therapies, including primidone, an anticonvulsant, and propranolol, a beta-adrenergic receptor antagonist, are effective in the treatment of essential tremor [2]. However, these agents reduce tremor amplitude by no more than 50%, and present a significant adverse side effect profile including dizziness, generalized fatigue, and bradycardia [3]. Additionally, about 30% of patients receive no therapeutic benefit from oral medications, leaving a relatively large population of individuals with pronounced ET untreated. Surgical options exist, including thalamotomy or implantation of either unilateral or bilateral thalamic deep brain stimulators, with Level C recommendation as 'possibly effective', but can only be performed in patients under the age of 75 [4]. Both pharmacologic and surgical options for the management of essential tremor, though effective for some, have their own potential for adverse events.

Local administration of intramuscular injections of botulinum toxin (BoNT) reduces excessive involuntary muscle activity and has emerged as an effective treatment for many movement disorders that are associated with muscle overactivity, including limb tremors. This article evaluates the current knowledge and evidence for the administration of botulinum toxin for limb tremors, including the process of muscle selection. This review will focus on techniques for botulinum toxin administration in limb tremors, as well as the safety/efficacy.

2. Review of the Literature

A tremor, which is an oscillatory movement produced by alternating or synchronous contractions of antagonistic muscles, is the most common movement disorder. Pharmacotherapy is usually not sufficient to control high-amplitude tremors, which can impair activities of daily living. Postural tremors respond more robustly to BoNT than do either kinetic or action tremors. In 1991, Jankovic, et al. reported the results of an open trial of BoNT in the treatment of 51 individuals with dystonic tremor, essential tremor, Parkinsonian tremor, peripherally induced tremor, and midbrain tremor [5]. They performed local injection for both head and limb tremor, noting that 67% of patients improved with an average latency from injection to response of 6.8 days. The average maximum duration of improvement was 10.5 weeks. This pilot study launched further investigation into the application of BoNT for selected movement disorders.

Shortly after this publication, Trosch and Pullman conducted an open-label study to determine the utility of BoNT injection in the management of severe hand tremors. They focused on forearm and arm tremors in 26 patients (12 with Parkinson disease, 14 with essential tremor), and used two clinical rating scales, subjective evaluations of function improvement and global disability, measures of weakness, and computer-assisted quantitative assessments of tremor to evaluate the effect of toxin injection after six weeks [6]. Although no change in clinical scores was noted, patients' disability scores (as measured by the Webster Tremor and Global Disability Scales) showed statistically significant differences between pre- and post-injection. Additionally, although amplitude differences were minimal, patients reported moderate to marked subjective improvement in functional benefit after injection. Thus, the study concluded that, while no major changes in clinical ratings or objective measures were noted, BoNT injections may subjectively improve tremor in some patients, particularly those with essential tremor.

In 1996, Jankovic, et al. performed the first randomized, double-blind, placebo-controlled study to evaluate BoNT-A in essential hand tremor. They studied 25 patients who were randomized to 50 units of botulinum type A compared to placebo. They evaluated rest, postural, and kinetic tremor at two- to four-week intervals over a 16-week period, using various tremor severity rating scales, accelerometry, and subjective improvement and disability scores [7]. They noted a significant improvement on the tremor severity scale at four weeks in the toxin group as compared to placebo control, with prolonged maintenance of the effect of toxin without significant effects on functional rating scales. Tremor evaluation using postural accelerometry showed a >30% reduction in amplitude in nine of 12 toxin-treated patients.

In 2000, Pacchetti et al. reported an open-label study of BoNT in 20 patients with disabling ET who did not respond to pharmacologic therapy, using activity of daily living self-questionnaires and tremor severity scales to establish patients' functional disability and tremor severity [8]. They noted a significant reduction in both severity and functional rating scales scores, as well as tremor amplitude reduction as measured with accelerometry and electromyography (EMG). They concluded that BoNT is safe and effective in reducing disability due to essential tremor.

In 2001, Brin et al. performed a multicenter, double-blind, placebo-controlled trial of botulinum toxin type A in essential hand tremor, studying 133 patients with ET, who were randomized to receive 50 or 100 units of botulinum toxin type A into both the wrist flexors and extensors, followed by a four-month follow-up [9]. The study showed significant improvement in postural tremor, with only minimal improvements in kinetic tremor and functional assessments.

3. Process of Muscle Selection in Toxin Administration for Limb Tremors

Early studies relied heavily on the clinical and electrophysiologic evaluation of patients' tremors to localize the muscles involved. In Jankovic's trial in 1991, careful clinical evaluation of the extremity was performed as it was held against gravity (to evaluate for postural tremor), during goal-directed movements (to evaluate kinetic tremor), or while performing specific activities such as writing (task-specific tremor). Surface electrode recording was performed on the limb in question, and muscle selection involved both agonist and antagonist groups (i.e., wrist extensors in addition to wrist flexors). Toxin was distributed into four to six different sites that were anatomically related to the muscles involved in the production of the tremor [5].

Trosch et al., working in 1994, also relied on clinical examination and EMG for tremor analysis. They used surface EMG of the flexor and extensor carpi radialis and ulnaris (FCU, FCR, ECR, and ECU), pronator teres, supinator, brachioradialis, flexor digitorum superficialis (FDS), extensor digitorum communis (EDC), biceps, and triceps muscles for each patient. Muscles that discharged rhythmically on needle EMG were injected, with almost every patient receiving wrist flexor and extensor injection [6]. Jankovic et al. used the clinical examination coupled with direct current amplification of EMG for the determination of accelerometry output for muscle selection in their randomized, double-blind, placebo-controlled study to evaluate toxin use in essential hand tremor [7]. Brin, et al. randomized patients to receive either 50 or 100 units, and used EMG guidance for BoNT administration [9]. Brin et al. and Jankovic et al. employed a fixed BoNT dosing schedule and a predetermined set of muscles. This is often currently not the case in practice, as dosages and selection of muscles injected are generally chosen individually based on tremor pattern. Pacchetti et al., in 2002, performed accelerometry and surface EMG to identify muscles with tremorogenic activity during impaired positions. They did not use EMG guidance for targeting muscles [8].

In 1997, O'Brien noted the importance of being proficient in electromyographic guidance and electrical stimulation for the improvement of the efficacy of therapy with BoNT injections [10]. More precise targeting of desired muscles for injection can be performed using these techniques, and assists the injector in preventing undesired adverse events. In using EMG guidance, the electromyographer's objective is to record motor unit potentials that are in close proximity to the needle tip, and, in so doing, to confirm the placement of toxin in the target tissue. Crisp, full-sized, bi- or triphasic motor unit potentials with fast rise times indicate that placement is near a contracting fascicle. This technique, coupled with clinical examination, was employed in early studies evaluating the efficacy of BoNT in the management of limb tremors.

4. Techniques for Botulinum Toxin Administration for Limb Tremors

More recent work on the use of botulinum toxin formulations has allowed for a different set of techniques in clinical decision-making and muscle selection with regards to toxin injection. Rahimi et al., in 2015, evaluated the use of sensor-based biomechanical patterns in assisting with incobotulinumtoxinA injection in upper extremity tremors of patients with Parkinson's disease [11]. They performed a 38-week open-label study on 528 patients with upper extremity tremor associated with Parkinson's disease, using kinematic technology to guide muscle selection in the injection of incobotulinumtoxinA. Specific kinematic measures of tremor amplitude allowed for detailed segmentation of tremor (with sensors placed at the fingers, hand, wrist, elbow, and shoulder) into components based on the direction at each joint in the upper extremity. Using specific MatLab® software, a detailed analysis of the directional contribution of each segment of the extremity was generated. Focusing on individual joints, a movement disorders neurologist used clinical judgment to determine the botulinum toxin dosage based on the kinematic measurement of tremor amplitude and the directional contribution of the tremor at each joint. This methodology tailored toxin injection to patient-specific tremor components. For the initial treatment, all participants were injected in the flexor carpi ulnaris and extensor carpi ulnaris muscles. At week 16, the Unified Parkinson's Disease Rating Scale (UPDRS) and Fahn–Tolosa–Marin (FTM) scale (measuring tremor severity) scores showed improvement. The authors proposed that kinematics is a simple method for standardizing the assessment and treatment of upper extremity tremors in Parkinson's disease, which allows for optimal BoNT injection and more personalized tremor therapy for this select patient population.

In 2016 Samotus et al. used kinematically determined biomechanical patterns in a study of incobotulinumtoxinA injection of 24 patients with essential tremor, who were injected every four months [1]. Motor tracking devices were placed over the forearm, wrist, elbow, and shoulder joints, which captured tremor severity in angular root mean square (RMS) amplitudes and degrees of freedom. Dosage of toxin was determined based on the injector's interpretation of tremor severity and distribution of tremor, using kinematic recordings. Additional refinement of the technique was performed by comparing the change in tremor as measured kinematically between pre-injection to six weeks post- (peak effect of botulinum toxin) and 16 weeks post-treatment. Again, as in prior studies, the most frequently injected muscles were the FCR and ECR. This study was the first to use whole-limb kinematics to segment complex movements at multiple joints that were implicated in the tremor production. This helped target toxin injection more effectively and objectively, with targeted injections for each patient based on the unique tremor kinematics. Additional use of this kinematic technology to refine injection site selection and toxin dosage for subsequent injections was helpful for the improvement of essential tremor in these patients. The assessment of tremor movements in multiple degrees of freedom at the upper extremity joints was also useful in targeting toxin as it allowed for selection of the tremulous muscles, as opposed to only injecting the flexor and extensor wrist muscles with use of surface EMG electrodes, or a combination of surface EMG electrodes and electrical stimulation. This study concluded that the use of individualized injection parameters resulted in an improvement of tremor and disability in patients with essential tremor.

Jog and the Essential Tremor Study Team performed a prospective, randomized, double-blind, placebo-controlled multicenter study of 30 patients with essential tremor who underwent incobotulinumtoxinA versus placebo injection using TremorTrek® kinematic technology to evaluate tremor amplitude (and thus judge severity) and localize muscles of involvement. They concluded that kinematic analysis-based incobotulinumtoxinA therapy decreased tremor severity and improved hand function as compared to a placebo, with marked improvement in tolerability and reduced incidence of muscle weakness [12].

Because botulinum toxin works directly at the neuromuscular junction, it is important to obtain accurate placement reaching the end plate zone (usually located at the midpoint of the muscle fiber), which helps to increase clinical response by as much as 50% [13]. The dose of botulinum toxin is usually divided between several injection sites, depending on muscle size, with reports of up to eight injection sites per muscle. Use of anatomical localization via palpation and EMG guidance has been described, though additional techniques specific to the evaluation of tremor have been employed, as described above. Precision of muscle selection with EMG and electrical stimulation has allowed for a reduced amount of toxin to be used to produce the same benefit, which has also allowed for reduced frequency of neutralizing antibody formation. Incorporation of neuromuscular ultrasound to further target muscles of interest has allowed for even more precise localization in BoNT injection. While most experienced injectors believe that careful muscle targeting improves outcomes, the American Academy of Neurology (AAN) evidence-based guidelines published in 2008 concluded that there was insufficient Class 1 evidence to recommend any muscle targeting technique for limb injections of botulinum toxin [14]. The above guidelines were put forth using an extensive literature review with two class II studies evaluating botulinum toxin administration in upper extremity essential tremor. The class of evidence for the use of botulinum toxin for the treatment of tremor is rated as level C by the AAN. Controlled comparative trials are underway to further evaluate this issue.

5. Safety/Efficacy of Toxin Use in Limb Tremors

The side effects of BoNT are related in part to undesired diffusion of the drug from the muscle of interest to nearby muscles/structures. This can result in inadvertent weakness of muscles that were not targeted by the clinician. Patients should be educated on the risk of possible excess weakness, usually noted within the first few weeks after toxin injection.

Contraindications to treatment with BoNT include pregnancy, known impairment of neuromuscular transmission, and myopathy, as well as the presence of prior pareses [15]. The most common adverse effects are mainly injection-site- and dose-dependent. Systemic effects are infrequent and occur after administration of 10 times the dose typically used in practice. Additionally, the formation of neutralizing antibodies is possible; studies have reported the incidence to be 0.5% to 5% of patients treated with botulinum toxin (depending on toxin subtype) [16,17].

Factors associated with the formation of neutralizing Ab resistance include total BoNT dose administered and frequency of injection. This led to the accepted dogma and FDA labeling requiring a 12-week interval between injection sessions. Notably, most of these studies of resistance were conducted with an earlier formulation of ona-BoNT containing five times the amount of protein in current formulations. More recent data show a far lower incidence of neutralizing Ab formation. This issue has increasing importance given the potential advantage of the use of "booster injections" at shorter intervals, especially in limb tremor, where careful titration of low doses may be optimal. These issues are being evaluated in controlled prospective trials.

In many of the aforementioned trials, there was a high incidence of dose-dependent adverse events, including finger weakness, pain at injection sites, hematoma formation, and paresthesias. In many of the older studies, patients self-reported a high incidence of excessive weakness, which made true rater blinding difficult to achieve. This has improved with more focused muscle targeting using kinematics (as reported in the more recent literature). Additionally, focusing toxin injection on the flexor compartment (and avoiding injection of the extensor carpi muscles, unless they were the ones causing excessive disability) allowed for preservation of finger strength in more patients, further improving patient functional outcomes in performing daily activities such as writing, using a spoon, holding a cup, and pouring liquids.

In summary, BoNT injection should be considered for patients with limb ET who have not achieved relief with oral pharmacotherapy, or in whom the drug side effect profile is poorly tolerated. After careful evaluation of the tremor, experienced clinicians, using a specific injection pattern and muscle targeting techniques such as EMG, electrical stimulation, and ultrasound, can target the toxin to the muscles of interest. These targeting techniques (along with careful anatomic palpation) allow for more effective toxin delivery, and thus minimize the possibility of toxin diffusion and neutralizing antibody formation. Novel techniques, such as quantification of tremor components and amplitude using kinematic techniques, show promise in providing even more precise localization, improved efficacy, and reduced unwanted weakness. Though no controlled data exist, one can speculate that the combination of kinematic studies, muscle visualization, ultrasonography, and confirmation with electrical stimulation will allow for an even more targeted injection approach.

Acknowledgments: There are no sources of funding of the study to disclose.

Conflicts of Interest: The authors declare no conflict of interest.

References

1. Samotus, O.; Rahimi, F.; Lee, J.; Jog, M. Functional Ability Improved in Essential Tremor by IncobotulinumtoxinA Injections Using Kinematically Determined Biomechanical Patterns—A New Future. *PLoS ONE* **2016**, *11*, e0153739. [CrossRef] [PubMed]
2. Zesiewicz, T.A.; Shaw, J.D.; Allison, K.G.; Staffetti, J.S.; Okun, M.S.; Sullivan, K.L. Update on treatment of Essential Tremor. *Curr. Treat. Options Neurol.* **2013**, *15*, 410–423. [CrossRef] [PubMed]
3. Rajput, A. Medical Treatment of Essential Tremor. *J. Cent. Nervous Syst. Dis.* **2014**, *29*. [CrossRef] [PubMed]
4. Baizabal-Carvallo, J.F.; Kagnoff, M.N.; Jimenez-Shahed, J.; Fekete, R.; Jankovic, J. The safety and efficacy of thalamic deep brain stimulation in essential tremor: 10 years and beyond. *J. Neurol. Neurosurg. Psychiatry* **2013**, *85*, 567–572. [CrossRef] [PubMed]

5. Jankovic, J.; Schwartz, K. Botulinum toxin treatment of tremors. *Neurology* **1991**, *41*, 1185. [CrossRef] [PubMed]
6. Trosch, R.M.; Pullman, S.L. Botulinum toxin a injections for the treatment of hand tremors. *Mov. Disord.* **1994**, *9*, 601–609. [CrossRef] [PubMed]
7. Jankovic, J.; Schwartz, K.; Clemence, W.; Aswad, A.; Mordaunt, J. A randomized, double-blind, placebo-controlled study to evaluate botulinum toxin type A in essential hand tremor. *Mov. Disord.* **1996**, *11*, 250–256. [CrossRef] [PubMed]
8. Pacchetti, C.; Mancini, F.; Bulgheroni, M.; Zangaglia, R.; Cristina, S.; Sandrini, G.; Nappi, G. Botulinum toxin treatment for functional disability induced by essential tremor. *Neurol. Sci.* **2002**, *21*, 349–353. [CrossRef]
9. Brin, M.F.; Lyons, K.E.; Doucette, J.; Adler, C.H.; Caviness, J.N.; Comella, C.L.; Dubinsky, R.M.; Friedman, J.H.; Manyam, B.V.; Matsumoto, J.Y.; et al. A randomized, double masked, controlled trial of botulinum toxin type A in essential hand tremor. *Neurology* **2001**, *56*, 1523–1528. [CrossRef] [PubMed]
10. O'Brien, C.F. Injection techniques for Botulinum Toxin Using Electromyography and Electrical Stimulation. *Muscle Nerve Suppl.* **1997**, *6*, S170–S180. [CrossRef]
11. Rahimi, F.; Samotus, O.; Lee, J.; Jog, M. Effective Management of Upper Limb Parkinsonian Tremor by IncobotulinumtoxinA Injections Using Sensor-based Biomechanical Patterns. *Tremor Other Hyperkinet. Mov.* **2015**, *30*, 348. [CrossRef]
12. Jog, M.; Lee, J.; Althaus, M.; Scheschonka, A.; Dersch, H.; Team, E.T.; Simpson, D. Efficacy and Safety of incobotulinumtoxinA (Inco/A) for Essentia Tremor of the Upper Limb using Kinematics-guided clinical decision support: A randomized, double-blind, placebo-controlled trial. In Proceedings of the Movement Disorders Society Meeting, Vancouver, BC, Canada, 4–8 June 2017.
13. Shaari, C.M.; Sanders, I. Quantifying how location and dose of botulinum toxin injections affect muscle paralysis. *MuscVésinet Nerve* **1993**, *16*, 964–969. [CrossRef] [PubMed]
14. Simpson, D.M.; Blitzer, A.; Brashear, A.; Comella, C.; Dubinsky, R.; Hallett, M.; Jankovic, J.; Karp, B.; Ludlow, C.L.; Miyasaki, J.M.; et al. Assessment: Botulinum neurotoxin for the treatment of movement disorders (an evidence-based review): Report of the Therapeutics and Technology Assessment Subcommittee of the American Academy of Neurology. *Neurology* **2008**, *70*, 1699–1706. [CrossRef] [PubMed]
15. Newman, W.J.; Davis, T.L.; Padaliya, B.B.; Covington, C.D.; Gill, C.E.; Abramovitch, A.I.; Charles, P.D. Erratum: Botulinum toxin type a therapy during pregnancy. *Mov. Disord.* **2004**, *19*, 1384–1385. *Mov. Disord.* **2005**, *20*, 121. [CrossRef]
16. Yablon, S.A.; Brashear, A.; Gordon, M.F.; Elovic, E.P.; Turkel, C.C.; Daggett, S.; Liu, J.; Brin, M.F. Formation of neutralizing antibodies in patients receiving botulinum toxin type a for treatment of poststroke spasticity: A pooled-data analysis of three clinical trials. *Clin. Ther.* **2007**, *29*, 683–690. [CrossRef] [PubMed]
17. Naumann, M.; Albanese, A.; Heinen, F.; Molenaers, G.; Relja, M. Safety and efficacy of botulinum toxin type a following long-term use. *Eur. J. Neurol.* **2006**, *13* (Suppl. S4), 35–40. [CrossRef] [PubMed]

toxins

MDPI

Article

Botulinum Toxin for the Treatment of Hand Tremor

Nicki Niemann and Joseph Jankovic *

Parkinson's Disease Center and Movement Disorders Clinic, Department of Neurology, Baylor College of Medicine, Houston, TX 77030, USA; niemann@bcm.edu

* Correspondence: josephj@bcm.edu; Tel.: +1-713-798-2273; Fax: +1-713-798-6808

Received: 26 June 2018; Accepted: 15 July 2018; Published: 19 July 2018

Abstract: The aim of this study is to review our longitudinal experience with onabotulinumtoxinA (onaBoNT-A) injections for medically refractory hand tremor. We performed a retrospective review of our database of patients treated with onaBoNT-A for hand tremor evaluated between 2010 and 2018 in at least 2 sessions with follow-up. The majority were injected into the forearm flexors (FF), although treatment was individualized. During the specified period, 91 patients (53 essential tremor, 31 dystonic tremor, 6 Parkinson's disease tremor, and 1 cerebellar outflow tremor) met our inclusion criteria. The mean age (SD) was 64.8 years (12.8), and mean duration of follow-up was 29.6 months (25.1) with mean of 7.7 (6.3) treatment visits. FF were injected in 89 (97.8%) patients, exclusively in 74 (81.3%), and 15 (16.5%) were injected in FF and other muscles. EMG guidance was used in 5 patients (5.5%). On a 0–4 "peak effect" rating scale (0 = no effect, 4 = marked improvement in severity and function), 80.2% and 85.7% of patients reported moderate or marked improvement (score 3 or 4) at their first and last follow-up visit, respectively. There was no statistically significant difference in the outcomes between first and last visit: average "peak effect" rating score (3.2 versus 3.4), "global" rating score (3.0 versus 3.2), latency of response (4.5 versus 3.8 days), and total duration of response (12.7 versus 12.8 weeks), except onaBoNT-A dose (65.0 versus 78.6 U/limb, $p = 0.002$). Of 1095 limb injections, there were 134 (12.2%) non-disabling and transient (mean 36 days) adverse events (132 limb weakness, 2 pain). OnaBoNT-A injections are safe and effective in the treatment of hand tremor.

Keywords: hand tremor; botulinum toxin; treatment; electromyography; kinematics; essential tremor; Parkinson's disease; dystonic tremor

Key Contribution: Botulinum toxin injections administered using surface anatomy are safe and associated with clinically meaningful and sustained improvement of hand tremor, regardless of etiology.

1. Introduction

Tremor is defined as an involuntary, rhythmic, oscillatory movement of a body part [1]. Hand tremor is a common movement disorder, often associated with impairment in quality of life [2]. Essential tremor (ET) is the most common cause of postural and kinetic hand tremor; 4.6% of individuals 65 years or older are thought to have ET [3]. Parkinson's disease (PD) affects 0.43–1.90% of individuals 60 years or older [4] with the majority experiencing rest or postural tremor [5,6]. While rest tremor is typically associated with PD, most PD patients also have a postural or re-emergent tremor, which is the most disabling form of PD-related tremor [6,7]. The prevalence of dystonic tremor is unknown [8], although hand tremor has been reported in up to 70% of patients in a series of patients with dystonia of various types [9]. There are many other causes of tremor besides ET, PD, and dystonia, which can affect not only hands but also other body parts [1]. Treatment of tremor with oral medications often provides insufficient relief, especially when the tremor is severe, and is frequently associated with systemic side effects [10,11]. Deep brain stimulation (DBS) is a highly effective treatment for tremor in ET and PD, but is invasive and can be associated with stimulation-induced and long-term side effects [12,13]. Functional lesional neurosurgery, especially focused ultrasound, has garnered more interest recently in the treatment of tremor but this intervention is not readily available and is associated with potentially serious adverse effects, particularly when performed bilaterally [14–16].

Botulinum toxin (BoNT) has been increasingly used in the treatment of focal tremors with reported good outcomes and long-term safety [17,18]. One of the main advantages of this treatment over above-noted strategies is the lack of systemic side effects. The aim of the present study is to describe our long-term experience with onabotulinumtoxinA (onaBoNT-A) in the treatment of medically refractory hand tremor using an individualized approach.

2. Results

We identified a total of 91 patients who were treated with onaBoNT-A for hand tremor at least twice and had adequate follow-up during the period from 1st January 2010 to 1st January 2018. Of these patients, 23 (25.3%) received their initial injection prior to 1st January 2010. Diagnoses included ET (53 patients with 395 visits), PD (6 patients with 27 visits), dystonia (31 patients with 269 visits), and cerebellar outflow tremor (1 patient with 13 visits) (Figure 1). The male to female ratio was 1.1:1 (48 male and 43 female) and the mean age of all participants was 64.8 years at the time of their initial injection visit (Table 1). The mean duration of symptoms prior to the first onaBoNT-A injection was 23.2 years. The mean duration of follow-up from the first to the last injection visit was 29.6 months during which time patients underwent a mean of 7.7 injections.

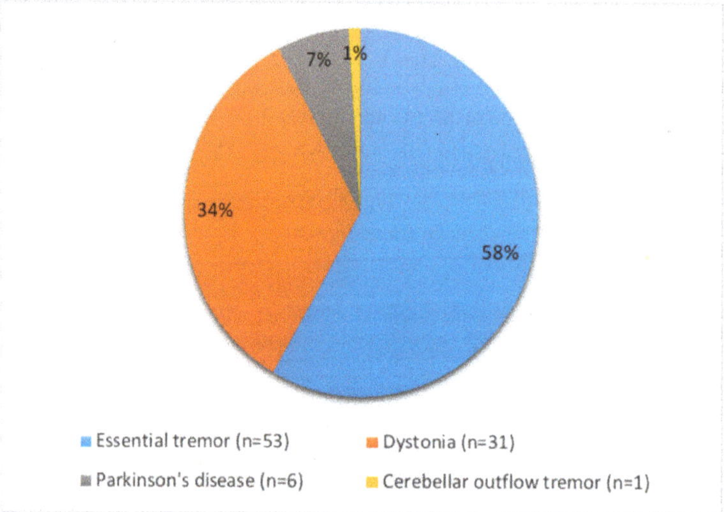

Figure 1. Etiology of hand tremor in patients treated with onabotulinumtoxinA (onaBoNT-A) injections from 1st January 2010 to 1st January 2018.

Table 1. Botulinum toxin in hand tremor: Demographics and baseline data ($n = 91$).

	Mean	SD	Range
Age at first injection (years)	64.8	12.8	18–93
Tremor duration at first injection (years)	23.2	17.5	0.5–75
Follow-up period (months)	29.6	25.1	3–88
Number of onaBoNT-A sessions	7.7	6.3	2–31
OnaBoNT-A units per session †	71.8	37.3	22.5–225
OnaBoNT-A units † (per treatment indication)			
ET ($n = 53$)	71.3	36.7	22.5–225
PD ($n = 6$)	47.9	11.5	37.5–67.5
Dystonia ($n = 31$)	77.3 *	41.0	27.5–187.5
COT ($n = 1$)	70	-	-

SD = Standard deviation, ET = Essential tremor, PD = Parkinson's disease, onaBoNT-A = onabotulinumtoxin-A, COT = Cerebellar outflow tremor. * $p = 0.49$ for comparison with ET. † mean dose per limb (first and last visit combined).

Forearm flexors were injected in 89 (97.8%) patients, 74 (81.3%) received injections exclusively to the forearm flexors, and 15 (16.5%) received injections to the forearm flexors and at least one other upper extremity muscle compartment (hand muscles, forearm extensors, arm flexors, arm extensors, and/or shoulder abductors); 2 (2.2%) received no forearm flexor injections. The specific muscles injected according to tremor etiology are listed in Table 2. EMG was used in 5 (5.5%) patients while the rest were injected using surface anatomy. The mean dose of onaBoNT-A increased significantly from 65.0 to 78.6 ($p = 0.002$) between the first and last visit; the mean dose was 71.8 U per limb. There was no statistically significant difference between outcomes from the first and last visit with respect to all other outcome measures: peak effect score was 3.2 versus 3.4 ($p = 0.17$), global rating was 3.0 versus 3.2 ($p = 0.06$), and latency of response was 4.5 versus 3.8 days ($p = 0.10$) (Table 3). Using the peak effect rating scale, 80.2% and 85.7% of patients rated their improvement as either moderate or marked (score of 3 or 4) at their first and last visit, compared to 74.7% and 80.2% of patients on the global effect rating scale at the first and last visit, respectively. A separate analysis comparing outcomes on the global rating and peak effect rating scale within each group (e.g., ET outcomes after first versus last injection) and between groups (e.g., ET versus dystonia) did not reveal any statistically significant differences (data not shown). The mean duration of maximum response at the first and last injection was 12.1 and 12.7 weeks ($p = 0.70$), respectively. The mean total duration of response at the first and last injection was 12.7 and 12.8 weeks ($p = 0.87$), respectively, but this is likely an underestimate as the effects of the prior injection had not fully worn off in 27 (29.7%) and 41 (45.1%) patients at the time of follow-up after the first and last visit. Of the total 1095 limbs injected, 134 (12.2%) were associated with some adverse effect (120 hand grip weakness, 1 focal finger flexor weakness, 11 elbow flexor weakness, and 2 pain), none of which were considered to be severe or disabling. The mean duration of side effects was 36 days (range 7–120).

Table 2. Injection strategy at the last visit according to tremor etiology ($n = 91$).

Treatment Indication (Muscles Injected/Limbs Injected)					
	ET	PD	Dystonia	COT	Total
Deltoid	0/99	0/6	1/37	1/1	2/143
Biceps	10/99	0/6	3/37	1/1	14/143
Triceps	1/99	0/6	0/37	0/1	1/143
Pronator teres	4/99	0/6	5/37	0/1	9/143
FCU	94/99	6/6	34/37	1/1	135/143
FCR	92/99	6/6	26/37	1/1	125/143
FDS	3/99	0/6	4/37	0/1	7/143
ADM	0/99	0/6	1/37	0/1	1/143
APB	1/99	0/6	11/37	0/1	12/143
ED	0/99	0/6	1/37	0/1	1/143
EPB	0/99	0/6	1/37	0/1	1/143
UNS extensor	0/99	0/6	1/37	0/1	1/143

ET = Essential tremor, PD = Parkinson's disease, COT = Cerebellar outflow tremor, FCU = Flexor carpi ulnaris, FCR = Flexor carpi radialis, FDS = Flexor digitorum superficialis, ADM = Abductor digiti minimi, APB = Abductor pollicis brevis, ED = extensor digitorum, EPB = Extensor pollicis brevis, UNS extensor = unspecified extensor muscle.

Table 3. Outcomes following onaBoNT-A injections for hand tremor ($n = 91$).

	First Injection (n)	Last Injection (n)	p *
Mean onaBoNT-A units	65.0 ± 31.2 (91)	78.6 ± 51.1 (91)	0.002
Mean global rating	3.0 ± 1.3 (91)	3.2 ± 1.2 (91)	0.06
Mean peak effect	3.2 ± 1.3 (91)	3.4 ± 1.1 (91)	0.18
Moderate or marked benefit (score of 3 or 4)			
Global rating	74.7%	80.2%	-
Peak effect	80.2%	85.7%	-
Mean latency of response, days	4.5 ± 4.3 (81)	3.8 ± 3.0 (78)	0.10
Mean total duration of response, weeks †	12.7 ± 3.6 (46)	12.8 ± 2.8 (37)	0.87

OnaBoNT-A = onabotulinumtoxin-A. * $p < 0.05$ indicating a statistically significant result. † Data not included for patients with persistent response (27 versus 41) or lack of data (18 versus 13) at the time of follow-up after the first and last injection.

At the end of the study period (1st January 2018), 41 (45.1%) patients were still receiving onaBoNT-A injections. The remaining 50 (54.9%) patients were no longer receiving injections in our clinic: 5 (5.5%) were lost to follow-up, 14 (15.4%) were dissatisfied and discontinued treatment usually after only 2–3 injections, and 4 (4.4%) transitioned to alternative therapy; the reason for discontinuation was financial or unknown in 24 (26.4%) and 3 (3.3%) died of unrelated causes. Additional 30 patients (ET, $n = 14$; dystonia, $n = 10$; other, $n = 6$) did not meet our inclusion criteria as they discontinued onaBoNT-A injections after just 1 visit, either for unknown reasons ($n = 15$), lack of benefit ($n = 10$), adverse effects ($n = 2$), or other reasons ($n = 3$).

3. Discussion

In this study we provide longitudinal, follow-up, data for 91 patients treated with onaBoNT-A for hand tremor over an average period of 2.5 years. To our knowledge, this is the longest duration of follow-up data reported regarding the use of BoNT for hand tremor, although we previously reported our long-term experience with BoNT in the treatment of dystonia over a period of more than 20 years [19]. The mean age of our patient population and the male predominance is similar to those reported in recently published studies of BoNT in the treatment of tremor [20–25]. There was a relatively long period of time between onset of symptoms and first injection (mean 23.2 years, up to 75 years). In contrast to our experience with BoNT for dystonia [19], we found no significant difference in the outcome measures (peak effect, global effect, latency of response, or duration of response) between the first and last visit. We found no difference in response to BoNT injections based on underlying etiology of the tremor as measured by the peak effect and global rating. There was, however, a modest but significant increase in the average dose of onaBoNT-A, from 65.0 U to 78.6 U (difference of 13.6 U; $p = 0.002$). The most plausible reason for the 21% increase in average BoNT dose per limb between the first and last visit is that the initial dose is often quite conservative and relatively lower than the estimated maintenance dose to minimize potential adverse effects such as hand weakness. We have observed sustained benefit during the follow-up period (mean, 29.6 months; range, 3–88 months) with a significant proportion of patients reporting moderate or marked improvement of tremor severity and function (score of 3 or 4) on the peak effect rating scale (80.2% versus 85.7%) and global effect rating scale (74.7% versus 80.2%) at the first and last visit. Of the 50 (54.9%) patients who had discontinued treatment with BoNT injections during the study period, 32 (35.2%) did so for unknown or unavoidable reasons, while only 14 (15.4%) were dissatisfied with treatment.

In the earliest study of onaBoNT-A in the treatment of tremor from our center, 10 patients with hand tremor (mixed etiology) received a mean dose of 95 ± 38 U predominantly divided between the forearm flexor and forearm extensor compartment [26]. The peak effect hand tremor was lower (2.0 ± 1.7 versus 3.2 ± 1.3) and the rate of focal weakness was higher (40.0% versus 12.1%) compared to the data reported in the present study. This is consistent with data from the first two double-blind, placebo-controlled trials of BoNT in the treatment of ET [27,28]. In both studies, a pre-determined set of muscles (forearm flexors and extensors) was injected with a fixed dose of BoNT, yielding clinically significant improvement of tremor, however with dose-dependent hand and finger weakness in up to 92% of patients. Because of the high frequency of extensor finger weakness we have since changed our injection technique to favor the forearm flexors while largely avoiding the forearm extensors, thereby reducing the frequency of clinically significant (extensor) wrist and finger weakness while maintaining tremor reduction (Figure 2) [29].

Several well-designed studies have evaluated the use of kinematic tremor analysis coupled with EMG-guidance in the application of BoNT [20,21,23,30–32]. Kinematic analysis allows the clinician to objectively characterize tremor at the wrist, elbow and shoulder joint, thereby creating an individual "tremor profile" which can be re-assessed at future visits thus allowing for optimization of the injection pattern. In a study involving 30 patients with ET who were randomized to receive a single injection of either incoBoNT-A ($n = 19$) or placebo ($n = 11$) using a kinematic analysis-based approach the mean total dose of incoBoNT-A was 116.3 ± 53.0 U distributed between multiple muscle compartments [23]. There was a significant reduction in wrist tremor amplitude and in the Fahn-Tolosa-Marin (FTM) tremor rating scale part B at week 4 and 8 post-injection. The injections were associated with approximately 15–20% reduced grip strength in the treatment group at week 4 and finger extensor weakness in 2 (10.5%) patients. There was no long-term data provided in this study but the same investigators conducted an open-label, long-term (96 weeks) study of kinematic analysis-guided incoBoNT-A injections for ET ($n = 24$) and PD ($n = 28$) upper limb tremor [32]. In this study, a mean of 9.4 ± 2.3 versus 10.2 ± 2.6 muscles were injected with a mean of 180.3 ± 74.8 versus 188.5 ± 78.1 U incoBoNT-A in PD and ET, respectively, at the time of the last injection visit. There was a statistically significant reduction of rest and action tremor on items 20 and 21 of the Unified Parkinson's Disease Rating Scale (UPDRS), FTM tremor rating scale part A–C, and tremor amplitude. A total of 6 patients (11.5% [4 PD and 2 ET]) withdrew from the study due to disabling weakness and another 5 patients (9.6% [3 PD and 2 ET]) withdrew due to lack of benefit. While the rate of significant weakness fluctuated throughout the study, 5.0–29.4% of PD and ET patients experienced significant finger extensor weakness after each injection session.

In a double-blind, placebo-controlled, cross-over study of 30 patients with PD-related rest and action tremor, Mittal and colleagues injected incoBoNT-A with EMG guidance to identify muscles with tremor activity [22]. IncoBoNT-A or placebo (saline) was injected at the start of the trial with cross-over to the opposite treatment arm at week 12; outcome was assessed at week 4 and 8 after each injection. A mean of 9 (range 7–12) injections into forearm and hand muscles with a mean of 100 U (range, 85–110) incoBoNT-A per patient per visit were performed. IncoBoNT-A injections were associated with significant reduction of tremor affecting activities of daily living as well as rest and action tremor (UPDRS items 16, 20, and 21) with low rates of non-disabling (10%) and disabling (6.6%) hand weakness. Using a similar study design, the same authors performed incoBoNT-A injections in 28 patients (of 33 enrolled) with hand ET [25]. IncoBoNT-A were injected into a mean of 9 (range, 8–14) hand and forearm muscles (80–120 U). IncoBoNT-A treatment led to significant reduction of tremor (FTM tremor rating scale part B and the National Institute of Health Collaborative Genetic Criteria tremor score severity) at weeks 4 and 8 ($p < 0.05$). IncoBoNT-A treatments were safe and well-tolerated, although mild hand weakness occurred in 21% and 1 patient withdrew from the study due to disabling hand weakness.

Although EMG, ultrasound, and kinematic-guided analysis can be utilized to successfully treat hand tremor with BoNT, no muscle targeting technique has yet been proven to be superior [33,34]. The results described in our study, using palpation and surface anatomy, seem similar to those obtained using kinematic analysis and/or EMG-guided injections [24,27,32,35]. Thus, it is unclear if a technology-guided approach is necessary and whether it yields better outcomes. Indeed, 21.2% of 52 patients treated using kinematic analysis and EMG-guided injections by Samotus et al. [32] withdrew because of adverse effects or lack of benefit, compared to only 15.4% of our 91 patients, although the two populations are not comparable. Technology-guided injections are useful in some instances, such as when the target muscles are difficult to identify, however, it is nearly impossible to sample all 20 forearm muscles plus other, more proximal, muscles to identify all the muscles that contribute to the tremor and target them for BoNT. Even when EMG is used to target the identified muscle the precise site of the tip of the electrode is impossible to validate with any certainty (even with ultrasound) and it is likely that the effects of BoNT will diffuse beyond the boundaries of the intended target [17]. Furthermore, EMG may sometimes be misleading, particularly in patients injected for dystonia, as it may not differentiate between the primary (agonist) and the compensatory (antagonist) muscle contraction, potentially resulting in injection of the wrong muscle. In this regard, evaluation for mirror movements may be helpful [36], particularly in patients with dystonic tremor. Finally, and perhaps most importantly, technology-guided injections are more time-consuming, more painful and more costly [37] without meaningfully improving the outcomes [38].

In our longitudinal study we demonstrated that a comparatively low dose of onaBoNT-A injected into a very limited number of muscles (forearm flexors were injected exclusively in 81.3% of patients) guided by palpation and surface anatomy produced clinically meaningful and sustained improvement of tremor in the majority of patients with low rates of non-disabling focal weakness (12.1%). Although we mainly injected the forearm flexors, the injection pattern should always be individualized and optimized based on the characteristics of the patient's tremor. For an instance, injection of the biceps brachii or pronator teres muscle may be considered in the treatment of the classical supination/pronation tremor in PD [39].

The main strength of our report is that it provides a "real world" account of long-term experience with the use of BoNT in hand tremor using a pragmatic, clinical approach. However, we acknowledge that our study has some limitations, particularly due to its open-label and retrospective design. Further, of 30 patients who discontinued treatment with BoNT after only 1 session, 12 (40%) did so due to either troublesome side effects or lack of benefit. We would not, however, consider these as "failures" since 2 or more treatment visits are often required to optimize the outcome. We do not think that bias and placebo response account for the reported outcomes as patients had sustained improvement over time, noticed wearing off between doses, and returned repeatedly for injections, many traveling long distances. Furthermore, it is important to point out that nearly all our patients were previously treated with optimal medical therapies but because of poor response or undesirable side effects were selected for treatment with BoNT. Prospective studies comparing different methods of muscle selection, localization, and injection techniques may provide further validation of our results.

4. Conclusions

In conclusion, onaBoNT-A injections are safe and associated with clinically meaningful and sustained improvement of hand tremor in a mixed population of patients with medically refractory hand tremor.

5. Materials and Methods

5.1. Study Description

We conducted a retrospective analysis of our medical records of patients treated with onaBoNT-A injections for hand tremor in the Parkinson's Disease Center and Movement Disorders Clinic (PDCMDC) at Baylor College of Medicine (BCM). The study was approved by the BCM Institutional Review Board (IRB), number H-42714, approved January 31st, 2018.

5.2. Data Collection

Patients treated with BoNT for tremor were identified through review of the electronic medical record (EMR) at BCM. The medical history, past treatments, examination and the indication for BoNT treatment was determined by review of the medical record. The "Botulinum Toxin Data Form" ("BoNT Data Form"), which captures injection data (muscle selection, dose, type of BoNT, and response to prior injection) was completed at the initial and all subsequent injection visits. The "peak effect", one of the two main outcome measures, was defined as the maximum improvement of tremor following BoNT injection, and was assessed by a 0–4 rating scale (0 = no effect; 1 = mild effect, but no functional improvement; 2 = moderate improvement, but no change in functional disability; 3 = moderate change in both severity and function; and 4 = marked improvement in severity and function). The "global rating", the other outcome measure, was defined as the peak effect score minus 1 point for a mild side effect, such as transient pain or mild weakness, and minus 2 points for a disabling side effect, such as marked weakness causing impairment of function. The "latency of response" was the time from injection of BoNT until the first noticeable response (in days), "duration of maximum response" was the period of time during which the patient experienced peak effect (in weeks), and "total duration of response" represented the time from the first noticeable response to complete wearing off (in weeks). The type, severity, and duration (in days) of side effects were also recorded.

5.3. Selection Criteria

Inclusion criteria for this study were: (1). Presence of troublesome hand tremor that is refractory to medical therapy, including optimized trial of propranolol, primidone, topiramate for ET; levodopa, dopamine agonists or anticholinergics for PD tremor; and anticholinergics for dystonic tremor, (2) chemodenervation using onaBoNT-A injections of the arm(s) for hand tremor, (3) minimum of two BoNT injection visits between 1st January 2010 (introduction of EMR at BCM), and 1st January 2018 with follow-up data, (4) follow-up within 1 year after the first and last injection, and (5) age older than 18 years at the time of the first injection. Patients first treated prior to introduction of the EMR were included in this study, but their "initial visit" was recorded as their first BoNT injection visit after introduction of the EMR. Injection and outcome data were analyzed for the first and last visit while information regarding side effects (type and duration) were captured for all visits. This approach was chosen for simplicity since some patients had more than a dozen injection visits during the study period which would make it difficult to analyze all outcomes at each visit separately. We further recorded the reason for discontinuation of onaBoNT-A injections (if known).

5.4. Botulinum Toxin Injection

We individualized the target muscle and dosage based on the amplitude and character of the tremor, starting at a relatively low dose and usually optimizing the treatment over subsequent 2–3 visits.

The majority of patients received an initial injection of approximately 25–75 units (U) of onaBoNT-A per limb divided between flexor carpi radialis (2/3) and flexor carpi ulnaris (1/3) (Figure 2). We do not routinely utilize electromyography (EMG) or ultrasound, but rely on palpation and surface anatomy for guidance in most BoNT injections.

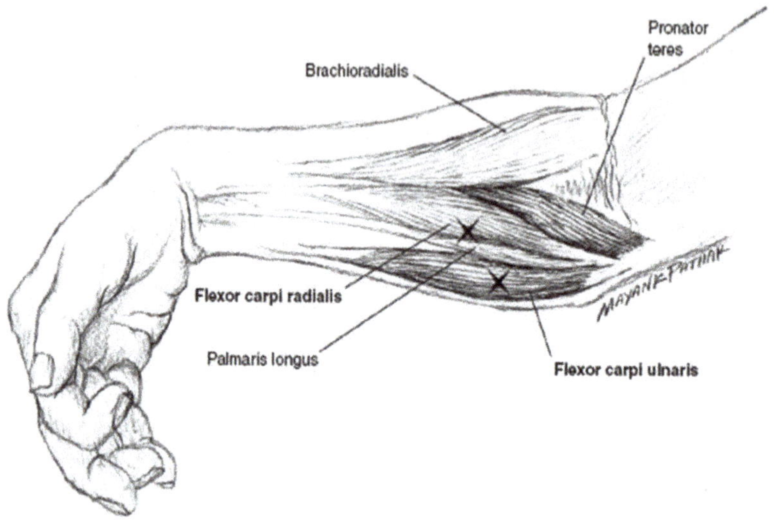

Figure 2. Localization of the forearm flexors most commonly injected in hand tremor. Reprinted with permission from [29], Copyright Cambridge University Press, 2003.

5.5. Statistical Analysis

Using descriptive statistics, we analyzed the following information: age at first injection visit, disease duration, number of injection visits, duration of treatment with onaBoNT-A, average dose of onaBoNT-A per limb, peak effect, global rating, latency of response, duration of maximum response, and total duration of response. A paired *t*-test was used to compare continuous data outcomes (e.g., BoNT dose) at the first and last injection visit. Ordinal outcomes (e.g., peak effect) were compared using nonparametric tests.

Author Contributions: Conceptualization, J.J.; Methodology, N.N., J.J.; Validation, N.N., J.J.; Formal Analysis, N.N.; Investigation, N.N.; Resources, J.J.; Data Curation, N.N.; Writing-Original Draft Preparation, N.N.; Writing-Review & Editing, N.N., J.J.; Visualization, N.N.; Supervision, J.J.; Project Administration, N.N., J.J.

Funding: This research received no external funding.

Conflicts of Interest: Nicki Niemann: The author declare no conflict of interest. Joseph Jankovic: Dr. Jankovic has received research and/or training grants from: Adamas Pharmaceuticals, Inc.; Allergan, Inc.; Biotie Therapies; CHDI Foundation; Civitas/Acorda Therapeutics; Dystonia Coalition; Dystonia Medical Research Foundation; F. Hoffmann-La Roche Ltd.; Huntington Study Group; Kyowa Haako Kirin Pharma, Inc.; Medtronic Neuromodulation; Merz Pharmaceuticals; Michael J. Fox Foundation for Parkinson Research; National Institutes of Health; Neurocrine Biosciences; NeuroDerm Ltd.; Parkinson's Foundation; Nuvelution; Parkinson Study Group; Pfizer Inc.; Prothena Biosciences Inc.; Psyadon Pharmaceuticals, Inc.; Revance Therapeutics, Inc.; Sangamo BioSciences, Inc.; St. Jude Medical; Teva Pharmaceutical Industries Ltd. Dr. Jankovic has served as a consultant or as an advisory committee member for: Adamas Pharmaceuticals, Inc.; Allergan, Inc.; Merz Pharmaceuticals; Pfizer Inc.; Prothena Biosciences; Revance Therapeutics, Inc.; Teva Pharmaceutical Industries Ltd. Dr. Jankovic has received royalties or other payments from: Cambridge; Elsevier; Future Science Group; Hodder Arnold; Medlink: Neurology; Lippincott Williams and Wilkins; Wiley-Blackwell. The funders had no role in the design of the study; in the collection, analyses, or interpretation of data; in the writing of the manuscript, and in the decision to publish the results.

References

1. Bhatia, K.P.; Bain, P.; Bajaj, N.; Elble, R.J.; Hallett, M.; Louis, E.D.; Raethjen, J.; Stamelou, M.; Testa, C.M.; Deuschl, G.; et al. Consensus Statement on the classification of tremors. From the task force on tremor of the International Parkinson and Movement Disorder Society. *Mov. Disord.* **2018**, *33*, 75–87. [CrossRef] [PubMed]
2. Louis, E.D.; Machado, D.G. Tremor-related quality of life: A comparison of essential tremor vs. Parkinson's disease patients. *Park. Relat. Disord.* **2015**, *21*, 729–735. [CrossRef] [PubMed]
3. Louis, E.D.; Ferreira, J.J. How common is the most common adult movement disorder? Update on the worldwide prevalence of essential tremor. *Mov. Disord.* **2010**, *25*, 534–541. [CrossRef] [PubMed]
4. Pringsheim, T.; Jette, N.; Frolkis, A.; Steeves, T.D. The prevalence of Parkinson's disease: A systematic review and meta-analysis. *Mov. Disord.* **2014**, *29*, 1583–1590. [CrossRef] [PubMed]
5. Thenganatt, M.A.; Jankovic, J. The relationship between essential tremor and Parkinson's disease. *Park. Relat. Disord.* **2016**, *22*, S162–S165. [CrossRef] [PubMed]
6. Dirkx, M.F.; Zach, H.; Bloem, B.R.; Hallett, M.; Helmich, R.C. The nature of postural tremor in Parkinson disease. *Neurology* **2018**, *90*, e1095–e1103. [CrossRef] [PubMed]
7. Jankovic, J. How Do I Examine for Re-Emergent Tremor? *Mov. Disord. Clin. Pract.* **2016**, *3*, 216–217. [CrossRef]
8. Fasano, A.; Bove, F.; Lang, A.E. The treatment of dystonic tremor: A systematic review. *J. Neurol. Neurosurg. Psychiatry* **2014**, *85*, 759–769. [CrossRef] [PubMed]
9. Pandey, S.; Sarma, N. Tremor in dystonia. *Park. Relat. Disord.* **2016**, *29*, 3–9. [CrossRef] [PubMed]
10. Jiménez, M.C.; Vingerhoets, F.J.G. Tremor revisited: Treatment of PD tremor. *Park. Relat. Disord.* **2012**, *18*, 93–95. [CrossRef]
11. Schneider, S.A.; Deuschl, G. The treatment of tremor. *Neurotherapeutics* **2014**, *11*, 128–138. [CrossRef] [PubMed]
12. Buhmann, C.; Huckhagel, T.; Engel, K.; Gulberti, A.; Hidding, U.; Poetter-Nerger, M.; Goerendt, I.; Ludewig, P.; Braass, H.; Choe, C.U.; et al. Adverse events in deep brain stimulation: A retrospective long-term analysis of neurological, psychiatric and other occurrences. *PLoS ONE* **2017**, *12*, e0178984. [CrossRef] [PubMed]
13. Baizabal-Carvallo, J.F.; Jankovic, J. Movement disorders induced by deep brain stimulation. *Park. Relat. Disord.* **2016**, *25*, 1–9. [CrossRef] [PubMed]
14. Schreglmann, S.R.; Krauss, J.K.; Chang, J.W.; Martin, E.; Werner, B.; Bauer, R.; Hägele-Link, S.; Bhatia, K.P.; Kägi, G. Functional lesional neurosurgery for tremor: Back to the future? *J. Neurol. Neurosurg. Psychiatry* **2018**, *89*, 727–735. [CrossRef] [PubMed]
15. Elble, R.J.; Shih, L.; Cozzens, J.W. Surgical treatments for essential tremor. *Expert Rev. Neurother.* **2018**, *18*, 303–321. [CrossRef] [PubMed]
16. Mohammed, N.; Patra, D.; Nanda, A. A meta-analysis of outcomes and complications of magnetic resonance-guided focused ultrasound in the treatment of essential tremor. *Neurosurg. Focus* **2018**, *44*. [CrossRef] [PubMed]
17. Ramirez-Castaneda, J.; Jankovic, J.; Comella, C.; Dashtipour, K.; Fernandez, H.H.; Mari, Z. Diffusion, spread, and migration of botulinum toxin. *Mov. Disord.* **2013**, *28*, 1775–1783. [CrossRef] [PubMed]
18. Jankovic, J. An update on new and unique uses of botulinum toxin in movement disorders. *Toxicon* **2018**, *147*, 84–88. [CrossRef] [PubMed]
19. Ramirez-Castaneda, J.; Jankovic, J. Long-term efficacy, safety, and side effect profile of botulinum toxin in dystonia: A 20-year follow-up. *Toxicon* **2014**, *90*, 344–348. [CrossRef] [PubMed]
20. Samotus, O.; Rahimi, F.; Lee, J.; Jog, M. Functional ability improved in essential tremor by incobotulinumtoxinA injections using kinematically determined biomechanical patterns—A new future. *PLoS ONE* **2016**, *11*, e0153739. [CrossRef] [PubMed]
21. Rahimi, F.; Samotus, O.; Lee, J.; Jog, M. Effective management of upper limb parkinsonian tremor by incobotulinumtoxinA injections using sensor-based biomechanical patterns. *Tremor Other Hyperkinet. Mov.* **2015**, *5*. [CrossRef]
22. Mittal, S.O.; Machado, D.; Richardson, D.; Dubey, D.; Jabbari, B. Botulinum toxin in Parkinson disease tremor: A randomized, double-blind, placebo-controlled study with a customized injection approach. *Mayo Clin. Proc.* **2017**, *92*, 1359–1367. [CrossRef] [PubMed]

23. Jog, M.; Lee, J.; Althaus, M.; Scheschonka, A.; Dersch, H.; Simpson, D.M.; ET Study Team. Efficacy and safety of incobotulinumtoxinA (inco/A) for essential tremor using kinematics-guided clinical decision support: A randomized, double-blind, placebo-controlled trial. *Mov. Disord.* **2017**, *32* (suppl. 2). Available online: http://www.mdsabstracts.org/abstract/efficacy-and-safety-of-incobotulinumtoxina-incoa-for-essential-tremor-using-kinematics-guided-clinical-decision-support-a-randomized-double-blind-placebo-controlled-trial/ (accessed on 18 July 2018).
24. Kim, S.D.; Yiannikas, C.; Mahant, N.; Vucic, S.; Fung, V.S. Treatment of proximal upper limb tremor with botulinum toxin therapy. *Mov. Disord.* **2014**, *29*, 835–838. [CrossRef] [PubMed]
25. Mittal, S.O.; Machado, D.; Richardson, D.; Dubey, D.; Jabbari, B. Botulinum toxin in essential hand tremor—A randomized double-blind placebo-controlled study with customized injection approach. *Park. Relat. Disord.* **2018**. [CrossRef] [PubMed]
26. Jankovic, J.; Schwartz, K.S. Botulinum toxin treatment of tremors. *Neurology* **1991**, *41*, 1185–1188. [CrossRef] [PubMed]
27. Jankovic, J.; Schwartz, K.; Clemence, W.; Aswad, A.; Mordaunt, J. A randomized, double-blind, placebo-controlled study to evaluate botulinum toxin type A in essential hand tremor. *Mov. Disord.* **1996**, *11*, 250–256. [CrossRef] [PubMed]
28. Brin, M.F.; Lyons, K.E.; Doucette, J.; Adler, C.H.; Caviness, J.N.; Comella, C.L.; Dubinsky, R.M.; Friedman, J.H.; Manyam, B.V.; Matsumoto, J.Y.; et al. A randomized, double masked, controlled trial of botulinum toxin type A in essential hand tremor. *Neurology* **2001**, *56*, 1523–1528. [CrossRef] [PubMed]
29. Jankovic, J. The use of botulinum toxin in tic disorders and essential hand and head tremor. In *Manual of Botulinum Toxin Therapy*, 2nd ed.; Cambridge University Press: Cambridge, UK, 2013; pp. 160–167.
30. Rahimi, F.; Bee, C.; Debicki, D.; Roberts, A.C.; Bapat, P.; Jog, M. Effectiveness of BoNT A in Parkinson's disease upper limb tremor management. *Can. J. Neurol. Sci.* **2013**, *40*, 663–669. [CrossRef] [PubMed]
31. Samotus, O.; Kumar, N.; Rizek, P.; Jog, M. Botulinum toxin type A injections as monotherapy for upper limb essential tremor using kinematics. *Can. J. Neurol. Sci.* **2018**, *45*, 11–22. [CrossRef] [PubMed]
32. Samotus, O.; Lee, J.; Jog, M. Long-term tremor therapy for Parkinson and essential tremor with sensor-guided botulinum toxin type A injections. *PLoS ONE* **2017**, *12*, e0178670. [CrossRef] [PubMed]
33. Zakin, E.; Simpson, D. Botulinum toxin in management of limb tremor. *Toxins* **2017**, *9*, 365. [CrossRef] [PubMed]
34. Karp, B.; Alter, K. Muscle selection for focal limb dystonia. *Toxins* **2017**, *10*, 20. [CrossRef] [PubMed]
35. Pacchetti, C.; Mancini, F.; Bulgheroni, M.; Zangaglia, R.; Cristina, S.; Sandrini, G.; Nappi, G. Botulinum toxin treatment for functional disability induced by essential tremor. *Neurol. Sci.* **2000**, *21*, 349–353. [CrossRef] [PubMed]
36. Sitburana, O.; Wu, L.J.; Sheffield, J.K.; Davidson, A.; Jankovic, J. Motor overflow and mirror dystonia. *Park. Relat. Disord.* **2009**, *15*, 758–761. [CrossRef] [PubMed]
37. Wu, C.; Xue, F.; Chang, W.; Lian, Y.; Zheng, Y.; Xie, N.; Zhang, L.; Chen, C. Botulinum toxin type A with or without needle electromyographic guidance in patients with cervical dystonia. *Springerplus* **2016**, *5*. [CrossRef] [PubMed]
38. Jankovic, J. Needle EMG guidance for injection of botulinum toxin. Needle EMG guidance is rarely required. *Muscle Nerve* **2001**, *24*, 1568–1570. [CrossRef] [PubMed]
39. Sheffield, J.K.; Jankovic, J. Botulinum toxin in the treatment of tremors, dystonias, sialorrhea and other symptoms associated with Parkinson's disease. *Expert Rev. Neurother.* **2007**, *7*, 637–647. [CrossRef] [PubMed]

toxins

MDPI

Article

Transitioning from Unilateral to Bilateral Upper Limb Tremor Therapy for Parkinson's Disease and Essential Tremor Using Botulinum Toxin: Case Series

Olivia Samotus [1,2], Jack Lee [1] and Mandar Jog [1,2,*]

1 Department of Clinical Neurological Sciences, London Health Sciences Centre—Lawson Health Research Institute, 339 Windermere Road, A10-026, London, ON N6A 5A5, Canada; osamotus@uwo.ca (O.S.); jack.lee@lhsc.on.ca (J.L.)
2 Schulich School of Medicine and Dentistry, University of Western, 1151 Richmond Street, London, ON N6A 3K7, Canada
* Correspondence: mandar.jog@lhsc.on.ca; Tel.: +1-(519)-663-3814

Received: 23 August 2018; Accepted: 22 September 2018; Published: 27 September 2018

Abstract: Botulinum toxin type A (BoNT-A) injections guided by kinematic analysis for unilateral upper limb essential tremor (ET) and Parkinson's disease (PD) tremor therapy has demonstrated efficacy, improvements in quality of life (QoL) and arm functionality. In this open-label pilot trial, 5 ET and 2 PD participants decided to switch from receiving long-term unilateral arm treatment to now bilateral BoNT-A arm therapy in their other tremulous arm which worsened over time. Injection patterns were based on kinematic analysis. Efficacy endpoints including kinematic analysis, Fahn-Tolosa-Marin tremor rating scale, QoL questionnaire, and maximal grip strength were collected over 2 treatments and 2 follow-up visits totaling 18-weeks. BoNT-A decreased wrist tremor amplitude by 84.6% and 89.6% 6-weeks following the 1st injection in the newly-treated limb in ET and PD participants, respectively. PD participants started with worse QoL but demonstrated an additional improvement in QoL by 29.9% for switching to bilateral treatment, whereas ET participants did not. Left and right arm tremor also did not share commonalities in severity or dose. This preliminary finding suggests trends for transitioning to bilateral therapy and warrants further studies to evaluate efficacy of bilateral tremor BoNT-A therapy in a larger cohort of PD and ET patients.

Keywords: Parkinson's disease; essential tremor; tremor; movement disorders; Botulinum toxin; kinematics; upper limb biomechanics; joint biomechanics; diagnostic guidance; clinical decision support

Key Contribution: Two PD and five ET participants transitioned from receiving serial unilateral BoNT-A injections to bilateral therapy for their upper limb tremor. All participants experienced a reduction in tremor severity, however PD participants found a QoL improvement where ET participants remained unchanged since ET participants had better QoL to start with as compared to PD. As this study demonstrates a glimpse to the possible benefits of bilateral BoNT-A therapy, tremor patients with worse QoL and more severe bilateral tremor may benefit more from bilateral rather than unilateral arm treatment.

---

1. Introduction

One-third of Parkinson's disease (PD) patients experience tremor-related quality of life (QoL) problems that interfere with daily activities, such as eating and dressing, which induce psychosocial stress in more than 25% of patients [1]. Tremor is a functional interference and social embarrassment for those with essential tremor (ET) and hence many seek therapy. ET and PD tremor amplitudes are generally asymmetric in severity and frequency [2,3] however it is typical to observe worsening of PD tremor severity over the disease progression where ET severity increase is correlated to patient age and duration of tremor and thus severity gradually worsens with time [4]. Traditional oral medications, such as levodopa for PD tremor and beta-blockers and anticonvulsants for ET, provide suboptimal benefit although are frequently coupled with significant adverse events [5–7] and many of these patients stop their oral treatments within the first year [8,9].

Visually assessed, targeted therapy by botulinum toxin type A (BoNT-A) injections for one arm have been shown to produce reasonable reduction of ET and PD wrist tremor severities although significant muscle weakness and limited functional benefit has warranted many patients to discontinue treatment [10–14]. Samotus et al. have demonstrated the importance of utilizing objective tremor analysis by measuring the severity and direction of tremor along the whole arm using motion sensor devices to guide the clinical determination of BoNT-A injection muscle groups to treat, thereby limiting the likelihood of muscle weakness over serial treatments [15–17]. Furthermore, a significant reduction in ET and PD tremor has been shown when treating the side of the arm with the most bothersome upper limb following the first treatment, which was sustained by a 76% and 70% improvement, respectively, up to 96 weeks compared to baseline tremor severity measures [17]. In addition, ET and PD patients experience improvement in arm function as functional disability caused by tremor was significantly reduced by 46.3% and 31.3%, respectively [17]. While ET participants showed a 46.1% improvement in QoL when treated in their most disabling limb, PD participants demonstrated no change in QoL [17].

This is the first proof of principle study to date to demonstrate that ET and PD participants who already received beneficial unilateral BoNT-A therapy can transition to bilateral BoNT-A injections for their upper limb tremor for further improvement. The decision to transition was based upon each participant's discretion and muscle injection patterns were based on kinematic tremor analysis.

2. Results

2.1. Study Population

A total of 7 (5 ET and 2 PD) participants who were no longer satisfied with their BoNT-A treatment chose to transition from unilateral to bilateral upper limb injections as they felt tremor in their untreated arm to be bothersome. These participants were part of the same cohort of individuals published in previous tremor papers from the London Movement Disorders Centre [15–17]. Clinical scores, demographics, number of injection cycles and the injection parameters in the first treated limb of the 7 participants are summarized in Table 1. All participants were right-handed and initially received BoNT-A therapy in their most bothersome tremor arm which was the right arm; a mean of 6 $\pm$ 3 additional injection cycles were administered following the 96-week study [17] before transitioning to bilateral therapy (initiation of treatment in their left arm). All participants had greater tremor severity in their original treated (right) arm at the start of the 96-week study. Three ET participants received monotherapy of BoNT-A and were not on any other tremor related medication.

The mean number of muscles and the dosages allocated to elbow and shoulder muscle groups were similar between both upper limbs for all participants. However, the mean wrist dose for the newly treated (left) arm was 46.4 $\pm$ 17.3 U compared to the optimized mean wrist dose of 72.1 $\pm$ 36.2 U in the right arm for all participants (Supplementary Tables S1 and S2). For all transition participants, a similar mean total dose was administered for the two treatment cycles in the left arm, 133.6 $\pm$ 47.3 U and 135.0 $\pm$ 48.0 U at the 1st injection (T1) and 2nd injection (T3), respectively (Figure 1). Mean BoNT-A dosages in the wrist muscles were lower in the newly treated arm (8.4 $\pm$ 4.9 U) compared to the original treated arm (10.8 $\pm$ 6.3 U) (Supplementary Tables S3 and S4). Dosages allocated to the elbow and shoulder muscles were also lower in the newly treated arm (16.6 $\pm$ 8.7 U) compared to the original treated arm (23.0 $\pm$ 5.8 U).

Table 1. Participant demographics and injection dosages, number of muscles and number of treatment cycles administered in the optimized, original treated right arm prior to transition into bilateral therapy.

ID	Diagnosis	Gender	Age	Medications (Daily Dose)	Dominant Limb	First Injected Limb	7th Injection–96 Weeks		
							Total Dose (Units)	# of Muscles Treated	# of Additional Unilateral Injections after 96-Weeks but before Transition
1	PD	M	35	Stalevo (400 mg)	R	R	300	13	10
2	ET	F	74	Primidone (125 mg)	R	R	85	7	8
3	ET	M	78	Primidone (125 mg)	R	R	200	8	9
4	PD	M	68	Sinemet (750 mg)	R	R	200	11	7
5	ET	F	65	-	R	R	280	13	6
6	ET	F	80	-	R	R	165	11	2
7	ET	M	73	-	R	R	115	9	3

Number (#).

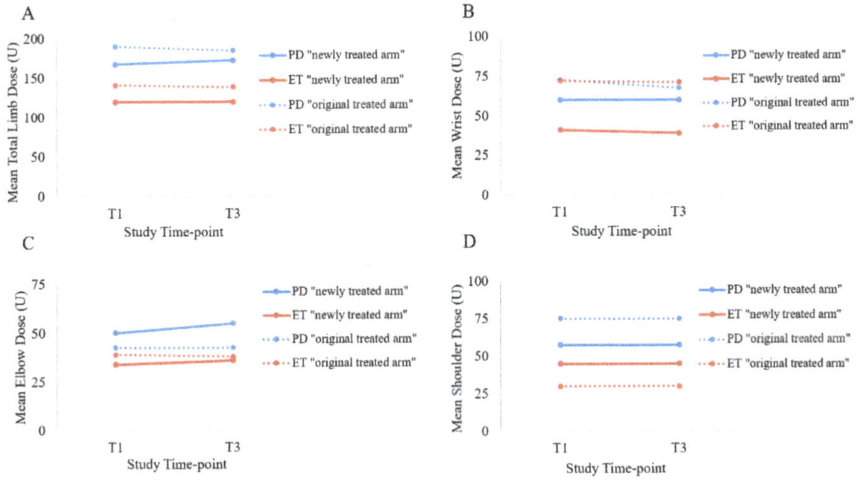

Figure 1. Mean BoNT-A dosages in the whole arm (**A**), wrist (**B**), elbow (**C**), and shoulder (**D**) joints are plotted for each limb for Parkinson's disease (PD) and essential tremor (ET) participants.

2.2. Fahn-Tolosa-Marin (FTM) Tremor Rating and Arm Functionality

Prior to treating the left arm (untreated), ET tremor severity was similar from L1 (week 0 of the original unilateral 96-week study [17]) to first transition visit (T1), indicating no increase in left arm tremor amplitude (Figure 2A). As for the PD participants' newly treated (left) arm, tremor severity (FTM part A) worsened by 83.3% (mean + 1.5 point difference) from week 0 (L1) to transition initiation (T1).

Following the second treatment (T4) in the newly treated (left) arm, a mean 26.3% tremor reduction (−1.0 FTM part A point difference) from mild-moderate (3.8 ± 1.8) at pre-treatment (T1) to slight-mild (2.8 ± 1.6) tremor severity was observed in the ET group (Figure 2A). A 31.3% (mean −2.0 point difference) improvement in fine motor tasks (FTM part B) was observed at T4 (2.5 ± 2.3) compared to T1 (4.5 ± 2.3) (Figure 2B). In the previously treated and optimized (right) limb, tremor severity and fine motor skills did not change over the two treatment cycles (Figure 2A,B). A reported 31.8% (mean −2.8 point difference) and a 11.4% (mean −1.0 point difference) improvement in FTM part C scores were observed at time of re-injection (T3; 6.0 ± 3.2) and following the 2nd injection (T4; 7.8 ± 4.3), respectively, compared to pre-injection (T1; 8.8 ± 5.6) demonstrating a trending improvement in daily activities for ET participants (Figure 2C).

In the PD group, a 72.7% reduction (mean −4.0 point difference) in tremor severity was observed from 5.5 ± 1.9 points at T1 to 1.5 ± 1.6 points at T4 demonstrating a reduction in severity from mild-moderate to a slight tremor severity (Figure 2A). A 44.4% improvement (mean −2.0 point difference) in fine motor skills (FTM part B) was observed from 4.5 ± 2.3 points at T1 to 2.5 ± 2.3 points at T4 in the PD group (Figure 2B). Functional disability caused by tremor (FTM part C) was reduced by 28.0% (mean −3.5 point difference) from 12.5 ± 5.6 points at T1 to 9.0 ± 3.2 points at time of re-injection (T3) (Figure 2C).

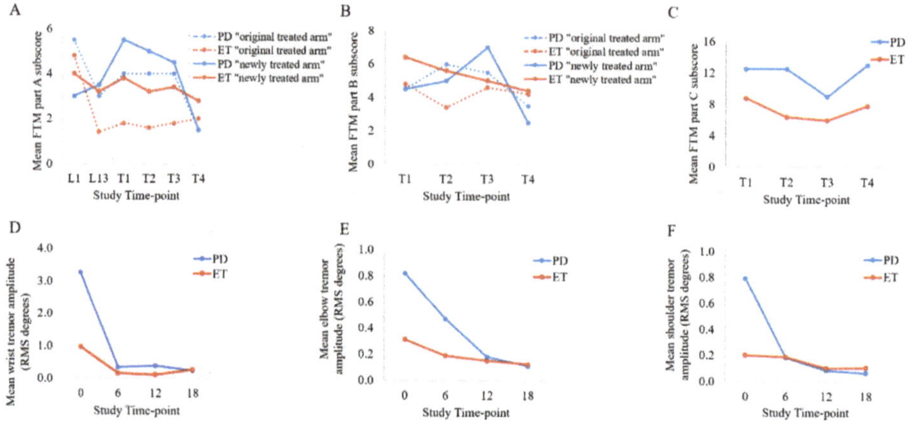

Figure 2. Mean Fahn-Tolosa-Marin (FTM) sub-scores for part A (**A**), part B (**B**), and part (**C**) and mean root mean square (RMS) tremor amplitudes at the wrist (**D**), elbow (**E**) and shoulder (**F**) joints for PD and ET participants across a period of 18 weeks. T1 and T3 study visits were injection visits 12-weeks apart and T2 and T4 were follow-up visits 6-weeks following an injection. For tremor severity (FTM part A), time-points at L1 and L13 indicating week 0 and week 96, respectively, of the previously published unilateral tremor-BoNT-A treatment study were included.

2.3. *Kinematic Tremor Analysis*

Four (1 PD and 3 ET) and two (1 PD and 1 ET) participants experienced their most severe wrist tremor amplitude during "posture" and "load" tasks, respectively, in the newly treated (left) arm as compared to their original treated (right) arm which was pre-dominantly most severe during the "load" tasks (Table 2). Similarly, five (2 PD and 3 ET) participants experienced their highest elbow tremor during "posture" in the newly treated arm while majority of the elbow tremor in the original treated arm was captured during "load" tasks. For shoulder tremor, the original treated arm most severe tremor was captured during "load" tasks, while for the newly treated arm there was no obvious task specific trend.

Prior to the treatment in the newly treated (left) arm, the PD participants (3.3 ± 1.9 RMS-degrees) exhibited a higher wrist tremor severity as compared to the ET group (1.0 ± 0.9 RMS-degrees). For ET participants in the newly treated arm, mean wrist RMS tremor amplitude was reduced by 84.6% (mean −0.8 RMS-degree difference) from 1.0 ± 0.9 RMS-degree at T1 to 0.1 ± 0.1 RMS-degree following the 1st injection (T2) and was maintained by a tremor reduction of 73.4% (0.2 ± 0.3 RMS-degrees) at following the 2nd injection (T4) (Figure 2D). Mean elbow and shoulder tremor amplitudes were reduced by 60.2% and 47.5%, respectively, following the 2nd injection (T4) as compared to pre-injection (T1) (Figure 2E,F). Similar changes in tremor severity were observed in the two PD participants, a mean reduction of 92.6%, 86.6% and 91.8% in wrist, elbow and shoulder tremor amplitude was observed following the 2nd injection compared to T1 (Figure 2D,F).

Table 2. The task with the highest tremor amplitude observed at each arm joint in the newly treated arm (left) and in the original treated arm (right).

ID	Diagnosis	Task with Highest Tremor Amplitude in the "Newly Treated Arm" (Left Arm)			Task with Highest Tremor Amplitude in the "Original Treated Arm" (Right Arm) *		
		Wrist	Elbow	Shoulder	Wrist	Elbow	Shoulder
1	PD	Posture-1	Posture-2	Posture-2	Load-1	Posture-2	Load-1
2	ET	Posture-1	Posture-2	Posture-2	Load-2	Load-2	Posture-2
3	ET	Load-1	Load-2	Load-2	Load-1	Load-2	Load-2
4	PD	Posture-2	Posture-2	Posture-1	Load-1	Load-2	Load-2
5	ET	Load-2	Load-1	Load-1	Rest-2	Posture-1	Load-2
6	ET	Posture-1	Load-2	Load-2	Load-1	Load-2	Load-2
7	ET	Posture-1	Posture-1	Rest-2	Posture-2	Load-1	Posture-2

* Tremor analysis of the original treated arm was performed during the conduct of the previously published report by Samotus O. et al., 2017.

2.4. Quality of Life Measures and Safety Outcomes

For the ET cohort that had bilateral tremor with predominant severity originally in the treated right arm, the transition into bilateral tremor treatment resulted in an additional improvement in QoL score (QUEST) by 13.3% (mean −2.0 point difference) from 15.0 ± 10.1 at time of 1st bilateral treatment (T1) to 13.0 ± 9.4 6-weeks following the 1st injection (T2), although a 17.3% (mean +2.6 point difference) worsening in QoL was observed following the 2nd injection at T4 (17.6 ± 13.8) (Figure 3A). For the PD participants, QoL was improved by 29.9% (mean −13.0 point difference) from 43.5 ± 4.9 at T1 to 30.5 ± 4.9 QUEST score at T4.

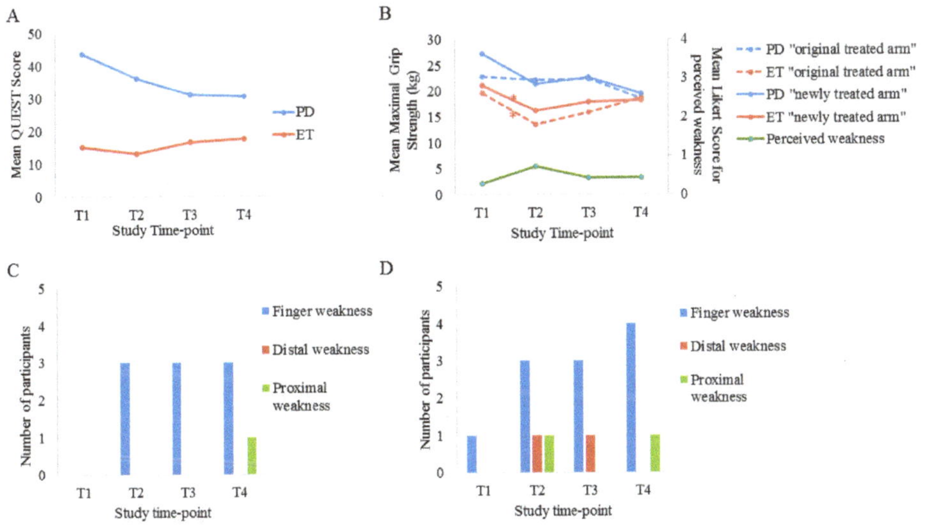

Figure 3. Mean quality of life for essential tremor questionnaire (QUEST) scores (**A**), changes in mean maximal grip strength and participant-perceived muscle weakness (**B**), and number of participants with a manual muscle testing (MMT), rating ≤ 3 in the newly treated arm (**C**) and in the original treated arm (**D**) across the transition 18-week period involving two BoNT-A treatments at T1 and T3 were plotted. Tremor impact on QoL was reduced demonstrated by a reduced QUEST score.

In the ET population, the mean maximal grip strength in the newly treated arm was reduced by 23.1% (mean −4.9 kg difference) from 21.1 ± 9.1 kg at T1 to 16.2 ± 9.2 kg following the 1st injection at T2, however this reduction in maximum grip strength was not noticeable at time of re-injection at

T3 (mean −3.1 kg difference; 17.9 ± 9.1 kg) or after at T4 (mean −2.8 kg difference; 18.3 ± 10.7 kg) (Figure 3B). In the original treated arm, which had received serial treatments prior to bilateral treatment, a reduction in mean grip strength by 31.4% (mean −6.2 kg difference) from 19.7 ± 7.1 kg at T1 to 13.5 ± 9.0 kg at T2, was observed in ET. In the PD group, the mean maximal grip strength in the newly treated arm was reduced by 21.5% (mean −5.8 kg difference) from 27.2 ± 14.8 kg at T1 to 21.3 ± 13.7 kg following the first injection at T2 and was further reduced to 19.5 ± 12.5 kg following the second injection at T4. In the original treated arm, mean maximal grip strength was similar from T1 to T3 although following the 2nd injection at T4, a 19.0% reduction in mean grip strength (−4.3 kg difference) was observed compared to 22.8 ± 12.0 kg at T1.

When questioning participants of their perceived change in hand and arm strength, the mean Likert score for participant-perceived weakness reported only slight perceived weakness in injected muscles following the 1st injection (T2) (Figure 3B). At the re-injection visit (T3), perceived muscle weakness was scored as none to slight mild weakness 6-weeks following the 2nd injection (T4).

Based on MMT of the newly treated (left) arm, three participants (1 PD and 2 ET) experienced finger weakness following the first treatment, at re-injection and following the second treatment (T2–T4) (Figure 3C). An ET participant was felt to have proximal (triceps) weakness following the second treatment (T4). In the original treated arm, 3 participants (1 PD and 2 ET) experienced finger weakness during the first treatment cycle (T2–T3) and 4 participants (1 PD and 3 ET) experienced middle finger weakness following the second treatment (T4) (Figure 3D). An ET participant experienced wrist flexor/extensor weakness at T2 and T3 and an ET participant experienced triceps weakness at T4.

3. Discussion

In this open-label, pilot, clinical phase II study, 5 ET and 2 PD participants chose to switch to bilateral tremor treatment as they perceived their untreated left arm to be now bothersome enough to warrant treatment. Prior to bilateral treatment, ET participants had been treated for their right arm tremor and already experienced significant functional and quality of life (QoL) improvement in their arm function as reported by all FTM and QUEST scores with sustained benefit over 96 weeks [17]. Once bilateral treatments were introduced, the tremor severity was vastly reduced at the wrist, elbow, and shoulder in the left arm. FTM functional scale reported an additional mild improvement, however scores for QoL did not further improve (Figures 2A and 3A). Given that these 5 ET participants prior to any BoNT-A therapy had asymmetric bilateral tremor (tremor was worse on right side), the participants still desired treatment to possibly hide and suppress the visual cues of their left arm tremor which had become more prominent in comparison to their treated right arm.

For the 2 PD participants in the newly treated (left) arm, tremor severity also was vastly reduced (Figure 2C). At the start of bilateral treatment, the two PD participants had worse QoL (QUEST) scores as compared to their ET counterparts, which may explain the large additional improvement in QoL (29.9% increase) following two treatment cycles (Figure 3A). Likewise, the PD participants had a measurable worsening of their left arm tremor leading up to the bilateral treatment, while this was not the case for the ET group who perceived their left arm to be more noticeable in tremor severity. Thus, the decision of the 2 PD participants to receive bilateral therapy could be due to their priority to further improve arm function and overall quality of life, and less likely due to tremor visibility.

When comparing the initial BoNT-A injection dose-response in the right arm (96-week study) to the left arm (current study), the decrease in tremor amplitude measured by kinematics and visual rating (FTM part A) show similar reduction in severity. Likewise, the decrease in maximal grip strength in the left arm, which majority of participants did not perceive as bothersome, and the reported non-debilitating finger weakness was expectantly like the initial weakness response experienced by participants in the right arm (Figure 2B–D) [17]. The ET and PD participants tolerability to additional muscles treated with BoNT-A for bilateral arm treatment did not impact their muscle weakness profile.

When comparing the tremor characteristics for each participant between the left and right arm, no global pattern in arm position or tasks was to be found. Furthermore, tremor at the wrist, elbow, and shoulder for each arm was unique for participants (Table 2). Thus, for optimal BoNT-A injection parameter customization, several arm positions or tasks must be conducted as tremor severity is variable depending on arm positioning. The individualized wrist, elbow, and shoulder dosing for muscles in each arm requires a high level of customization which is feasible by objective tremor analysis and is overwhelming and time consuming when done by visual (clinical) assessment (Supplemental Tables S1–S4). When comparing the left and right arm initial injection dosage within each participant, no obvious dose pattern was present for individual muscle targets; for the wrist specifically, some muscles were not treated if the tremor analysis showed minimal muscle group involvement for one arm but was present in the other arm (Supplemental Tables S3 and S4).

Given this was a small case series on select participants with asymmetric bilateral arm tremor (worse tremor in the right) and who were not naïve to BoNT-A, the trend suggests the use of bilateral tremor therapy provides greater benefit in QoL for those with worsening or equally severe tremor on both sides. It would be interesting to explore the use of bilateral BoNT-A therapy in a larger cohort of both BoNT-A-naïve ET and PD patients, and for these individuals to present with equally bothersome tremor on both sides to compare efficacy and tolerability outcomes to our present study. The findings from such a study would also be interesting to compare to the previous unilateral study to see if QoL and functional improvements are superior with fewer treatment cycles required and how patients perceive their arm weakness if treatment in both arms were initiated jointly. Presently, the overall combined dose for both arms ranged from 120–450 U and none of the 7 tremor participants experienced bothersome muscle weakness side-effects during bilateral treatment. One of the other limitations in this current report is the 18 weeks of available data; it would be of significant real-world value to conduct a longer study to see if the QoL and functional benefits witnessed are maintained following the first two treatment cycles in both arms.

Ultimately, this pilot bilateral tremor study gives us the first glimpse of the opportunity for treating patients with BoNT-A aided by tremor analysis. Presence of bilateral tremor alone might not necessitate the need to treat both sides, but instead require careful clinical consideration of objective tremor severity, handedness, and of course the patient's expectation of outcome; whether its visible suppression of tremor, or their desire for improvement in quality of life and hand function when performing bimanual tasks.

4. Materials and Methods

4.1. Study Design and Participants

An extension of a previously published single-centre, single-injector, open-label, clinical phase II pilot study by the London Movement Disorders Centre [15–17] was approved by the Western University Health Sciences Research Ethics Board (REB) on 9 September 2015, the REB study number is: 101749. Participants who received benefit in the original 96-weeks [17], continued to receive unilateral BoNT-A therapy and were identified to have bilateral tremor with bothersome tremor present on the untreated side. For the ET participants, they had presentation of bilateral tremor at the start of the unilateral study [17], however, majority of these ET participants had significantly more severe tremor in their dominant right hand, which received unilateral therapy, as compared to their left hand. These participants were given the choice to start receiving injections in their other upper (left) limb if participants perceived their tremor to be bothersome/disabling. 7 out of 21 participants (5 ET and 2 PD participants) decided to receive BoNT-A injection therapy in their other upper (left) limb. This report described a total of four study visits every 6 weeks totaling 18-weeks where participants received injections 12-weeks apart at transition visits 1 (T1) and 3 (T3) and follow-ups were conducted 6-weeks post-injection at transition visits 2 (T2) and 4 (T4). First participant's first visit and last participant's last visit occurred between August 2016 and May 2018. All participants provided written informed consent. The study and all related trials for this intervention are registered on the clinicaltrials.gov registry (ClinicalTrials.gov Identifier: NCT02427646).

4.2. Clinical Outcome Measures and Kinematic Tremor Analysis

Severity of tremor and limb functionality were reported using the Fahn-Tolosa-Marin (FTM) tremor rating scale, quality of life (QoL) measures were reported using the quality of life for essential tremor questionnaire (QUEST) [18,19]. Muscle weakness as a side effect to BoNT-A injections was monitored using a Baseline® hydraulic hand dynamometer (Item#: 12-0240, White Plains, NY, USA) to measure maximal grip strength [20]. A Likert style participant-rated scale ranging from 0: no weakness, 1: mild, 2: moderate, 3: marked and 4: severe weakness with functional loss in injected muscles was administered to assess perceived muscle weakness reported by all participants at each visit. In addition, manual muscle testing (MMT) was used to assess strength in the fingers, wrist, and elbow flexor/extensor muscles where a score of 3+ or higher representing the ability to hold muscle position against gravity and resist slight pressure [21].

Severity of upper limb tremor was captured with kinematic sensors while participants performed a series of six scripted tasks each held for 20 s over three trials, as previously described [15]. Wrist tremor was analyzed in multiple degrees of freedom (DOFs) which resulted in the decomposition of tremor muscle groups such as wrist flexion-extension (F/E), radial-ulnar (R/U), and pronation-supination (P/S). Kinematics was utilized to monitor change in tremor severity over the 18-week study. All participants were assessed while "ON" their medication and during the same time of day to reduce tremor variability.

4.3. Treatment

Participants received two treatments 12 weeks apart, bilateral, intramuscular injections of BoNT-A (incobotulinumtoxinA; Xeomin®, Merz Pharmaceuticals, Frankfurt, Germany) of a total dose ranging between 30–300 U into muscles of the wrist, elbow and/or shoulder. Injection parameters previously used for the originally treated right arm (injector's experience with visual and kinematic guidance to allocate dosages based on highest total tremor amplitude at each arm joint) were optimized for several cycles prior to the patient's transition to bilateral therapy [17]. For the newly treated left arm, kinematic analysis was conducted to determine the initial injection parameters for the transition arm by identifying the task that produced the highest tremor amplitude per arm joint. The initial BoNT-A dose per muscle for the left arm was based on kinematic tremor analysis; a dosing algorithm was created based on the relationship of total joint dose and highest joint tremor severity from the earlier unilateral tremor-toxin study [17]. Dosages per muscle for the second treatment cycle were adjusted by the injector based on changes in kinematic tremor severity from pre- to post-injection time-points, clinical judgement and with patient feedback, such as noticeable muscle weakness as previously described by Samotus et al. [17].

4.4. Analysis

No formal sample size calculation was performed, all analysis was exploratory, and clinical and kinematic data are presented as case reports. Mean clinical scale scores and RMS tremor amplitudes from the ET and PD population groups were plotted for all transition study visits (T1–T4). Changes in mean clinical scores and RMS tremor amplitudes, as mean percent change and mean point/RMS degree changes, were compared from baseline (T1) to each post-treatment time-point (week 6 (T2), 12 (T3) and 18 (T4)), between re-injection visits (baseline (T1) and week 12 (T3)) and between peak effect of BoNT-A (weeks 6 (T2) and 18 (T4)). FTM part A scores from weeks 0 (L1) and 96 (L13) were plotted from data previously published in Samotus et al. to report any changes in tremor severity prior to initiation of transition treatment [17].

5. Patents

Two patents, PCT/CA2013/000804 pending to MDDT Inc. (London, ON, Canada), and a patent PCT/CA2014/050893 pending to MDDT Inc., resulted from the work reported in this manuscript.

Supplementary Materials: The following are available online http://www.mdpi.com/2072-6651/10/10/394/s1, Table S1: Optimization of Botulinum toxin type A (BoNT-A) parameters over the two injection treatments in the optimized, original treated limb (right arm) (A) and in the newly treated limb (left arm) (B), Table S2: Optimization of BoNT-A parameters over the two injection treatments in the newly treated limb (left arm), Table S3: The muscles and BoNT-A dosing parameters over the two injection treatments in the original treated limb (right arm), Table S4: The muscles and BoNT-A dosing parameters over the two injection treatments in the newly treated limb (left arm).

Author Contributions: Conceptualization, O.S., J.L., and M.J.; methodology, O.S., J.L. and M.J.; formal analysis, O.S. and J.L.; investigation, O.S., J.L. and M.J.; resources, O.S., J.L. and M.J.; writing—original draft preparation, O.S.; writing—review and editing, O.S., J.L. and M.J.; visualization, O.S., J.L. and M.J.; supervision, O.S., J.L. and M.J.; project administration, O.S., J.L. and M.J.; funding acquisition, O.S., J.L. and M.J.

Funding: The present study was partially funded by a research grant from Merz Pharma Canada and government-industry matched grant from MITACS (#IT03924).

Acknowledgments: We would like to acknowledge the contribution by the participants and by the post-doctoral engineering and volunteer research staff at the National Parkinson Foundation Centre of Excellence, London Movement Disorders Centre located within the London Health Sciences Centre, London, ON, Canada.

Conflicts of Interest: M.J. reports a research grant from Merz Pharma, during the conduct of the study. Outside of this study, M.J. also is a scientific advisor and receives research financial support from the following companies: AbbVie, Allergan Inc., Boston Scientific, Ipsen, MDDT Inc., Medtronic, Merz Pharma, Novartis, and Teva Pharmaceuticals. In addition, M.J., who is commercializing this medical device, TremorTek, has a patent PCT/CA2013/000804 pending to MDDT Inc., and a patent PCT/CA2014/050893 pending to MDDT Inc. J.L. is a former research associate and now is a MDDT Inc. employee. M.J. and J.L. are both shareholders of MDDT Inc. O.S. reports a MITACS (Merz Pharma) grant during the conduct of the study.

Abbreviations

BoNT-A	botulinum toxin type A
DOF	degree of freedom
ET	essential tremor
FTM	Fahn-Tolosa-Marin
MMT	manual muscle testing
PD	Parkinson's disease
QoL	quality of life
QUEST	Quality of Life in Essential Tremor Questionnaire
RMS	root mean square

References

1. Louis, E.D.; Machado, D.G. Tremor-related quality of life: A comparison of essential tremor vs. Parkinson's disease patients. *Parkinsonism Relat. Disord.* **2015**, *21*, 729–735. [CrossRef] [PubMed]
2. Hedera, P.; Cibulčík, F.; Davis, T.L. Pharmacotherapy of essential tremor. *J. Cent. Nerv. Syst. Dis.* **2013**, *5*, 43–55. [CrossRef] [PubMed]
3. Machowska-Majchrzak, A.; Pierzchała, K.; Łabuz-Roszak, B.; Bartman, W. The usefulness of accelerometric registration with assessment of tremor parameters and their symmetry in differential diagnosis of parkinsonian, essential and cerebella tremor. *Neurologia i Neurochirurgia Polska* **2012**, *46*, 145–156. [CrossRef] [PubMed]
4. Elble, R.J. What is Essential Tremor? *Curr. Neurol. Neurosci. Rep.* **2013**, *13*, 353. [CrossRef] [PubMed]
5. Schadt, C.R.; Duffis, E.I.; Charles, P.D. Pharmacological treatment of disabling tremor. *Expert Opin. Pharmacother.* **2005**, *6*, 419–428. [CrossRef] [PubMed]
6. Katzenschlager, R.; Sampaio, C.; Costa, J.; Lees, A. Anticholinergics for symptomatic management of Parkinson's disease. *Cochrane Database Syst. Rev.* **2003**, *2*, CD003735. [CrossRef]
7. Rajput, A.H.; Rajput, A. Medical treatment of essential tremor. *J. Cent. Nerv. Syst. Dis.* **2014**, *6*, 29–39. [CrossRef] [PubMed]
8. Koller, W.C.; Vetere-Overfield, B. Acute and chronic effects of propranolol and primidone in essential tremor. *Neurology* **1989**, *39*, 1587–1588. [CrossRef] [PubMed]
9. Louis, E.D.; Rios, E.; Henchcliffe, C. How are we doing with the treatment of essential tremor (ET)? Persistence of ET patients on medication: Data from 528 patients in three settings. *Eur. J. Neurol.* **2010**, *17*, 882–884. [CrossRef] [PubMed]

10. Zesiewicz, T.A.; Elble, R.; Louis, E.D.; Hauser, R.A.; Sullivan, K.L.; Dewey, R.B.; Ondo, W.G.; Gronseth, G.S.; Weiner, W.J. Practice parameter: Therapies for essential tremor—Report of the quality standards subcommittee of the American academy of neurology. *Neurology* **2005**, *64*, 2008–2020. [CrossRef] [PubMed]
11. Kim, S.D.; Yiannikas, C.; Mahant, N.; Vucic, S.; Fung, V.S.C. Treatment of proximal upper limb tremor with botulinum toxin therapy. *Mov. Disord.* **2014**, *29*, 835–838. [CrossRef] [PubMed]
12. Trosch, R.M.; Pullman, S.L. Botulinum toxin A injections for the treatment of hand tremors. *Mov. Disord.* **1994**, *9*, 601–609. [CrossRef] [PubMed]
13. Pullman, S.L.; Greene, P.; Fahn, S.; Pedersen, S.F. Approach to the treatment of limb disorders with botulinum toxin A. Experience with 187 patients. *Arch. Neurol.* **1996**, *53*, 617–624. [CrossRef] [PubMed]
14. Jankovic, J.; Schwartz, K.; Clemence, W.; Aswad, A.; Mordaunt, J. A randomized, double-blind, placebo-controlled study to evaluate botulinum toxin type A in essential hand tremor. *Mov. Disord.* **1996**, *11*, 250–256. [CrossRef] [PubMed]
15. Rahimi, F.; Samotus, O.; Lee, J.; Jog, M. Effective Management of Upper Limb Parkinsonian Tremor by IncobotulinumtoxinA Injections Using Sensor-based Biomechanical Patterns. *Tremor Other Hyperkinet Mov.* **2015**, *5*, 348. [CrossRef]
16. Samotus, O.; Rahimi, F.; Lee, J.; Jog, M. Functional Ability Improved in Essential Tremor by IncobotulinumtoxinA Injections Using Kinematically Determined Biomechanical Patterns—A New Future. *PLoS ONE* **2016**, *11*, e0153739. [CrossRef] [PubMed]
17. Samotus, O.; Lee, J.; Jog, M. Long-term tremor therapy for Parkinson and essential tremor with sensor-guided botulinum toxin type A injections. *PLoS ONE* **2017**, *12*, e0178670. [CrossRef] [PubMed]
18. Fahn, S.; Tolosa, E.; Marin, C. Clinical rating scale for tremor. In *Parkinson's Disease and Movement Disorders*, 2nd ed.; Jankovic, J., Tolosa, E., Eds.; Williams and Wilkins: Baltimore, MD, USA, 1993; pp. 271–280.
19. Tröster, A.I.; Pahwa, R.; Fields, J.A.; Tanner, C.M.; Lyons, K.E. Quality of life in Essential Tremor Questionnaire (QUEST): Development and initial validation. *Parkinsonism Relat. Disord.* **2005**, *11*, 367–373. [CrossRef] [PubMed]
20. MacDermid, F. Measurement of Health Outcomes Following Tendon and Nerve Repair. *J. Hand. Ther.* **2005**, *18*, 297–312. [CrossRef] [PubMed]
21. Cutter, N.C.; Kevorkian, C.G. *Handbook of Manual Muscle Testing*, 1st ed.; McGraw-Hill Health Professions Division: New York, NY, USA, 1999; ISBN 0070331502.

toxins

MDPI

Article

Early AbobotulinumtoxinA (Dysport®) in Post-Stroke Adult Upper Limb Spasticity: ONTIME Pilot Study

Raymond L Rosales [1,2,*], Jovita Balcaitiene [3], Hugues Berard [3], Pascal Maisonobe [3], Khean Jin Goh [4], Witsanu Kumthornthip [5], Mazlina Mazlan [6], Lydia Abdul Latif [6], Mary Mildred D. Delos Santos [1], Chayaporn Chotiyarnwong [5], Phakamas Tanvijit [5], Odessa Nuez [7] and Keng He Kong [7]

1. Centre for Neurodiagnostic and Therapeutic Services (CNS), Metropolitan Medical Centre, Manila 1012, Philippines; marymildred8888@yahoo.com
2. Department of Neurology & Psychiatry, Faculty of Medicine and Surgery, University of Santo Tomas, Manila 1008, Philippines
3. Ipsen Group, Boulogne-Billancourt, 92100 Paris, France; jovita.balcaitiene@gmail.com (J.B.); hugues.berard@ipsen.com (H.B.); pascal.maisonobe@ipsen.com (P.M.)
4. Division of Neurology, Department of Medicine, University of Malaya Medical Centre, Kuala Lumpur 59100, Malaysia; gohkj@ummc.edu.my
5. Department of Rehabilitation Medicine, Siriraj Hospital, Mahidol University, Bangkok 10700, Thailand; wkumthornthip@yahoo.com (W.K.); hedhom2000@hotmail.com (C.C.); siphakamas@gmail.com (P.T.)
6. Department of Rehabilitation Medicine, Faculty of Medicine, University of Malaya, Kuala Lumpur 50603, Malaysia; mazlinamazlan@ummc.edu.my (M.M.); lydia@ummc.edu.my (L.A.L.)
7. Department of Rehabilitation Medicine, Tan Tock Seng Hospital, Novena 308433, Singapore; nuez_odessa_setiota@ttsh.com.sg (O.N.); keng_he_kong@ttsh.com.sg (K.H.K.)

* Correspondence: raymond.rosales@ust.edu.ph or rlrosalesmd88@gmail.com; Tel.: +632-2547432

Received: 29 May 2018; Accepted: 11 June 2018; Published: 21 June 2018

Abstract: The ONTIME study investigated whether early post-stroke abobotulinumtoxinA injection delays appearance or progression of upper limb spasticity (ULS) symptoms. ONTIME (NCT02321436) was a 28-week, exploratory, double-blind, randomized, placebo-controlled study of abobotulinumtoxinA 500U in patients with ULS (Modified Ashworth Scale [MAS] score $\geq$ 2) 2–12 weeks post-stroke. Patients were either symptomatic or asymptomatic (only increased MAS) at baseline. Primary efficacy outcome measure: time between injection and visit at which re-injection criteria were met (MAS $\geq$ 2 and $\geq$1, sign of symptomatic spasticity: pain, involuntary movements, impaired active or passive function). Forty-two patients were randomized (abobotulinumtoxinA 500U: n = 28; placebo: n = 14) with median 5.86 weeks since stroke. Median time to reach re-injection criteria was significantly longer for abobotulinumtoxinA (156 days) than placebo (32 days; log-rank: p = 0.0176; Wilcoxon: p = 0.0480). Eleven (39.3%) patients receiving abobotulinumtoxinA did not require re-injection for $\geq$28 weeks versus two (14.3%) in placebo group. In this exploratory study, early abobotulinumtoxinA treatment significantly delayed time to reach re-injection criteria compared with placebo in patients with post-stroke ULS. These findings suggest an optimal time for post-stroke spasticity management and help determine the design and sample sizes for larger confirmatory studies.

Keywords: abobotulinumtoxinA; botulinum toxin type A; upper limb spasticity; post-stroke; early use; ONTIME

Key Contribution: ONTIME is an exploratory study that provides evidence that early abobotulinumtoxinA prolongs time to fulfill re-injection criteria versus placebo in patients with upper limb spasticity. This supportive evidence will aid the design and sample size calculation for larger confirmatory studies.

1. Introduction

Spasticity, arising from involuntary activation of muscles, may lead to pain, disability, functional impairment, and eventually, contractures [1]. Post-stroke spasticity (PSS) occurs in one third of stroke survivors [1], and has consistently been demonstrated to negatively impact patients' quality of life and increase the number of falls and fractures, as well as caregiver burden [2–4]. Additionally, direct costs are quadrupled in stroke survivors with spasticity vs. those without [5]. 'Symptomatic' patients with upper limb spasticity (ULS) present with symptoms such as impaired passive and active function, pain, and associated reactions [6]. Time to development of symptomatic PSS ranges from 3 to 18 months [6–10]; however, some studies have shown muscle tone changes in the affected limb within 3 weeks post-stroke [11–13].

Botulinum toxin A (BoNT-A) safety and efficacy in chronic focal spasticity treatment is well established [14–16]. BoNT-A is not usually initiated until muscle overactivity is demonstrated [17], thus, data regarding early PSS treatment are limited. However, as far back as 2010, an international consensus statement advocated the role of early BoNT-A injection in preventing contracture development, with potential to unmask active functional improvement [15]. Early BoNT-A may improve hypertonicity, passive function, and pain in upper and lower limb spasticity [18]; however, the impact of BoNT-A on symptomatic spasticity progression has not been evaluated. The ABCDE-S study investigated efficacy of early (≤12 weeks post-stroke) abobotulinumtoxinA on muscle tone in patients with post-stroke ULS [13]. ONTIME is an exploratory study, and the first to investigate whether early abobotulinumtoxinA not only improves muscle tone, but also delays the time to symptom development or progression in PSS. This study will also provide additional supportive data to determine the design and sample size for further confirmatory studies.

Objectives

Primary objective: assessment of time between upper limb (UL) injection of abobotulinumtoxinA (≤12 weeks post-stroke) and the appearance or progression of symptomatic ULS. For this, ONTIME used a composite index, consisting of pre-selected, clinic-based, observable re-injection criteria, focused on hypertonicity and functional symptoms of spasticity.

Secondary objectives: assessments of muscle tone in primary targeted muscle group (PTMG), UL active motor function, time to reach re-injection criteria stratified by baseline symptomatic/asymptomatic spasticity and global assessment of change. Concomitant non-drug therapy sessions were recorded.

2. Results

2.1. Baseline Characteristics and Patient Disposition

Forty-two patients with ULS were recruited and randomized (abobotulinumtoxinA 500U, $n = 28$; placebo, $n = 14$). Safety and intention-to-treat (ITT) populations included all randomized and injected patients ($n = 42$). The per-protocol population included 40 (95.2%) patients. Two (4.8%) patients withdrew from the study: one patient (abobotulinumtoxinA) withdrew consent, and one (placebo) was lost to follow-up and excluded (Figure 1).

Baseline characteristics were well-matched between treatment groups (Table S1). Mean time post-stroke was 6.18 and 6.52 weeks for abobotulinumtoxinA and placebo, respectively. Elbow flexors were the most commonly selected PTMG. Patients mostly presented with baseline symptomatic spasticity (76.2%), i.e., affected by impaired passive function (64.3%; Likert score ≥ 1), active function (57.1%), involuntary movements (47.6%), and/or pain (38.1%; Numeric Pain Rating Scale [NPRS] score ≥ 4), in addition to hypertonicity (MAS ≥ 2; Table S1). Symptom presentation varied between treatment groups and both groups recorded mild pain (mean NPRS score: 3.1) (Table S1).

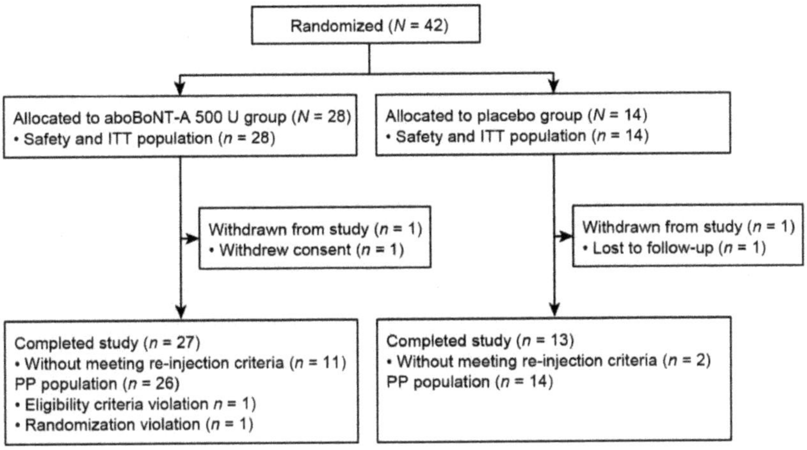

Figure 1. Patient disposition. aboBoNT-A, abobotulinumtoxinA; ITT, intention-to-treat; PP, per-protocol.

2.2. Time to Re-Injection

Median (95% confidence interval [CI]) time between injection and meeting re-injection criteria was significantly longer for abobotulinumtoxinA (156.0 [86.0–206.0] days) vs. placebo (32.0 [29.0–114.0] days; log-rank: $p = 0.0176$; Wilcoxon: $p = 0.0480$).

For abobotulinumtoxinA, 20/28 patients (71.4%) did not meet re-injection criteria until after Week 12, vs. 5/14 (35.7%) for placebo (Figure 2). At study end, 11 (39.3%) patients in the abobotulinumtoxinA group had not met re-injection criteria, vs. 2 (14.3%) for placebo.

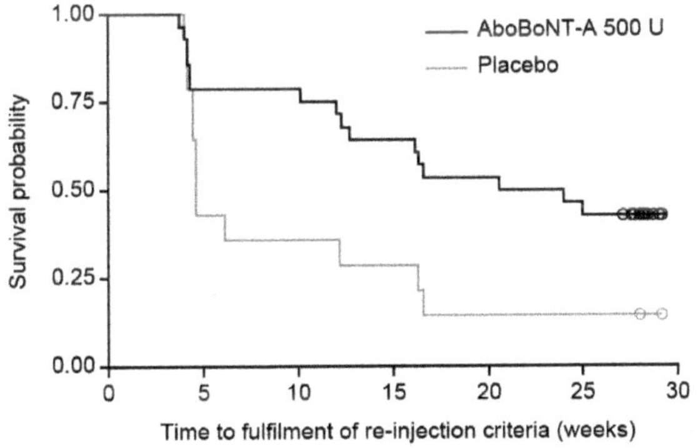

Figure 2. Time to fulfilment of re-injection criteria—KM analysis (ITT population). Circles indicate patients who had not met re-injection criteria at their last study visit. AboBoNT-A, abobotulinumtoxinA; ITT, intention to treat; KM, Kaplan–Meier.

For the symptomatic spasticity cohort, a significant difference was observed between abobotulinumtoxinA and placebo (130.0 [30.0–206.0] vs. 32.0 [28.0–85.0] days, respectively; log-rank: $p = 0.0384$; Wilcoxon: $p = 0.0798$). The asymptomatic cohort had insufficient patients ($n = 10$) for robust statistical testing.

2.3. Assessment of Change in Muscle Tone

Differences in muscle tone between abobotulinumtoxinA and placebo were statistically significant at first post-baseline assessment (Week 4) to Week 12, with the maximal decrease in muscle tone observed at Weeks 6 and 8 with abobotulinumtoxinA (Figure 3). At Week 12, difference in MAS score was −0.83 (−1.39, −0.26; $p = 0.0052$). After Week 12, no robust calculation could be completed due to low placebo group patient numbers.

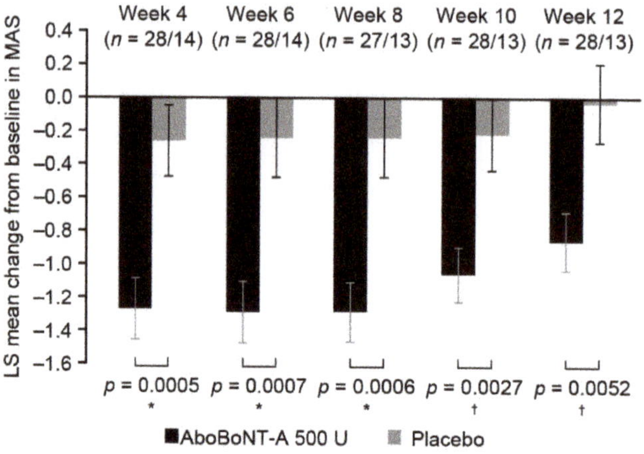

Figure 3. MAS change from baseline to each visit (ITT population). Values are presented as the least squares mean changes from baseline (standard error) in MAS score. * $p \leq 0.01$ and † $p \leq 0.001$, *p*-values are based on an analysis of variance performed at each visit. AboBoNT-A, abobotulinumtoxinA; LS, least squares; MAS, Modified Ashworth Scale; *n*, number of patients in aboBoNT-A group/placebo group at each visit.

2.4. Assessment of Motor Function Recovery

No statistically significant differences in motor recovery scores were observed. As most placebo group patients met re-injection criteria at Week 4 (Figure 2), motor function was not assessed at subsequent visits. At Week 4, change from baseline was numerically higher for abobotulinumtoxinA vs. placebo (6.4 [2.5] vs. 5.6 [4.4], $p = 0.8754$) and motor function improved with abobotulinumtoxinA until Week 12 (11.1 [3.5]).

2.5. Changes in Global Assessment

No statistically significant association between treatment and global assessment of changes at last visit was identified ($p = 0.6128$); however, numerically higher proportions of patients treated with abobotulinumtoxinA were assessed as 'better' or 'much better' (Table 1). Placebo group data were limited, due to meeting re-injection criteria.

Table 1. Global assessment of change at last visit (ITT population).

Results, *n* (%)	AbobotulinumtoxinA 500 U (*N* = 28)			Placebo (*N* = 14)		
	Symptomatic Spasticity (*n* = 16)	Asymptomatic Spasticity (*n* = 6)	All (*n* = 22)	Symptomatic Spasticity (*n* = 4)	Asymptomatic Spasticity (*n* = 2)	All (*n* = 6)
Much better	1 (6.3)	1 (16.7)	2 (9.1)	0	0	0
Better	14 (87.5)	4 (66.7)	18 (81.8)	3 (75.0)	2 (100.0)	5 (83.3)
No change	0	1 (16.7)	1 (4.5)	1 (25.0)	0	1 (16.7)
Worse	1 (6.3)	0	1 (4.5)	0	0	0
Much worse	0	0	0	0	0	0
Cochran-Mantel-Haenszel *p*-value = 0.6128						

No data are available for 14 patients as they met re-injection criteria at Week 4. Cochran–Mantel–Haenszel *p*-value represents the strength of the association between treatment and global assessments of changes at the last visit, adjusted for symptomatic status at baseline. ITT, intention-to-treat.

2.6. Concomitant Therapy

Thirty-nine (92.9%; 89.3% for abobotulinumtoxinA vs. 100% for placebo) patients received concomitant non-drug therapies for PSS in their affected UL, including physiotherapy (85.7%) and occupational therapy (31.0%). Mean duration of physiotherapy was 157.9 days with abobotulinumtoxinA and 126.1 days with placebo (Table S2). Patients receiving abobotulinumtoxinA had a longer duration of therapy vs. placebo, as most placebo group patients met re-injection criteria before Week 12.

Concomitant medications received during the study are described in Table S3.

2.7. Safety Assessment

Twenty-three treatment-emergent adverse events (TEAEs) occurred in 12 patients (Table 2); most were mild-to-moderate intensity. One abobotulinumtoxinA group patient reported two severe TEAEs (pain and hypertensive crisis), neither were considered related to treatment by the investigator. Three abobotulinumtoxinA group patients reported four serious adverse events (AEs) during the study. Two patients reported head injury following a fall, one reported asthma exacerbation, and one reported pneumonia. All patients recovered and none were considered related to study treatment. No AEs led to premature withdrawal and no deaths were reported. All variations in vital signs were considered within normal range.

Table 2. Summary of adverse events (safety population).

	AbobotulinumtoxinA 500 U (*N* = 28)	**Placebo (*N* = 14)**	**All patients (*N* = 42)**
Any adverse events	8 (28.6), *17*	4 (28.6), *6*	12 (28.6), *23*
Any serious adverse events	3 (10.7), *4*	0	3 (7.1), *4*
Any TEAEs	7 (25.0), 16	4 (28.6), *6*	11 (26.2), *22*
Intensity of TEAEs			
Severe	1 (3.6), *2*	0	1 (2.4), *2*
Moderate	6 (21.4), *11*	1 (7.1), *1*	7 (16.7), *12*
Mild	3 (10.7), *3*	3 (21.4), *5*	6 (14.3), *8*
Related TEAEs	0	0	0
	Reported TEAEs:		
Head injury	2 (7.1), *2*	0	2 (4.8), *2*
Insomnia	2 (7.1), *2*	0	2 (4.8), *2*
Fall	1 (3.6), *1*	1 (7.1), *1*	2 (4.8), *2*
Urinary tract infection	1 (3.6), *1*	1 (7.1), *2*	2 (4.8), *3*
Asthma	1 (3.6), *1*	0	1 (2.4), *1*
Constipation	1 (3.6), *1*	0	1 (2.4), *1*
Cough	1 (3.6), *1*	0	1 (2.4), *1*
Hypertensive crisis	1 (3.6), *1*	0	1 (2.4), *1*
Hypokalemia	1 (3.6), *1*	0	1 (2.4), *1*
Pain	1 (3.6), *1*	0	1 (2.4), *1*
Pneumonia	1 (3.6), *1*	0	1 (2.4), *1*
Pyrexia	1 (3.6), *1*	0	1 (2.4), *1*
Tachycardia	1 (3.6), *1*	0	1 (2.4), *1*
Vomiting	1 (3.6), *1*	0	1 (2.4), *1*
Dizziness	0	1 (7.1), *1*	1 (2.4), *1*
Epistaxis	0	1 (7.1), *1*	1 (2.4), *1*
Neuralgia	0	1 (7.1), *1*	1 (2.4), *1*

All values are presented as the number of patients (percentage of patients), *number of occurrences*. Medical Dictionary for Regulatory Activities (MedDRA) Version 18.0. TEAE, treatment-emergent adverse event.

3. Discussion

The ONTIME exploratory study assessed whether abobotulinumtoxinA 500U, administered 2–12 weeks after stroke, delays development of symptomatic spasticity in adult patients with increased muscle tone (MAS $\geq$ 2). Baseline MAS $\geq$ 2 was based on results from a previous study [11].

AbobotulinumtoxinA significantly prolonged time to fulfilment of re-injection criteria compared with placebo, with abobotulinumtoxinA-treated patients having an additional 124 days before they met re-injection criteria. At Week 28, 39.3% of patients (n = 11) who received abobotulinumtoxinA had not reached re-injection criteria, vs. 14.3% (n = 2) for placebo. These substantial benefits of abobotulinumtoxinA over placebo were observed despite any potential influence of the high level of concomitant non-drug therapy use in each group. AEs were similar between groups and there were no related TEAEs.

While based on goals, a physician's decision to inject BoNT-A is not driven by increased muscle tone alone but by signs of impaired function, pain, or both, which can differ in presentation among patients. Thus, the novel composite re-injection criteria used in ONTIME, combining hypertonicity and associated symptoms of spasticity, may make the present results particularly relevant to clinical practice. Spasticity-related clinical accompaniments of the composite re-injection criteria were included, based on previous findings that identified pain, involuntary movements, and impaired active and passive function as key treatment goal areas for patients with post-stroke ULS [19]. In this present study, 76% of patients were symptomatic at baseline (2–12 weeks post-stroke), with 38–64% exhibiting ≥1 item of symptomatic spasticity, in addition to hypertonicity. The prevalence and heterogenic presentation of symptoms observed highlights the need for composite, patient-centered outcome measurements and the importance of early intervention.

The long time to reach re-injection criteria observed during the ONTIME study (156.0 days for abobotulinumtoxinA vs. 32.0 days for placebo) is supported by the ABCDE-S study, which also assessed single injections of abobotulinumtoxinA 500U to hypertonic upper limb muscles [13]. In both ONTIME and ABCDE-S, significant improvements in MAS for abobotulinumtoxinA vs. placebo were sustained for up to 6 months (Week 24) [13]. The proportion of patients not requiring retreatment by the end of this present study (Week 28, 39.3%) is around five-fold greater than observed in a recent study of adults receiving repeated abobotulinumtoxinA injection for upper limb spasticity at least 6 months post-stroke or post-traumatic brain injury (7.9% at Week 24 or later, after first open-label injection) [20,21]. This suggests a prolonged duration of effect for early intervention with abobotulinumtoxinA. Among cohort differences (e.g., chronic spasticity in a Caucasian population, repeated and >500U abobotulinumtoxinA, and trial design), it should be noted that retreatment in the Gracies et al. (2017) study was by clinicians' judgement [21], while ONTIME employed a composite index based on patient-centered functional assessments in addition to hypertonicity to evaluate need for re-injection.

While the ONTIME study suggests early abobotulinumtoxinA injection delays symptomatic spasticity development, the effects may not be restorative to maladaptive changes in the brain, due to the finite duration of treatment effect. However, early treatment may modify disease progression before secondary local biomechanical changes occur [22–24]. Disease modification at the level of cortical reorganization was demonstrated through functional magnetic resonance imaging in BoNT-A therapy for chronic PSS [25], suggesting preventive potential—and a possible paradigm shift towards early intervention. As spasticity is a form of maladaptive plasticity that progresses over time [13,26], early therapeutic intervention may provide an opportunity to prevent or reduce neurological changes leading to disabling spasticity [23]. Furthermore, early intervention with BoNT-A, combined with adjunctive therapies [27,28], could maximize the impact of treatment on function and tone reduction [18,29]. Although this is a novel approach in spasticity treatment, early intervention using disease-modifying therapies is recognized in current clinical practice guidelines for multiple sclerosis [30], another disease in which a BoNT-A treatment algorithm has been developed for associated spasticity [31].

Early intervention with abobotulinumtoxinA and longer time to symptomatic spasticity progression may positively impact patients' lives with fewer injections and healthcare provider visits. In addition to patient benefit (demonstrated here by positive impact on global assessment of changes), early abobotulinumtoxinA has shown reduced caregiver burden in previous studies [32,33]. Extending the symptom-free period could have pharmacoeconomic implications, reducing dependency on caregivers and healthcare systems. Cost-effectiveness of BoNT-A in early PSS is a secondary endpoint in an ongoing study [34].

As ONTIME was an exploratory study, the sample size was chosen on the basis of determining the sample size estimation for further confirmatory studies, thus the generalization of efficacy and safety results should be approached with caution. ONTIME study limitations include low numbers of asymptomatic patients at baseline. Additionally, although a trend for improving motor recovery with abobotulinumtoxinA was observed until Week 12, a robust effect was not established due to limited placebo group data. If Fugl–Meyer assessments were performed in all patients until Week 12, or the trial extended, an improvement in active motor function may have occurred. Difficulties in demonstrating motor function improvements with BoNT-A vs. placebo have been experienced previously [18,26]. Future studies should have a longer duration (>24 weeks post-intervention) to observe long-term effects of early abobotulinumtoxinA [29].

4. Conclusions

The ONTIME exploratory study demonstrated that early administration of abobotulinumtoxinA, 2–12 weeks post-stroke in patients with spastic paresis, significantly increased time to re-injection criteria fulfilment, compared with placebo, due to prolonged MAS improvements and delayed appearance of spasticity symptoms. Due to the trial design, it was not possible to demonstrate significant differences in motor function. Safety results corresponded to the known profile of abobotulinumtoxinA, and no new safety signals were identified. These results demonstrate that early abobotulinumtoxinA has a good safety profile, may modify the disease course, delay symptom presentation, and lead to healthcare savings. These data provide a basis for future trials to select sample sizes that can confirm these results.

5. Materials and Methods

Full details of the ONTIME study (NCT02321436) protocol have been published [35]. ONTIME was conducted in accordance with the Declaration of Helsinki, International Conference on Harmonisation Good Clinical Practice Guidelines, and local regulatory requirements, with approval from relevant independent ethics committee/institutional review boards. Written informed consent was obtained from patients prior to study entry.

5.1. Primary Research Question

This study asked whether early abobotulinumtoxinA treatment, in patients with post-stroke ULS, delays time between injection and fulfilment of re-injection criteria (Class I evidence).

5.2. Study Design and Participants

ONTIME was a Phase IV, prospective, exploratory, double-blind, randomized, placebo-controlled trial, conducted at four centers in Malaysia, Thailand, Singapore, and the Philippines, initiated in December 2014 and completed in March 2016.

Inclusion criteria included age 18–80 years, 2–12 weeks after first ischemic/hemorrhagic stroke onset, presence of ULS defined as MAS $\geq$ 2 [36] in PTMG. The investigator selected PTMG at first visit, in agreement with the patient/caregiver. Patients were classified into asymptomatic (increased muscle tone, MAS $\geq$ 2; Criterion A) and symptomatic cohorts. Symptomatic spasticity (Table S1) was defined as the presence of $\geq$1 of the following items (Criterion B), in addition to increased muscle tone:

- Impaired passive function (score $\geq$ 1 on a 4-point Likert scale: 0 = no impact, 1 = mild impact, 2 = moderate impact, 3 = severe impact).
    - 'In general, how much does spasticity impact the following activities of daily living and/or your rehabilitation program: hygiene (i.e., hand, nails, armpit, elbows), dressing the affected limb, positioning the affected limb, splint application or removal?'

- Impaired active function (score $\geq$ 1 on a 4-point Likert scale, as above).
    - 'In general, how much does spasticity impact the following activities of daily living and/or your rehabilitation program: reaching, grasping, releasing, gripping, holding, bimanual function, manipulating objects, dexterity, fine motor skills, lifting and carrying?' [19]
- Presence of involuntary movements, which occur during standing up, walking, and transfers (if unable to stand up/walk) (score $\geq$ 1 on a 4-point Likert scale: 0 = no involuntary movements, 1 = involuntary movements with mild impact on posture and ambulation, 2 = involuntary movements with moderate impact on posture and ambulation, 3 = involuntary movements with severe impact on posture and ambulation).
- Pain (score $\geq$ 4 on the NPRS: 0 = no pain to 10 = severe disabling pain, with impacts on movement; score of 4 indicates moderate pain) [37].
- Question to each patient was oriented to obtain a relevant answer. Answers were spontaneous and not condition-dependent (e.g., active/passive movements or during night/day). A support could be used to help patients assess pain.
    - Average pain intensity over 1 week was collected.

Further details of inclusion and exclusion criteria are detailed in the published protocol [35].

5.3. *Recruitment and Randomization*

Patients were randomized, using an interactive web response system (IWRS) service, to abobotulinumtoxinA or placebo in a 2:1 ratio (maximizing patient numbers receiving active treatment, with sufficient placebo patients to power statistical analyses). The double-blind status of treatment allocation was ensured via separate lists for randomization and treatment numbering. Products were similar in size, color, smell, taste, and appearance. In exceptional instances of an AE, the blind could be broken on an individual basis following review with the Central Department of Pharmacovigilance at Ipsen, or if necessary, by the investigator obtaining a patients' treatment identification from the IWRS.

5.4. *Interventions*

Patients received intramuscular injections, administered using a 25-gauge needle, of abobotulinumtoxinA 500U or equal volume placebo into selected muscles. AbobotulinumtoxinA and placebo were provided as white lyophilized powders for reconstitution (Dysport®, Ipsen Pharma SAS, Paris, France), packed in vials containing 500U BoNT-A hemagglutinin complex or excipients of the investigational product, respectively. Vials were reconstituted with 2.5 mL of preservative-free sodium chloride for injection (0.9%; 200 mL). Doses were administered per muscle according to investigators' judgements. Recommended dosing regimens were previously published [35]. Most patients participated in occupational and physiotherapy practices.

5.5. *Efficacy Assessments*

5.5.1. Primary Efficacy Assessment

The primary efficacy outcome measure was the time between initial injection (baseline) and visit at which both re-injection criteria were fulfilled (Criterion A: increased muscle tone in PTMG [MAS $\geq$ 2]; and Criterion B: presence of $\geq$1 items of symptomatic spasticity).

Re-injection criteria, evaluated at every visit from Week 4, assessed appearance/reappearance of symptomatic spasticity. 'Appearance' was assessed for patients asymptomatic and 'reappearance' for patients symptomatic at baseline.

5.5.2. Secondary Efficacy Assessments

Secondary assessments included change in muscle tone (MAS) in PTMG, assessed at baseline and each subsequent visit. Active motor function in affected UL was evaluated using Fugl–Meyer assessment (total score, 0–66) for: upper extremity (scored 0–36), wrist (0–10), hand (0–14), and in terms of coordination/speed (0–6) [35,38]. Global assessment of change was investigator-evaluated (5-point Likert scale, ranging from 'much better' to 'much worse'). Fugl–Meyer and global assessment of change were assessed at baseline and each subsequent visit up to, but not including, visit when re-injection criteria were met. Non-drug therapy for ULS was recorded at baseline and each subsequent visit.

5.6. *Safety Assessments*

AEs were monitored and recorded from provision of informed consent until end of participation. TEAEs were reported, events classified as mild, moderate, or severe, and assessed for any causal relationship. Physical examinations and measurement of vital signs were performed by physicians at baseline and all subsequent visits.

5.7. *Study Schedule*

The study schedule has been published previously [35]. The first visit recorded patient demographics, type of stroke, medical and surgical history, and severity of stroke-induced disability (modified Rankin Scale). Visits were scheduled every 2 weeks (±3 days) from Week 4–12, then every 4 weeks (±1 week) to Week 28. Visits up to Week 12 were mandatory, regardless of whether re-injection criteria were met. For patients not fulfilling re-injection criteria by Week 12, subsequent visits were required until re-injection criteria were met or study end.

5.8. *Statistical Analysis*

The sample size ($N = 42$) was chosen for exploratory purposes and not intended for definitive conclusions about efficacy. Statistical analyses were performed using SAS v9.2. Efficacy analyses were performed on the ITT population. Primary endpoint was analyzed by Kaplan–Meier (KM) survival analysis. Median survival time and 95% CIs were estimated for each treatment group using KM product-limit estimation. Data for patients not meeting re-injection criteria at Week 28 were censored at the patient's last study visit. Treatment differences between abobotulinumtoxinA and placebo groups were tested using two-sided, stratified log-rank and Wilcoxon tests ($\alpha = 5\%$; spasticity status as stratification factor). p-values are for exploratory purpose only.

Treatment effect for muscle tone change was assessed using analysis of variance (ANOVA; treatment and symptomatic spasticity status as fixed effects); data are shown as adjusted means, 95% CI, and corresponding p-values. Treatment differences in active motor function between abobotulinumtoxinA and placebo groups were assessed using a mixed ANCOVA model on change from baseline (treatment group and symptomatic spasticity status as fixed effects; score value at baseline as covariate). For global assessment of change, differences between treatment groups at last visit were assessed using the Cochran–Mantel–Haenszel statistic, controlling for symptomatic spasticity status. Homogeneity of treatment effect across strata (symptomatic/asymptomatic) was assessed by the Breslow–Day test. Safety analyses were based on safety population and AEs coded using Medical Dictionary for Regulatory Activities (MedDRA) v18.0.

5.9. *Changes in Conduct of the Study and Planned Analyses*

In January 2015, the protocol was amended to correct national legal minimum age in Thailand and clarify data collection methods. A minor statistical update to secondary MAS endpoint analysis was made to replace use of covariance analysis by ANOVA.

Supplementary Materials: The following are available online at http://www.mdpi.com/2072-6651/10/7/253/s1, Table S1: Baseline characteristics for patients in the ONTIME study (ITT population), Table S2: Concomitant non-drug therapy use (safety population), Table S3: Concomitant post-stroke medications by therapeutic class (safety population).

Author Contributions: Statistical analysis conducted by: P.M. Study concept and design: J.B., P.M., H.B., and R.L.R. Acquisition: analysis, or interpretation of data: J.B., P.M., and R.L.R. Writing and review of manuscript: R.L.R., J.B., H.B., P.M., K.J.G., W.K., M.M., L.A.L., M.M.D.D.S., C.C., P.T., O.N., and K.H.K.

Funding: This study was funded by Ipsen Pharma.

Acknowledgments: All members of the ONTIME study group are authors on this paper. The authors thank all of the patients who participated in the ONTIME study and acknowledge the work of the study project managers at Ipsen, Marion Genoulaz and Elodie Blouquit, and the support of the clinical research organization, EPS. In addition, the authors thank Cassandra Hines, MSc and Catherine Jones of Watermeadow Medical, Macclesfield, UK for providing medical writing and editing support, which was funded by Ipsen Pharma, in accordance with Good Publication Practice (GPP3) guidelines.

Conflicts of Interest: R.L.R., K.J.G., W.K., and K.H.K. have received consultancy fees from Ipsen. R.L.R. has received scientific advisory board, consulting, and speaker fees from Ipsen, Allergan, and Pfizer. K.J.G. has received honorarium as a moderator for 4th Pompe Disease Symposium, 4th and 5th November 2016, Shanghai, China from Sanofi Genzyme. W.K. was a speaker and injector for hands-on workshops in Thailand and Vietnam, sponsored by Allergan. C.C. and P.T. served as speakers and injectors for a hands-on workshop in Thailand, sponsored by Allergan. W.K., C.C., and P.T. have received research funding as investigators in a trial sponsored by Ipsen, outside of this study. M.M., L.A.L., M.M.D.D.S., and O.N. have nothing to disclose. H.B., and P.M. are full-time employees of Ipsen. J.B. was a full-time employee of Ipsen at the time of manuscript submission.

References

1. Rosales, R.L. *Botulinum Toxin Therapy Manual for Dystonia and Spasticity*; Intech Open Access Publishers: Rijeka, Croatia, 2016.
2. Doan, Q.V.; Brashear, A.; Gillard, P.J.; Varon, S.F.; Vandenburgh, A.M.; Turkel, C.C.; Elovic, E.P. Relationship between disability and health-related quality of life and caregiver burden in patients with upper limb poststroke spasticity. *PM R* **2012**, *4*, 4–10. [CrossRef] [PubMed]
3. Zorowitz, R.D.; Gillard, P.J.; Brainin, M. Poststroke spasticity: Sequelae and burden on stroke survivors and caregivers. *Neurology* **2013**, *80*, S45–S52. [CrossRef] [PubMed]
4. Esquenazi, A. The human and economic burden of poststroke spasticity and muscle overactivity. *JCOM* **2011**, *18*, 607–614.
5. Lundström, E.; Smits, A.; Borg, J.; Terént, A. Four-fold increase in direct costs of stroke survivors with spasticity compared with stroke survivors without spasticity. *Stroke* **2010**, *41*, 319–324. [CrossRef] [PubMed]
6. Kong, K.H.; Chua, K.S.; Lee, J. Symptomatic upper limb spasticity in patients with chronic stroke attending a rehabilitation clinic: Frequency, clinical correlates and predictors. *J. Rehabilit. Med.* **2010**, *42*, 453–457. [CrossRef] [PubMed]
7. Kong, K.H.; Lee, J.; Chua, K.S. Occurrence and temporal evolution of upper limb spasticity in stroke patients admitted to a rehabilitation unit. *Arch. Phys. Med. Rehabilit.* **2012**, *93*, 143–148. [CrossRef] [PubMed]
8. Watkins, C.L.; Leathley, M.J.; Gregson, J.M.; Moore, A.P.; Smith, T.L.; Sharma, A.K. Prevalence of spasticity post stroke. *Clin. Rehabilit.* **2002**, *16*, 515–522. [CrossRef] [PubMed]
9. Leathley, M.J.; Gregson, J.M.; Moore, A.P.; Smith, T.L.; Sharma, A.K.; Watkins, C.L. Predicting spasticity after stroke in those surviving to 12 months. *Clin. Rehabilit.* **2004**, *18*, 438–443. [CrossRef] [PubMed]
10. Wissel, J.; Manack, A.; Brainin, M. Toward an epidemiology of poststroke spasticity. *Neurology* **2013**, *80*, S13–S19. [CrossRef] [PubMed]
11. Wissel, J.; Schelosky, L.D.; Scott, J.; Christe, W.; Faiss, J.H.; Mueller, J. Early development of spasticity following stroke: A prospective, observational trial. *J. Neurol.* **2010**, *257*, 1067–1072. [CrossRef] [PubMed]
12. Welmer, A.K.; Widen Holmqvist, L.; Sommerfeld, D.K. Location and severity of spasticity in the first 1–2 weeks and at 3 and 18 months after stroke. *Eur. J. Neurol.* **2010**, *17*, 720–725. [CrossRef] [PubMed]
13. Rosales, R.L.; Kong, K.H.; Goh, K.J.; Kumthornthip, W.; Mok, V.C.; Delgado-De Los Santos, M.M.; Chua, K.S.; Abdullah, S.J.; Zakine, B.; Maisonobe, P.; et al. Botulinum toxin injection for hypertonicity of the upper extremity within 12 weeks after stroke: A randomized controlled trial. *Neurorehabilit. Neural Repair* **2012**, *26*, 812–821. [CrossRef] [PubMed]

14. Simpson, D.M.; Hallett, M.; Ashman, E.J.; Comella, C.L.; Green, M.W.; Gronseth, G.S.; Armstrong, M.J.; Gloss, D.; Potrebic, S.; Jankovic, J.; et al. Practice guideline update summary: Botulinum neurotoxin for the treatment of blepharospasm, cervical dystonia, adult spasticity, and headache: Report of the Guideline Development Subcommittee of the American Academy of Neurology. *Neurology* **2016**, *86*, 1818–1826. [CrossRef] [PubMed]
15. Sheean, G.; Lannin, N.A.; Turner-Stokes, L.; Rawicki, B.; Snow, B.J.; Cerebral Palsy Institute. Botulinum toxin assessment, intervention and after-care for upper limb hypertonicity in adults: International consensus statement. *Eur. J. Neurol.* **2010**, *17*, 74–93. [CrossRef] [PubMed]
16. Wissel, J.; Ward, A.B.; Erztgaard, P.; Bensmail, D.; Hecht, M.J.; Lejeune, T.M.; Schnider, P.; Altavista, M.C.; Cavazza, S.; Deltombe, T.; et al. European consensus table on the use of botulinum toxin type A in adult spasticity. *J. Rehabilit. Med.* **2009**, *41*, 13–25. [CrossRef] [PubMed]
17. Royal College of Physicians; British Society of Rehabilitation Medicine; Chartered Society of Physiotherapy. Association of Chartered Physiotherapists Interested in Neurology. In *Spasticity in Adults: Management Using Botulinum Toxin*; National guidelines, Royal College of Physicians: London, UK, 2009.
18. Rosales, R.L.; Efendy, F.; Teleg, E.S.; Delos Santos, M.M.; Rosales, M.C.; Ostrea, M.; Tanglao, M.J.; Ng, A.R. Botulinum toxin as early intervention for spasticity after stroke or non-progressive brain lesion: A meta-analysis. *J. Neurol. Sci.* **2016**, *371*, 6–14. [CrossRef] [PubMed]
19. Ashford, S.; Fheodoroff, K.; Jacinto, J.; Turner-Stokes, L. Common goal areas in the treatment of upper limb spasticity: A multicentre analysis. *Clin. Rehabilit.* **2016**, *30*, 617–622. [CrossRef] [PubMed]
20. Gracies, J.M.; Brashear, A.; Marciniak, C.; Jech, R.; Banach, M.; Marque, P.; Grandoulier, A.S.; Vilain, C.; Picaut, P. Duration of effect of abobotulinumtoxinA (Dysport) in adult patients with upper limb spasticity (ULS) post stroke or traumatic brain injury. *Toxicon* **2016**, *123*, S35. [CrossRef]
21. Gracies, J.M.; O'Dell, M.; Vecchio, M.; Hedera, P.; Kocer, S.; Rudzinska-Bar, M.; Rubin, B.; Timerbaeva, S.L.; Lusakowska, A.; Boyer, F.C.; et al. Effects of repeated abobotulinumtoxinA injections in upper limb spasticity. *Muscle Nerve* **2018**, *57*, 245–254. [CrossRef] [PubMed]
22. Fheodoroff, K.; Jacinto, J.; Geurts, A.; Molteni, F.; Franco, J.H.; Santiago, T.; Rosales, R.; Gracies, J.M. How can we improve current practice in spastic paresis? *Eur. Neurol. Rev.* **2016**, *11*, 79–86. [CrossRef]
23. Rosales, R.L.; Kanovsky, P.; Fernandez, H.H. What's the "catch" in upper-limb post-stroke spasticity: Expanding the role of botulinum toxin applications. *Parkinsonism Relat. Disord.* **2011**, *17*, S3–S10. [CrossRef] [PubMed]
24. Rosales, R.L. Dystonia, spasticity and botulinum toxin therapy: Rationale, evidences and clinical context. In *Dystonia—The Many Facets*; Rosales, R.L., Ed.; InTech: Chicago, IL, USA, 2012. [CrossRef]
25. Veverka, T.; Hlustik, P.; Hok, P.; Otruba, P.; Tudos, Z.; Zapletalova, J.; Krobot, A.; Kanovsky, P. Cortical activity modulation by botulinum toxin type A in patients with post-stroke arm spasticity: Real and imagined hand movement. *J. Neurol. Sci.* **2014**, *346*, 276–283. [CrossRef] [PubMed]
26. Hesse, S.; Mach, H.; Frohlich, S.; Behrend, S.; Werner, C.; Melzer, I. An early botulinum toxin A treatment in subacute stroke patients may prevent a disabling finger flexor stiffness six months later: A randomized controlled trial. *Clin. Rehabilit.* **2012**, *26*, 237–245. [CrossRef] [PubMed]
27. Kinnear, B.Z.; Lannin, N.A.; Cusick, A.; Harvey, L.A.; Rawicki, B. Rehabilitation therapies after botulinum toxin-A injection to manage limb spasticity: A systematic review. *Phys. Ther.* **2014**, *94*, 1569–1581. [CrossRef] [PubMed]
28. Mills, P.B.; Finlayson, H.; Sudol, M.; O'Connor, R. Systematic review of adjunct therapies to improve outcomes following botulinum toxin injection for treatment of limb spasticity. *Clin. Rehabilit.* **2016**, *30*, 537–548. [CrossRef] [PubMed]
29. Rosales, R. Botulinum toxin therapy as an early intervention for post-stroke spasticity: Beyond a functional viewpoint. *J. Neurol. Sci.* **2017**, *382*, 187–188. [CrossRef] [PubMed]
30. Noyes, K.; Weinstock-Guttman, B. Impact of diagnosis and early treatment on the course of multiple sclerosis. *Am. J. Manag. Care* **2013**, *19*, s321–s331. [PubMed]
31. Dressler, D.; Bhidayasiri, R.; Bohlega, S.; Chahidi, A.; Chung, T.M.; Ebke, M.; Jacinto, L.J.; Kaji, R.; Kocer, S.; Kanovsky, P.; et al. Botulinum toxin therapy for treatment of spasticity in multiple sclerosis: Review and recommendations of the IAB-Interdisciplinary Working Group for Movement Disorders task force. *J. Neurol.* **2017**, *264*, 112–120. [CrossRef] [PubMed]

32. Bhakta, B.B.; Cozens, J.A.; Chamberlain, M.A.; Bamford, J.M. Impact of botulinum toxin type A on disability and carer burden due to arm spasticity after stroke: A randomised double blind placebo controlled trial. *J. Neurol. Neurosurg. Psychiatr.* **2000**, *69*, 217–221. [CrossRef]
33. Simpson, D.M.; Gracies, J.M.; Graham, H.K.; Miyasaki, J.M.; Naumann, M.; Russman, B.; Simpson, L.L.; So, Y. Assessment: Botulinum neurotoxin for the treatment of spasticity (an evidence-based review): Report of the Therapeutics and Technology Assessment Subcommittee of the American Academy of Neurology. *Neurology* **2008**, *70*, 1691–1698. [CrossRef] [PubMed]
34. Lindsay, C.; Simpson, J.; Ispoglou, S.; Sturman, S.G.; Pandyan, A.D. The early use of botulinum toxin in post-stroke spasticity: Study protocol for a randomised controlled trial. *Trials* **2014**, *15*, 12. [CrossRef] [PubMed]
35. Kong, K.H.; Balcaitiene, J.; Berard, H.; Maisonobe, P.; Goh, K.J.; Kumthornthip, W.; Rosales, R.L. Effect of early use of AbobotulinumtoxinA after stroke on spasticity progression: Protocol for a randomised controlled pilot study in adult subjects with moderate to severe upper limb spasticity (ONTIME pilot). *Contempor. Clin. Trials Commun.* **2017**, *6*, 9–16. [CrossRef] [PubMed]
36. Bohannon, R.W.; Smith, M.B. Interrater reliability of a modified Ashworth scale of muscle spasticity. *Phys. Ther.* **1987**, *67*, 206–207. [CrossRef] [PubMed]
37. McCaffery, M.; Beebe, A. *Pain: Clinical Manual for Nursing Practice*; Mosby: St. Louis, MO, USA, 1989; p. 353.
38. Fugl-Meyer, A.R.; Jaasko, L.; Leyman, I.; Olsson, S.; Steglind, S. The post-stroke hemiplegic patient. 1. a method for evaluation of physical performance. *Scand. J. Rehabilit. Med.* **1975**, *7*, 13–31.

toxins

MDPI

Article

Botulinum Toxin Injections and Electrical Stimulation for Spastic Paresis Improve Active Hand Function Following Stroke

Jong-Min Lee [1], Jean-Michel Gracies [2], Si-Bog Park [3], Kyu Hoon Lee [3], Ji Yeong Lee [1] and Joon-Ho Shin [1,*]

1 Department of NeuroRehabilitation, National Rehabilitation Center, Ministry of Health and Welfare, 58 Samgaksan-ro, Gangbuk-gu, Seoul 01022, Korea; ljm21c2000@naver.com (J.-M.L.); wldud3575@hanmail.net (J.Y.L.)

2 Service de Rééducation Neurolocomotrice, Albert Chenevier-Henri Mondor Hospital, 94000 Créteil, France; jean-michel.gracies@aphp.fr

3 Department of Rehabilitation Medicine, Hanyang University College of Medicine, Seoul 04763, Korea; sibopark@hanyang.ac.kr (S.-B.P.); dumitru1@hanyang.ac.kr (K.H.L.)

* Correspondence: asfreelyas@gmail.com; Tel.: +82-2-901-1884; Fax: +82-901-1590

Received: 22 September 2018; Accepted: 21 October 2018; Published: 25 October 2018

Abstract: Botulinum toxin type A (BTX-A) injections improve muscle tone and range of motion (ROM) among stroke patients with upper limb spasticity. However, the efficacy of BTX-A injections for improving active function is unclear. We aimed to determine whether BTX-A injections with electrical stimulation (ES) of hand muscles could improve active hand function (AHF) among chronic stroke patients. Our open-label, pilot study included 15 chronic stroke patients. Two weeks after BTX-A injections into the finger and/or wrist flexors, ES of finger extensors was performed while wearing a wrist brace for 4 weeks (5 days per week; 30-min sessions). Various outcomes were assessed at baseline, immediately before BTX-A injections, and 2 and 6 weeks after BTX-A injections. After the intervention, we noted significant improvements in Box and Block test results, Action Research Arm Test results, the number of repeated finger flexions/extensions, which reflect AHF, and flexor spasticity. Moreover, significant improvements in active ROM of wrist extension values were accompanied by marginally significant changes in Medical Research Council wrist extensor and active ROM of wrist flexion values. In conclusion, BTX-A injections into the finger and/or wrist flexors followed by ES of finger extensors improve AHF among chronic stroke patients.

Keywords: spasticity; spastic paresis; botulinum toxin; electrical stimulation; stroke management; rehabilitation; hand

Key Contribution: Botulinum toxin type A injections into the finger and/or wrist flexor muscles followed by electrical stimulation of finger extensors targeting spastic paresis improve active hand function and impairment among patients with chronic stroke.

1. Introduction

Upper limb spasticity (ULS) is a common impairment after stroke, which can cause abnormal posture, pain, reduced movement, and functional impairment [1–4]. Various interventions, including occupational therapy, physical therapy, oral medications, orthoses, and focal neurolysis, have been used in the management of ULS.

Intramuscular injection of botulinum toxin type A (BTX-A) is the recommended first-line treatment for focal ULS [5–9]. Botulinum toxin type A, which is produced by anaerobic, gram-positive, spore-forming microorganisms from the genus *Clostridium*, is the most potent toxin among various serotypes, and its safety is well established [10,11]. Its neurospecific activity, reversibility, and limited diffusion on local injection make it a safe and successful agent for symptoms characterized by hyperfunction of peripheral nerve terminals [12,13]. Although BTX-A injections have been shown to improve muscle tone, range of motion, and physical global assessment findings, evidence regarding their efficacy for improving active upper limb function (e.g., moving/manipulating objects) is lacking [14,15]. Indeed, systematic reviews have demonstrated that BTX-A has greater effects on passive function than on active function, and some studies have failed to show any improvements in active function with BTX-A treatment [4,16]. These results might hinder active treatment with BTX-A, because the ultimate goal of rehabilitation is functional improvement.

Several explanations for the discrepancy between impairment and function have been proposed. First, most previous treatments have targeted spasticity per se, while factors other than hypertonicity are likely to be associated with active function, including stretch-sensitive paresis, overactivity of agonistic muscles, and learned non-use [2,3,15]. Second, optimal adjunct therapies following BTX-A injections have not been used, despite the need for adjuvant therapy to improve efficacy [17,18]. The combination of modified constraint-induced movement therapy or active task-specific training with BTX-A injections has been shown to improve upper limb function among patients with chronic spastic hemiparesis [19,20]. However, these approaches are not available for individuals with moderate-to-severe muscle weakness, prompting the need for commonly or easily applicable optimal adjunctive therapies to augment hand function. Third, although hand function is critical for upper limb function as an end-effector, few studies have targeted active function of the hand itself [21]. As hand spasticity is particularly disruptive, improvements in shoulder or elbow function may not be adequate to ensure overall functional improvement [22]. In addition, appropriate outcome measures related to both impairment and function, especially active hand function, have not been used [23–25]. Although previous studies have used various outcome measures for upper limb function (e.g., disability assessment scale, motor activity log, and global self-assessment), none have focused on active hand function [20,24,26]. Fourth, standardized techniques for administering BTX-A are yet to be established, and thus there are variations in muscle selection, injection methods, and medication doses.

Many patients having ULS exhibit difficulty with finger extension, which is critical for gripping, grasping, and releasing movements. Thus, we hypothesized that relief of finger flexor spasticity following BTX-A treatment would help patients regain finger extensor strength, which would in turn improve hand function. Based on the findings of previous studies, we further hypothesized that electrical stimulation (ES) is a simple yet effective form of adjuvant therapy, as it facilitates muscle reeducation, including antagonist strengthening and agonist lengthening [27,28]. Therefore, in the present preliminary study, we aimed to determine whether BTX-A injections targeting finger flexor spasticity with concomitant ES of finger extensors can improve active hand function and impairment among patients with chronic stroke.

2. Results

Among the 15 included patients, 7 experienced cerebral infarction and 8 experienced intracerebral hemorrhage. Thirteen patients experienced lesions in the right hemisphere. The mean time from stroke was 12.8 ± 3.7 months. All 15 patients completed the study, and none experienced adverse events.

2.1. Primary Outcomes

After the intervention, there were significant improvements in Box and Block (BB) ($\chi^2 = 6.50$, $p = 0.039$), Action Research Arm Test (ARAT)-total ($\chi^2 = 6.29$, $p = 0.043$), and ARAT-gross movement scores ($\chi^2 = 8.64$, $p = 0.013$), which reflect active hand function (Table 1). Post-hoc analysis confirmed that there were significant improvements in these outcomes in the T1–T3 phase. In addition, significant improvements in ARAT-total and ARAT-gross movement scores were observed in the T2–T3 and T1–T2 phases, respectively.

Table 1. Changes in primary outcome measures over time.

Outcome					p †		
	T1	T2	T3	p *	T1–T2	T2–T3	T1–T3
BB test	3.07 ± 3.85	3.60 ± 4.91	4.67 ± 5.25	0.039	0.473	0.120	0.028
ARAT-total	11.33 ± 8.03	11.27 ± 7.71	12.73 ± 7.67	0.043	1.000	0.036	0.044
ARAT-grasp	2.87 ± 3.82	3.00 ± 3.98	3.27 ± 3.75	0.276	0.854	0.334	0.276
ARAT-grip	2.13 ± 2.07	1.67 ± 1.92	2.53 ± 1.92	0.120	0.141	0.059	0.257
ARAT-gross movement	5.67 ± 2.16	5.93 ± 2.15	6.27 ± 2.37	0.013	0.046	0.096	0.021
ARAT-pinch	0.67 ± 1.23	0.67 ± 0.98	0.67 ± 0.98	1.000	1.000	1.000	1.000

Data are presented as mean ± standard deviation. Outcomes were assessed at immediately before (T1), 2 weeks (T2), and 6 weeks of BTX-A injections (T3). * Friedman test; † Post-hoc Wilcoxon signed-rank test between T1 and T2, between T2 and T3, and between T1 and T3. ARAT: Action Research Arm Test, BB: Box and Block.

2.2. Secondary Outcomes

Repeat-finger extensor/extension (FE) values showed significant increases (χ^2 = 10.00, p = 0.007) in the T1–T3 and T2–T3 phases. Active-FE values showed marginally significant increases during the T2–T3 phase (χ^2 = 5.615, p = 0.060).

Flexor spasticity significantly decreased (Modified Ashworth Scale for wrist flexor/flexion (MAS-WF): χ^2 = 8.40, p = 0.015; MAS for finger flexor/flexion (MAS-FF): χ^2 = 20.18, p < 0.001), and post-hoc tests revealed significant differences in the T1–T2 and T1–T3 phases, but not in the T2–T3 phase (Table 2). Significant increases in active range of motion for wrist extensor/extension (AROM-WE) values (χ^2 = 9.08, p = 0.011) were accompanied by marginally significant increases in Medical Research Council WE (MRC-WE) (χ^2 = 6.00, p = 0.05) and AROM-WF (χ^2 = 6.00, p = 0.05) values. Post-hoc analyses demonstrated that AROM-WE values were higher at T3 than at T1 or T2 and that MRC-WE values significantly increased from T1 to T3. No significant changes were noted for other secondary outcomes, such as the Quick Disabilities of Arm, Shoulder, and Hand (QDASH) score (χ^2 = 3.636, p = 0.162).

Table 2. Changes in secondary outcome measures over time.

Outcome					p †		
	T1	T2	T3	p *	T1–T2	T2–T3	T1–T3
Active-FE	1.73 ± 0.88	2.00 ± 0.85	2.20 ± 0.94	0.060	0.102	0.180	0.053
Distance-FP (cm)	2.58 ± 3.12	3.80 ± 3.02	3.67 ± 2.58	0.212	0.023	0.655	0.027
Repeat-FE	2.07 ± 1.58	2.27 ± 1.16	3.13 ± 1.77	0.007	0.558	0.017	0.008
Thumb opposition	0.07 ± 0.26	0.13 ± 0.35	0.33 ± 0.62	0.223	0.317	0.180	0.102
MAS-WF	2.13 ± 0.35	1.80 ± 0.41	1.73 ± 0.46	0.015	0.025	0.317	0.014
MAS-WE	0.20 ± 0.41	0.13 ± 0.35	0.07 ± 0.26	0.223	0.317	0.317	0.157
MAS-FF	2.33 ± 0.49	1.67 ± 0.49	1.60 ± 0.51	<0.001	0.002	0.317	0.001
MAS-FE	0.07 ± 0.26	0.00 ± 0.00	0.00 ± 0.00	0.368	0.317	1.000	0.317
MRC-WF	2.40 ± 0.91	2.40 ± 0.91	2.53 ± 0.83	0.135	1.000	0.157	0.157
MRC-WE	2.27 ± 0.88	2.40 ± 0.74	2.53 ± 0.83	0.050	0.157	0.157	0.046
MRC-FF	2.60 ± 0.51	2.60 ± 0.51	2.67 ± 0.49	0.717	1.000	0.317	0.564
MRC-FE	1.47 ± 0.64	1.60 ± 0.63	1.67 ± 0.62	0.097	0.157	0.317	0.083
AROM-WF (°)	46.67 ± 26.37	46.67 ± 26.37	49.33 ± 23.44	0.050	1.000	0.102	0.102
AROM-WE (°)	32.67 ± 26.04	33.67 ± 25.53	38.00 ± 24.55	0.011	0.396	0.024	0.023
AROM-RD (°)	4.67 ± 7.42	5.33 ± 6.40	6.67 ± 7.24	0.174	0.564	0.157	0.083
AROM-UD (°)	4.67 ± 6.40	5.33 ± 6.40	5.33 ± 6.40	0.368	0.317	1.000	0.317
Grip strength (kg)	0.27 ± 1.03	0.13 ± 0.52	0.33 ± 1.05	0.223	0.317	0.180	0.317
QDASH	56.88 ± 17.22	54.65 ± 14.88	53.87 ± 16.54	0.162	0.220	0.529	0.058

Data are presented as mean ± standard deviation. Outcomes were assessed at immediately before (T1), 2 weeks (T2), and 6 weeks of BTX-A injections (T3). * Friedman test; † Post-hoc Wilcoxon signed-rank test between T1 and T2, between T2 and T3, and between T1 and T3. FE: finger extensor/extension, FP: fingertip to the palm, MAS: Modified Ashworth Scale, WF: wrist flexor/flexion, WE: wrist extensor/extension, FF: finger flexor/flexion, MRC: Medical Research Council, AROM: active range of motion, RD: radial deviation, UD: ulnar deviation, QDASH: Quick Disabilities of Arm, Shoulder, and Hand, °: degree.

3. Discussion

In the present study, we attempted to examine the efficacy of BTX-A treatment targeting finger flexor spasticity and concomitant ES for improving active hand function in the chronic phase of stroke. We found that BTX-A injections into the flexor muscles of the fingers and wrist followed by ES improved active hand function, as indicated by significant improvements in BB, ARAT (ARAT-total, ARAT-gross movement), and Repeat-FE scores. These findings are in contrast to those of previous studies, which failed to demonstrate improvements in active function after BTX-A treatment among patients with chronic stroke [29–31].

These discrepancies may be explained by our concept of intervention, as we considered treatment according to spastic paresis rather than flexor muscle spasticity only [2,3]. Overactivity of flexor muscles due to spasticity impedes finger and wrist extension, aggravating stretch-sensitive paresis and inhibiting voluntary recruitment of extensors. Similarly, a previous study demonstrated co-activation of spastic flexors and weak extensors [32]. Rehabilitation strategies often focus on finger/wrist flexors, as most hand functions are related to flexor movement (e.g., grasping, pinching, and manipulating objects). However, many patients with ULS following stroke exhibit difficulty with finger extension, which is needed to initiate hand grip and grasp. Thus, we attempted to restore the balance between the flexors and extensors of the wrist/fingers by targeting asymmetrical spastic paresis in two main steps (BTX-A injections and ES with a wrist brace).

Botulinum toxin type A injections to finger/wrist flexors reduced involuntary activation of the flexor muscles and further led to "therapeutic weakness" [33]. However, such weakness is only observed when the doses of BTX-A administered at the flexor digitorum superficialis and profundus are much larger than the doses recommended by the current consensus report [34,35]. Therapeutic weakening of the agonistic finger/wrist flexors allowed for restoration of antagonistic finger/wrist extensor function by reducing reciprocal inhibition from the flexors, stretch-induced paresis, agonistic flexor overactivity, and reflex tone [2,3,36].

Improved balance between agonist and antagonist muscles was accomplished with proprioceptive discharge reduction via group-IA afferents [37,38]. Botulinum toxin type A decreased afferent input of the muscle spindles and their stretch sensitivity. Presynaptic acetylcholine release block with BTX-A was more profound and earlier in gamma-motoneurons than in alpha-motoneurons. From the viewpoint of cortical activity, this BTX-A effect on proprioception is important because abnormal spindle activity generating irregular proprioceptive input may result in abnormal intracortical inhibition and cortical excitability [39]. Similarly, BTX-A-induced spasticity relief was associated with central sensorimotor activation change, which was likely mediated by an altered afferent input from spastic muscles [40]. Moreover, BTX-A reduced the activation of the contralateral putamen and thalamus via modulation of basal ganglia activation [41].

On the other hand, fascicle selection was tailored to each patient, and a flexible dosing regimen was utilized to ensure the appropriate level of weakness without inadvertent over-weakness. This may explain why we observed significant changes in ARAT-gross movement and MAS-WF/finger flexor/flexion (FF) values, but not MRC-WF/FF values or functional deterioration, between T1 and T2.

We subsequently utilized ES to facilitate target muscle (finger/wrist extensor) contraction, which has been difficult to achieve owing to increased flexor tone. ES enabled reeducation, stretching, and strengthening of the extensor muscles [28]. This selective facilitation of agonistic extensor muscles resulted in significant improvements in AROM-WE between T2 and T3, rather than improvements in AROM-WF. Concordantly, active function-related improvements were observed in ARAT-total, ARAT-gross movement, Repeat-FE, and Active-FE values during this phase, but not between T1 and T2.

Such differences between T1–T2 and T2–T3 may explain the discrepancies between active and passive functions following BTX-A treatment [42]. Our findings suggest that spasticity control is insufficient for restoring active function and that concomitant interventions selectively facilitating agonist muscles are necessary to improve outcomes. Notably, cyclic ES of both finger flexors and extensors following BTX-A injections has not been shown to be associated with functional improvements [25], suggesting that such interventions should target agonist function rather than antagonist spasticity per se.

In addition, we utilized a wrist brace to maximize finger extension during ES while reducing unwanted wrist or metacarpophalangeal joint hyperextension. Full finger extension is difficult during concomitant wrist extension owing to passive tension that results from the muscle insertion pattern of two-joint finger flexor muscles. The wrist brace maintained the wrist/metacarpophalangeal joints in a neutral position to allow sufficient extension of the distal or proximal interphalangeal joints, and it may have decreased stretch-sensitive paresis of the finger extensors.

In the present study, we attempted to utilize comprehensive hand-relevant outcome measures for both impairment (MRC, MAS, and AROM) and active function (ARAT and BB). We also utilized measures specific to hand function, particularly finger extension (Active FE, Distance-FP, Repeat-FE, and grip strength). These various measures assessed at different time points helped classify the effects of our intervention in terms of spastic paresis. Recently, goal attainment scales have been used to determine individualized, focal changes following BTX-A injections [43]. However, such scales do not measure objective outcomes but rather measure subjective achievement according to the opinions of the physicians and patients [44]. Therefore, we believe that the objective scales utilized in the present study are more appropriate than goal attainment scales for determining focal functional changes in clinical trials.

According to the QDASH results, no improvement in subjective upper limb function was observed, and this is likely due to the small yet significant objective change over the course of the intervention. Further studies should examine whether both subjective and objective improvements in upper limb function can be observed in select groups of patients, such as those in the subacute phase of stroke and those with some level of strength in the wrist/finger extensors.

The present study had several limitations. First, as this was not a randomized controlled trial, it is difficult to conclude whether our intervention would outperform other interventions or whether the combination of BTX-A injections and ES is more effective than either approach alone. Second, we did not measure outcomes at 12 weeks, when the effects of BTX-A can no longer be observed [45]. Finally, we did not take into account thumb function. Considering that thumb function accounts for 40% of hand performance, future studies should investigate the efficacy of our intervention with regard to thumb function [46].

4. Conclusions

Our findings indicate that BTX-A injections into the finger and/or wrist flexor muscles followed by ES of finger extensors improve active hand function and impairment among patients with chronic stroke. The present results support the notion that interventions targeting spastic paresis, rather than spasticity per se, may improve active hand function.

5. Materials and Methods

The present open-label, pilot study included 15 patients (14 men; 14 right-handed individuals; mean age, 44.7 ± 15.0 years; age range, 22–74 years; Table 3) from the stroke unit of a rehabilitation hospital between March 2016 and February 2017. Patients engaged in inpatient rehabilitation programs at the time of enrollment were allowed to continue therapy throughout the intervention, and anti-spasticity medications were continued at current or reduced doses or were discontinued. The study was approved by the ethics review board of our rehabilitation hospital (NRC-2016-02-011), and all participants provided written informed consent prior to enrollment. The study was registered with ClinicalTrials.gov (number NCT 03549975, 29 March 2016).

Table 3. Clinical characteristics of the study population.

Patient	Stroke Type	Lesion Side	Time from Stroke (Months)	Dominant Hand	Injection Site (Dosage in Units)
1	Ischemic	Rt.	11.5	Rt.	FCU (25), FDP 2/3/4/5 (10/20/20/10), FDS 2/3/4/5 (20/30/25/15), FPL (25)
2	Ischemic	Rt.	10.9	Rt.	FCU (25), FDP 2/3/4 (15/20/15), FDS 2/3/4/5 (25/25/30/15), FPL (30)
3	Hemorrhagic	Rt.	13.2	Rt.	FCU (40), FDP 2/3/4 (10/15/15), FDS 2/3/4/5 (25/30/35/20), FPB (10), FPL (30), PT (50)
4	Hemorrhagic	Rt.	17.4	Rt.	AP (10), BB (40), brachialis (50), FDP 2/3/4/5 (10/15/15/5), FDS 2/3/4/5 (25/35/40/15), FPL (40)
5	Ischemic	Rt.	18.9	Rt.	AP (10), brachialis (55), FDP 2/3/4 (10/10/10), FDS 2/3/4/5 (30/40/35/20), FPL (40), PT (40)
6	Ischemic	Rt.	10.2	Rt.	FCU (30), FDP 2/3/4/5 (10/20/10/10), FDS 2/3/4/5 (25/25/20/15), FPB (5), FPL (25), PT (20)
7	Hemorrhagic	Lt.	12.6	Rt.	Brachialis (60), FCU (40), FDP 2/3/4 (10/10/15), FDS 2/3/4/5 (25/35/30/15), FPL (20), PT (40)
8	Ischemic	Lt.	13	Rt.	Brachialis (60), deltoid (20), FDP 2/3/4/5 (15/15/10/10), FDS 2/3/4/5 (30/40/30/10), FPB (10), FPL (30), PT (20)
9	Hemorrhagic	Rt.	10.3	Lt.	Brachialis (60), deltoid (20), FDP 2/3/4/5 (15/15/10/10), FDS 2/3/4/5 (30/40/30/10), FPB (10), FPL (30), PT (20)
10	Hemorrhagic	Rt.	20.3	Rt.	AP (10), FCU (30), FDS 2/3/4 (10/15/10), FPB (10), FPL (20), lumbricals (10)
11	Ischemic	Rt.	8.6	Rt.	AP (10), FCU (30), FDP 2/3/4/5 (5/10/10/5), FDS 2/3/4/5 (20/30/20/10), FPL (20)
12	Ischemic	Rt.	7.2	Rt.	AP (10), BB (40), FDP 2/3/5 (10/10/5), FDS 2/3/4/5 (30/35/20/10), FPL (30)
13	Hemorrhagic	Rt.	9.8	Rt.	AP (15), FDP 2/3/4 (5/10/5), FDS 2/3/4/5 (10/20/15/5), FPL (15)
14	Hemorrhagic	Rt.	12.8	Rt.	FDP 2/3/4/5 (30/30/35/25), FDS 2/3/4 (10/15/15), FPL (30), opponens (5)
15	Hemorrhagic	Rt.	14.9	Rt.	Brachialis (50), brachioradialis (20), FCU (30), FDP 2/3/4 (15/15/15), FDS 2/3/4/5 (35/40/30/20), FPL (30)

AP: adductor pollicis, BB: biceps brachii, FCU: flexor carpi ulnaris, PT: pronator teres, FDP: flexor digitorum profundus, FDS: flexor digitorum superficialis, FPB: flexor pollicis brevis, FPL: flexor pollicis longus, Rt.: right, Lt.: left.

5.1. Inclusion and Exclusion Criteria

The inclusion criteria were as follows: (1) age older than 18 years; (2) hemiplegic ULS secondary to unilateral ischemic or hemorrhagic stroke; (3) finger and wrist flexor spasticity graded at least 1+ on the MAS; and (4) stroke occurrence at least 6 months prior to enrollment. The exclusion criteria were as follows: (1) fixed contracture of the wrist or hand; (2) previous ULS treatment with neurolytic therapy, surgery, or BTX-A injection; (3) presence of any active implanted device; (4) presence of any neurological disorder causing motor deficit or spasticity, other than stroke; (5) inability to cooperate for all outcome measure-related tasks secondary to cognitive impairment or aphasia; (6) pregnancy, planned pregnancy, or lactation; and (7) contraindication for BTX-A treatment.

5.2. Intervention

5.2.1. BTX-A Administration

Patients received BTX-A (onabotulinumtoxin A, Botox; Allergan Inc., Irvine, KY, USA) injections at week 0. The dilution of BTX-A was standardized, such that each vial of BTX-A (100 U) was diluted with 2 mL of normal saline (5 U/0.1 mL). A physician with experience in BTX-A treatment performed clinical evaluations of ULS and freely selected the target muscle and dose according to the pattern and severity of ULS in each patient. BTX-A injections were then administered under ultrasonographic guidance (ACCUVIX XG; Medison, Seoul, Korea). Injections at the flexor digitorum superficialis and profundus were administered by tailoring fascicle selection to each patient and by adopting a flexible dosing regimen. In each patient, the total BTX-A dose did not exceed 360 U. The dosages and injection sites are listed in Table 3.

5.2.2. ES with a Wrist Brace

After 2 weeks of BTX-A injections, patients received ES of finger extensors while wearing a wrist brace for 4 weeks. ES was administered 5 days per week during 30-min sessions by trained occupational therapists, using a Novastim CU-FS1 unit (CU, Medical, Seoul, Korea). During ES, each patient was seated in a chair with the affected arm resting on a table and with a small pillow supporting the pronated forearm. Cyclic ES was administered to induce muscle contractions, using biphasic pulses (frequency, 50 Hz; pulse duration, 200 μs) delivered for 6 s (ramp up, 1 s; ramp down, 2 s), with a 12-s burst-off. Two surface electrodes (5 × 5 cm) were placed over the extensor digitorum communis. The amplitude of stimulation was adjusted to elicit adequate finger extension for a sufficient range of motion against gravity, without pain.

The wrist brace (National Rehabilitation Center, Seoul, Korea) used during ES was made of soft fabric, and it covered the area from the wrist to the metacarpophalangeal joint. Two metal bars were attached to the volar and dorsal regions of the brace to immobilize the wrist in a neutral position. This immobilization ensured that ES could induce selective distal or proximal interphalangeal joint extension while overcoming unwanted simultaneous wrist or metacarpophalangeal joint extension. A Velcro strap was used to restrain the dorsal and volar sides of the brace.

5.3. *Outcome Measures*

We recorded baseline characteristics, including sex, age, stroke type, brain lesion side, time since stroke, and handedness. Primary and secondary outcomes were assessed at baseline (week −1, T0), immediately before BTX-A injections (week 0, T1), and 2 weeks (week 2, T2) and 6 weeks (week 6, T3) after BTX-A injections, by an experienced research occupational therapist. For further screening, we evaluated changes in outcomes between T0 and T1. Patients exhibiting changes between these two time points were excluded from the study. We examined the effects of BTX-A at 2 weeks, as previous studies have indicated that BTX-A shows maximum efficacy between 1 and 2 weeks after treatment [47]. Outcomes at T3 represented the combined effects of BTX-A and ES with a wrist brace (Figure 1).

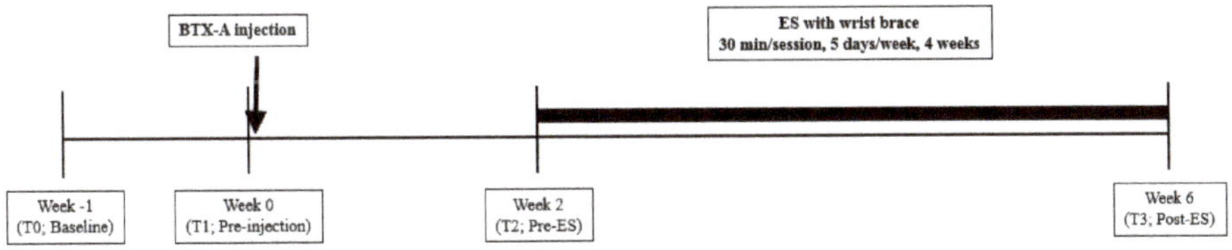

Figure 1. Experimental design. Primary and secondary outcomes are assessed at baseline (week 1, T0), immediately before BTX-A injections (week 0, T1), and 2 weeks (week 2, T2) and 6 weeks (week 6, T3) after BTX-A injections, by an experienced research occupational therapist. Patients exhibiting changes in outcomes between T0 and T1 were excluded. BTX-A: botulinum toxin type A, ES: electrical stimulation.

5.3.1. Primary Outcomes

The primary outcomes were changes in patient results in the BB test and ARAT between T1 and T3, which represent changes in the active function of the upper limb following the present intervention. The BB test is a reliable and validated measure of unilateral gross manual dexterity, in which participants are required to pick up a 1-inch block, lift it over a partition, and then release it within a target area as many times as possible within 60 s [48]. The ARAT is a reliable and validated measure of arm function using observational methods with the following four subsections: grasp, grip, pinch, and gross movement. It comprises 19 items rated using a 4-point ordinal scale (0–3). Thus, the total scores on the ARAT range from 0 (failure to perform all movements; patients cannot perform any part of the test) to 57 (all movements are performed normally) [49].

5.3.2. Secondary Outcomes

Hand-specific active function was assessed according to active finger extension (Active-FE), the maximum distance from the fingertip to the palm (Distance-FP), the number of repeated finger flexion/extension movements within 20 s (Repeat-FE), the rating of active thumb opposition (Thumb-opposition), and grip strength as measured using the Jamar dynamometer (Sammons Preston, Bolingbrook, IL, USA). Active-FE was rated using a 5-point ordinal scale (0 = no movement, 4 = functional extension of all digits) by reviewing a video clip [50]. Distance-FP (cm) values were obtained by measuring the distance from the middle fingertip to the mid-palmar crease [51]. Thumb-opposition was rated using a 7-point scale (1 = to the distal phalanx of the index finger, 7 = to the medial phalanx of the small finger) [51].

Upper limb impairment was assessed according to MAS scores for the wrist and finger flexors/extensors (MAS-WF/WE/FF/FE), MRC grades for wrist and finger flexor/extensor strength (MRC-WF/WE/FF/FE), and active range of motion for wrist flexion/extension (AROM-WF/WE) and radial/ulnar deviation (AROM-RD/UD) as determined through goniometric measurement. Modified Ashworth Scale grades of spasticity were converted from 1+, 2, 3, and 4 to 2, 3, 4, and 5, respectively [52].

Subjective general upper limb function was evaluated using the self-reported QDASH scale. The QDASH scale consists of 11 items regarding physical function and symptoms during the previous week, and the total scores range from 0 (no disability) to 100 (most severe disability) [53].

5.4. Statistical Analysis

For all outcome measures, the Friedman test was used to determine the overall change from pre-intervention (T1) to post-intervention (T2)/follow-up (T3). When the Friedman test yielded significant results, various pairwise comparisons were performed using post-hoc Wilcoxon signed-rank tests in order to determine the effect of each intervention (BTX-A/ES). All statistical analyses were performed using SPSS 20.0 (IBM SPSS Statistics, IBM Corporation, Armonk, NY, USA). The level of statistical significance was set at $p < 0.05$.

Author Contributions: Conceptualization, J.-M.L., J.-M.G. and J.-H.S.; methodology, J.-H.S.; software, J.Y.L.; validation, S.-B.P. and K.H.L.; formal analysis, J.-M.L.; investigation, J.Y.L.; resources, S.-B.P.; data curation, K.H.L.; writing—original draft preparation, J.-M.L.; writing—review and editing, J.-H.S.; visualization, J.-M.L.; supervision, J.-H.S.; project administration, J.-H.S.; funding acquisition, J.-H.S.

Funding: This research was funded by the Translational Research Center for Rehabilitation Robots, National Rehabilitation Center, Ministry of Health and Welfare, Republic of Korea, grant number NRCTR-IN14002, NRCTR-IN15002.

Conflicts of Interest: Jean-Michel Gracies served as a consultant on advisory boards for and received research grant support from Allergan, Ipsen, and Merz. The funders had no role in the design of the study; in the collection, analyses, or interpretation of data; in the writing of the manuscript; or in the decision to publish the results.

References

1. Sommerfeld, D.K.; Eek, E.U.-B.; Svensson, A.-K.; Holmqvist, L.W.; von Arbin, M.H. Spasticity after stroke: Its occurrence and association with motor impairments and activity limitations. *Stroke* **2004**, *35*, 134–139. [CrossRef] [PubMed]
2. Gracies, J.M. Pathophysiology of spastic paresis. I: Paresis and soft tissue changes. *Muscle Nerve* **2005**, *31*, 535–551. [CrossRef] [PubMed]
3. Gracies, J.M. Pathophysiology of spastic paresis. II: Emergence of muscle overactivity. *Muscle Nerve* **2005**, *31*, 552–571. [CrossRef] [PubMed]
4. Foley, N.; Pereira, S.; Salter, K.; Fernandez, M.M.; Speechley, M.; Sequeira, K.; Miller, T.; Teasell, R. Treatment with botulinum toxin improves upper-extremity function post stroke: A systematic review and meta-analysis. *Arch. Phys. Med. Rehabil.* **2013**, *94*, 977–989. [CrossRef] [PubMed]

5. Esquenazi, A.; Albanese, A.; Chancellor, M.B.; Elovic, E.; Segal, K.R.; Simpson, D.M.; Smith, C.P.; Ward, A.B. Evidence-based review and assessment of botulinum neurotoxin for the treatment of adult spasticity in the upper motor neuron syndrome. *Toxicon* **2013**, *67*, 115–128. [CrossRef] [PubMed]
6. Wissel, J.; Ward, A.B.; Erztgaard, P.; Bensmail, D.; Hecht, M.J.; Lejeune, T.M.; Schnider, P. European consensus table on the use of botulinum toxin type A in adult spasticity. *J. Rehabil. Med.* **2009**, *41*, 13–25. [CrossRef] [PubMed]
7. Simpson, D.; Gracies, J.; Graham, H.; Miyasaki, J.; Naumann, M.; Russman, B.; Simpson, L.; So, Y. Assessment: Botulinum neurotoxin for the treatment of spasticity (an evidence-based review) Report of the Therapeutics and Technology Assessment Subcommittee of the American Academy of Neurology. *Neurology* **2008**, *70*, 1691–1698. [CrossRef] [PubMed]
8. Demetrios, M.; Khan, F.; Turner-Stokes, L.; Brand, C.; Mc-Sweeney, S. Multidisciplinary rehabilitation following botulinum toxin and other focal intramuscular treatment for post-stroke spasticity. *Cochrane Database Syst. Rev.* **2012**, *6*, 12. [CrossRef]
9. Simpson, D.M.; Hallett, M.; Ashman, E.J.; Comella, C.L.; Green, M.W.; Gronseth, G.S.; Armstrong, M.J.; Gloss, D.; Potrebic, S.; Jankovic, J. Practice guideline update summary: Botulinum neurotoxin for the treatment of blepharospasm, cervical dystonia, adult spasticity, and headache Report of the Guideline Development Subcommittee of the American Academy of Neurology. *Neurology* **2016**, *86*, 1818–1826. [CrossRef] [PubMed]
10. Pirazzini, M.; Rossetto, O.; Eleopra, R.; Montecucco, C. Botulinum neurotoxins: Biology, pharmacology, and toxicology. *Pharmacol. Rev.* **2017**, *69*, 200–235. [CrossRef] [PubMed]
11. Pirazzini, M. Novel Botulinum Neurotoxins: Exploring Underneath the Iceberg Tip. *Toxins* **2018**, *10*, 190.
12. Hallett, M.; Albanese, A.; Dressler, D.; Segal, K.R.; Simpson, D.M.; Truong, D.; Jankovic, J. Evidence-based review and assessment of botulinum neurotoxin for the treatment of movement disorders. *Toxicon* **2013**, *67*, 94–114. [CrossRef] [PubMed]
13. Naumann, M.; Dressler, D.; Hallett, M.; Jankovic, J.; Schiavo, G.; Segal, K.R.; Truong, D. Evidence-based review and assessment of botulinum neurotoxin for the treatment of secretory disorders. *Toxicon* **2013**, *67*, 141–152. [CrossRef] [PubMed]
14. Shaw, L.; Rodgers, H.; Price, C.; van Wijck, F.; Shackley, P.; Steen, N.; Barnes, M.; Ford, G.; Graham, L. BoTULS: A multicentre randomised controlled trial to evaluate the clinical effectiveness and cost-effectiveness of treating upper limb spasticity due to stroke with botulinum toxin type A. *Health Technol. Assess.* **2010**, *14*, 1–113. [CrossRef] [PubMed]
15. Gracies, J.M.; Brashear, A.; Jech, R.; McAllister, P.; Banach, M.; Valkovic, P.; Walker, H.; Marciniak, C.; Deltombe, T.; Skoromets, A.; et al. Safety and efficacy of abobotulinumtoxinA for hemiparesis in adults with upper limb spasticity after stroke or traumatic brain injury: A double-blind randomised controlled trial. *Lancet Neurol.* **2015**, *14*, 992–1001. [CrossRef]
16. Dong, Y.; Wu, T.; Hu, X.; Wang, T. Efficacy and safety of Botulinum Toxin type A for upper limb spasticity after stroke or traumatic brain injury: A systematic review with meta-analysis and trial sequential analysis. *Eur. J. Phys. Rehabil. Med.* **2016**, *53*. [CrossRef]
17. Rosales, R.L.; Efendy, F.; Teleg, E.S.; Santos, M.M.D.; Rosales, M.C.; Ostrea, M.; Tanglao, M.J.; Ng, A.R. Botulinum toxin as early intervention for spasticity after stroke or non-progressive brain lesion: A meta-analysis. *J. Neurol. Sci.* **2016**, *371*, 6–14. [CrossRef] [PubMed]
18. Mills, P.B.; Finlayson, H.; Sudol, M.; O'Connor, R. Systematic review of adjunct therapies to improve outcomes following botulinum toxin injection for treatment of limb spasticity. *Clin. Rehabil.* **2016**, *30*, 537–548. [CrossRef] [PubMed]
19. Sun, S.-F.; Hsu, C.-W.; Sun, H.-P.; Hwang, C.-W.; Yang, C.-L.; Wang, J.-L. Combined botulinum toxin type A with modified constraint-induced movement therapy for chronic stroke patients with upper extremity spasticity: A randomized controlled study. *Neurorehabil. Neural Repair* **2010**, *24*, 34–41. [CrossRef] [PubMed]
20. Meythaler, J.M.; Vogtle, L.; Brunner, R.C. A preliminary assessment of the benefits of the addition of botulinum toxin a to a conventional therapy program on the function of people with longstanding stroke. *Arch. Phys. Med. Rehabil.* **2009**, *90*, 1453–1461. [CrossRef] [PubMed]
21. Broeks, J.G.; Lankhorst, G.J.; Rumping, K.; Prevo, A.J. The long-term outcome of arm function after stroke: Results of a follow-up study. *Disabil. Rehabil.* **1999**, *21*, 357–364. [CrossRef] [PubMed]

22. Mayer, N.H.; Esquenazi, A.; Childers, M.K. Common patterns of clinical motor dysfunction. *Muscle Nerve* **1997**, *20*, 21–35. [CrossRef]
23. Picelli, A.; Lobba, D.; Midiri, A.; Prandi, P.; Melotti, C.; Baldessarelli, S.; Smania, N. Botulinum toxin injection into the forearm muscles for wrist and fingers spastic overactivity in adults with chronic stroke: A randomized controlled trial comparing three injection techniques. *Clin. Rehabil.* **2014**, *28*, 232–242. [CrossRef] [PubMed]
24. Brashear, A.; Gordon, M.F.; Elovic, E.; Kassicieh, V.D.; Marciniak, C.; Do, M.; Lee, C.-H.; Jenkins, S.; Turkel, C. Intramuscular injection of botulinum toxin for the treatment of wrist and finger spasticity after a stroke. *N. Engl. J. Med.* **2002**, *347*, 395–400. [CrossRef] [PubMed]
25. Weber, D.J.; Skidmore, E.R.; Niyonkuru, C.; Chang, C.-L.; Huber, L.M.; Munin, M.C. Cyclic functional electrical stimulation does not enhance gains in hand grasp function when used as an adjunct to onabotulinumtoxinA and task practice therapy: A single-blind, randomized controlled pilot study. *Arch. Phys. Med. Rehabil.* **2010**, *91*, 679–686. [CrossRef] [PubMed]
26. Gracies, J.M.; Bayle, N.; Goldberg, S.; Simpson, D.M. Botulinum toxin type B in the spastic arm: A randomized, double-blind, placebo-controlled, preliminary study. *Arch. Phys. Med. Rehabil.* **2014**, *95*, 1303–1311. [CrossRef] [PubMed]
27. Billian, C.; Gorman, P.H. Upper extremity applications of functional neuromuscular stimulation. *Assist. Technol.* **1992**, *4*, 31–39. [CrossRef] [PubMed]
28. Chae, J.; Bethoux, F.; Bohinc, T.; Dobos, L.; Davis, T.; Friedl, A. Neuromuscular stimulation for upper extremity motor and functional recovery in acute hemiplegia. *Stroke* **1998**, *29*, 975–979. [CrossRef] [PubMed]
29. Simpson, D.; Alexander, D.; O'brien, C.; Tagliati, M.; Aswad, A.; Leon, J.; Gibson, J.; Mordaunt, J.; Monaghan, E. Botulinum toxin type A in the treatment of upper extremity spasticity A randomized, double-blind, placebo-controlled trial. *Neurology* **1996**, *46*, 1306. [CrossRef] [PubMed]
30. Smith, S.; Ellis, E.; White, S.; Moore, A. A double-blind placebo-controlled study of botulinum toxin in upper limb spasticity after stroke or head injury. *Clin. Rehabil.* **2000**, *14*, 5–13. [CrossRef] [PubMed]
31. Sheean, G.L. Botulinum treatment of spasticity: Why is it so difficult to show a functional benefit? *Curr. Opin. Neurol.* **2001**, *14*, 771–776. [CrossRef] [PubMed]
32. Kamper, D.; Rymer, W. Impairment of voluntary control of finger motion following stroke: Role of inappropriate muscle coactivation. *Muscle Nerve* **2001**, *24*, 673–681. [CrossRef] [PubMed]
33. Li, S.; Francisco, G.E. New insights into the pathophysiology of post-stroke spasticity. *Front. Hum. Neurosci.* **2015**, *9*, 192. [CrossRef] [PubMed]
34. Picelli, A.; Baricich, A.; Cisari, C.; Paolucci, S.; Smania, N.; Sandrini, G. The Italian real-life post-stroke spasticity survey: Unmet needs in the management of spasticity with botulinum toxin type A. *Funct. Neurol.* **2017**, *32*, 89–96. [CrossRef] [PubMed]
35. Simpson, D.M.; Patel, A.T.; Alfaro, A.; Ayyoub, Z.; Charles, D.; Dashtipour, K.; Esquenazi, A.; Graham, G.D.; McGuire, J.R.; Odderson, I. OnabotulinumtoxinA Injection for Poststroke Upper-Limb Spasticity: Guidance for Early Injectors from a Delphi Panel Process. *PM R* **2017**, *9*, 136–148. [CrossRef] [PubMed]
36. Filippi, G.M.; Errico, P.; Santarelli, R.; Bagolini, B.; Manni, E. Botulinum A toxin effects on rat jaw muscle spindles. *Acta Oto-Laryngol.* **1993**, *113*, 400–404. [CrossRef]
37. Manni, E.; Bagolini, B.; Pettorossi, V.E.; Errico, P. Effect of botulinum toxin on extraocular muscle proprioception. *Doc. Ophthalmol.* **1989**, *72*, 189–198. [CrossRef] [PubMed]
38. Wöber, C.; Schnider, P.; Steinhoff, N.; Trattnig, S.; Zebenholzer, K.; Auff, E. Posturographic findings in patients with idiopathic cervical dystonia before and after local injections with botulinum toxin. *Eur. Neurol.* **1999**, *41*, 194–200. [CrossRef] [PubMed]
39. Kaňovský, P.; Rosales, R.L. Debunking the pathophysiological puzzle of dystonia–with special reference to botulinum toxin therapy. *Parkinsonism Relat. Disord.* **2011**, *17*, S11–S14. [CrossRef] [PubMed]
40. Veverka, T.; Hluštík, P.; Hok, P.; Otruba, P.; Zapletalová, J.; Tüdös, Z.; Krobot, A.; Kaňovský, P. Sensorimotor modulation by botulinum toxin A in post-stroke arm spasticity: Passive hand movement. *J. Neurol. Sci.* **2016**, *362*, 14–20. [CrossRef] [PubMed]
41. Dresel, C.; Bayer, F.; Castrop, F.; Rimpau, C.; Zimmer, C.; Haslinger, B. Botulinum toxin modulates basal ganglia but not deficient somatosensory activation in orofacial dystonia. *Mov. Disord.* **2011**, *26*, 1496–1502. [CrossRef] [PubMed]

42. Zakin, E.; Simpson, D. Evidence on botulinum toxin in selected disorders. *Toxicon* **2018**, *147*, 134–140. [CrossRef] [PubMed]
43. McCrory, P.; Turner-Stokes, L.; Baguley, I.J.; De Graaff, S.; Katrak, P.; Sandanam, J.; Davies, L.; Munns, M.; Hughes, A. Botulinum toxin A for treatment of upper limb spasticity following stroke: A multi-centre randomized placebo-controlled study of the effects on quality of life and other person-centred outcomes. *J. Rehabil. Med.* **2009**, *41*, 536–544. [CrossRef] [PubMed]
44. Fheodoroff, K.; Ashford, S.; Jacinto, J.; Maisonobe, P.; Balcaitiene, J.; Turner-Stokes, L. Factors influencing goal attainment in patients with post-stroke upper limb spasticity following treatment with botulinum toxin A in real-life clinical practice: Sub-analyses from the Upper Limb International Spasticity (ULIS)-II Study. *Toxins* **2015**, *7*, 1192–1205. [CrossRef] [PubMed]
45. Shaw, L.C.; Price, C.I.; van Wijck, F.M.; Shackley, P.; Steen, N.; Barnes, M.P.; Ford, G.A.; Graham, L.A.; Rodgers, H. Botulinum Toxin for the Upper Limb after Stroke (BoTULS) Trial: Effect on impairment, activity limitation, and pain. *Stroke* **2011**, *42*, 1371–1379. [CrossRef] [PubMed]
46. Emerson, E.T.; Krizek, T.J.; Greenwald, D.P. Anatomy, physiology, and functional restoration of the thumb. *Ann. Plast. Surg.* **1996**, *36*, 180–191. [CrossRef] [PubMed]
47. Asutay, F.; Atalay, Y.; Asutay, H.; Acar, A.H. The Evaluation of the Clinical Effects of Botulinum Toxin on Nocturnal Bruxism. *Pain Res. Manag.* **2017**, *2017*, 5. [CrossRef] [PubMed]
48. Desrosiers, J.; Bravo, G.; Hébert, R.; Dutil, É.; Mercier, L. Validation of the Box and Block Test as a measure of dexterity of elderly people: Reliability, validity, and norms studies. *Arch. Phys. Med. Rehabil.* **1994**, *75*, 751–755. [PubMed]
49. Van der Lee, J.H.; Beckerman, H.; Lankhorst, G.J.; Bouter, L.M. The responsiveness of the Action Research Arm test and the Fugl-Meyer Assessment scale in chronic stroke patients. *J. Rebab. Med.* **2001**, *33*, 110–113.
50. Rodriquez, A.A.; McGinn, M.; Chappell, R. Botulinum toxin injection of spastic finger flexors in hemiplegic patients. *Am. J. Phys. Med. Rehabil.* **2000**, *79*, 44–47. [CrossRef] [PubMed]
51. Ring, H.; Rosenthal, N. Controlled study of neuroprosthetic functional electrical stimulation in sub-acute post-stroke rehabilitation. *J. Rehabil. Med.* **2005**, *37*, 32–36. [CrossRef] [PubMed]
52. Bohannon, R.W.; Smith, M.B. Interrater reliability of a modified Ashworth scale of muscle spasticity. *Phys. Ther.* **1987**, *67*, 206–207. [CrossRef] [PubMed]
53. Gummesson, C.; Ward, M.M.; Atroshi, I. The shortened disabilities of the arm, shoulder and hand questionnaire (Quick DASH): Validity and reliability based on responses within the full-length DASH. *BMC Musculoskelet. Disord.* **2006**, *7*, 44. [CrossRef] [PubMed]

toxins

MDPI

Article

"Appropriate Treatment" and Therapeutic Window in Spasticity Treatment with IncobotulinumtoxinA: From 100 to 1000 Units

Giancarlo Ianieri *, Riccardo Marvulli, Giulia Alessia Gallo, Pietro Fiore and Marisa Megna

Department of Basic Sciences, Neuroscience and Sense Organs, University of Bari "Aldo Moro", G. Cesare Place 11, 70125 Bari, Italy; ricmarv81@hotmail.it (R.M.); giulia.gallo1985@gmail.com (G.A.G.); p_fiore@hotmail.it (F.P.); marisa.megna@uniba.it (M.M.)

* Correspondence: igc@neurol.uniba.it; Tel.: +39-080-559-5519

Received: 12 February 2018; Accepted: 23 March 2018; Published: 28 March 2018

Abstract: Many neurological diseases (ischemic and hemorrhagic stroke, multiple sclerosis, infant cerebral palsy, spinal cord injuries, traumatic brain injury, and other cerebrovascular disorders) may cause muscle spasticity. Different therapeutic strategies have been proposed for the treatment of spasticity. One of the major treatments for tone modulation is botulinum toxin type A (BTX-A), performed in addition to other rehabilitation strategies based on individualized multidisciplinary programs aimed at achieving certain goals for each patient. Therapeutic plans must be precisely defined as they must balance the reduction of spastic hypertonia and retention of residual motor function. To perform and optimize the treatment, an accurate clinical and instrumental evaluation of spasticity is needed to determine how this symptom is invalidating and to choose the best doses, muscles and times of injection in each patient. We introduce an "appropriate treatment" and no "standard or high dosage treatment" concept based on our retrospective observational study on 120 patients lasting two years, according to the larger Therapeutic Index and Therapeutic Window of Incobotulinumtoxin A doses from 100 to 1000 units. We studied the efficiency and safety of this drug considering the clinical spasticity significance for specialist physicians and patients.

Keywords: spasticity; botulinum toxin type A; appropriate treatment; Therapeutic Index

Key Contribution: To underline larger Therapeutic Index and Therapeutic Window of IncobotulinumtoxinA doses (from 100 to 1000 units) considering clinical spasticity significance for specialist physicians and patients.

---

1. Introduction

Spasticity is the most common complication of many neurological diseases followed by ischemic and hemorrhagic stroke, multiple sclerosis, infant cerebral palsy, spinal cord injuries, traumatic brain injury, and other cerebrovascular disorders [1].

Comprehending the various mechanisms of muscle tone alteration and the quantitative evaluation of muscle rheological modifications can lead to the development of more precise and targeted therapeutic interventions for the treatment of spasticity [2,3]. Anatomically, there is a reduction in type II fibers and an increase in type I fibers. Clinically, it is an involuntary motor disorder, characterized by hypertonic muscle tone with increased excitability of the muscle relaxation reflex and increased tendon reflexes. Muscle weakness or paresis in the limbs is associated with spasticity and contributes to loss of motor dexterity and functional capacity [4]. Spasticity, if left untreated, can hinder the functional result by promoting persistent abnormal postures which produce muscle-tendon contractions and bone deformities. Substantial complications resulting from spasticity include movement impairment, difficulty in managing hygiene and self-care, poor self-esteem, body image alteration, pain, and pressure ulcers. In addition, patients with severe spasticity may suffer poor social interaction drastically worsening quality of life [5,6].

For these clinical problems and their related high social costs, various therapeutic strategies have been proposed for the treatment of spasticity including surgical, medical, and rehabilitation procedures. One of the major treatments for muscle tone modulation is botulinum toxin type A (BTX-A) administered intramuscularly [5,7]. BTX-A, by modulating the release of acetylcholine from synaptic vesicles, brings a reduction in muscle tone and, if associated with appropriate rehabilitation treatment, can stop the cascade of events that causes muscle fibrosis with subsequent retraction and joint blocks. BTX-A is indicated when spasticity is focal or segmental and interferes with active or passive operation. The primary purpose of spastic muscle treatment is to maintain length and to allow normal limb placement to avoid secondary shortening of soft tissues. In general, treatment with BTX-A is performed in addition to other rehabilitation strategies based on individualized multidisciplinary programs aimed at achieving tailored goals for each patient. Therapeutic plans must be precisely defined as they must balance the reduction of spastic hypertonia and retention of residual motor function. Although there is no consensus on when BTX-A therapy should begin or how long it should last, BTX-A intramuscular infiltrations are considered the first line of medical treatment for focal/segmental spasticity [8].

Proper use of botulinum toxin both in terms of dosage and injection requires careful monitoring of spastic hypertonia over time. The most commonly used muscular tone measurement is the Modified Ashworth Scale (MAS), where resistance to the passive muscle extension is rated in five points on an ordinal scale. MAS has been criticized for non-standardization of extension speed in manual trials, it does not quantify an absolute resistance, it is physician-dependent, only applies to distal body segments, and has low sensitivity to small variations in muscle tone [9]. We have also discussed the reliability and validity of this scale. MAS is reliable for measuring the muscle tone of some muscle groups such as the elbow, wrist, and knee flexors [10]. Considering the difficulties in distinguishing between the increase in muscle tone and soft tissue rigidity, as well as lack of correlation with functional changes after each treatment, appropriate clinical and instrumental measurements should be used to obtain reliable and accurate values of their rheological properties (tone, elasticity, and stiffness). A tool with these portable and reliable features is MyotonPRO®, a painless and non-invasive device which can provide quantitative and objective evaluations of muscle properties [11,12].

A proper assessment of muscle properties is important to make appropriate clinical decisions and to monitor therapy results in patients with spasticity.

The aim of this retrospective observational study is to objectify the efficacy and safety of 100 to 1000 units botulinum toxin treatment to modulate spasticity according to the individual patient's needs.

2. Results

Patients were initially divided into three groups according to the botulinum toxin A dosage, as reported in the Methods section. During the observation period, some patients switched to another group because the dosage used increased (Table 1).

Table 1. Number of patients in each group at the beginning of study and after 9 months when there were no other switches. In the first group largest number of patients switched to another group (the second one).

Time	GR A 100–400 U	GR B 400–700 U	GR C 700–1000 U
t 0 (beginning)	30	40	50
t 1 (after 9 months)	20	42	58

In group A, average doses increased during the study, but there was no statistical significance. At the third injection, dosage was increased in 10 patients (33%) due to poor clinical effects or to treat more muscles, so they switched to group B. In the following injections, these patients improved their clinical and instrumental measurement of spasticity (Figures 1 and 2).

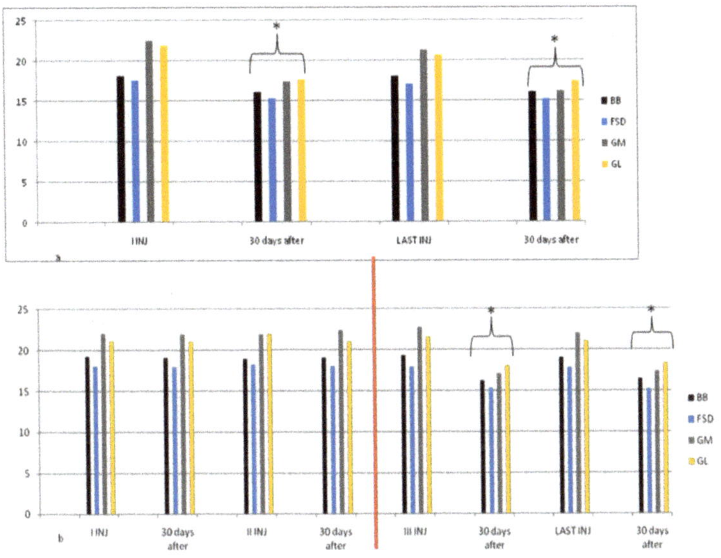

Figure 1. Myometric muscle tone evaluation in group A. This figure shows a statistically significant reduction in muscle tone after 30 days from the first and from the last injection in 20 patients treated with dosage up to 400 UI (**a**); For 10 patients of this group, muscle tone reduction was lower in the first and second cycle of injections; when we increased dosage (up to 700 UI, red line) due to increased units for each muscle or having injected other muscles not evaluated with myotonPRO®, reduction was statistically significant after 30 days for each cycle of injection (**b**). * $p < 0.05$. BB = Biceps Brachii, FSD = Flexorum Superficial Digitorum, GM = Gastrocnemius Medialis, GL = Gastrocnemius Lateralis.

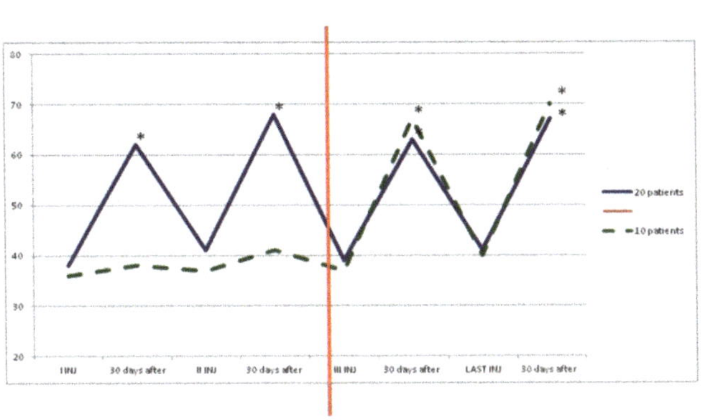

Figure 2. Functional Independence Measure (FIM) value in group A. The dark blue line shows statistical improvement of FIM in 20 patients treated with dosage up to 400 UI. Instead, the green and dashed line shows a statistical improvement of FIM in other 10 patients of this group when we increased dosage (up to 700 UI, red line) due to increased units for each muscle or to having injected other muscles. * $p < 0.05$. We considered the first three and last cycles of injection because statistical improvement of data occurred after dosage increased in 10 patients and it was constant until the end in both subgroups.

In group B, average increase in dosage was not statistically significant during the study. After the first injection, eight patients (20%) showed no clinical and instrumental improvement, so we increased dosage (we treated muscles with greater dosage rather than treating more muscles) and they switched to group C. In the following injections, these eight patients improved their clinical and instrumental measurement of spasticity (Figures 3 and 4).

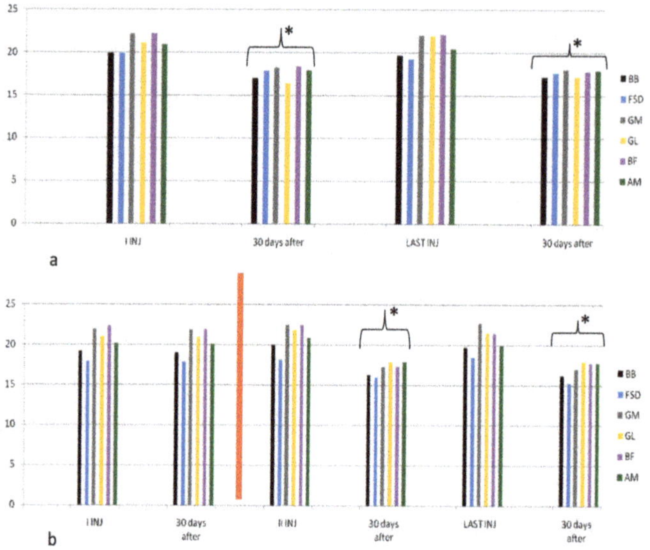

Figure 3. Myometric muscles tone evaluation in group B. This figure shows a statistically significant reduction in muscle tone after 30 days from the first and from the last injection in 32 patients treated with dosage from 400 UI to 700 UI (**a**); For 8 patients of this group, muscle tone reduction was lower in the first and second cycle of injections; when we increased dosage (up to 1000 UI, red line) due to increased units for each muscle (rather than having injected other muscles), reduction was statistically significant after 30 days for each cycle of injection (**b**). * $p < 0.05$. BF = Biceps Femoris, AM = Adductor Magnus.

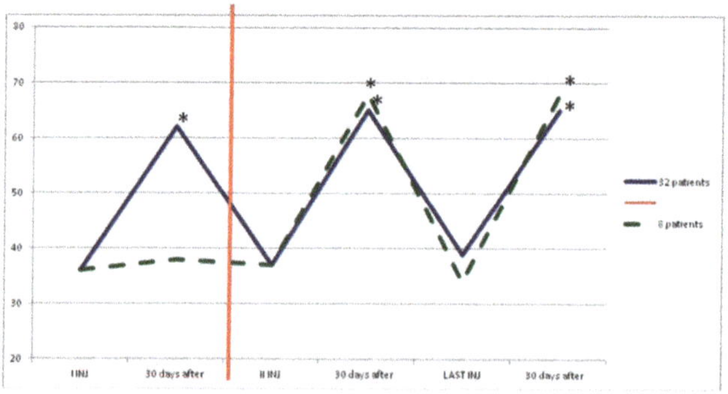

Figure 4. FIM value in group B. The dark blue line shows statistical improvement of FIM in 32 patients treated with dosage up to 700 UI. Instead, the green and dashed line shows a statistical improvement of FIM in other 10 patients of this group when we increased dosage (up to 1000 UI, red line) due to increased units for each muscle or having injected other muscles. * $p < 0.05$.

In the group C, average doses at the end of study were statistically significant compared to the beginning (from 775.65 ± 30.45 to 986.65 ± 13.67, p <0.05). During the study all patients improved their clinical and instrumental measurement of spasticity (Figures 5 and 6).

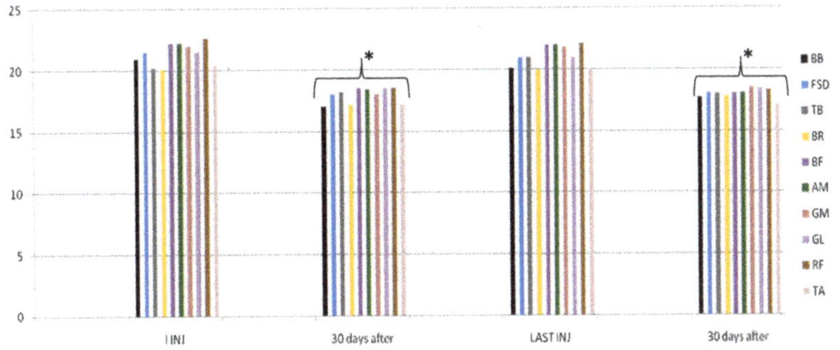

Figure 5. Myometric muscle tone evaluation in group C. In each cycle of treatment, a statistically significant reduction in muscle tone after 30 days from injection was found; this figure shows data of first and last cycle of treatment. * $p < 0.05$. TB = Triceps Brachii, BR = Brachioradialis, RF = Rectus Femoris, TA = Tibialis Anterior.

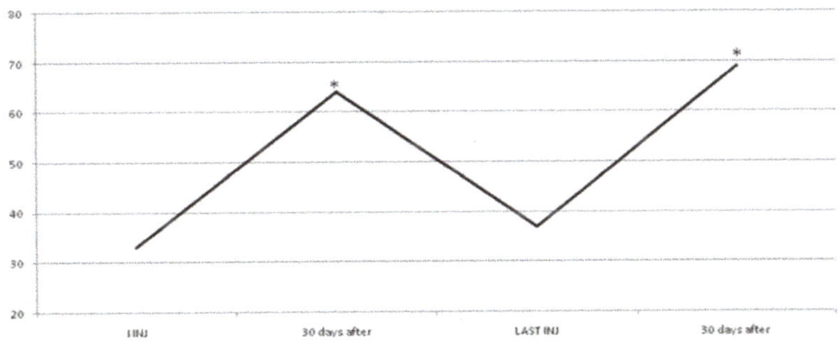

Figure 6. FIM value in group C. FIM value in all 50 patients treated with dosage from 700 UI to 1000 UI showed a statistically significant improvement (* $p < 0.05$). This figure shows values of first and last cycle of treatment.

Adverse Events

We found a good safety profile for long-term use of Incobotulinumtoxin A, also in patients treated with dosage up to 1000 UI. The adverse events reported were rare (Table 2).

Considering all injection sessions, only four cases (3.3%) of excessive local muscle weakness were found, two cases (1.6%) of transient generalized weakness lasting 20 and 10 days respectively and only one case of mild dysphagia (0.8%). More specifically:

- local muscle weakness: no case in group A, two cases in group B (5%) and two cases in group C (4%);
- transient generalized weakness: no cases in group A and B, two cases in group C (4%);
- mild dysphagia: no case in group A and B, one case in group C (2%; in the first cycle of injection, we also treated in this patient the left sternocleidomastoid muscle with 50 U of IncobotulinumtoxinA 1% saline due to muscle dystonia; this probably caused an adverse event because in the second cycle we treated the same muscle with 35 U of drug with good clinical response of dystonia and no dysphagia).

No patients abandoned treatment over the study.

Table 2. Summary of adverse events in each group. AE were rare and transient.

	1°GR 100–400 U BTX A	2°GR 400–700 U BTX A	3°GR 700–1000 U BTX A
Local muscle weakness	-	5%	4%
Transientgeneralized weakness	-	-	4%
Bradycardia	-	-	-
Dysphagia	-	-	2%
Dysphonia	-	-	-
Dyspnea	-	-	-
Constipation	-	-	-

3. Discussion

This study demonstrated long term treatment efficacy of IncobotulinumtoxinA in the management of muscle spasticity using variable doses.

According to the severity of spasticity, clinically and instrumentally evaluated, and to the number of muscles treated, we injected different botulinum toxin A doses measuring spasticity improvement after each injection cycle. In 10 of 30 patients in group A and 8 of 40 patients in group B, the dose administered was increased after the third and first injection respectively due to a non-significant clinical and instrumental effect; in group A, we increased units for each muscle or we increased number of muscles treated; in group B, we only increased units for each muscle. Different studies demonstrated that improper injection techniques or a denatured toxin resulted in therapeutic failure [13–15]. In the 18 patients of our study, injection technique or toxin A reconstitution were the same as the other patients, so therapeutic failure was due to incorrect dosage or clinical evaluation of the patient. After the total units administered were changed, spasticity improved after each injection in all of the 18 patients.

Changing dosage and using higher doses than approved is possible following a ratio known as Therapeutic Index (TI) or Therapeutic Ratio (TR) [16]. In clinical practice, the TI is the range of doses at which a medication appears to be effective in clinical trials for a median of participants without unacceptable adverse events. For most drugs, this range is wide enough, and the maximum concentration of the drug and the area under the concentration–time curve achieved when the recommended doses of a drug are prescribed lies sufficiently above the minimum therapeutic concentration and sufficiently below the toxic concentration [17]. Thus, it can be expected that at the recommended prescribed doses, drugs present clinical efficacy with an adequate safety margin. A higher TI means a safer drug. A drug is generally considered having a good safety profile if its TI exceeds the value of 10 [16,18]. Patients with multifocal spasticity require higher total doses of botulinum toxin A and several studies have demonstrated IncobotulinumtoxinA having a high TI. With escalating total doses, a higher number of spasticity patterns were successfully treated, leading to increasing improvements in muscle tone, shown by consistent decreases in clinical and instrumental evaluation. In this study, the use of doses from 100 to 1000 UI demonstrate that IncobotulinumtoxinA has a wide therapeutic window, indicating the drug has a good safety profile, since, even at high doses [13] side effects were mild and transient.

In this study we used myometric evaluation (Myoton PRO®) to objectively assess muscle tone. In an objective, simple, repeatable and non-invasive way, we evaluated even minimum changes in muscle tone; we obtained a broader pathophysiological vision of rheological properties of muscle tissue in different neurological, orthopedic, and sports pathologies [19]. In fact, during any pharmacological and/or physiokinesis and/or instrumental spasticity treatment, we studied therapeutic efficacy and we monitored the desired clinical effects without any alterations either in the omolateral antagonist muscles or in the contralateral agonists and antagonist muscles [20]. For example, wrist and finger control is very compromised after stroke; evaluating properties of the muscles responsible for these functions can help the physiatrist to realize the severity of the disability that the patient is encountering [21]. Instead, evaluation of triceps muscle tone may provide useful indications of load and balance alterations while standing and walking, with consequent repercussions on the entire musculoskeletal system [22,23].

In daily clinical practice, a number of organizational and methodological aspects must always be taken into account when planning a treatment strategy that includes the administration of botulinum toxin A [24]. These aspects include goals and treatment methods, clinical evaluation methods (MAS, myometry, FIM) injection programs (injecting muscles, injection technique, number of injection site for muscle, dose, and dilution), and other therapies (including targeted rehabilitation programs) to be integrated into the therapeutic plan [24,25]. Muscle weakness in the limbs and paresis is associated with spasticity and contributes to loss of motor dexterity and functional capacity. Spasticity, if untreated, can hinder the functional result by promoting persistent abnormal postures which produce muscular-tendon contractions and bone deformities [26]. Moreover, spasticity complications include movement impairment, difficulty in managing hygiene and self-care, poor self-esteem, body image alteration, pain, and pressure ulcers [26,27].

This study highlights the safety of high dose treatment with IncobotulinumtoxinA [28]. Few (less than 5%) and of no clinical relevance were the adverse events found. With different and high doses particularly, we obtained a safe and effective treatment for patients with chronic upper and lower limb spasticity following brain injury; using doses above 400 U enables treating a greater number of muscles and clinical spasticity patterns, resulting in increased improvements of muscle tone, goal attainment, and global efficacy, without compromising patients' safety or tolerability [13,28]. High IncobotulinumtoxinA dosage offers the potential for comprehensive, well-tolerated and effective spasticity treatment of more clinical patterns, which allows greater focus on patients' needs and goals with respect to lower doses in chronic spasticity [14,15,29].

Finally, our study also shows that repeated and long-term treatment (two years) with IncobotulinumtoxinA does not lead to any reduction in clinical efficacy due to antibodies forming against the active substance and/or excipients of the pharmacological preparation [30]. In fact, the possible development of botulinum toxin A antibodies related to injection frequency and dosage is a source of variability for possible adverse events [24]. In this study, several sets of high dose toxin exclude the adverse events and the development of antibodies against the toxin stimulated by higher doses. Certainly, using a highly purified botulinum toxin A formulation (IncobotulinumtoxinA), free from complexing proteins, is associated with a relatively low risk of immunogenicity and represents a therapeutic advantage for a long-term treatment with higher doses [13–15,29,30].

4. Conclusions

Botulinum toxin chemo-denervation has become popular because it is effective due to its local selectivity and its effects are repeatable and safe without important adverse events or the development of antibodies. To perform and optimize the treatment, an accurate clinical and instrumental evaluation of spasticity is needed to determine how this symptom is invalidating and to choose the best doses, muscles, and times of injection in each patient. Considering larger Therapeutic Index and Therapeutic Window (from 100 to 1000 UI) of IncobotulinumtoxinA, we can better modulate spasticity by considering its clinical significance for each patient. Therefore, we could introduce the concept of an "appropriate treatment" instead of a "standard or high dosage treatment"; this allows us to underline the actual clinical needs of each patient.

5. Materials and Methods

This was a retrospective observational study lasting two years. One hundred and twenty adult patients (Table 1) with spasticity due to ischemic/hemorrhagic stroke, multiple sclerosis, spinal cord injuries, traumatic brain injury, and other cerebrovascular disorders were recruited. All subjects gave their informed consent for inclusion before participating in the study. The study was conducted in accordance with the Declaration of Helsinki, and the protocol number of the Ethics Committee was 5590. All patients signed the informed consent form. Exclusion criteria were: age above 80 or below 18, muscle fibrosis/tendon retraction detected by ultrasound, concomitant treatment with other muscle relaxants, peripheral myopathy/neuropathy, cognitive deterioration (Mini-Mental State Examination $\geq$ 24) and positive history of allergy to the drug.

5.1. Study Design

Patients were initially divided into three groups (data homogeneity are in Table 3) according to the botulinum toxin A dosage used at the beginning of study (IncobotulinumtoxinA, Xeomin®, Merz Pharma, 100 U/mL in normal saline):

(1) Group A (30 patients) up to 400 U
(2) Group B (40 patients) from 400 U to 700 U
(3) Group C (50 patients) from 700 U to 1000 U (maximum dose 600 U per limb).

The doses were chosen depending on the severity of spasticity clinically evaluated and on the number of muscles treated.

Table 3. Patient demographics and baseline characteristics in the three groups; data demonstrate homogeneity of the samples.

	GR A 100–400 U BTX A	GR B 400–700 U BTX A	GR C 700–1000 U BTX A
N° patients	30	40	50
Age	64 ± 6.2	63 ± 8.4	66 ± 3.2
Sex M/F	17/13	23/17	28/22
Clinical: Hemip.dx	4	8	5
Hemip. sx	13	14	22
Monoparesis	4	1	0
Paraparesis	8	6	7
Tetraparesis	1	11	16

Treated muscles were Biceps Brachii, Brachioradialis, Triceps Brachii, Superficial FlexorumDigitorum, Ulnar FlexorumCarpis and Opponenspollicis for upper limb, Rectus Femoris, Biceps FemorisAdductor Magnus, Tibialis Anterior, Flexor Hallucis Longus, Gastrocnemius Medialis and Lateralis, Soleus, Tibialis Posterior and Flexor Digitorum for lower limb, with different average dosage (see Tables 4 and 5).

Table 4. This table shows how many patients of each group had a specific muscle treated and its percentage. In the first group, soleus was injected in 100% of patients; in the second group, the most treated muscle was biceps brachii, while in the third one they were triceps surae muscles.

Muscles Treated	GR A 100–400 U N° Patients	GR B 400–700 U N° Patients	GR C 700–1000 U N° Patients
Biceps brachii	28 93.3%	40 100%	43 86%
Brachioradialis	-	32 80%	41 82%
Triceps brachii	-	1 2.5%	38 76%
Superficial flexorumdigitorum	26 86.6%	34 85%	43 86%
Ulnar flexorumcarpis	-	22 55%	41 82%

Table 4. *Cont.*

Muscles Treated	GR A 100–400 U N° Patients	GR B 400–700 U N° Patients	GR C 700–1000 U N° Patients
Opponens pollicis	-	34 85%	43 86%
Rectus femoris	-	-	40 80%
Adductor magnus	-	26 65%	38 76%
Tibialis anterior	-	-	16 32%
Flexor alluci longus	-	18 45%	34 68%
Gastrocnemius medialis	27 90%	39 97.5%	50 100%
Gastrocnemius lateralis	27 90%	39 97.5%	50 100%
Soleus	30 100%	39 97.5%	50 100%
Tibialis posterior	-	26 65%	45 90%
Flexor digitorum brevis	-	16 40%	36 72%
Biceps Femoris	-	26 65%	36 72%

Table 5. Minimum, Maximum, Average ± SD dosage of each muscle in the three groups at the beginning of the study. In the first group, soleus received the highest dose compared to the other muscles (average 73.3 ± 2.5 UI). In the second group, muscles with highest doses were biceps brachii, superficial flexorum digitorum, gastrocnemius medialis, gastrocnemius lateralis, soleus, and tibialis posterior. In the third group, muscles with high doses were adductor magnus and those listed in the previous group.

Muscles	GR A 100–400 U Min-Max (Average ± SD)	GR B 400–700 U Min-Max (Average ± SD)	GR C 700–1000 U Min-Max (Average ± SD)
Biceps brachii	50–80 (60.2 ± 10.3)	70–90 (82.3 ± 10.1)	80–100 (91.2 ± 10.1)
Brachioradialis		50–60 (55.5 ± 10.4)	70–80 (75.3 ± 2.2)
Triceps brachii		50–60 (55.2 ± 10.1)	80–90 (85.6 ± 2.2)
Superficial flexorumdigitorum	50–80 (60.6 ± 10.2)	50–90 (75.3 ± 10.3)	100–150 (122.3 ± 20.1)
Ulnar flexorumcarpis		50–60 (55.5 ± 2.2)	80–100 (85.6 ± 2.1)
Opponenspollicis		20–30 (22.2 ± 10.3)	30–40 (33.4 ± 1.1)
Rectus femoris			70–80 (74.2 ± 1.1)
Adductor magnus		50–60 (55.3 ± 10.2)	100–150 (132.3 ± 20.2)
Tibialis anterior			50–60 (55.3 ± 2.4)
Flexor alluci longus		40–50 (44.2 ± 3.3)	50–60 (54.2 ± 1.3)
Gastrocnemius medialis	60–80 (73.4 ± 10.5)	80	100–150 (132.4 ± 10.4)
Gastrocnemius lateralis	60–80 (72.5 ± 10.4)	80	100–150 (122.4 ± 11.6)
Soleus	70–80 (76.3 ± 2.5)	80–90 (88.3 ± 1.3)	100–150 (135.7 ± 17.4)
Tibialis posterior		70–80(84.9 ± 3.3)	100–120 (111.2 ± 2.4)
Flexor digitorum brevis		50–60 (55.6 ± 3.4)	80–100 (89.9 ± 5.6)
Biceps Femoris		70–90 (84.6 ± 9.7)	100–150 (145.7 ± 14.9)

During the study, patients received rehabilitation (stretching of injected muscles, active and passive limb mobilization, walking training, and global muscle strengthening) daily for the first 30 days after injection, then followed by three days a week until the next injection.

5.2. Outcome Measures

The evaluation method applied included the Functional Independence Measure (FIM, an international standard of disability measurement that differentiates motor from cognitive impairment; in our study we considered only motor impairment [31,32]) and myometric measurement (MyotonPRO®, tool that determines an objective value of muscle tone, elasticity and stiffness); furthermore, we took into consideration (muscle) tone values of superficial muscles [33,34]).

All assessments for each patient were performed at recruitment (during the 1st injection session), at every injection session, and during follow ups (one month after each session).

5.3. Statistical Analysis

Statistical analysis was carried out using the IBM SPSS Statistics program for Windows. Myometric measurements were analyzed with TWO WAY ANOVA method while FIM measurements with the t-student test. The alpha level for significance was set at $p < 0.05$. Data are expressed as average. In group A and group B we considered two patient subgroups according to dosage used at the beginning and the end of study.

Acknowledgments: We did not receive sources of funding, grants or funds for covering the costs to publish in open access.

Author Contributions: Giancarlo Ianieri and Riccardo Marvulli conceived and designed the experiments; Riccardo Marvulli and Giulia Alessia Gallo performed the experiments; Giancarlo Ianieri, Marisa Megna, Pietro Fiore analyzed the data; all the authors wrote the paper.

Conflicts of Interest: The authors declare no conflict of interest.

References

1. Jost, W.H.; Hefter, H.; Reissig, A.; Kollewe, K.; Wissel, J. Efficacy and safety of botulinum toxin type A (Dysport) for the treatment of post-stroke arm spasticity: Results of the German-Austrian open-label post-marketing surveillance prospective study. *J. Neurol. Sci.* **2014**, *337*, 86–90. [CrossRef] [PubMed]
2. Hefter, H.; Jost, W.H.; Reissig, A.; Zakine, B.; Bakheit, A.M.; Wissel, J. Classification of posture in poststroke upper limb spasticity: A potential decision tool for botulinum toxin A treatment? *Int. J. Rehabil. Res.* **2012**, *35*, 227–233. [CrossRef] [PubMed]
3. Simpson, D.M.; Gracies, J.M.; Graham, H.K.; Miyasaki, J.M.; Naumann, M.; Russman, B.; Simpson, L.L.; So, Y. Therapeutics and Technology Assessment Subcommittee of the American Academy of Neurology. Assessment: Botulinum neurotoxin for the treatment of spasticity (an evidence-based review): Report of the Therapeutics and Technology Assessment Subcommittee of the American Academy of Neurology. *Neurology* **2008**, *70*, 1691–1698. [CrossRef] [PubMed]
4. Simpson, D.M.; Hallett, M.; Ashman, E.J.; Comella, C.L.; Green, M.W.; Gronseth, G.S.; Armstrong, M.J.; Gloss, D.; Potrebic, S.; Jankovic, J.; et al. Practice guideline update summary: Botulinum neurotoxin for the treatment of blepharospasm, cervical dystonia, adult spasticity, and headache: Report of the Guideline Development Subcommittee of the American Academy of Neurology. *Neurology* **2016**, *86*, 1818–1826. [CrossRef] [PubMed]
5. Royal College of Physicians, British Society of Rehabilitation Medicine. Chartered Society of Physiotherapy, Association of Chartered Physiotherapists Interested in Neurology. Spasticity in Adults: Management Using Botulinum Toxin: National Guidelines. Available online: www.rcplondon.ac.uk/sites/default/files/documents/spasticity-in-adults-management-botulinum-toxin.pdf (accessed on 1 January 2016).
6. Kocabas, H.; Salli, A.; Demir, A.H.; Ozerbil, O.M. Comparison of phenol and alcohol neurolysis of tibial nerve motor branches to the gastrocnemius muscle for treatment of spastic foot after stroke: A randomized controlled pilot study. *Eur. J. Phys. Rehabil. Med.* **2010**, *46*, 5–10. [PubMed]
7. Bensmail, D.; Hanschmann, A.; Wissel, J. Satisfaction with botulinum toxin treatment in post-stroke spasticity: Results from two cross-sectional surveys (patients and physicians). *J. Med. Econ.* **2014**, *17*, 618–625. [CrossRef] [PubMed]

8. Yang, D.J.; Park, S.K.; Uhm, Y.H.; Park, S.H.; Chun, D.W.; Kim, J.H. The correlation between muscle activity of the quadriceps and balance and gait in stroke patients. *J. Phys. Ther. Sci.* **2016**, *28*, 2289–2292. [CrossRef] [PubMed]
9. Mohammad, H.; Shahram, A.; Seyed, A.H. Validity of Modified Ashworth Scale as a Measure of Wrist Spasticity in Stroke Patients. *Iran. Rehabil. J.* **2011**, *9*, 26–30.
10. Fleuren, J.F.; Voerman, G.E.; Erren-Wolters, C.V.; Snoek, G.J.; Rietman, J.S.; Hermens, H.J.; Nene, A.V. Stop using the Ashworth Scale for the assessment of spasticity. *J. Neurol. Neurosurg. Psychiatry* **2010**, *81*, 46–52. [CrossRef] [PubMed]
11. Von Werder, S.C.; Disselhorst-Klug, C. The role of biceps brachii and brachioradialis for the control of elbow flexion and extension movements. *J. Electromyogr. Kinesiol.* **2016**, *28*, 67–75. [CrossRef] [PubMed]
12. Van Deun, B.; Hobbelen, J.S.; Cagnie, B.; Van Eetvelde, B.; Van Den Noortgate, N.; Cambier, D. Reproducible Measurements of Muscle Characteristics Using the MyotonPRO Device: Comparison Between Individuals with and without Paratonia. *J. Geriatr. Phys. Ther.* **2016**. [CrossRef] [PubMed]
13. Wissel, J.; Bensmail, D.; Ferreira, J.J.; Molteni, F.; Satkunam, L.; Moraleda, S.; Rekand, T.; McGuire, J.; Scheschonka, A.; Flatau-Baqué, B.; et al. Safety and efficacy of incobotulinumtoxinA doses up to 800 U in limb spasticity: The TOWER study. *Neurology* **2017**, *88*, 1321–1328. [CrossRef] [PubMed]
14. Merz Pharma UK Ltd. XEOMIN® 100 U Summary of Product Characteristics. Available online: www.medicines.org.uk/emc/medicine/20666 (accessed on 6 January 2016).
15. Merz Pharmaceuticals, LLC. Xeomin® US Prescribing Information. Available online: www.xeomin.com/wp-content/uploads/xeomin-full-prescribing-information.pdf (accessed on 6 January 2016).
16. Tamargo, J.; Le Heuzey, J.Y.; Mabo, P. Narrow therapeutic index drugs: A clinical pharmacological consideration to flecainide. *Eur. J. Clin. Pharmacol.* **2015**, *71*, 549–567. [CrossRef] [PubMed]
17. Reiffel, J.A. Formulation substitution and other pharmacokinetic variability: Underappreciated variables affecting antiarrhythmic efficacy and safety in clinical practice. *Am. J. Cardiol.* **2000**, *85*, 46D–52D. [CrossRef]
18. Reiffel, J.A. Issues in the use of generic antiarrhythmic drugs. *Curr. Opin. Cardiol.* **2001**, *16*, 23–29. [CrossRef] [PubMed]
19. Ianieri, G.; Saggini, R.; Marvulli, R.; Tondi, G.; Aprile, A.; Ranieri, M.; Benedetto, G.; Altini, S.; Lancioni, G.E.; Goffredo, L.; et al. New approach in the assessment of the tone, elasticity and the muscular resistance: Nominal scales vs MYOTON. *Int. J. Immunopathol. Pharmacol.* **2009**, *22* (Suppl. 3), 21–24. [CrossRef] [PubMed]
20. Marvulli, R.; Megna, M.; Romanelli, E.; Mastromauro, L.; Conte, E.; Lancioni, G.; Dargenio, M.; De Venuto, G.; Gallo, G.A.; Lerario, R.; et al. Effectiveness of the Treatment with Botulinum Toxin Type A (BTX-A) in the Management of the Spasticity in Patients with Amyotrophic Lateral Sclerosis (ALS). *Clin. Immunol. Endocr. Metab. Drugs* **2016**, *3*. [CrossRef]
21. Marvulli, R.; Mastromauro, L.; Romanelli, E.; Lopopolo, A.; Dargenio, M.; Fornarelli, F.; Conte, E.; Fiore, P.; Megna, M.; Ianieri, G. How Botulinum Toxin Type A—Occupational Therapy (OT)-Functional Electrical Stimulation (FES) Modify Spasticity and Functional Recovery in Patients with Upper Limb Spasticity Post Stroke. *Clin. Immunol. Endocr. Metab. Drugs* **2016**, *3*, 62–67. [CrossRef]
22. Munari, D.; Pedrinolla, A.; Smania, N.; Picelli, A.; Gandolfi, M.; Saltuari, L.; Schena, F. High-intensity treadmill training improves gait ability, VO2peak and cost of walking in stroke survivors: Preliminary results of a pilot randomized controlled trial. *Eur. J. Phys. Rehabil. Med.* **2016**. Epub ahead of print. Available online: https://www.minervamedica.it/en/journals/europa-medicophysica/article.php?cod=R33Y9999N00A16083004 (accessed on 27 March 2018).
23. Picelli, A.; Bacciga, M.; Melotti, C.; LA Marchina, E.; Verzini, E.; Ferrari, F.; Pontillo, A.; Corradi, J.; Tamburin, S.; Saltuari, L.; et al. Combined effects of robot-assisted gait training and botulinum toxin type A on spastic equinus foot in patients with chronic stroke: A pilot, single blind, randomized controlled trial. *Eur. J. Phys. Rehabil. Med.* **2016**, *52*, 759–766. [PubMed]
24. Demetrios, M.; Khan, F.; Turner-Stokes, L.; Brand, C.; McSweeney, S. Multidisciplinary rehabilitation following botulinum toxin and other focal intramuscular treatment for post-stroke spasticity. *Cochrane Database Syst. Rev.* **2013**, *6*, CD009689. [CrossRef] [PubMed]

25. Picelli, A.; Tamburin, S.; Cavazza, S.; Scampoli, C.; Manca, M.; Cosma, M.; Berto, G.; Vallies, G.; Roncari, L.; Melotti, C.; et al. Relationship between ultrasonographic, electromyographic, and clinical parameters in adult stroke patients with spastic equinus: An observational study. *Arch. Phys. Med. Rehabil.* **2014**, *95*, 1564–1570. [CrossRef] [PubMed]
26. Synnot, A.; Chau, M.; Pitt, V.; O'Connor, D.; Gruen, R.L.; Wasiak, J.; Clavisi, O.; Pattuwage, L.; Phillips, K. Interventions for managing skeletal muscle spasticity following traumatic brain injury. *Cochrane Database Syst. Rev.* **2017**, *11*, CD008929. [CrossRef] [PubMed]
27. Gao, F.; Grant, T.H.; Roth, E.J.; Zhang, L.Q. Changes in passive mechanical properties of the gastrocnemius muscle at the muscle fascicle and joint levels in stroke survivors. *Arch. Phys. Med. Rehabil.* **2009**, *90*, 819–826. [CrossRef] [PubMed]
28. Dressler, D.; Saberi, F.A.; Kollewe, K.; Schrader, C. Safety aspects of incobotulinumtoxinA high-dose therapy. *J. Neural Transm.* **2015**, *122*, 327–333. [CrossRef] [PubMed]
29. Fabbri, M.; Leodori, G.; Fernandes, R.M.; Bhidayasiri, R.; Marti, M.J.; Colosimo, C.; Ferreira, J.J. Neutralizing Antibody and Botulinum Toxin Therapy: A Systematic Review and Meta-analysis. *Neurotox. Res.* **2016**, *29*, 105–117. [CrossRef] [PubMed]
30. Dressler, D. Five-year experience with incobotulinumtoxinA (Xeomin®): The first botulinum toxin drug free of complexing proteins. *Eur. J. Neurol.* **2012**, *19*, 385–389. [CrossRef] [PubMed]
31. Velozo, C.A.; Seel, R.T.; Magasi, S.; Heinemann, A.W.; Romero, S. Improving measurement methods in rehabilitation: Core concepts and recommendations for scale development. *Arch. Phys. Med. Rehabil.* **2012**, *93* (Suppl. 8), S154–S163. [CrossRef] [PubMed]
32. Gerrard, P.; Goldstein, R.; Divita, M.A.; Ryan, C.M.; Mix, J.; Niewczyk, P.; Kazis, L.; Kowalske, K.; Zafonte, R.; Schneider, J.C. Validity and reliability of the FIM instrument in the inpatient burn rehabilitation population. *Arch. Phys. Med. Rehabil.* **2013**, *94*, 1521–1526.e4. [CrossRef] [PubMed]
33. Lo, W.L.A.; Zhao, J.L.; Li, L.; Mao, Y.R.; Huang, D.F. Relative and Absolute Interrater Reliabilities of a Hand-Held Myotonometer to Quantify Mechanical Muscle Properties in Patients with Acute Stroke in an Inpatient Ward. *Biomed. Res. Int.* **2017**. [CrossRef] [PubMed]
34. Jarocka, E.; Marusiak, J.; Kumorek, M.; Jaskólska, A.; Jaskólski, A. Muscle stiffness at different force levels measured with two myotonometric devices. *Physiol. Meas.* **2012**, *33*, 65–78. [CrossRef] [PubMed]

toxins

MDPI

Review

Botulinum Toxin in the Field of Dermatology: Novel Indications

Yoon Seob Kim, Eun Sun Hong and Hei Sung Kim *

Department of Dermatology, Incheon St. Mary's Hospital, College of Medicine, The Catholic University of Korea, Seoul 06591, Korea; kysbbubbu@hotmail.com (Y.S.K.); dmsun99@gmail.com (E.S.H.)

* Correspondence: hazelkimhoho@gmail.com; Tel.: +82-32-280-5105; Fax: +82-32-506-9514

Academic Editor: Siro Luvisetto

Received: 20 November 2017; Accepted: 14 December 2017; Published: 16 December 2017

Abstract: Since its approval by the US Food and Drug Administration in 2002 for glabellar wrinkles, botulinum toxin (BTX) has been widely used to correct facial wrinkles. As a result, many consider BTX synonymous with cosmetic dermatology. Recent studies indicate that BTX elicits biological effects on various skin cell types via the modulation of neurotransmitter release, and it seems that BTX has a wider zone of dermatologic influence than originally understood. Clinicians and researchers are now beginning to explore the potential of BTX beyond the amelioration of facial lines and encouraging results are seen with BTX in a variety of skin conditions. In this paper, we review novel dermatological indications of BTX which includes (but not limited to) scar prevention, facial flushing, post-herpetic neuralgia and itch. These areas show great promise, but there is definite need for larger, double-blinded, randomized control trials against established treatments before BTX becomes a clinical reality.

Keywords: botulinum toxin; biological effect; various cell types; neurotransmitter; dermatology; novel indication

---

1. Introduction

Botulinum toxin (BTX) is a potent neurotoxin produced by the bacterium *Clostridium botulinum*. Seven distinct isoforms (BTX-A, B, C, D, E, F, and G) have been described, with BTX-A and BTX-B being commercially available. BTX blocks the release of acetylcholine and a number of other neurotransmitters from presynaptic vesicles by deactivating SNARE proteins and has a long history of therapeutic application in neurological conditions with a strong efficacy and safety profile. As widely known, the skin interacts with the nervous system and there is increasing evidence that the neurological system directly participates in cutaneous inflammation and wound healing [1,2]. With that said, BTX has been used experimentally in a number of dermatological conditions which include scar prevention, facial flushing, post-herpetic neuralgia and itch with good results. The general mechanism which underlies these novel indications includes suppression of mast cell activity, and the inhibition of substance P, calcitonin gene-related peptide (CGRP) and glutamate release. In this review, we analyze the possible off-label applications of BTX based on published data.

2. Off-Label Use of BTX in Dermatology

2.1. BTX in Hypertrophic Scar Treatment

Scars are defined as marks that remain after the healing of a wound. They cause significant cosmetic concern, especially when located on conspicuous areas such as the head and neck.

Hypertrophic scars and keloids represent an aberrant response to the wound healing process and are characterized by dysregulated growth and excessive collagen formation [3].

BTX has been reported as a treatment measure for hypertrophic scars and keloids in a number of studies [4–7] (Table 1). In one study [4], BTX injection (2.5 IU/cm^3) was performed once a month for three months, leading to a significant decrease in erythema, itching, and pliability of the scar. In another study [7], 12 keloid patients received BTX injection (70–140 IU per session, every 3 months for a maximum of 9 months) and achieved more than 50% improvement in symptoms, size, height, and induration of the scar. In a randomized controlled trial (RCT) [5], the efficacy of BTX (5 IU/cm^3, 3 sessions, repeated every 8 weeks) was compared with that of steroid injection (triamcinolone, kenacort 10 mg/cc, 6 sessions, repeated every 4 weeks) in keloids, where BTX led to a more significant reduction of subjective complaints (itch and pain of the scar).

The molecular mechanism of BTX on hypertrophic scars and keloids is not yet perfectly explained, but BTX has been shown to inhibit the proliferation of fibroblasts derived from hypertrophic scar tissues. In addition, BTX is reported to suppress the expression of transforming growth factor (TGF)-β1, collagen I and III, α-smooth muscle actin and myosin II protein in keloid fibroblasts [8–11].

One particularly favorable aspect of BTX is its ability to control the subjective symptoms of hypertrophic scars. BTX can immobilize the local muscles of a scar and reduce skin tension caused by the muscle pull [12]. This relieves trapped nerve fibers in keloids, neutralizing the itch and pain associated with small-fiber neuropathy [13]. Another advantage of BTX is the absence of skin atrophy and telangiectasia which is often seen after steroid injection.

The limitations of BTX on hypertrophic scars and keloids would be the high cost of the drug (with the dosages mentioned in prior studies) and its potential effect on the surrounding muscles. Due to these limitations, many suggest the use of BTX as an adjuvant rather than first line treatment for hypertrophic scars.

2.2. *BTX in Scar Prevention*

Nowadays, many acknowledge the role of active scar prevention important in post-operative scar management. A key factor that determines the final cosmetic appearance of a surgical scar is the tension that acts on the wound edges during the healing phase [14,15]. By blocking acetylcholine neurotransmitter release from peripheral nerves, BTX allows near-complete elimination of dynamic muscle tension on the healing wound. The tension relieving properties, together with the direct inhibitory effects of BTX on fibroblasts and TGF-β1 expression support its usage in surgical scar prevention [16–18]. The anti-inflammatory effect of BTX and its action of the cutaneous vasculature calms down the inflammatory phase (immediate to 2–5 days) of the wound healing process which may also contribute to scar prevention.

A number of studies have reported the effectiveness of BTX in scar prevention [19–22] (Table 2). In a split-scar RCT [19], the safety and efficacy of early postoperative BTX injection was assessed in 15 thyroidectomy scar patients. A single treatment with either BTX (20–65 IU) or 0.9% saline (control) was applied to fresh scars (within 10 days of thyroidectomy), where the BTX-treated halves showed a significantly better outcome in terms of scar scales and patient satisfaction compared to the saline treated sides. In 2006, Gassner [21] tested whether postoperative injection of BTX improved facial scars following forehead lacerations and excisions. BTX (15–45 IU) was injected to post-op scars within 24 h after wound closure to produce enhanced wound healing and improved cosmesis compared to placebo (normal saline) injection.

BTX is best used for op scars. It would be optimal to inject BTX intraoperatively or shortly (preferably within days) after the surgery. To note, BTX should be avoided in open wounds as it delays wound closure.

Table 1. Representative studies of botulinum toxin (BTX) in hypertrophic scar treatment.

First Author [Ref.], Year	Type of Study	*n*	Treatment Regimen	Outcome Measures	Follow-Up	Results (Including Adverse Effects)
Elhefnawy [4], 2016	Prospective, single arm (BTX)	20	BTX once a month for 3 months. BTX concentration: 5 IU/0.1 mL; Injected dose: 2.5 IU/cm^3, not exceeding 100 IU/session	Overall assessment made by the patient and physician (5-point scale). Lesions were assessed for erythema, itching, and pliability; each item was assessed on a 5-point scale	6 months	Therapeutic satisfaction was "good" in 14 patients, "excellent" in 6; The mean erythema score decreased from 3.2 to 1.0, mean pliability score from 3.3 to 0.8 and the mean itching score from 2.7 to 0.7; All findings were statistically significant. No recurrence or complications.
Shaarawy [5], 2015	Randomized, double-blinded, comparative study (BTX vs. IL steroid injection)	24	Group A (12 patients; Triamcinolone, Kenacort® 10 mg/cc; repeated every 4 weeks for 6 sessions/or till complete remission) Group B (12 patients; BTX 5 IU/cm^3 repeated every 8 weeks for three sessions/or till complete remission of keloid)	Objective parameters (hardness, elevation, and redness) and subjective complaints (itching, pain and tenderness) on a scale of 0–3; Volume of keloid; Patient satisfaction (3-point scale)	7 months	Significant decrease in scar volume after treatment with a volume reduction of 82.7% (group A) and 79.2% (group B). Significant softening, significant decrease in height and significant decrease in redness with little difference between the groups. All patients mentioned a significant reduction of their subjective complaints which was more prominent in group B (BTX group). Skin atrophy and telangiectasia was evident in 3 patients of group A.
Xiao [6], 2009	Prospective, single arm (BTX)	19	BTX once a month for a total of 3 months. BTX injection dose: 2.5 IU/cm^3, not exceeding 100 IU/session.	Physician and patient satisfaction (5-point scale); Clinical symptoms in terms of erythema, pliability and itching sensation (each graded on a 5-point scale)	6 months	Patient satisfaction: good (63.1%), excellent (36.8%) Physician satisfaction: good (78.9%), excellent (10.5%) Mean erythema score decreased from 3.41 to 1.23; The pliability score decreased from 3.85 to 0.78; and the itching score decreased from 3.50 to 0.83. All reductions were statistically significant. Besides the injection pain, no other complication was detected in this study.
Zhibo [7], 2009	Prospective, single arm (BTX)	12	BTX at 3 months interval for a maximum of 9 months. BTX concentration: 35 IU/mL; injected dose: 70–140 IU/session	Improvement was judged based on a decrease in size and flattening of the lesion with a 5-point scale; Patient satisfaction	1 year	Therapeutic outcome: excellent (25%), good (41.7%), fair (33.3%). The level of patient satisfaction was very high. There were no serious adverse sequelae.

BTX: Onabotulinum toxin unless otherwise stated, IL: intra-lesional.

Table 2. Representative studies of BTX in scar prevention.

First Author [Ref.], Year	Type of Study	*n*	Treatment Regimen	Outcome Measures	Follow-Up	Results (Including Adverse Effects)
Kim [19], 2014	A split-scar, double-blind, RCT (BTX vs. saline)	15	Treatment with either BTX or 0.9% normal saline on scar halves. A single treatment delivered within 10 days of thyroidectomy. BTX concentration: 5 IU/mL; Injection dose: 20–65 IU	Modified Stony Brook Scar Evaluation Scale (SBSES) Patient satisfaction (4-point scale)	6 months	A significant improvement in SBSES score was noted for the BTX-treated halves ($p < 0.001$), with minimal change on the saline-treated side. The mean calculated difference in SBSES scores (final/initial) between the BTX-treated side and the saline-treated side was also significant ($p < 0.001$). Subjects were significantly more satisfied with the overall outcome of the BTX-treated side at 6 months' follow-up, according to a four-point grading scale ($p = 0.000$; 95% CI 1.24 to 2.36)
Ziade [20], 2013	RCT (BTX vs. no injection)	BTX group: 15 (4 lost for FU) Control group: 15 (2 lost for FU)	BTX group: A single treatment delivered within 72 h following op. BTX concentration: 10 IU/mL; Injection dose: 15–40 IU. Control group: No injection	Patient Scar Assessment Scale (PSAS) Observer Scar Assessment Scale (OSAS) Vancouver Scar Scale (VSS), Visual Analogue Scale (VAS)	12 months	No statistically significant differences were found between the two groups for the PSAS, OSAS and VSS scores. The median VAS rated by the six evaluators was 8.25 for the botulinum toxin-treated group compared with 6.35 for the control group ($p < 0.001$).
Gassner [21], 2006	RCT (BTX vs. saline)	BTX group: 22 (6 excluded) Control group: 20 (5 excluded)	BTX group: A single injection within 24 h after wound closure. BTX concentration: 75 IU/mL; Injection dose: 15–45 IU. Control group: A single injection within 24 h after wound closure. Injection dose: 0.2–0.6 mL of saline	Visual Analogue Scale (VAS)	6 months	The overall median VAS score for the BTX-treated group was 8.9 compared with 7.2 for the placebo group ($p = 0.003$), indicating enhanced healing and improved cosmesis of the experimentally immobilized scars.
Wilson [22], 2006	Prospective, single-arm	55 (15 dropped out)	BTX was injected once at the end of the operation. BTX concentration: 10 IU/mL; Injection dose: 1.5 IU per cm of wound length.	Objective assessment Subjective assessment	12–16 months	The outcome was considered highly satisfactory in 36 patients (90%). Thirty patients rated the improvement as marked (75%), six rated it as significant (15%), and four rated it as unchanged (10%). In 3 cases (7.5%), the scars re-widened, while in one case (2.5%), residual scar depression persisted.

BTX: Onabotulinum toxin unless otherwise stated.

2.3. BTX in Rosacea and Facial Flushing

Rosacea is a common inflammatory dermatosis characterized by persistent erythema, telangiectasia, papules, pustules, and facial flush. Oral medication, topicals, and laser therapy are routinely performed but often fail to relieve the facial flush. Persistent facial flushing is also a troublesome menopausal symptom.

A number of reports demonstrate the possible action of BTX on rosacea and menopausal hot flashes [23–26] (Table 3). In a prospective pilot study [23], the effect of BTX on the Dermatology Life Quality Index (DLQI) of patients with facial flushing was examined. BTX was injected once up to a total dose of 30 units on the cheeks which led to a significant decrease in DLQI at 2 months follow-up. Odo et al. [26] reported BTX (6.2 IU of abo-BTX per injection point, 40 points over the face, chest, neck, and scalp) to significantly reduce the mean number of menopausal hot flashes at day 60. The effect of abo-BTX was also investigated in 15 patients with rosacea. 15–45 IU of BTX was injected to the face which resulted in a statistically significant improvement in erythema at 3 months follow-up [24]. Adverse effects were rarely reported in the studies.

One possible mechanism by which BTX improves flushing is the potent blockade of acetylcholine release from autonomic peripheral nerves of the cutaneous vasodilatory system [27,28]. It is also well-known that BTX inhibits the release of inflammatory mediators such as substance P and calcitonin gene-related peptide (CGRP) [29]. The reduction and control of local skin inflammation may allow the erythema to fade out.

Larger, controlled, randomized studies are warranted to determine the optimal dose and duration of BTX activity on rosacea and facial flushing. BTX injection for facial flushing has additional benefits as it also improve the fine lines and wrinkles by diminishing the pull of the facial depressors.

2.4. BTX in Postherpetic Neuralgia

Postherpetic neuralgia (PHN) is the most frequent chronic complication of herpes zoster and the most common neuropathic pain resulting from infection. It is conventionally defined as dermatomal pain (usually a score of 40 or higher on a Likert scale ranging from 0-no pain to 100-worst possible pain), persisting at least 90 days after the appearance of the acute herpes zoster rash. PHN causes considerable suffering and results in a health care burden at both the individual and societal levels [30].

Treatment approaches include nonsteroidal anti-inflammatory drugs, gabapentin, opioids, and tricyclic antidepressants as well as topical anesthetics and capsaicin cream, but pain can be resistant to all of these drugs.

A number of reports have been made on the efficacy of BTX in PHN [31–33] (Table 4). Xiao et al. [33] performed a randomized, double-blind, placebo-controlled study on 60 PHN patients with the following arms: the BTX group, the 0.5% lidocaine group, and the 0.9% saline group. All patients were treated once (as for BTX, a dose of 200 IU at maximum), and were followed-up for 3 months. The BTX treated patients were found to have the most significant improvement in Visual Analog Scale (VAS) and sleep quality compared to those of the other two groups. Apalla et al. [32] also performed a RCT where 30 PHN patients received either BTX (200 IU in total) or placebo. BTX patients showed a significant reduction in VAS pain scores as well the sleep scores which lasted for approximately 16 weeks. In a prospective study, Ding et al. [31] treated 58 PHN with BTX (50 to 100 IU in total) to find promising results (reduced frequency of pain attacks, lower pain severity, reduction in the quantity of painkillers consumed by patients) with very few adverse reactions.

The mechanism involved in the pain-relieving effect of BTX is still unclear, but it is thought that both the peripheral and central mechanism play a role [33]. The peripheral effects of BTX injection come through the inhibition of neuropeptide release from the peripheral nociceptive nerves [34,35]. In addition, BTX has been suggested to exert central nervous system (CNS) effects through axonal transport to the CNS after peripheral application [36,37].

Although promising, cost would be one of the main considerations to BTX use in PHN. Also, unlike other therapeutic modalities, BTX induces antitoxin antibodies which can limit the clinical effectiveness of the drug after repetitive, long-term use.

Table 3. Representative studies of BTX in rosacea and facial flushing.

First Author [Ref.], Year	Type of Study	*n*	Treatment Regimen	Outcome Measures	Follow-Up	Results (Including Adverse Effects)
Eshghi [23], 2016	Prospective single arm (BTX)	24	A single treatment with BTX. 1 IU of BTX was injected intracutaneously in every square cm, to a total dose of 30 IU on both sides of cheeks.	The Dermatology Life Quality Index (DLQI)	2 months	The mean of DLQI improved from 8.08 ± 1.17 (baseline) to 4.5 ± 1.21 (2 months follow-up) ($p < 0.005$)
Bloom [24], 2015	Prospective, single arm (Abo-BTX)	25 (15 completed the study)	A single treatment with abo-BTX. Abo-BTX concentration: 100 IU/mL; Injected dose: 15–45 IU to the nose, cheeks, forehead, and chin	Facial erythema assessed by a non-treating physician using a standardized grading system (0–3)	3 months	The treatment resulted in statistically significant improvement in erythema grade at 1 ($p < 0.05$), 2 ($p < 0.001$), and 3 months ($p < 0.05$) after treatment when compared with baseline.
Geddoa [25], 2013	Prospective, single arm (BTX)	22 (18 included in the final analysis)	A single treatment with BTX for 20 patients and two sessions of treatment for 2. BTX concentration: 10 IU/mL; Injected dose: 1–2 IU/cm^2 with maximum total dose of 100 IU (neck and/or chest)	Dermatology Life Quality Index (DLQI)	4 weeks	The mean change in DLQI (before-after treatment) was 3.56 ± 4.6, suggesting a significant improvement in quality of life at 4 weeks following treatment ($p < 0.004$)
Odo [26], 2011	RCT (Abo-BTX vs. saline)	60 women with menopausal hot flushes Group BTX: 30 (25 completed) Group Control: 30 (23 completed)	A single treatment with either abo-BTX or saline. Group BTX: Abo-BTX concentration: 500 IU/3.2 mL; Injected dose: 6.2 IU at each selected point in the skin (40 injection points to the face, chest, neck, and scalp) Group Control: saline solution injected at a volume of 0.04 mL per injection point	Intensity of sweating, number of hot flashes, and Starch-Iodine test. Number of women reporting episodes of night sweating and mood changes	6 months	The sweating and hot flashes were less severe than before abo-BTX treatment, especially at 2 months follow-up; In the control group, there was no significant difference in mean intensity of sweating or in the mean number of hot flashes. Other menopausal symptoms such as night sweats were found better 2 months after abo-BTX treatment than in the control group ($p < 0.001$).

BTX: Onabotulinum toxin unless otherwise stated, Abo-BTX: Abobotulinum toxin.

Table 4. Representative studies of BTX in postherpetic neuralgia (PHN).

First Author [Ref.], Year	Type of Study	n	Treatment Regimen	Outcome Measures	Follow-Up	Results (Including Adverse Effects)
Ding [31], 2017	Prospective, single arm (BTX)	58	A single session of treatment was performed. BTX concentration: 4 IU/mL; Injection dose: 50–100 IU in total	Pain severity (VAS) Neuropathy pain scale (NPS) Quality of Life Scale (SF-36) PHN seizure severity, seizure duration, and frequency of attacks. The use of painkillers	6 months	At 6 months follow-up, a significant decrease in seizure frequency, seizure duration, VAS score, NPS score, SF-36 score and the required amount of painkiller was observed ($p < 0.05$). After BTX injection, 4 patients complained of pain around the injection area which disappeared within a week.
Apalla [32], 2013	Double-blinded RCT (BTX vs. saline)	BTX group: 15 Control group: 15	BTX group: A single treatment delivered. BTX concentration: 25 IU/mL; Injection dose: each patient received 40 injections in total (5 IU/point). Control group: A single treatment with saline.	Pain severity (VA) Quality of sleep	4 months	Thirteen patients from the experimental arm achieved at least 50% reduction in VAS score, compared with none of the placebo group ($p < 0.001$). BTX patients showed significant reduction in VAS pain scores between baseline and week 2, which persisted for a median period of 16 weeks. BTX patients showed significant reduction in sleep scores between baseline and week 2, which remained unchanged until week 16 ($p < 0.001$). Treatment was well-tolerated.
Xiao [33], 2010	Double-blinded RCT (BTX vs. 0.5% lidocaine vs. saline)	BTX group: 20 (19 completed) Lidocaine group: 20 (19 completed) Control group: 20 (18 completed)	BTX group: A single injection. BTX concentration: 5 IU/mL; Injection dose: 200 IU at maximum. Lidocaine group: A single session of treatment of the same volume as BTX. Control group: A single injection of the same volume as BTX	Visual Analogue Scale (VAS) Quality of Life Percent of Opioid use	3 months	Compared with pretreatment, VAS pain scores decreased at day 7 and 3 months posttreatment in all 3 groups. However, the VAS pain scores of the BTX group decreased more significantly compared with lidocaine and placebo groups at day 7 and 3 months posttreatment ($p < 0.01$). Sleep time improved in all 3 groups but was most significant in the BTX group compared with the lidocaine and placebo groups ($p < 0.01$). The percentage of subjects using opioids posttreatment in the BTX was the lowest (21.1%), compared with the lidocaine (52.6%) and placebo (66.7%) groups ($p < 0.01$).

BTX: Onabotulinum toxin unless otherwise stated, PHN: post-herpetic neuralgia.

2.5. BTX in Pruritus

Pruritus (also known as itch) is an unpleasant sensation of the skin leading to the desire to scratch. Among the 4 subtypes (pruriceptive, neurogenic, neuropathic, and psychogenic itch), the pruriceptive itch is a peripherally induced pruritus arising from the skin and mucosa and is often seen in dermatological disease.

A number of reports have been made on the efficacy of BTX in pruriceptive pruritus [38–40] (Table 5). Recalcitrant pruritus is a hallmark of lichen simplex, a localized variant of atopic dermatitis. In an open pilot study [40], BTX (abo-BTX, 20–80 IU) was injected intradermally into 5 circumscribed lichenoid lesions with recalcitrant pruritus. Within a week, all patients reported to have noticeable alleviation of itching and at 12 weeks, all were still free from the uncontrollable urge to scratch. Itch is also a common and well-recognized problem in burns [38]. Nine patients with recalcitrant itching secondary to burns were treated with BTX (dosage not specified) where the burn itch fell to 0 out of 10 in 4 weeks. The average duration of symptom free period was reported as nine months.

As clinical evidence has revealed the antipruritic effect of BTX, Arendt-Nielsen et al. [39], investigated the effect of subcutaneous administration of BTX on experimentally histamine-induced itch in human skin. In this double-blind, placebo-controlled study, 14 healthy men received BTX and isotonic saline on the volar surface of either forearm. Histamine prick tests were performed four times at the treatment sites (before treatment, and days 1, 3, and 7 after treatment) where BTX reduced the histamine-induced itch intensity, and itch area compared with saline at all time points.

Several possible mechanisms can be responsible for the reduction of pruriceptive itch. Acetylcholine mediates itch in pruritic skin conditions such as atopic dermatitis [41] and BTX inhibits the release of acetylcholine from presynaptic vesicles [42]. BTX is also known to interact with molecules associated with itch and flare such as substance P (releases histamine via the activation of mast cells, promotes vasodilation) and CGRP (a potent vasodilator) [36,43–45]. BTX inhibits the release of such mediators, thus reducing the sensation of itch. Lastly, BTX has also been shown to stabilize mast cells and inhibit their degranulation [46].

Pruritogenic pruritus is usually accompanied by skin inflammation. Since BTX is capable of reducing neurogenic inflammation [29], it is natural to expect improvement of the primary skin disease (e.g., atopic dermatitis, psoriasis) as well, which has in fact been reported through animal studies [47,48], human studies [49] and case reports [50,51]. Although promising in pruritogenic itch (and also in inflammatory dermatoses), we feel that BTX would be best used as an adjunct to conventional therapy. It should be applied focally, considering that the product can induce muscle weakening.

2.6. BTX in Dermatological Conditions Associated with Hyperhidrosis

A number of skin disease are caused by and/or have symptoms that are exacerbated by hyperhidrosis, a condition that can be treated successfully with BTX.

Pompholyx or dyshidrotic eczema is a common vesiculo-bullous disease of the palms and/or soles. A hallmark of this disease is its tendency to relapse in response to various provoking factors which includes wet work, occlusion and hyperhidrosis. An intra-individual study of 10 patients [52] (Table 6) investigated the use of BTX (mean dose of 162 IU per palm) for pompholyx, using the using the untreated site as control. 70% of patients reported a marked improvement of both sweating and itching on the treated site after 6 weeks. In another side-by-side trial [53], dyshidrotic hand eczema was treated with BTX (100 IU per palm) as an adjunct to topical steroids. Six patients who completed the study were found to have improved symptoms of pompholyx and reduced number of relapses by BTX injection.

The anhidrotic effect of BTX in pompholyx can be explained by its action on smooth muscles surrounding the sweat glands and through the inhibition of acetylcholine release. Inhibition of substance P release also explains the reduction in pruritus [54,55].

Hidradenitis suppurativa (HS) is a chronic inflammatory dermatosis of the apocrine glands which typically affects the axillae and groin. Patients afflicted by HS have severe discomfort and treatment is extremely challenging. It is well-known that a moist environment in folds, especially in the axilla and groin, provides ideal conditions for the flourishing of bacteria and is a precipitating factor of HS.

In 2005, HS on the axillae was first reported to be successfully treated with BTX (abo-BTX, 250 IU) with 10 months of complete remission [56] (Table 6). Khoo et al. [57] also confirmed the efficacy of BTX in HS where a 46-year-old woman with Hurley stage 2 HS responded well to axillary BTX treatment (50 IU per side) with a remission period of 12 months. The patient had been recalcitrant to conventional treatments and also underwent surgical drainage.

The exact mechanism by which BTX affects the disease process in HS is unclear but it is likely that the effect of BTX on sweat production reduces the population of skin flora and its potential inflammatory effect [56,57]. A second hypothesis is that by inhibiting apocrine secretion, BTX prevents the rupture and spread of follicular material from the pilosebaceous unit [57].

BTX has been studied in inverse psoriasis (Table 6) which is also thought to be exacerbated by excessive sweating. A pilot study of 15 patients with flexural psoriasis [49] showed that 50–100 IU of BTX improved subjective symptoms and objective photographic evidence of disease in 87% of patients at 2, 4, and 12 weeks follow-up. It is hypothesized that the beneficial effects of BTX in inverse psoriasis is largely due to the reduction of local sweating in folds [49]. Patients with psoriasis are also known to have a higher concentration of substance P receptors in their skin [58,59], meaning that BTX can reduce pruritus and vasodilation by inhibiting neuropeptide liberation (and preventing substance P binding to multiple receptors).

Hailey–Hailey disease is an autosomal dominant acantholytic disorder with mutation of the *ATP2C1* gene, clinically manifesting as macerated flexural erythema. Heat and sweat aggravate the disease, worsening the discomfort and pruritic symptoms.

Several case reports [60,61] (Table 6) have evidenced improvement of Hailey–Hailey disease with the use of BTX (50–125 IU per side). In one study, the effect of BTX was found to be comparable to that of laser ablation and dermabrasion [61].

BTX can rationally ameliorate the symptoms of Hailey–Hailey disease via its inhibition of acetylcholine and substance P release from the nerve endings [54,55] (Table 6). Although more clinical evidence is needed to prove effectiveness, BTX may be considered as a possible treatment modality for Hailey–Hailey disease recalcitrant to conventional treatment.

2.7. BTX in Oily Skin

Sebum contributes to the delivery of fat-soluble antioxidants to the skin surface and has antimicrobial activity, thereby functioning as a skin barrier. However, excess sebum blocks the pores, provides nourishment to bacteria, and can result in skin inflammation (e.g., acne, seborrheic dermatitis).

Recently, insights into the effect of BTX on sebum production have been published [62,63] (Table 7). Min et al. [62] randomly assigned 42 volunteers with forehead wrinkles to receive 10 or 20 units of BTX, which was administered in five standard injection sites. Treatment with BTX exhibited significant sebum reduction at the injection site of both groups, with a sebum gradient surrounding the injection point. The efficacy did not improve significantly with higher injection doses and the sebum production recovered to normal levels at 16-week follow-up for both treatment groups. Rose and Goldberg [63] also evaluated the safety and efficacy of BTX on the oily skin of 25 subjects. A 10-point injection was made with BTX (abo-BTX, total amount of 30-45 IU) on the forehead to find significantly lower sebum production and high patient satisfaction.

The mechanism by which intradermal BTX injection results in decreased sebum production is not entirely clear because the role of the nervous system and acetylcholine on sebaceous glands is not well defined. However, it is most likely that the arrector pili muscles and the local muscarinic receptors in the sebaceous glands are targets for the neuro-modulatory effects of BTX. Li et al. [64] demonstrated that nicotinic acetylcholine receptor $\alpha 7$ (nAchR$\alpha 7$) is expressed in human sebaceous glands in vivo, and acetylcholine signal increased lipid synthesis in vitro in a dose-dependent manner. Further study is needed to determine the best candidates, optimal injection techniques and doses.

Table 5. Representative studies of BTX in itch.

First Author [Ref.], Year	Type of Study	*n*	Treatment Regimen	Outcome Measures	Follow-Up	Results (Including Adverse Effects)
Akhtar [38], 2012	Prospective, single arm (BTX)	9	Treatment with BTX once on the burn scar. BTX concentration: 10–25 IU/mL; Injection dose: not stated	Severity of itch (0–10 scale)	11.3 months on average	On average, the burn covered 24% of the total body surface area and 87.5% of patients rated their burn itch as being severe (>7 on the itch scale). Following the administration of BTX, this fell to 0 out of 10 in 4 weeks. The average duration of symptom free period was 9 months (3–18 months).
Gazerani [39], 2009	Double-blind, split arm, RCT (BTX vs. saline)	14	BTX treated arm: 5 IU of BTX was injected into the skin once. Control arm: The same volume of 0.9% saline as in the BTX treated side was injected. After BTX and saline injection, a skin prick test with histamine was performed on both sites.	Itch ratings (0–10 scale), itch area, neurogenic inflammation (visible flare area) Blood flow (Laser Doppler imaging) Cutaneous temperature (Infrared thermography	1 week	BTX reduced the histamine-induced itch intensity ($p < 0.001$), and itch area ($p = 0.011$) compared with saline at all time points after treatment. The duration of itch was also shorter for BTX treated areas ($p < 0.001$), with a peak effect at day 7. The flare area was smaller in the BTX treated arm compared with the saline treated arm at all time points after treatment ($p = 0.002$). Findings from blood flow ($p < 0.001$), and temperature measurements ($p < 0.001$), clearly showed suppressive effects of BTX on vasomotor reactions, with the maximal effect on day 3 and 7.
Heckmann [40], 2002	Prospective, single arm (Abo-BTX)	4	Abo-BTX was injected to a total of 6 lichen simplex chronicus (LSC) patches once. Abo-BTX concentration: 100 IU/mL; Injection dose: 20–80 IU.	Sensation of pruritus (VAS 0–10)	4 months	After a week, all patients reported a noticeable alleviation of itching. Three patients felt no more itching at all; in one patient pruritus was reduced to less than 50% according to the VAS used before and after treatment. After 4 weeks, 5 of 6 lesions had cleared without any other treatment. After 12 weeks, 3 patients were still free of symptoms. One patient who had one lesion on the shin developed a new lesion on the dorsum of his foot which was cleared in 2 weeks after BTX treatment.

BTX: Onabotulinum toxin unless otherwise stated, Abo-BTX: abobotulinumtoxin, VAS: Visual Analogue Scale.

Table 6. BTX in dermatologic disease associated with hyperhidrosis.

First Author [Ref.], Year	Type of Study	n	Treatment Regimen	Outcome Measures	Follow-Up	Results (Including Adverse Effects)
Pompholyx						
Swartling [52], 2002	A side-by-side prospective controlled trial (BTX vs. no treatment)	10	BTX group: BTX was injected once. BTX concentration: 100 IU/mL; Injection dose: a mean of 162 IU. Control group: No treatment.	Effect of treatment (5-point scale) VAS for itch Disease activity score Extent of the dermatitis	5–6 weeks	In the self-assessment, 7 of the 10 patients in the study experienced good or very good effect of the treatment. After injection with BTX, the VAS score for itching decreased by 39% on the treated side compared to an increase by 52% on the untreated side. Comparing treated vs. untreated sides, it was found that with BTX injection, a decrease in the disease activity score (54% vs. 29%), occurrence of vesicles (74 vs. 27), infiltration (54 vs. 18), erythema (53 vs. 30), and extent of the disease (58 vs. 31). No changes or only minor changes were seen in the objective parameters of scaling, crusting, and excoriations.
Wollina [53], 2002	A side-by-side prospective controlled trial (BTX vs. control)	8 (6 completed the study)	Topical steroid was applied to both hands in combination with BTX on one hand and no additional treatment on the other. A single injection of BTX was given. BTX concentration: 50 IU/mL; BTX was injection in aliquots of 5 IU per point; Injection dose: Not mentioned.	Dyshidrotic Eczema Area and Severity Index (DASI)	8 weeks	Six patients completed the study. The mean DASI score changed from 28 to 17 with topical therapy alone and from 36 to 3 with adjuvant BTX ($p < 0.01$). Itching and vesicles were inhibited earlier when using the combination of steroids and BTX. There was one relapse in the steroid group and none in the BTX group.
Hidradenitis suppurativa						
Khoo [57], 2014	Case report (BTX)	3 (only one described in detail)	Over the course of 3 years, a Hurley Stage II HS patient received 4 BTX treatments. 50 IU of BTX administered to each axilla per treatment. BTX concentration: 25 IU/mL			The patient showed good clinical response within 3 months of her first treatment, and, following her second treatment, went into clinical remission. She was still in remission when discharged from follow-up 1 year after her fourth treatment.
O'Reilly [56], 2005	Case report (Abo-BTX)	1	BTX was injected once to both axilla. Injection dose: 250 IU of abo-BTX in total.			There was no evidence of active inflammation on follow-up at a fortnight after administration. The patient had complete remission of symptoms until approximately 10 months later, when the first symptoms of mild inflammation re-appeared.

Table 6. *Cont.*

First Author [Ref.], Year	Type of Study	*n*	Treatment Regimen	Outcome Measures	Follow-Up	Results (Including Adverse Effects)
Psoriasis						
Zanchi [49], 2008	Prospective, single-arm (BTX)	15	BTX was injected once to the inverse psoriasis sites. BTX concentration: 20 IU/mL; Dose injected: 50–100 IU in total.	Photographic assessment of the psoriatic area Subjective symptomatology (10-point VAS)	12 weeks	The location of the psoriasis was as follows: armpits (7 patients), sub-mammary sulcus (6), intergluteal folds (7), inguinal folds (5) and umbilicus (1). Subjective symptomatology according to the 10-point VAS scale improved in all patients. Mean VAS scores were 9.1 at the pre-treatment assessment, with post-treatment mean scores of 4.2 after 2 weeks, 2.1 after 4 weeks and 2.4 after 12 weeks. Erythema extension, intensity and infiltration improved in 13 of 15 patients (87%). The change in the erythematous area was evident from the first post-treatment assessment at 2 weeks and continued to improve until the assessment at 4 weeks. At the final visit (12 weeks post-treatment), improvement had been maintained.
Hailey–Hailey disease						
Lopez-Ferrer [60], 2012	Case report (BTX)	3	Case 1: 80 IU of BTX was first administered on each axilla. A total of 200 IU of BTX was injected every 2 months for maintenance. Case 2: 80–300 IU of BTX was injected to the groin, below the left breast, the left axilla, and the side of the neck. Case 3: 200–300 IU of BTX was injected to the axilla, sub-mammary region, and groin.			The Hailey–Hailey disease improved in all 3 patients after BTX injection. BTX injection had to be repeated for maintaining remission.
Konrad [61], 2001	Case report with side-by side comparison (BTX alone vs. BTX + Erbium: YAG vs. BTX + dermabrasion	1	Both sub-mammary areas were treated with BTX at a concentration of 20 IU/mL. Four days later, surgical (right side) or laser therapy (left side) was performed on an area of 5×5 cm^2.			Wound healing was faster after laser (7 days) versus dermabrasion (14 days). Those areas treated only with BTX showed remission of hyperhidrosis within 3 days and clearance of Hailey-Hailey within 2 weeks. During a follow-up of 12 months, no relapse was seen for dermabrasion, laser ablation and BTX. Final cosmetic results were comparable.

BTX: Onabotulinum toxin unless otherwise stated, Abo-BTX: Abobotulinumtoxin, VAS: Visual Analogue Scale.

Table 7. Representative studies of BTX in oily skin.

First Author [Ref.], Year	Type of Study	*n*	Treatment Regimen	Outcome Measures	Follow-Up	Results (Including Adverse Effects)
Min [62], 2015	Prospective (BTX 10 IU vs. BTX 20 IU)	42 (41 completed the study) 20 received 10 IU of BTX 20 received 20 IU	Treatment with BTX once on the forehead. BTX concentration: 40 IU/mL; Injection dose: A final volume of 10 IU or 20 IU was injected evenly in 5 injection sites.	Sebum production (sebumeter)	16 weeks	Treatment with BTX exhibited significant sebum alteration at the injection site of both groups (10 IU, 20 IU), with a sebum gradient surrounding the injection point. The efficacy did not improve at higher injection doses, with the four-unit regimen generally not being more potent than the two-unit regimen. The sebum production recovered to normal levels at the 16-week follow-up for both treatment groups, indicating that a higher dosage (4 units) did not results in a longer duration until relapse compared with the two-unit dose.
Rose [63], 2012	Prospective, single-arm (Abo-BTX)	25	Abo-BTX was injected once on the forehead. Abo-BTX concentration: 100 IU/mL; Injection dose: A total of 30–45 IU delivered to 10 injection sites.	Sebum production (sebumeter) Patient satisfaction (4-point scale)	3 months	Treatment with BTX resulted in significantly lower sebum production at 1 week and 1, 2, and 3 months after injection ($p < 0.001$). Twenty-one patients (91%) reported that they were satisfied (50–75% improvement) with intradermal BTX as a treatment for oily skin.

BTX: Onabotulinum toxin unless otherwise stated, Abo-BTX: abobotulinumtoxin.

3. Conclusions

In this review, we highlighted the promising outcomes of BTX in several off-label indications of interest for dermatologists. There is overwhelming evidence that BTX exhibits biological effects on many human cell types, but much is yet to be learned about the drug and its mechanism of action. Knowing that the skin closely interacts with the nervous system, future studies should investigate the link between BTX and the cutaneous neuroimmune system to better understand its therapeutic potential in dermatology. A consensus on the dose regimen and injection technique is also desirable for standardized treatment. Generally, high doses of BTX were applied, with an average total of 300 IU for hypertrophic scars, 50 IU for scar prevention, 50–100 IU for facial flush/rosacea, 100 IU for PHN, 150 IU for pompholyx, 100 IU for HS, 75 IU for inverse psoriasis and 250 IU for Hailey-Hailey disease. Lastly, with the limitations of BTX treatment (high cost, muscle weakening, risk of tachyphylaxis and production of antibodies), BTX may be optimally used as an adjunct in recalcitrant cases to conventional therapy.

Acknowledgments: This study was supported by the National Research Foundation of Korea (NRF) grant funded by the Korea government (MSIT) (Grant No.: 2017R1C1B5016144) and the 2016 Amore-Pacific grant.

Conflicts of Interest: The authors declare no conflict of interest.

References

1. Steinhoff, M.; Stander, S.; Seeliger, S.; Ansel, J.C.; Schmeiz, M.; Luger, T. Modern aspects of cutaneous neurogenic inflammation. *Arch. Dermatol.* **2003**, *139*, 1479–1488. [CrossRef]
2. Ansel, J.C.; Kaynard, A.H.; Armstrong, C.A.; Olerud, J.; Bunnett, N.; Payan, D. Skin-nervous system interactions. *J. Investig. Dermatol.* **1996**, *106*, 198–204. [CrossRef]
3. Berman, B.; Maderal, A.; Raphael, B. Keloids and hypertrophic scars: Pathophysiology, classification, and treatment. *Dermatol. Surg.* **2017**, *43* (Suppl. 1), S3–S18. [CrossRef]
4. Elhefnawy, A.M. Assessment of intralesional injection of botulinum toxin type A injection for hypertrophic scars. *Indian J. Dermatol. Venereol. Leprol.* **2016**, *82*, 279–283. [CrossRef]
5. Shaarawy, E.; Hegazy, R.A.; Abdel Hay, R.M. Intralesional botulinum toxin type A equally effective and better tolerated than intralesional steroid in the treatment of keloids: A randomized controlled trail. *J. Cosmet. Dermatol.* **2015**, *14*, 161–166. [CrossRef]
6. Xiao, Z.; Zhang, F.; Cui, Z. Treatment of hypertrophic scars with intralesional botulinum toxin type A injections: A preliminary report. *Aesthet. Plast. Surg.* **2009**, *33*, 409–412. [CrossRef]
7. Zhibo, X.; Miaobo, Z. Intralesional botulinum toxin type A injection as a new treatment measure for keloids. *Plast. Reconstr. Surg.* **2009**, *124*, 275e–277e. [CrossRef] [PubMed]
8. Xiao, Z.; Zhang, M.; Liu, Y.; Ren, L. Botulinum toxin type A inhibits connective tissue growth factor expression in fibroblasts derived from hypertrophic scar. *Aesthet. Plast. Surg.* **2011**, *35*, 802–807. [CrossRef] [PubMed]
9. Chen, M.; Yan, T.; Ma, K.; Lai, L.; Liu, C.; Liang, L.; Fu, X. Botulinum toxin type a inhibits alpha-smooth muscle actin and myosin ii expression in fibroblasts derived from scar contracture. *Ann. Plast. Surg.* **2016**, *77*, e46–e49. [CrossRef] [PubMed]
10. Jeong, H.S.; Lee, B.H.; Sung, H.M.; Park, S.Y.; Ahn, D.K.; Jung, M.S.; Suh, I.S. Effect of botulinum toxin type a on differentiation of fibroblasts derived from scar tissue. *Plast. Reconstr. Surg.* **2015**, *136*, 171e–178e. [CrossRef] [PubMed]
11. Wang, X.; Chen, X.; Xiao, Z. Effects of botulinum toxin type a on expression of genes in keloid fibroblasts. *Aesthet. Surg. J.* **2014**, *34*, 154–159. [CrossRef] [PubMed]
12. Viera, M.H.; Amini, S.; Valins, W.; Berman, B. Innovative therapies in the treatment of keloids and hypertrophic scars. *J. Clin. Aesthet. Dermatol.* **2010**, *3*, 20–26. [PubMed]
13. Uyesugi, B.; Lippincott, B.; Dave, S. Treatment of painful keloid with botulinum toxin type A. *Am. J. Phys. Med. Rehabil.* **2010**, *89*, 153–155. [CrossRef] [PubMed]
14. Lee, B.J.; Jeong, J.H.; Wang, S.G.; Lee, J.C.; Goh, E.K.; Kim, H.W. Effect of botulinum toxin type A on a rat surgical wound model. *Clin. Exp. Otorhinolaryngol.* **2009**, *2*, 20–27. [CrossRef] [PubMed]

15. Wolfram, D.; Tzankov, A.; Pulzl, P.; Piza-Katzer, H. Hypertrophic scars and keloids—A review of their pathophysiology, risk factors, and therapeutic management. *Dermatol. Surg.* **2009**, *35*, 171–181. [CrossRef] [PubMed]
16. Zhibo, X.; Miaobo, Z. Botulinum toxin type A affects cell cycle distribution of fibroblasts derived from hypertrophic scar. *J. Plast. Reconstr. Aesthet. Surg.* **2008**, *61*, 1128–1129. [CrossRef] [PubMed]
17. Zhibo, X.; Miaobo, Z. Potential therapeutical effects of botulinum toxin type A in keloid management. *Med. Hypotheses* **2008**, *71*, 623. [CrossRef] [PubMed]
18. Xiao, Z.; Zhang, F.; Lin, W.; Zhang, M.; Liu, Y. Effect of botulinum toxin type A on transforming growth factor beta 1 in fibroblasts derived from hypertrophic scar: A preliminary report. *Aesthet. Plast. Surg.* **2010**, *34*, 424–427. [CrossRef] [PubMed]
19. Kim, Y.S.; Lee, H.J.; Cho, S.H.; Lee, J.D.; Kim, H.S. Early postoperative treatment of thyroidectomy scars using botulinum toxin: A split-scar, double-blind, randomized controlled trial. *Wound Repair Regen.* **2014**, *22*, 605–612. [CrossRef] [PubMed]
20. Ziade, M.; Domergue, S.; Batifol, D.; Jreige, R.; Sebbane, M.; Goudot, P.; Yachouh, J. Use of botulinum toxin type A to improve treatment of facial wounds: A prospective randomized study. *J. Plast. Reconstr. Aesthet. Surg.* **2013**, *66*, 209–214. [CrossRef] [PubMed]
21. Gassner, H.G.; Brissett, A.E.; Otley, C.C.; Boahene, D.K.; Boggust, A.J.; Weaver, A.L.; Sherris, D.A. Botulinum toxin to improve facial wound healing: A prospective, blinded, placebo-controlled study. *Mayo Clin. Proc.* **2006**, *81*, 1023–1028. [CrossRef] [PubMed]
22. Wilson, A.M. Use of botulinum toxin type A to prevent widening of facial scars. *Plast. Reconstr. Surg.* **2006**, *117*, 1758–1766. [CrossRef] [PubMed]
23. Eshghi, G.; Khezrian, L.; Alirezaei, P. Botulinum toxin in treatment of facial flushing. *Acta Med. Iran* **2016**, *54*, 454–457. [PubMed]
24. Bloom, B.S.; Payongayong, L.; Mourin, A.; Goldberg, D.J. Impact of intradermal abobotulinumtoxin A on facial erythema of rosacea. *Dermatol. Surg.* **2015**, *41* (Suppl. 1), S9–S16. [CrossRef] [PubMed]
25. Geddoa, E.; Matar, H.E.; Paes, T.R. The use of botulinum toxin-a in the management of neck and anterior chest wall flushing: Pilot study. *Int. J. Dermatol.* **2013**, *52*, 1547–1550. [CrossRef] [PubMed]
26. Odo, M.E.; Odo, L.M.; Farias, R.V.; Primavera, R.A.; Leao, L.; Cuce, L.C.; Juliano, Y. Botulinum toxin for the treatment of menopausal hot flushes: A pilot study. *Dermatol. Surg.* **2011**, *37*, 1579–1583. [CrossRef] [PubMed]
27. Kellogg, D.L., Jr. In vivo mechanisms of cutaneous vasodilation and vasoconstriction in humans during thermoregulatory challenges. *J. Appl. Phys.* **2006**, *100*, 1709–1718. [CrossRef] [PubMed]
28. Kellogg, D.L., Jr.; Pergola, P.E.; Piest, K.L.; Kosiba, W.A.; Crandall, M.; Johnson, J.M. Cutaneous active vasodilation in humans is mediated by cholinergic nerve cotransmission. *Circ. Res.* **1995**, *77*, 1222–1228. [CrossRef] [PubMed]
29. Carmichael, M.M.; Dostrovsky, J.O.; Charlton, M.P. Peptide-mediated transdermal delivery of botulinum neurotoxin type A reduces neurogenic inflammation in the skin. *Pain* **2010**, *149*, 316–324. [CrossRef] [PubMed]
30. Johnson, R.W.; Rice, A.S. Clinical practice. Postherpetic neuralgia. *N. Engl. J. Med.* **2014**, *371*, 1526–1533. [CrossRef] [PubMed]
31. Ding, X.D.; Zhong, J.; Liu, Y.P.; Chen, H.X. Botulinum as a toxin for treating post-herpetic neuralgia. *Iran J. Public Health* **2017**, *46*, 608–611. [PubMed]
32. Apalla, Z.; Sotiriou, E.; Lallas, A.; Lazaridou, E.; Ioannides, D. Botulinum toxin a in postherpetic neuralgia: A parallel, randomized, double-blind, single-dose, placebo-controlled trial. *Clin. J. Pain* **2013**, *29*, 857–864. [CrossRef] [PubMed]
33. Xiao, L.; Mackey, S.; Hui, H.; Xong, D.; Zhang, Q.; Zhang, D. Subcutaneous injection of botulinum toxin A is beneficial in postherpetic neuralgia. *Pain Med.* **2010**, *11*, 1827–1833. [CrossRef] [PubMed]
34. Gazerani, P.; Pedersen, N.S.; Staahi, C.; Drewes, A.M.; Arendt-Nielsen, L. Subcutaneous botulinum toxin type A reduces capsaicin-induced trigeminal pain and vasomotor reactions in human skin. *Pain* **2009**, *141*, 60–69. [CrossRef] [PubMed]
35. Gazerani, P.; Staahi, C.; Drewes, A.M.; Arendt-Nielsen, L. The effects of botulinum toxin type A on capsaicin-evoked pain, flare, and secondary hyperalgesia in an experimental human model of trigeminal sensitization. *Pain* **2006**, *122*, 315–325. [CrossRef] [PubMed]

36. Aoki, K.R. Review of a proposed mechanism for the antinociceptive action of botulinum toxin type A. *Neurotoxicology* **2005**, *26*, 785–793. [CrossRef] [PubMed]
37. Antonucci, F.; Rossi, C.; Gianfranceschi, L.; Rossetto, O.; Caleo, M. Long-distance retrograde effects of botulinum neurotoxin A. *J. Neurosci.* **2008**, *28*, 3689–3696. [CrossRef] [PubMed]
38. Akhtar, N.; Brooks, P. The use of botulinum toxin in the management of burns itching: Preliminary results. *Burns* **2012**, *38*, 1119–1123. [CrossRef] [PubMed]
39. Gazerani, P.; Pedersen, N.S.; Drewes, A.M.; Arendt-Nielsen, L. Botulinum toxin type A reduces histamine-induced itch and vasomotor responses in human skin. *Br. J. Dermatol.* **2009**, *161*, 737–745. [CrossRef] [PubMed]
40. Heckmann, M.; Heyer, G.; Brunner, B.; Plewig, G. Botulinum toxin type A injection in the treatment of lichen simplex: An open pilot study. *J. Am. Acad. Dermatol.* **2002**, *46*, 617–619. [CrossRef] [PubMed]
41. Hallett, M. How does botulinum toxin work? *Ann. Neurol.* **2000**, *48*, 7–8. [CrossRef]
42. Huang, W.; Foster, J.A.; Rogachefsky, A.S. Pharmacology of botulinum toxin. *J. Am. Acad. Dermatol.* **2000**, *43*, 249–259. [CrossRef] [PubMed]
43. Arezzo, J.C. Possible mechanisms of the effects of botulinum toxin on pain. *Clin. J. Pain* **2002**, *18* (Suppl. 6), S125–S132. [CrossRef] [PubMed]
44. McMahon, H.T.; Foran, P.; Dolly, J.O.; Verhage, M.; Wiegant, V.M.; Nicholls, D.G. Tetanus toxin and botulinum toxins type A and B inhibit glutamate, gamma-aminobutyric acid, aspartate, and met-enkephalin release from synaptosomes. Clues to the locus of action. *J. Biol. Chem.* **1992**, *267*, 21338–21343. [PubMed]
45. Purkiss, J.; Welch, M.; Doward, S.; Foster, K. Capsaicin-stimulated release of substance P from cultured dorsal root ganglion neurons: Involvement of two distinct mechanisms. *Biochem. Pharmacol.* **2000**, *59*, 1403–1406. [CrossRef]
46. Park, T.H. The effects of botulinum toxin A on mast cell activity: Preliminary results. *Burns* **2013**, *39*, 816–817. [CrossRef] [PubMed]
47. Han, S.B.; Kim, H.; Cho, S.H.; Chung, J.H.; Kim, H.S. Protective effect of botulinum toxin type A against atopic dermatitis-like skin lesions in NC/Nga mice. *Dermatol. Surg.* **2017**. [CrossRef] [PubMed]
48. Ward, N.L.; Kavlick, K.D.; Diaconu, D.; Dawes, S.M.; Michaels, K.A.; Gilbert, E. Botulinum neurotoxin A decreases infiltrating cutaneous lymphocytes and improves acanthosis in the KC-Tie2 mouse model. *J. Investig. Dermatol.* **2012**, *132*, 1927–1930. [CrossRef] [PubMed]
49. Zanchi, M.; Favot, F.; Bizzarini, M.; Piai, M.; Donini, M.; Sedona, P. Botulinum toxin type A for the treatment of inverse psoriasis. *J. Eur. Acad. Dermatol. Venereol.* **2008**, *22*, 431–436. [CrossRef] [PubMed]
50. Saber, M.; Brassard, D.; Benohanian, A. Inverse psoriasis and hyperhidrosis of the axillae responding to botulinum toxin type A. *Arch. Dermatol.* **2011**, *147*, 629–630. [CrossRef] [PubMed]
51. Gilbert, E.; Ward, N.L. Efficacy of botulinum neurotoxin type A for treating recalcitrant plaque psoriasis. *J. Drugs Dermatol.* **2014**, *13*, 1407–1408. [PubMed]
52. Swartling, C.; Naver, H.; Lindberg, M.; Anveden, I. Treatment of dyshidrotic hand dermatitis with intradermal botulinum toxin. *J. Am. Acad. Dermatol.* **2002**, *47*, 667–671. [CrossRef] [PubMed]
53. Wollina, U.; Karamfilov, T. Adjuvant botulinum toxin A in dyshidrotic hand eczema: A controlled prospective pilot study with left-right comparison. *J. Eur. Acad. Dermatol. Venereol.* **2002**, *16*, 40–42. [CrossRef] [PubMed]
54. Humm, A.M.; Pabst, C.; Lauterburg, T.; Burgunder, J.M. Enkephalin and aFGF are differentially regulated in rat spinal motoneurons after chemodenervation with botulinum toxin. *Exp. Neurol.* **2000**, *161*, 361–372. [CrossRef] [PubMed]
55. Ishikawa, H.; Mitsui, Y.; Yoshitomi, T.; Mashimo, K.; Aoki, S.; Mukuno, K.; Shimizu, K. Presynaptic effects of botulinum toxin type A on the neuronally evoked response of albino and pigmented rabbit iris sphincter and dilator muscles. *Jpn. J. Opthalmol.* **2000**, *44*, 106–109. [CrossRef]
56. O'Reilly, D.J.; Pleat, J.M.; Richards, A.M. Treatment of hidradenitis suppurativa with botulinum toxin A. *Plast. Reconstr. Surg.* **2005**, *116*, 1575–1576. [CrossRef] [PubMed]
57. Khoo, A.B.; Burova, E.P. Hidradenitis suppurativa treated with clostridium botulinum toxin A. *Clin. Exp. Dermatol.* **2014**, *39*, 749–750. [CrossRef] [PubMed]
58. Staniek, V.; Doutremepuich, J.; Schmitt, D.; Claudy, A.; Misery, L. Expression of substance P receptors in normal and psoriatic skin. *Pathobiology* **1999**, *67*, 51–54. [CrossRef] [PubMed]
59. Nakamura, M.; Toyoda, M.; Morohashi, M. Pruritogenic mediators in psoriasis vulgaris: Comparative evaluation of itch-associated cutaneous factors. *Br. J. Dermatol.* **2003**, *149*, 718–730. [CrossRef] [PubMed]

60. Lopez-Ferrer, A.; Alomar, A. Botulinum toxin A for the treatment of familial benign pemphigus. *Actas Dermosifiliogr.* **2012**, *103*, 532–535. [CrossRef] [PubMed]
61. Konrad, H.; Karamfilov, T.; Wollina, U. Intracutaneous botulinum toxin A versus ablative therapy of Hailey-Hailey disease—A case report. *J. Cosmet. Laser Ther.* **2001**, *3*, 181–184. [CrossRef] [PubMed]
62. Min, P.; Xi, W.; Grassetti, L.; Trisliana Perdanasari, A.; Torresetti, M.; Feng, S.; Su, W.; Pu, Z.; Zhang, Y.; Han, S.; et al. Sebum production alteration after botulinum toxin type A injections for the treatment of forehead rhytides: A prospective randomized double-blind dose-comparative clinical investigation. *Aesthet. Surg. J.* **2015**, *35*, 600–610. [CrossRef] [PubMed]
63. Rose, A.E.; Goldberg, D.J. Safety and efficacy of intradermal injection of botulinum toxin for the treatment of oily skin. *Dermatol. Surg.* **2013**, *39*, 443–448. [CrossRef] [PubMed]
64. Li, Z.J.; Park, S.B.; Sohn, K.C.; Lee, Y.; Seo, Y.J.; Kim, C.D.; Kim, Y.S.; Lee, J.H.; Im, M. Regulation of lipid production by acetylcholine signalling in human sebaceous glands. *J. Dermatol. Sci.* **2013**, *72*, 116–122. [CrossRef] [PubMed]

toxins

MDPI

Review

Antipruritic Effects of Botulinum Neurotoxins

Parisa Gazerani

Department of Health Science and Technology, Aalborg University, Frederik Bajers Vej 7A2, A2-208, 9220 Aalborg East, Denmark; gazerani@hst.aau.dk; Tel.: +45-9940-2412

Received: 5 March 2018; Accepted: 27 March 2018; Published: 29 March 2018

Abstract: This review explores current evidence to demonstrate that botulinum neurotoxins (BoNTs) exert antipruritic effects. Both experimental and clinical conditions in which botulinum neurotoxins have been applied for pruritus relief will be presented and significant findings will be highlighted. Potential mechanisms underlying antipruritic effects will also be discussed and ongoing challenges and unmet needs will be addressed.

Keywords: botulinum neurotoxins; itch; pruritus; antipruritic; clinical; experimental

Key Contribution: This review highlights the potential utility of BoNTs to relieve pruritus. Presented information; discussion of limitations and promising results are valuable for both researchers and clinicians in the field.

1. Introduction

Botulinum neurotoxins (BoNTs) are protein neurotoxins that are produced by anaerobic, spore-forming bacteria of the *Clostridium* genus, including *Clostridium botulinum*, *Clostridium butyrricum*, *Clostridium barati*, and *Clostridium argentinensis* [1]. An updated review of biology, pharmacology, and toxicology of BoNTs can be found in M. Pirazzini et al.'s excellent recent review [2]. Since its first therapeutic use in humans in the 1980s [3], clinical use of BoNTs has significantly increased [4]. BoNTs have been used for therapeutic purposes in a diverse range of medical conditions, such as ophthalmology, neurology, gastroenterology, urology, and psychiatry [2,4–6]. Advanced understanding of the mechanism of action of BoNTs has led to increasing use of these molecules with novel, unique, and desirable pharmacological properties [2]. BoNTs have also been tested in many dermatological conditions, several of which with off-label uses [7,8]. This review focuses on the antipruritic effects of BoNTs as presented in clinical and experimental conditions which specifically addressed potential itch-relieving mechanisms. The aim is to highlight the value of BoNTs in an expanded evaluation as potential antipruritic agents in future practice. It is worth mentioning that one case [9] in the literature presented that an application of OnabotulinumtoxinA (100 U) provoked itchiness in a patient when it was used for neuromuscular pain. In that instance, pruritus was treated with oral hydroxyzine and camphor-menthol topical lotion [9].

2. Pruritus

Itchiness (pruritus) is a common unpleasant sensation that elicits a desire to scratch [10]. Acute itch [11] serves as a warning and self-protective mechanism to prevent potentially harmful irritations. However, chronic itch is a challenging and significant clinical problem [12] which is often associated with skin diseases, systemic diseases, metabolic disorders, and psychiatric disorders [13]. Although scratching temporarily relieves acute itch, persistent itch-scratch cycles often exacerbate skin problems, disrupt sleep, and reduce the quality of life in chronic itch patients [14]. Recent studies have documented a high prevalence of chronic pruritus (13–17%) with a lifetime prevalence of 22–26% [15]. On the basis of international consensus, a threshold of six weeks has been set for the definition of chronic pruritus. Chronic pruritus is a major challenge to overcome [16] and requires interdisciplinary cooperation despite many interfering factors. Successful treatment usually involves dermatologists, internists, general practitioners, neurologists, gynecologists, and psychiatrists [16]. An understanding of the molecular mechanisms underlying itch has advanced the identification of itch-specific pathways and transmitters for selective targeting [17].

Itch can broadly be categorized as either histaminergic and non-histaminergic [18]. Histamine is released by mast and epithelial cells and binds to H1–H4 receptors, leading to the activation of downstream target molecules within sensory neurons [17,19,20]. Histamine has been identified as the main mediator of itch in several pruritic conditions, such as urticaria and allergic diseases. Antipruritic treatment strategies [12] have been successfully used to target histaminergic pathways [21].

Non-histaminergic itch has attracted more attention in recent years because many chronic itch conditions are resistant to antihistamines, necessitating the need to consider alternative treatments. Cowhage (*Mucuna pruriens*) is a tropical legume known to cause itch, pricking, stinging, and burning sensations that otherwise do not respond to antihistamines. This characteristic has made cowhage a useful tool for studying non-histaminergic mechanisms underlying itch. When cowhage spicules are inserted, the cysteine protease mucunain is released. When the mucanin reaches the nerve endings of primary sensory neurons in the epidermis, it activates protease-activated receptors (PAR) 2 and 4, which are members of the G protein-coupled receptor family [22]. Interestingly, PAR2 and tryptase (an endogenous PAR2 agonist, the most abundant secretory granule-derived serine proteinase released by mast cells causing itch), have been found highly elevated in patients with atopic dermatitis (AD) [23]. Mas-related G protein-coupled receptors (Mrgprs) are involved in the response to non-histaminergic pruritogens [24]. MrgprA3 is expressed in a sub-population of sensory neurons known as peptidergic C-fibers and encodes pruritic effects of chloroquine, which is an antimalarial drug [25,26]. These receptors [27,28] are also responsive to histamine, bovine adrenal medulla 8–22 (BAM8–22), cowhage spicules, and capsaicin. Interestingly, mice lacking MrgprA3 neurons are resistant to pruritogens such as histamine, BAM8–22, SLIGRL, α-methyl-5HT, ET-1, and chloroquine [26]. However, MrgprA3-ablated mice scratch in response to β-alanine [29]. Therefore, MrgrpA3 positive sensory neurons are different from those neurons responding to β-alanine for itch. MrgprD is the receptor activated by β-alanine [30], and mice lacking MrgprD do not scratch following an intradermal injection of β-alanine [29]. Transient receptor potential (TRP) channels are also involved in itch. Histaminergic itch transmission through TRPV1 has been reported [31]. TRPA1 is a downstream target of MrgprA3 and MrgprC11. Ablation of TRPA1 blocks itch in a dry skin mouse model of chronic itch. Mice lacking TRPA1 exhibit no scratch following subcutaneous injections of chloroquine and BAM8–22, but do scratch in response to α-methyl-5HT [17,32]. Voltage-gated sodium channel (NaV) 1.7 has also been found to mediate itch. A monoclonal antibody targeting NaV 1.7 could abolish both acute and chronic itch in mice [33].

Immune cells of skin interact with nerve endings and play an important role in pathological itch. Cytokines released from T helper 2 cells are found elevated in several pruritus conditions [34]. Interleukin-31 (IL-31) is known to play a role in AD [35]. Intradermal injection of IL-31 in mice provokes scratching [36] that is also correlated with elevated expression of IL-31RA in the DRG (dorsal root ganglion) [37].

Taken together, novel findings on peripheral receptors and mediators [38] present that itch is mediated by several different subpopulations of primary sensory neurons. Some itch-provoking substances activate overlapping populations of neurons, while others only activate distinct populations (e.g., chloroquine vs. β-alanine; MrgprA3 vs. MrgprD). Depending on pruritogen, method of delivery, and species, itch-related responses are variable [17]. One must also consider that a cross-talk exists between the neurons and immune cells in the skin [38].

In addition to advancements in peripheral mechanisms of itch, several hypotheses have been proposed for central mechanisms of itch [17,38]. Gastrin-releasing peptide (GRP) and GRP receptors were the first central components of itch identified in the spinal cord [39]. Ablation of inhibitory interneurons (B5-I) in mice resulted in the development of skin lesions and scratching in mice [40]. B5-I interneurons are activated following certain transient receptor potential (TRP) channels signaling and release dynorphin that can block itch signaling [41]. Spinal interneurons that express neuropeptide Y also exist which mediate mechanical itch [42]. Cross-talk between neurons and central glia has also been suggested in modulating itch [43]. For example, in a mouse model of contact dermatitis and AD, spinal reactive astrogliosis has been reported [44]. Toll-like receptor 4 has been found to contribute to this type of astrogliosis in a dry skin mouse model of itch [45]. Apart from astrocytes activation, spinal microglial activation has also been found in mouse models; for example, after intradermal injection of compound 48/80 (histamine-dependent) and 5′-guanidinonaltrindole [46]. Microglial activation can be subsided by intrathecal minocycline (a microglial modulator) which can reduce scratching and symptoms of dermatitis in a mouse model of AD [47].

In short, identification of peripheral and central components of itch [17,38] has pushed the field forward for novel and effective targeting. Several established models of itch exist which are applicable in both animals and humans. These models are useful in understanding itch pathways and also in testing novel antipruritics [48]. Many compounds are in early stages of development and several are going through final phases of antipruritic pipelines.

BoNTs were initially used for muscle hyperactivity [49]. Soon after the identification of broader biological effects (e.g., neuronal and non-neuronal effects in dermal fibroblasts, sebocytes and vascular endothelial cells), additional indications garnered attention and further mechanisms underlying BoNTs effects were proposed [50,51]. The antipruritic effect of Botulinum Toxin Type A (BoNTA) was identified in an open-label pilot study of lichen simplex in 2002 [52]. Its antipruritic effect in dyshidrotic hand dermatitis was also reported in the same year [53,54]. Since then [6], BoNTs have been subjected to investigation for many other pruritic conditions, such as Hailey-Hailey disease and inversed psoriasis. First, one must understand how BoNTs can exert potential effects against itch. An acceptable rationale for application of BoNTs in itch is that acetylcholine mediates itch and BoNTA inhibits the release of acetylcholine from presynaptic vesicles. However, other mechanisms also play a role in antipruritic effects of BoNTs. In the section below, proposed underlying mechanisms of BoNTs in reducing itch are described. Since botulinum toxin type A (BoNTA) is the most used in the current literature, the rest of this manuscript focuses on this neurotoxin unless otherwise stated.

3. Botulinum Toxin Type A (BoNTA)

BoNTA inhibits vesicular release of neurotransmitters by interfering with exocytotic release. BoNTA is composed of a heavy chain with a receptor-binding site and a translocation domain as well as a light chain with endopeptidase activity. This permits cleavage of synaptosomal-associated protein 25 (SNAP-25) which is an essential molecule for membrane fusion [55]. BoNTA was first known to block acetylcholine release at the neuromuscular junction [56]. It has been used for disorders with abnormal muscle contraction because of its ability to relax spastic muscles [49]. However, it became evident that BoNTA also inhibits the release of other transmitters, such as glutamate, substance P (SP), and calcitonin gene-related peptide (CGRP) [57]. The anti-itch effect of BoNTA is also a result of inhibition of acetylcholine release and other mediators involved in itch [8,9]. As such, evidence from analgesic properties of BoNTs in pain and nociception have also been inspirational for scientists [58–64].

4. Experimental Evidence for Antipruritic Effects of BoNTA in Healthy Humans

Our group was first to investigate the effect of subcutaneous administration of BoNTA on experimentally induced itch (histamine) in healthy subjects. Fourteen healthy men received BoNTA (5U, BOTOX®, Allergan, NJ, USA) on the volar forearm. Saline was used as control. Histamine prick tests were performed at the application sites before, one, three days, and a week after treatments. Itch intensity and neurogenic inflammation were evaluated. BoNTA significantly reduced histamine-evoked itch intensity, flare size, and vasomotor reactions to histamine [65].

Another study in healthy volunteers looked into the antipruritic effects of BoNTA in a non-histaminergic model where cowhage was used (clinicaltrials.gov; identifier: NCT02639052). In this study, 35 healthy subjects (16 men and 19 women; age 26.8 ± 6.8 years) were enrolled and intradermal BoNTA (10U, BOTOX®, Allergan, NJ, USA) was injected in a 4 × 4 cm area on volar arms. Saline was used as control. Itch intensity following application of cowhage was recorded before treatment and one week, one month, and three months post-treatment. BoNTA reduced cowhage-evoked itch at all time points, suggesting a long-lasting effect. This study was presented at the 9th World Congress on Itch [66].

5. Experimental Evidence for Antipruritic Effects of BoNTA in Animal Models

Animal studies have also been conducted to look deeper into the cellular-molecular mechanism(s) of antipruritic effects of BoNTA.

It is generally accepted that TRPV1 (transient receptor potential cation channel subfamily V member 1) is essential for histamine-dependent itch [31], whereas TRPA1 (transient receptor potential ankyrin 1) is required for histamine-independent itch, e.g., chloroquine-evoked itch, bile acids-induced cholestatic itch [67], and oxidative stress-induced itch [68,69]. A mice study [70] has investigated the effects of BoNTA on acute and chronic itch and the possible association of TRP channels to antipruritic mechanisms of BoNTA. Findings from this study demonstrated that BoNTA inhibited chloroquine-evoked itch which is considered an acute non-histaminergic model similar to that of compound 48/80-induced itch. Compound 48/80 is a potent histamine-releasing agent, primarily from mast cells, with a subsequent depletion of tissue histamine [71]. It was also presented that, following a single intradermal injection of BoNTA (0.1 U) into the nape of the neck, mRNA expression of TRPV1 and TRPA1 notably decreased in DRG and lasted for seven days. Protein expression of TRPA1 was highly elevated following AEW (acetone–diethylether–water) treatment—a dry skin itch model—and pretreatment with BoNTA could significantly abolish upregulation of TRPA1 expression in this model. Authors proposed that TRPV1 and TRPA1 play an important role in both acute and chronic itch and that BoNTA might exert its anti-itch effects through downregulated expression of TPRV1 and TPRA1 in DRG [70]. This study confirmed that antipruritic effects of BoNTA present independently of mice models and can be used both for histamine-dependent and histamine-independent itch and dry skin-induced chronic itch [70].

Another study studied AD in mice models [72]. AD is accompanied by debilitating itch and a complex interaction is believed to exist between immune cells and nerve fibers [73]. NC/Nga mouse is a relevant animal model to study AD [74] because these animals spontaneously develop AD-like skin lesions under conventional conditions. In this study [72], the authors examined the protective effect of BoNTA (intradermal injection on the rostral back) on AD lesions in NC/Nga mouse. The primary outcome was skin thickness and transepidermal water loss. Authors assessed skin thickness, water loss, skin severity scores, histological alterations of skin, e.g., mast cell count, skin interleukin (IL)-4 mRNA and protein expression, and total serum IgE levels [72].This study showed that BoNTA could significantly suppress AD severity, IL-4 expression level, and the number of infiltrating mast cells [72]. Study period was limited to 14 days and long-term effects were not investigated.

The effects of BoNTA on mast cell activity has also been studied in animal models [75,76]. In a study by Park [75], 10 Sprague Dawley rats were randomly divided into two groups receiving BoNT A and vehicle (control). A distally based 3 × 9 cm random pattern flap including the panniculus carnosus muscle was elevated. BoNTA was administered five days prior to flap elevation. Seven days after flap elevation, tissue samples (1 × 1 cm) were taken from the center of each flap. Findings [75] demonstrated that BoNTA decreased mast cell activity.

Another animal study looked into the mechanisms of BoNTA in targeting psoriasis. In a KC-Tie2 mouse model of psoriasis [77], researchers showed that intradermal injection of BoNTA improved psoriasiform skin inflammation and epidermal hyperplasia. It also decreased the number of infiltrating $CD4^+$ T cells and $CD11c^+$ dendritic cells (DCs) in parallel with reducing the number of blood vessels and their adjacent nerves [77]. The decreased number of blood vessels within the affected skin of the treated mice illustrates the role of nerves and blood vessels in an inflammatory skin disease such as psoriasis. This study illustrates the role of blood vessel and nerve communication in psoriasis and the potential role of BoNTA in blocking this communication. Authors proposed that the persistence of some plaques in psoriasis patients might be explained by local microenvironments within the tissue, including nerve-derived SP and CGRP [77]. BoNTA, a known inhibitor of CGRP and SP release, can help with the interruption of this cascade and may present significant improvement in disease severity as early as two weeks after treatment. Therefore, they proposed that BoNTA may serve as a supplemental agent to topical or biologic therapeutic regimens [77].

6. Clinical Evidence for Antipruritic Effects of BoNTs

BoNTs have been used in clinics for many dermatological conditions that can present with or without itch. For a review, see A. Campanati et al., Y.S. Kim et al., and A.S. Al-Ghamdi et al. [7,8,78]. A recent review has summarized the use of intradermal BoNTA in treating chronic refractory pruritus based on 11 studies between 1996 and 2016 [79].

Many applications are still off-label [7] and the cases presented below both summarize current clinical evidence and encourage additional well-designed studies to reach a consensus on safe applicability, optimal dose, and delivery route for the standardization of BoNTs use for antipruritic effects.

6.1. Post Herpetic Itch

Post herpetic itch (PHI) is considered a type of neuropathic itch and has been investigated less than postherpetic neuralgia (PHN) [80]. PHN is a long-term neuropathic pain that remains after the rash from shingles (also known as herpes zoster) has healed. Varicella-zoster virus (VZV) is the cause of herpes zoster. Besides shingles, degenerative nerve root compression (notalgia paresthetica), and sensory polyneuropathy can cause neuropathic itch [81]. Almost half of PHN patients report PHI. This finding suggests that mechanisms underlying PHI and PHN are most likely independent [82]. PHI is a common disorder that equally affects men and women. PHI is age-independent and occurs in both young and old patients. PHI often appears on the head and neck (V1 dermatome) [82].

BoNTA treatment has been successful to reverse pain in PHN [83]. Accordingly, the usefulness of BoNTA in PHI has been considered [84] and the effectiveness of BoNTA for a neuropathic itch caused by dermatomal damage to the thoracic nerves has been presented [84]. In this study, BoNTA injections (dose range 16–25 U) were given in several points within the involved dermatome. Double-blind, randomized, control trials are required in a larger sample size before the use of BoNTA in different types of neuropathic itch such as PHI can be considered. BoNTs could be considered in severe cases of intractable PHI, which are not responsive to other options [80].

6.2. Brachioradial Pruritus

Brachioradial pruritus (BRP) was first described in Florida in 1968 by Waisman [85] and is classified as a deep itch of the forearms and upper trunk which can worsen with either scratching or sunlight [86]. Brachioradial pruritus is considered another neurogenic itch which often occurs in the upper extremities, usually localized on the dorsolateral forearm overlying the proximal head of the brachioradialis muscle; however, upper arms and shoulders may also be affected [87,88]. BRP might be unilateral or bilateral and it is still considered a common "tropical" dermopathy [89]. It is still not known if BRP is a symptom of neuropathy, similar to chronic cervical radiculopathy, or a condition that occurs secondary to chronic ultraviolet damage. Larger studies for better understanding of BRP are warranted. BRP responds to ice packs but efficacy is only temporary [90]. Lamotrigine and gabapentin have also been found useful for BRP. Intradermal injections of BoNTA (100 IU) was reported in a 59-year-old Caucasian female with BRP for 12 years [86]. This patient had disabling itch and a burning sensation on the upper posterior arms, scapular regions, and neck. A diverse range of topical and systemic treatments, hypnotherapy, and Chinese herbal medicine did not improve the patient's condition. Application of icepacks was not beneficial in this case. However, this patient reported dramatic itch relief, lasting for up to six months, after four rounds of BoNTA injections. It was proposed that the effect of BoNTs for this condition and those similar to it, may have been due in part to its ability to block the release of neurotransmitters involved in itch, e.g., acetylcholine.

6.3. Notalgia Paresthetica

Notalgia paresthetica (NP) [91,92] is a sensory neuropathic syndrome with pruritus, pain, paresthesia, hypo-hyper-esthesia, and burning as common symptoms. NP is characterized by a brownish itchy patch in the affected area. This condition mainly occurs in the elderly or in association with musculoskeletal disorders driven by spinal nerve compression, particularly at the C4–C6 level [92]. NP is a difficult condition to treat and quality of life is rather low in these patients. Less efficient treatments for NP are partially attributable to its unidentified underlying mechanisms or pathogenesis.

In 2007, two NP patients were treated with BoNTA [84]. Later in 2010, Wallengren and Bartosik [93] reported limited effectiveness of BoNTA treatment in six NP patients. One double-blind randomized clinical trial for NP was reported in 2014 [94], in which the effectiveness of BoNTA was tested in 20 NP patients who were resistant to topical therapies. The study investigated pruritus, effects on hyperpigmentation, and global effectiveness as rated by both patients and investigators. Pruritus rated on VAS (visual analogue scale) did not show any itch reduction when it was compared between patients and controls (receiving saline) [94]. BoNTA treatment also did not improve hyperpigmentation or global efficacy indicators. In this study, injections of 0.1 mL (50 U/mL) for every 1–2 cm^2 of hyperpigmented area were given. Maximum dose reached to 200 U [94].

Injection of BoNTA is an option, but further research is required to confirm safety and efficacy of BoNTA for NP. Patient selection and dose also need to be determined.

6.4. Lichen Simplex Chronicus (LSC)

Lichen simplex chronicus (LSC) is also known as neurodermatitis circumscripta. LSC is an eczematous dermatosis, characterized by intense localized pruritus and thickening of the skin with variable scaling arising secondarily from repetitive scratching or rubbing. This condition can be intense or recurrent and often disrupts sleep, sexual function, and quality of life in affected individuals. Breaking the itch-scratch cycle is challenging. Exact incidence in general population is unknown, but one study demonstrated that 12% of aging patients with pruritic skin presented with LSC [95]. This disorder is observed more commonly in females than in males. BoNTA has been considered an option for LSC [52]. One pilot study investigated the effect of intradermal injection of Abobotulinumtoxin A in five lesions in three patients and found that pruritus diminished within three to seven days in all patients. By four weeks, all lesions had cleared completely with no recurrences [96]. Another case study reported a successful result with BoNTA in a 55-year-old woman with a six-year history of intense facial pruritus at the right side of face [97]. Despite the small sizes of these studies, the antipruritic effects of BoNTA in LSC is promising [78]; however, additional large studies are required to confirm its efficacy in LSC.

6.5. Vulvodynia

Vulvodynia is a complex disorder [98] affecting 16% of women in the general population. It is described by burning, stinging, itching, irritation, or rawness. The International Society for the Study of Vulvovaginal Disease (ISSVD) has defined vulvodynia as "vulvar pain occurring in the absence of an underlying recognizable disease." There are no clinical or histopathologic criteria for the diagnosis other than consideration and careful evaluation to exclude other causes of pain. Successful therapy often requires a multidisciplinary approach with more than one type of therapeutic intervention. BoNTA has been shown to be effective treatment for vulvodynia [99]. While several small open-label studies have shown improvement in symptoms with botulinum toxin at doses of 20–100 units, the only randomized double-blind, placebo-controlled trial demonstrated no improvement with 20 units over placebo in 64 women with vulvodynia [100].

6.6. Keloids and Hypertrophic Scars

Keloids and hypertrophic scars are structures formed during the wound healing process and present with dysregulated growth and a high level of collagen formation. To prevent these scars, silicone dressings, laser therapy, and immune response modulators are applied [101]. Intralesional (IL) corticosteroid therapy with triamcinolone acetonide is a common therapy in keloids treatment [102]. In 2000, Gassner and colleagues [103] suggested that BoNTA injections can paralyze muscles close to wounds and subsequently reduce pressure on wound edges. This first study was conducted in a primate model and confirmed the hypothesis. Another study used optical 3D profilometry as an objective evaluation of keloids following treatment by BoNTA [104]. Only four patients were included in this study and no changes was evident on fibroblast proliferation. In a rabbit ear hypertrophic scar model [105], BoNTA also was found to have less effect on hypertrophic index, fibroblast density, and collagen density when it was compared with IL triamcinolone acetonide and 5-fluorouracil [106]. However, other in vitro and experimental animal models support BoNTA as treatment of keloids and scars [107]. BoNTA delays fibroblast growth through the inhibition of the cell cycle which subsequently reduces hypertrophic scar development. BoNTA also decreases the expression of connective tissue growth factor and inhibits the growth of fibroblasts and scar expansion. BoNTA reduces the concentration of TGF-β1 in fibroblasts and decreases the infiltration of inflammatory cells during wound healing; it also reduces fibrosis [107].

In 2015, a large randomized double-blind study tested the effect of BoNTA compared with IL corticosteroid therapy in 24 patients with keloids [108]. In this study, patients were allocated to receive IL steroid every four weeks for six sessions and IL BoNTA 5 IU/cm every eight weeks for three sessions. Hardness, elevation, and redness, together with itching, pain, and tenderness were evaluated and patients were asked for their subjective satisfaction. No significant difference was observed between groups in most of the measured parameters. However, patients receiving BoNTA reported higher satisfaction with their therapy. Authors proposed that BoNTA might have reduced small-fiber neuropathy causing itching, pain, and allodynia [108].

A potential use for BoNTA in keloids and hypertrophic scars is predicted. But additional randomized double-blind controlled trials are needed to compare with current treatments to evaluate efficacy and safety profile. Efficacy in the prevention and treatment of hypertrophic scars might vary according to the scar's location on the body; hence, testing both facial and other body parts such as chest or back is proposed. Surgical and trauma wounds must also be differentiated. In addition, stratification according to ethnicity and age is essential as both elements affect wound healing.

6.7. Psoriasis

Psoriasis is a skin disorder strongly linked to both genetic and environmental factors. An immunological reaction mediated by T lymphocytes is thought to be the main player in the pathogenesis of psoriasis. Cutaneous inflammation and keratinocyte hyperproliferation are featured characteristics of such a response.

Inverse or flexural psoriasis is a specific form of psoriasis with red, dry, smooth, and shiny skin. Clinically, inverse psoriasis manifests with sharply demarcated erythematous plaques with infiltration that accompany sensations of itching and burning. Common locations of inverse psoriasis include armpits, groin, under the breasts, and in other flexion skin folds, such as around the genitals and buttocks. It is particularly troublesome for patients with deep skin folds and/or those who are overweight. Treatment of inverse psoriasis can be difficult. Steroid creams and ointments are considered effective; however, overuse of steroids can result in side effects, especially thinning of the skin and stretch marks. Skin folds, where inverse psoriasis is common, are susceptible to yeast and fungal infections. Topical immunomodulators, such as tacrolimus and pimecrolimus, have also been effective.

Administration of BoNTA has been proposed as a novel therapy in inverse psoriasis [109,110] in consideration of its mechanism of action in the neuroglandular junction, which reduces sweating. However, a link between high nerve fiber density in psoriatic skin and elevated CGRP and SP release has been reported. It has been demonstrated that psoriasis undergoes remission phases as a result of innervation loss or lack of nerve function, such as following a nerve injury. This can explain how BoNTA inhibits CGRP and SP release from nerve endings and can lead to subjective reports of improvement after administration of BoNTA.

Zanchi and colleagues [109] reported that in 15 patients with inverse psoriasis, BoNTA presented effectiveness; however, the effect was mainly evaluated by self-assessment in patients rating itch and pain on a visual analogue scale (VAS). In this study, psoriasis that was located in the armpits, submammary sulcus, intergluteal folds, inguinal folds, and umbilicus in patients was treated with BoNTA injections with a total dose of 50–100 U per patient relative to psoriasis extent and severity. Evaluations were performed before and after treatment in weeks 2, 4, and 12. The erythematous area was defined using objective photographic evidence and subjective patient assessment of pain and itch was assessed using a 10-point VAS. BoNTA therapy resulted in improvements in subjective patient symptomatology and objective reductions in erythema and maceration in the treated areas according to photographic evidence. However, findings from this study were questioned [111], pointing to the lack of quantitative assessment for improvement; for example, using psoriasis area and severity index (PASI) or obtaining histological evident before and after the treatment.

Overall, current evidence demonstrates that BoNTA is capable of reducing pain, itch, and inflammation in psoriasis-affected skin. Dermal and epidermal cytokines and peptides produced by keratinocytes, fibroblasts, lymphocytes, and macrophages are involved in the pathogenesis of psoriasis. Interleukin-1 (IL-1) stimulates the proliferation of keratinocytes and the production of cellular adhesion molecules which then stimulate the release of other cytokines (e.g., IL-6, IL-8). IL-6 stimulates the proliferation of B and T lymphocytes, which is an important factor in stimulating keratinocyte growth, and IL-8 exerts a powerful chemotaxis action towards leucocytes. In future randomized clinical trials evaluating the potential role of BoNTA in the treatment of psoriasis, special attention needs to be given to psoriasis as a variable pathology with several spontaneous relapses and remissions over time which can cause difficulties in evaluation of effectiveness. Amount and depth of injection are yet to be determined. Assessment of effectiveness must include both subjective and objective parameters including cutaneous sensory, vasomotor, and autonomic function. Safety, tolerability, and cost effectiveness should also be carefully evaluated before considering BoNTA as a routine clinical practice.

6.8. Pompholyx

Dyshidrotic eczema, also called pompholyx, is a common relapsing vesicular-bullous disease found on the palm or soles of feet [112]. The pathogenesis of this condition is still unresolved; however, one study examined the roles of aquaporin 3 and aquaporin 10, which are water channel proteins located in the epidermis, and concluded that overexpression of these channels may play a role [113]. Wet works, sweating, and occlusion are among the provoking factors. Pain, itch, and burning sensations together with discomfort in wearing gloves or shoes, bacterial infection, or mycosis are among the common symptoms.

An improvement in hand eczema was observed in patients with palmar hyperhidrosis following intradermal BoNTA [53]. This study was conducted in 10 patients with bilateral vesicular hand dermatitis where BoNTA injections (100 U BOTOX®) or saline (control) were given in either hand. Seven out of the 10 patients reported a good or very good effect of the treatment. Another study [54] applied topical corticosteroids on both hands in combination with intracutaneous injections of BoNTA (100 U BOTOX®) in six patients with more severely affected hands. A rapid improvement in pruritus and vesiculation was observed in the treated hand with combination therapy. A case study [114] has also demonstrated BoNTA effects in palmar pompholyx. No placebo-controlled trial is available. Therefore, effective and safe application of BoNTA for dyshidrotic eczema requires further validation.

6.9. Postburn Itch

Itching is a common secondary symptom related to burn injuries [115]. Research has proposed multiple mechanisms underlying itch as secondary to burn conditions. Several medications have been identified and used to manage this condition. BoNTA has also been considered as an option. In 2012, a study was conducted [116] to investigate the effectiveness of BoNTA and found that 87.5% of patients rated their postburn itch as severe (>7). Following the administration of BoNTA, itch intensity dropped to zero within four weeks. The average duration of the symptom-free period was nine months (range 3–18 months). BoNTA might be an option for burn-associated itch which are resistant to conventional therapies. This study [116] only included a small sample size and larger studies are warranted before establishment of this treatment at clinic.

6.10. Fox–Fordyce Disease

Fox–Fordyce disease (FFD), characterized by intensely pruritic papules in apocrine gland-bearing regions, is a rare disorder for which there is currently no definitive treatment or known cure [117]. FFD is a chronic, pruritic disorder caused by keratin plugging of the follicular infundibulum at the distal portion of the apocrine sweat duct and less often by plugging of apoeccrine ducts. This obstruction causes apocrine sweat retention and, over time, rupture of glands with secondary inflammatory dermal alterations. The etiology remains unclear although epidemiological data support a hormonal component, as women between 15 and 35 years of age are more commonly affected and this condition may remit after menopause.

The condition is often intensely pruritic and is usually associated with hypohidrosis. Pruritus is aggravated by emotional, physical, or pharmacological stimulations that enhance sweating. Therapeutic knowledge of FFD is derived from case reports but no large case series has been carried out. Topical and intralesional corticosteroids are often a first-line therapy. In medication-refractory cases, surgical interventions have proven to be successful. A case has been presented in which BoNTA injections resulted in the disappearance of pruritus and a partial clinical response after one session [117]. This response was sustained over time. The study's authors suggested that chemodenervation of cholinergic nerve terminals to the eccrine and apoeccrine glands, inhibiting their sweat secretion, might be considered as underlying mechanism for the effects seen in this case. Other cases of hyperhidrotic pruritic axillary granular parakeratosis responders to BoNTA have also been reported [118]. Clinical trials to evaluate optimal treatment regimen with BoNTA for FFD are required.

6.11. Hailey-Hailey Disease

Hailey-Hailey disease (familial benign pemphigus) is a rare genetic skin disease, often presented with blisters or vesicles and erythematous plaques in skin folds. Axilla, groin, neck, and inframammary folds are amongst the most common sites of disease manifestation. The disease's associated red scaly areas can be itchy. The topical and oral corticosteroids, oral retinoid, cyclosporine, and methotrexate used for treatment are often linked to side effects. There are cases of Hailey-Hailey disease treated with BoNTA with successful outcome [119,120]. Reduced sweating and local irritation help to improve lesions conditions as well as a reduction in itch. BoNTA can potentially be considered as a treatment option, in particular for those patients with limited response or intolerance to other treatments [120].

6.12. Rhinitis

Rhinitis is an inflammation of the nasal mucous membranes, presented with nasal discharge, nasal obstruction, sneezing, and itching [121,122]. It is a common disease affecting around 20% of general population and can be divided into infectious, allergic, occupational, drug-induced, hormonal, and idiopathic rhinitis (IR). The latter is also known as non-allergic, noninfectious perennial rhinitis, intrinsic, or vasomotor rhinitis. BoNTs have been used in both allergic [123] and idiopathic rhinitis (IR) [124,125].

Allergic rhinitis (AR) is a noninfectious inflammatory disorder in nasal mucosa provoked by an allergen exposure and an IgE-mediated immune response. The major mediator of nasal inflammation in AR is histamine which causes symptoms such as vascular permeability, mucus secretion, and stimulation of the sensory nerve fibers. Other mediators involved are neurokinin A, SP, CGRP, VIP, and neurotrophins. Current treatments include intranasal corticosteroids, antihistamines, mast cell stabilizers, and leukotriene receptor antagonists. AR can benefit from BoNTA injection, when it is given intranasally [124]. No serious adverse or systemic effects have been noted but burning after injection, nasal dryness, and epistaxis have been recorded. Nasal injection of BoNTA has shown comparable therapeutic effect to cetirizine in AR [126]. Arguments for the use of BoNTA in rhinitis are grounded in its modulatory effect on the secretory tone, which is related to the action of autonomic nervous system. A similar rationale has been used for the positive effects of BoNTA in Frey syndrome, hyperhidrosis, and sialorrhea. AR's symptoms result from the activation of inflammatory mediators and an imbalance in the autonomic nervous system. Histamine, prostaglandin, and leukotrienes enhance vascular permeability and produce edema, in addition to altering the balance of the autonomic nervous system [127]. Underlying mechanisms of IR remain to be elucidated; however, autonomic nervous system imbalance with a dominant parasympathetic tone in the nasal mucosa has been proposed. Nasal blockage and rhinorrhea are more common in IR, while itching and sneezing are mostly present in AR. All symptoms can be prevented by application of BoNTA.

Several other mechanisms for BoNTA effect in nasal mucosa have been proposed [124]. For example, BoNTA can induce apoptosis in the nasal glands, inhibit acetylcholine release from nasal mucosa nerve endings, decrease the release of neuropeptides (e.g., VIP and SP) from the trigeminal and parasympathetic nerve endings, and inhibit acetylcholine release from preganglionic cholinergic nerve endings in the sphenopalatine ganglion. As such, it has been suggested that targeting an upstream source of parasympathetic innervation at the sphenopalatine ganglion can potentially affect both nasal mucosa and nasal glands to yield an additive effect from the intraganglionic injection. A study proposed a technique to inject BoNTA into the posterior lateral nasal wall, which is located adjacent to the sphenopalatine ganglion. They conducted a pilot study with this technique applying a low dose of 25 units, resulting in only moderate discomfort to participants but yielding safe and effective results. Improved effects on congestion and itch had already been seen with dosages above 12 units. Accordingly, the authors suggested that low dose administration of BoNTA can be advantageous from a safety perspective.

BoNTA also may be considered in patients resistant to other treatments or intolerant to current treatments, e.g., nasal corticosteroids or systemic antihistamines. This treatment also allows for longer lasting effects, beneficial for patients. However, larger studies are required to identify the long-term effects and safety profile of BoNTA [126]. Further investigation is needed to identify whether BoNTA is to be used in clinic for rhinitis and which technique would yield the optimal outcome (e.g., posterior injection, turbinate injection, septal injection, or topical) [128]. RT001 is a novel topical gel formulation which contains a purified 150kDa BoNTA protein that has been used in a rat model [129]. The gel formula includes a prietary peptide to enhance transcutaneous and transmucosal flux of BoNTA. In the model, after a single intranasal administration of RT001, associated clinical signs of rhinitis, including inflammation, were significantly resolved within 5 days after treatment.

The optimal dose and patient selection also need to be determined. In addition, it is still unclear whether and how repetitive administration of BoNTA would influence the outcome. Desensitization following repeated application is still an open question. Another important point is that some outcome measures are difficult to be objectified, for instance, nasal pruritus. Hence, analyzing effectiveness calls for the development of some objective methods to complement existing subjective instruments.

7. Concluding Remarks and Future Perspectives

This review highlighted the potential for BoNTs with a major focus on BoNTA to relieve pruritus. A lack of a sufficient number of randomized controlled trials, limited sample size in the current literature, diverse range of outcome measures, and a lack of knowledge about placebo effects make it difficult to draw a firm conclusion on the antipruritic effects of BoNTs. In addition, for each condition, several critical components remain unidentified, including safe and effective dosage, route of delivery (also considering new formulations of BoNTs), single versus repeated application with optimal interval, and standardization of techniques used in outcome measures. In addition, a strategy for patient selection and precise identification of responders in terms of gender, age, and ethnic background would substantially aid in targeting the right group for optimal effect. The long-lasting effects of BoNTs make it desirable in terms of patients' compliance. However, measured use must also be considered in terms of cost and comparable effectiveness with other agents available for each pruritus condition. Most of the studies presented in the literature have suggested BoNTA as an option; however, not as a first-line therapy and predominantly for those patients either who are having recurrent problems or who are non-responders to other treatment options. It is likely only a matter of time before the full potential of BoNTs for pruritus is elucidated. However, for the time being, focus should be on more common conditions or those for which stronger evidence exists for successful use of BoNTs can be on those conditions that are more common and stronger evidence exist in the literature for successful use of BoNTs.

Conflicts of Interest: The author has no relevant affiliations or financial involvement with any organization or entity with a financial interest in or financial conflict with the subject matter or materials discussed in this manuscript. No writing assistance was utilized in the production of this manuscript.

References

1. Brin, M.F. Botulinum toxin: Chemistry, pharmacology, toxicity, and immunology. *Muscle Nerve Suppl.* **1997**, *6*, S146–S168. [CrossRef]
2. Pirazzini, M.; Rossetto, O.; Eleopra, R.; Montecucco, C. Botulinum neurotoxins: Biology, pharmacology, and toxicology. *Pharmacol. Rev.* **2017**, *69*, 200–235. [CrossRef] [PubMed]
3. Scott, A.B. Botulinum toxin injection into extraocular muscles as an alternative to strabismus surgery. *Ophthalmology* **1980**, *87*, 1044–1049. [CrossRef]
4. Dressler, D. Clinical applications of botulinum toxin. *Curr. Opin. Microbiol.* **2012**, *15*, 325–336. [CrossRef] [PubMed]
5. Luvisetto, S.; Gazerani, P.; Cianchetti, C.; Pavone, F. Botulinum toxin type a as a therapeutic agent against headache and related disorders. *Toxins* **2015**, *7*, 3818–3844. [CrossRef] [PubMed]
6. Wollina, U. Botulinum toxin: Non-cosmetic indications and possible mechanisms of action. *J. Cutan. Aesthet. Surg.* **2008**, *1*, 3–6. [CrossRef] [PubMed]
7. Campanati, A.; Martina, E.; Giuliodori, K.; Consales, V.; Bobyr, I.; Offidani, A. Botulinum toxin off-label use in dermatology: A review. *Skin Appendage Disord.* **2017**, *3*, 39–56. [CrossRef] [PubMed]
8. Kim, Y.S.; Hong, E.S.; Kim, H.S. Botulinum toxin in the field of dermatology: Novel indications. *Toxins* **2017**, *9*, 403. [CrossRef]
9. Ho, D.; Jagdeo, J. Pruritus associated with onabotulinumtoxina treatment of neuromuscular pain. *J. Drugs Dermatol.* **2015**, *14*, 199–200. [PubMed]
10. Ikoma, A.; Steinhoff, M.; Stander, S.; Yosipovitch, G.; Schmelz, M. The neurobiology of itch. *Nat. Rev. Neurosci.* **2006**, *7*, 535–547. [CrossRef] [PubMed]
11. Green, D.; Dong, X. The cell biology of acute itch. *J. Cell Biol.* **2016**, *213*, 155–161. [CrossRef] [PubMed]
12. Grundmann, S.; Stander, S. Chronic pruritus: Clinics and treatment. *Ann. Dermatol.* **2011**, *23*, 1–11. [CrossRef] [PubMed]
13. Stander, S.; Weisshaar, E.; Mettang, T.; Szepietowski, J.C.; Carstens, E.; Ikoma, A.; Bergasa, N.V.; Gieler, U.; Misery, L.; Wallengren, J.; et al. Clinical classification of itch: A position paper of the international forum for the study of itch. *Acta Derm. Venereol.* **2007**, *87*, 291–294. [CrossRef] [PubMed]

14. Kini, S.P.; DeLong, L.K.; Veledar, E.; McKenzie-Brown, A.M.; Schaufele, M.; Chen, S.C. The impact of pruritus on quality of life the skin equivalent of pain. *Arch. Dermatol.* **2011**, *147*, 1153–1156. [CrossRef] [PubMed]
15. Carr, C.W.; Veledar, E.; Chen, S.C. Factors mediating the impact of chronic pruritus on quality of life. *JAMA Dermatol.* **2014**, *150*, 613–620. [CrossRef] [PubMed]
16. Stander, S.; Zeidler, C.; Magnolo, N.; Raap, U.; Mettang, T.; Kremer, A.E.; Weisshaar, E.; Augustin, M. Clinical management of pruritus. *J. Dtsch. Dermatol. Ges.* **2015**, *13*, 101–115. [CrossRef] [PubMed]
17. Lee, J.S.; Han, J.S.; Lee, K.; Bang, J.; Lee, H. The peripheral and central mechanisms underlying itch. *BMB Rep.* **2016**, *49*, 474–487. [CrossRef] [PubMed]
18. LaMotte, R.H.; Dong, X.Z.; Ringkamp, M. Sensory neurons and circuits mediating itch. *Nat. Rev. Neurosci.* **2014**, *15*, 19–31. [CrossRef] [PubMed]
19. Bell, J.K.; McQueen, D.S.; Rees, J.L. Involvement of histamine h4 and h1 receptors in scratching induced by histamine receptor agonists in balb c mice. *Br. J. Pharmacol.* **2004**, *142*, 374–380. [CrossRef] [PubMed]
20. Strasser, A.; Wittmann, H.J.; Buschauer, A.; Schneider, E.H.; Seifert, R. Species-dependent activities of g-protein-coupled receptor ligands: Lessons from histamine receptor orthologs. *Trends Pharmacol. Sci.* **2013**, *34*, 13–32. [CrossRef] [PubMed]
21. Akiyama, T.; Carstens, E. Neural processing of itch. *Neuroscience* **2013**, *250*, 697–714. [CrossRef] [PubMed]
22. Nystedt, S.; Emilsson, I.E.; Wahlestedt, C.; Sundelin, J. Molecular-cloning of a potential proteinase activated receptor. *Proc. Natl. Acad. Sci. USA* **1994**, *91*, 9208–9212. [CrossRef] [PubMed]
23. Steinhoff, M.; Neisius, U.; Ikoma, A.; Fartasch, M.; Heyer, G.; Skov, P.S.; Luger, T.A.; Schmelz, M. Proteinase-activated receptor-2 mediates itch: A novel pathway for pruritus in human skin. *Exp. Dermatol.* **2004**, *13*, 529–591. [CrossRef]
24. Liu, Q.; Dong, X. The role of the mrgpr receptor family in itch. *Handb. Exp. Pharmacol.* **2015**, *226*, 71–88. [PubMed]
25. Han, L.; Ma, C.; Liu, Q.; Weng, H.J.; Cui, Y.; Tang, Z.; Kim, Y.; Nie, H.; Qu, L.; Patel, K.N.; et al. A subpopulation of nociceptors specifically linked to itch. *Nat. Neurosci.* **2013**, *16*, 174–182. [CrossRef] [PubMed]
26. Liu, Q.; Tang, Z.; Surdenikova, L.; Kim, S.; Patel, K.N.; Kim, A.; Ru, F.; Guan, Y.; Weng, H.J.; Geng, Y.; et al. Sensory neuron-specific gpcr mrgprs are itch receptors mediating chloroquine-induced pruritus. *Cell* **2009**, *139*, 1353–1365. [CrossRef] [PubMed]
27. Lembo, P.M.; Grazzini, E.; Groblewski, T.; O'Donnell, D.; Roy, M.O.; Zhang, J.; Hoffert, C.; Cao, J.; Schmidt, R.; Pelletier, M.; et al. Proenkephalin a gene products activate a new family of sensory neuron-specific gpcrs. *Nat. Neurosci.* **2002**, *5*, 201–209. [CrossRef] [PubMed]
28. Sikand, P.; Dong, X.; LaMotte, R.H. Bam8-22 peptide produces itch and nociceptive sensations in humans independent of histamine release. *J. Neurosci.* **2011**, *31*, 7563–7567. [CrossRef] [PubMed]
29. Liu, Q.; Sikand, P.; Ma, C.; Tang, Z.; Han, L.; Li, Z.; Sun, S.; LaMotte, R.H.; Dong, X. Mechanisms of itch evoked by beta-alanine. *J. Neurosci.* **2012**, *32*, 14532–14537. [CrossRef] [PubMed]
30. Shinohara, T.; Harada, M.; Ogi, K.; Maruyama, M.; Fujii, R.; Tanaka, H.; Fukusumi, S.; Komatsu, H.; Hosoya, M.; Noguchi, Y.; et al. Identification of a g protein-coupled receptor specifically responsive to beta-alanine. *J. Biol. Chem.* **2004**, *279*, 23559–23564. [CrossRef] [PubMed]
31. Shim, W.S.; Tak, M.H.; Lee, M.H.; Kim, M.; Kim, M.; Koo, J.Y.; Lee, C.H.; Kim, M.; Oh, U. Trpv1 mediates histamine-induced itching via the activation of phospholipase a2 and 12-lipoxygenase. *J. Neurosci.* **2007**, *27*, 2331–2337. [CrossRef] [PubMed]
32. Gamper, N. Itchy channels and where to find them. *J. Physiol.-Lond.* **2017**, *595*, 3257–3259. [CrossRef] [PubMed]
33. Lee, J.H.; Park, C.K.; Chen, G.; Han, Q.J.; Xie, R.G.; Liu, T.; Ji, R.R.; Lee, S.Y. A monoclonal antibody that targets a na(v)1.7 channel voltage sensor for pain and itch relief. *Cell* **2014**, *157*, 1393–1404. [CrossRef] [PubMed]
34. Storan, E.R.; O'Gorman, S.M.; McDonald, I.D.; Steinhoff, M. Role of cytokines and chemokines in itch. *Handb. Exp. Pharmacol.* **2015**, *226*, 163–176. [PubMed]
35. Nattkemper, L.A.; Martinez-Escala, M.E.; Gelman, A.B.; Singer, E.M.; Rook, A.H.; Guitart, J.; Yosipovitch, G. Cutaneous t-cell lymphoma and pruritus: The expression of il-31 and its receptors in the skin. *Acta Derm. Venereol.* **2016**, *96*, 894–898. [CrossRef] [PubMed]

36. Arai, I.; Tsuji, M.; Takeda, H.; Akiyama, N.; Saito, S. A single dose of interleukin-31 (il-31) causes continuous itch-associated scratching behaviour in mice. *Exp. Dermatol.* **2013**, *22*, 669–671. [CrossRef] [PubMed]
37. Arai, I.; Tsuji, M.; Miyagawa, K.; Takeda, H.; Akiyama, N.; Saito, S. Repeated administration of il-31 upregulates il-31 receptor a (il-31ra) in dorsal root ganglia and causes severe itch-associated scratching behaviour in mice. *Exp. Dermatol.* **2015**, *24*, 75–78. [CrossRef] [PubMed]
38. Sanders, K.M.; Nattkemper, L.A.; Yosipovitch, G. Advances in understanding itching and scratching: A new era of targeted treatments. *F1000Res* **2016**, *5*. [CrossRef] [PubMed]
39. Sun, Y.G.; Chen, Z.F. A gastrin-releasing peptide receptor mediates the itch sensation in the spinal cord. *Nature* **2007**, *448*, 700–703. [CrossRef]
40. Ross, S.E.; Mardinly, A.R.; McCord, A.E.; Zurawski, J.; Cohen, S.; Jung, C.; Hu, L.; Mok, S.I.; Shah, A.; Savner, E.M.; et al. Loss of inhibitory interneurons in the dorsal spinal cord and elevated itch in bhlhb5 mutant mice. *Neuron* **2010**, *65*, 886–898. [CrossRef] [PubMed]
41. Kardon, A.P.; Polgar, E.; Hachisuka, J.; Snyder, L.M.; Cameron, D.; Savage, S.; Cai, X.Y.; Karnup, S.; Fan, C.R.; Hemenway, G.M.; et al. Dynorphin acts as a neuromodulator to inhibit itch in the dorsal horn of the spinal cord. *Neuron* **2014**, *82*, 573–586. [CrossRef] [PubMed]
42. Bourane, S.; Duan, B.; Koch, S.C.; Dalet, A.; Britz, O.; Garcia-Campmany, L.; Kim, E.; Cheng, L.Z.; Ghosh, A.; Ma, Q.F.; et al. Gate control of mechanical itch by a subpopulation of spinal cord interneurons. *Science* **2015**, *350*, 550–554. [CrossRef] [PubMed]
43. Andersen, H.H.; Arendt-Nielsen, L.; Gazerani, P. Glial cells are involved in itch processing. *Acta Derm. Venereol.* **2016**, *96*, 723–727. [CrossRef] [PubMed]
44. Shiratori-Hayashi, M.; Koga, K.; Tozaki-Saitoh, H.; Kohro, Y.; Toyonaga, H.; Yamaguchi, C.; Hasegawa, A.; Nakahara, T.; Hachisuka, J.; Akira, S.; et al. Stat3-dependent reactive astrogliosis in the spinal dorsal horn underlies chronic itch. *Nat. Med.* **2015**, *21*, 927–931. [CrossRef] [PubMed]
45. Liu, T.; Han, Q.J.; Chen, G.; Huang, Y.; Zhao, L.X.; Berta, T.; Gao, Y.J.; Ji, R.R. Toll-like receptor 4 contributes to chronic itch, alloknesis, and spinal astrocyte activation in male mice. *Pain* **2016**, *157*, 806–817. [CrossRef] [PubMed]
46. Zhang, Y.; Dun, S.L.; Chen, Y.H.; Luo, J.J.; Cowan, A.; Dun, N.J. Scratching activates microglia in the mouse spinal cord. *J. Neurosci. Res.* **2015**, *93*, 466–474. [CrossRef] [PubMed]
47. Torigoe, K.; Tominaga, M.; Ko, K.C.; Takahashi, N.; Matsuda, H.; Hayashi, R.; Ogawa, H.; Takamori, K. Intrathecal minocycline suppresses itch-related behavior and improves dermatitis in a mouse model of atopic dermatitis. *J. Investig. Dermatol.* **2016**, *136*, 879–881. [CrossRef] [PubMed]
48. Hoeck, E.A.; Marker, J.B.; Gazerani, P.; H, H.A.; Arendt-Nielsen, L. Preclinical and human surrogate models of itch. *Exp. Dermatol.* **2016**, *25*, 750–757. [CrossRef] [PubMed]
49. Chen, S. Clinical uses of botulinum neurotoxins: Current indications, limitations and future developments. *Toxins (Basel)* **2012**, *4*, 913–939. [CrossRef] [PubMed]
50. Silberstein, S.D.; Aoki, K.R. Botulinum toxin type A: Myths, facts, and current research. *Headache* **2003**, *43* (Suppl. 1), S1. [CrossRef]
51. Aoki, K.R. Review of a proposed mechanism for the antinociceptive action of botulinum toxin type A. *Neurotoxicology* **2005**, *26*, 785–793. [CrossRef] [PubMed]
52. Heckmann, M.; Heyer, G.; Brunner, B.; Plewig, G. Botulinum toxin type a injection in the treatment of lichen simplex: An open pilot study. *J. Am. Acad. Dermatol.* **2002**, *46*, 617–619. [CrossRef] [PubMed]
53. Swartling, C.; Naver, H.; Lindberg, M.; Anveden, I. Treatment of dyshidrotic hand dermatitis with intradermal botulinum toxin. *J. Am. Acad. Dermatol.* **2002**, *47*, 667–671. [CrossRef] [PubMed]
54. Wollina, U.; Karamfilov, T. Adjuvant botulinum toxin a in dyshidrotic hand eczema: A controlled prospective pilot study with left-right comparison. *J. Eur. Acad. Dermatol. Venereol.* **2002**, *16*, 40–42. [CrossRef] [PubMed]
55. Breidenbach, M.A.; Brunger, A.T. New insights into clostridial neurotoxin-snare interactions. *Trends Mol. Med.* **2005**, *11*, 377–381. [CrossRef] [PubMed]
56. Dressler, D.; Saberi, F.A. Botulinum toxin: Mechanisms of action. *Eur. Neurol.* **2005**, *53*, 3–9. [CrossRef] [PubMed]
57. Aoki, K.R. Evidence for antinociceptive activity of botulinum toxin type a in pain management. *Headache* **2003**, *43* (Suppl. 1), S9–S15. [CrossRef] [PubMed]

58. Da Silva, L.B.; Karshenas, A.; Bach, F.W.; Rasmussen, S.; Arendt-Nielsen, L.; Gazerani, P. Blockade of glutamate release by botulinum neurotoxin type a in humans: A dermal microdialysis study. *Pain Res. Manag.* **2014**, *19*, 126–132. [CrossRef]
59. Gazerani, P.; Au, S.; Dong, X.D.; Kumar, U.; Arendt-Nielsen, L.; Cairns, B.E. Botulinum neurotoxin type a (bonta) decreases the mechanical sensitivity of nociceptors and inhibits neurogenic vasodilation in a craniofacial muscle targeted for migraine prophylaxis. *Pain* **2010**, *151*, 606–616. [CrossRef] [PubMed]
60. Da Silva, L.B.; Poulsen, J.N.; Arendt-Nielsen, L.; Gazerani, P. Botulinum neurotoxin type a modulates vesicular release of glutamate from satellite glial cells. *J. Cell. Mol. Med.* **2015**, *19*, 1900–1909. [CrossRef] [PubMed]
61. Gazerani, P.; Staahl, C.; Drewes, A.M.; Arendt-Nielsen, L. Effect of botulinum toxin type a (bonta) on capsaicin-evoked pain, flare, and secondary hyperalgesia in an experimental human model of trigeminal sensitization. *Cephalalgia* **2005**, *25*, 990.
62. Gazerani, P.; Pedersen, N.S.; Staahl, C.; Drewes, A.M.; Arendt-Nielsen, L. Subcutaneous botulinum toxin type a reduces capsaicin-induced trigeminal pain and vasomotor reactions in human skin. *Pain* **2009**, *141*, 60–69. [CrossRef] [PubMed]
63. Da Silva, L.B.; Kulas, D.; Karshenas, A.; Cairns, B.E.; Bach, F.W.; Arendt-Nielsen, L.; Gazerani, P. Time course analysis of the effects of botulinum neurotoxin type a on pain and vasomotor responses evoked by glutamate injection into human temporalis muscles. *Toxins* **2014**, *6*, 592–607. [CrossRef] [PubMed]
64. Wheeler, A.; Smith, H.S. Botulinum toxins: Mechanisms of action, antinociception and clinical applications. *Toxicology* **2013**, *306*, 124–146. [CrossRef] [PubMed]
65. Gazerani, P.; Pedersen, N.S.; Drewes, A.M.; Arendt-Nielsen, L. Botulinum toxin type a reduces histamine-induced itch and vasomotor responses in human skin. *Brit. J. Dermatol.* **2009**, *161*, 737–745. [CrossRef] [PubMed]
66. Leigh, A.; Nattkemper, L.A.; Stull, C.; Lavery, M.J.; Valdes-Rodriguez, R.; McGregory, M.; Ramsey, R.V.; Chen, Y.H.; Mochizuki, H.; Yosipovitch, G. Prolonged antipruritic effect of Botulinum toxin type A on cowhage induced itch. OP43, lecture abstracts, Abstracts from the 9th world congress on itch. *Acta Derm. Venereol.* **2017**, *97*, 1021.
67. Lieu, T.; Jayaweera, G.; Zhao, P.; Poole, D.P.; Jensen, D.; Grace, M.; McIntyre, P.; Bron, R.; Wilson, Y.M.; Krappitz, M.; et al. The bile acid receptor tgr5 activates the trpa1 channel to induce itch in mice. *Gastroenterology* **2014**, *147*, 1417–1428. [CrossRef] [PubMed]
68. Liu, T.; Ji, R.R. Oxidative stress induces itch via activation of transient receptor potential subtype ankyrin 1 in mice. *Neurosci. Bull.* **2012**, *28*, 145–154. [CrossRef] [PubMed]
69. Zhou, F.M.; Cheng, R.X.; Wang, S.; Huang, Y.; Gao, Y.J.; Zhou, Y.; Liu, T.T.; Wang, X.L.; Chen, L.H.; Liu, T. Antioxidants attenuate acute and chronic itch: Peripheral and central mechanisms of oxidative stress in pruritus. *Neurosci. Bull.* **2017**, *33*, 423–435. [CrossRef] [PubMed]
70. Cao, L.F.; Si, M.; Huang, Y.; Chen, L.H.; Peng, X.Y.; Qin, Y.Q.; Liu, T.T.; Zhou, Y.; Liu, T.; Luo, W.F. Long-term anti-itch effect of botulinum neurotoxin a is associated with downregulation of trpv1 and trpa1 in the dorsal root ganglia in mice. *Neuroreport* **2017**, *28*, 518–526. [CrossRef] [PubMed]
71. Rothschild, A.M. Mechanisms of histamine release by compound 48–80. *Br. J. Pharmacol.* **1970**, *38*, 253–262. [CrossRef] [PubMed]
72. Han, S.B.; Kim, H.; Cho, S.H.; Chung, J.H.; Kim, H.S. Protective effect of botulinum toxin type a against atopic dermatitis-like skin lesions in nc/nga mice. *Dermatol. Surg.* **2017**. [CrossRef] [PubMed]
73. Mollanazar, N.K.; Smith, P.K.; Yosipovitch, G. Mediators of chronic pruritus in atopic dermatitis: Getting the itch out? *Clin. Rev. Allergy Immunol.* **2016**, *51*, 263–292. [CrossRef] [PubMed]
74. Martel, B.C.; Lovato, P.; Baumer, W.; Olivry, T. Translational animal models of atopic dermatitis for preclinical studies. *Yale J. Biol Med.* **2017**, *90*, 389–402. [PubMed]
75. Park, T.H. The effects of botulinum toxin a on mast cell activity: Preliminary results. *Burns* **2013**, *39*, 816–817. [CrossRef] [PubMed]
76. Akhtar, N. Response to: The effects of botulinum toxin a on mast cell activity: Preliminary results. *Burns* **2013**, *39*, 817–818. [CrossRef] [PubMed]
77. Ward, N.L.; Kavlick, K.D.; Diaconu, D.; Dawes, S.M.; Michaels, K.A.; Gilbert, E. Botulinum neurotoxin a decreases infiltrating cutaneous lymphocytes and improves acanthosis in the kc-tie2 mouse model. *J. Investig. Dermatol.* **2012**, *132*, 1927–1930. [CrossRef] [PubMed]

78. Al-Ghamdi, A.S.; Alghanemy, N.; Joharji, H.; Al-Qahtani, D.; Alghamdi, H. Botulinum toxin: Non cosmetic and off-label dermatological uses. *J. Dermatol. Dermatol. Surg.* **2015**, *19*, 1–8. [CrossRef]
79. Boozalis, E.; Sheu, M.; Selph, J.; Kwatra, S.G. Botulinum toxin type a for the treatment of localized recalcitrant chronic pruritus. *J. Am. Acad. Dermatol.* **2018**, *78*, 192–194. [CrossRef] [PubMed]
80. Wood, G.J.; Akiyama, T.; Carstens, E.; Oaklander, A.L.; Yosipovitch, G. An insatiable itch. *J. Pain* **2009**, *10*, 792–797. [CrossRef] [PubMed]
81. Eisenberg, E.; Barmeir, E.; Bergman, R. Notalgia paresthetica associated with nerve root impingement. *J. Am. Acad. Dermatol.* **1997**, *37*, 998–1000. [CrossRef]
82. Mittal, A.; Srivastava, A.; Balai, M.; Khare, A.K. A study of postherpetic pruritus. *Indian Dermatol. Online J.* **2016**, *7*, 343–344. [CrossRef] [PubMed]
83. Argoff, C.E. A focused review on the use of botulinum toxins for neuropathic pain. *Clin. J. Pain* **2002**, *18*, S177–S181. [CrossRef]
84. Weinfeld, P.K. Successful treatment of notalgia paresthetica with botulinum toxin type A. *Arch. Dermatol.* **2007**, *143*, 980–982. [CrossRef] [PubMed]
85. Waisman, M. Solar pruritus of the elbows (brachioradial summer pruritus). *Arch. Dermatol.* **1968**, *98*, 481–485. [CrossRef] [PubMed]
86. Kavanagh, G.M.; Tidman, M.J. Botulinum a toxin and brachioradial pruritus. *Brit. J. Dermatol.* **2012**, *166*, 1147. [CrossRef] [PubMed]
87. Heyl, T. Brachioradial pruritus. *Arch. Dermatol.* **1983**, *119*, 115–116. [CrossRef] [PubMed]
88. Veien, N.K.; Hattel, T.; Laurberg, G.; Spaun, E. Brachioradial pruritus. *J. Am. Acad. Dermatol.* **2001**, *44*, 704–705. [CrossRef] [PubMed]
89. Walcyk, P.J.; Elpern, D.J. Brachioradial pruritus: A tropical dermopathy. *Br. J. Dermatol.* **1986**, *115*, 177–180. [CrossRef] [PubMed]
90. Bernhard, J.D.; Bordeaux, J.S. Medical pearl: The ice-pack sign in brachioradial pruritus. *J. Am. Acad. Dermatol.* **2005**, *52*, 1073. [CrossRef] [PubMed]
91. Alai, N.N.; Skinner, H.B.; Nabili, S.T.; Jeffes, E.; Shahrokni, S.; Saemi, A.M. Notalgia paresthetica associated with cervical spinal stenosis and cervicothoracic disk disease at c4 through c7. *Cutis* **2010**, *85*, 77–81. [PubMed]
92. Chiriac, A.; Podoleanu, C.; Moldovan, C.; Stolnicu, S. Notalgia paresthetica, a clinical series and review. *Pain Pract.* **2016**, *16*, E90–E91. [CrossRef] [PubMed]
93. Wallengren, J.; Bartosik, J. Botulinum toxin type a for neuropathic itch. *Br. J. Dermatol.* **2010**, *163*, 424–426. [CrossRef] [PubMed]
94. Maari, C.; Marchessault, P.; Bissonnette, R. Treatment of notalgia paresthetica with botulinum toxin A: A double-blind randomized controlled trial. *J. Am. Acad. Dermatol.* **2014**, *70*, 1139–1141. [CrossRef] [PubMed]
95. Morris, A.; Cardones, A.; Berger, T. Pruritic skin disease in the elderly. *J. Investig. Dermatol.* **2008**, *128*, 1606.
96. Apalla, Z.; Sotiriou, E.; Lallas, A.; Lazaridou, E.; Ioannides, D. Botulinum toxin a in postherpetic neuralgia: A parallel, randomized, double-blind, single-dose, placebo-controlled trial. *Clin. J. Pain* **2013**, *29*, 857–864. [CrossRef] [PubMed]
97. Salardini, A.; Richardson, D.; Jabbari, B. Relief of intractable pruritus after administration of botulinum toxin a (botox): A case report. *Clin. Neuropharmacol.* **2008**, *31*, 303–306. [CrossRef] [PubMed]
98. Eppsteiner, E.; Boardman, L.; Stockdale, C.K. Vulvodynia. *Best Pract. Res. Clin. Obstet. Gynaecol.* **2014**, *28*, 1000–1012. [CrossRef] [PubMed]
99. Yoon, H.; Chung, W.S.; Shim, B.S. Botulinum toxin a for the management of vulvodynia. *Int. J. Impot. Res.* **2007**, *19*, 84–87. [CrossRef] [PubMed]
100. Petersen, C.D.; Giraldi, A.; Lundvall, L.; Kristensen, E. Botulinum toxin type a-a novel treatment for provoked vestibulodynia? Results from a randomized, placebo controlled, double blinded study. *J. Sex. Med.* **2009**, *6*, 2523–2537. [CrossRef] [PubMed]
101. Berman, B.; Maderal, A.; Raphael, B. Keloids and hypertrophic scars: Pathophysiology, classification, and treatment. *Dermatol. Surg.* **2017**, *43*, S3–S18. [CrossRef] [PubMed]
102. Perdanasari, A.T.; Torresetti, M.; Grassetti, L.; Nicoli, F.; Zhang, Y.X.; Dashti, T.; Di Benedetto, G.; Lazzeri, D. Intralesional injection treatment of hypertrophic scars and keloids: A systematic review regarding outcomes. *Burns Trauma* **2015**, *3*, 14. [CrossRef] [PubMed]

103. Gassner, H.G.; Sherris, D.A.; Otley, C.C. Treatment of facial wounds with botulinum toxin a improves cosmetic outcome in primates. *Plast Reconstr. Surg.* **2000**, *105*, 1948–1953. [CrossRef] [PubMed]
104. Gauglitz, G.G.; Bureik, D.; Dombrowski, Y.; Pavicic, T.; Ruzicka, T.; Schauber, J. Botulinum toxin a for the treatment of keloids. *Skin Pharmacol. Phys.* **2012**, *25*, 313–318. [CrossRef] [PubMed]
105. Nabai, L.; Ghahary, A. Hypertrophic scarring in the rabbit ear: A practical model for studying dermal fibrosis. *Methods Mol. Biol.* **2017**, *1627*, 81–89. [PubMed]
106. Caliskan, E.; Gamsizkan, M.; Acikgoz, G.; Durmus, M.; Toklu, S.; Dogrul, A.; Kurt, A.; Tunca, M. Intralesional treatments for hypertrophic scars: Comparison among corticosteroid, 5-fluorouracil and botulinum toxin in rabbit ear hypertrophic scar model. *Eur. Rev. Med. Pharmacol.* **2016**, *20*, 1603–1608.
107. Prodromidou, A.; Frountzas, M.; Vlachos, D.E.G.; Vlachos, G.D.; Bakoyiannis, I.; Perrea, D.; Pergialiotis, V. Botulinum toxin for the prevention and healing of wound scars: A systematic review of the literature. *Plast. Surg.* **2015**, *23*, 260–264. [CrossRef]
108. Shaarawy, E.; Hegazy, R.A.; Hay, R.M.A. Intralesional botulinum toxin type a equally effective and better tolerated than intralesional steroid in the treatment of keloids: A randomized controlled trial. *J. Cosmet. Dermatol. US* **2015**, *14*, 161–166. [CrossRef] [PubMed]
109. Zanchi, M.; Favot, F.; Bizzarini, M.; Piai, M.; Donini, M.; Sedona, P. Botulinum toxin type-a for the treatment of inverse psoriasis. *J. Eur. Acad. Dermatol.* **2008**, *22*, 431–436. [CrossRef] [PubMed]
110. Brassard, D.; Benohanian, A.; Saber, M. A case of inverse psoriasis responding to botulinum toxin type A. *J. Am. Acad. Dermatol.* **2011**, *64*, Ab161.
111. Chroni, E.; Monastirli, A.; Tsambaos, D. Botulinum toxin for inverse psoriasis? *J. Eur. Acad. Dermatol. Venereol.* **2009**, *23*, 955. [CrossRef] [PubMed]
112. Molin, S.; Diepgen, T.L.; Ruzicka, T.; Prinz, J.C. Diagnosing chronic hand eczema by an algorithm: A tool for classification in clinical practice. *Clin. Exp. Dermatol.* **2011**, *36*, 595–601. [CrossRef] [PubMed]
113. Soler, D.C.; Bai, X.; Ortega, L.; Pethukova, T.; Nedorost, S.T.; Popkin, D.L.; Cooper, K.D.; McCormick, T.S. The key role of aquaporin 3 and aquaporin 10 in the pathogenesis of pompholyx. *Med. Hypotheses* **2015**, *84*, 498–503. [CrossRef] [PubMed]
114. Kontochristopoulos, G.; Gregoriou, S.; Agiasofitou, E.; Nikolakis, G.; Rigopoulos, D.; Katsambas, A. Letter: Regression of relapsing dyshidrotic eczema after treatment of concomitant hyperhidrosis with botulinum toxin-a. *Dermatol. Surg.* **2007**, *33*, 1289–1290. [CrossRef] [PubMed]
115. Nedelec, B.; LaSalle, L. Postburn itch: A review of the literature. *Wounds* **2018**, *30*, E118–E124. [PubMed]
116. Akhtar, N.; Brooks, P. The use of botulinum toxin in the management of burns itching: Preliminary results. *Burns* **2012**, *38*, 1119–1123. [CrossRef] [PubMed]
117. Gonzalez-Ramos, J.; Alonso-Pacheco, M.L.; Goiburu-Chenu, B.; Mayor-Ibarguren, A.; Herranz-Pinto, P. Successful treatment of refractory pruritic fox-fordyce disease with botulinum toxin type a. *Br. J. Dermatol.* **2016**, *174*, 458–459. [CrossRef] [PubMed]
118. Ravitskiy, L.; Heymann, W.R. Botulinum toxin-induced resolution of axillary granular parakeratosis. *SkinMed* **2005**, *4*, 118–120. [CrossRef] [PubMed]
119. Ho, D.; Jagdeo, J. Successful botulinum toxin (onabotulinumtoxina) treatment of hailey-hailey disease. *J. Drugs Dermatol.* **2015**, *14*, 68–70. [PubMed]
120. Bagherani, N.; Smoller, B.R. The efficacy of botulinum toxin type a in the treatment of hailey-hailey disease. *Dermatol. Ther.* **2016**, *29*, 394–395. [CrossRef] [PubMed]
121. Bousquet, J.; Khaltaev, N.; Cruz, A.A.; Denburg, J.; Fokkens, W.J.; Togias, A.; Zuberbier, T.; Baena-Cagnani, C.E.; Canonica, G.W.; van Weel, C.; et al. Allergic rhinitis and its impact on asthma (aria) 2008 update (in collaboration with the world health organization, ga(2)len and allergen). *Allergy* **2008**, *63* (Suppl. 86), 8–160. [CrossRef] [PubMed]
122. International consensus report on the diagnosis and management of rhinitis. International rhinitis management working group. *Allergy* **1994**, *49*, 1–34.
123. Zhang, E.Z.; Tan, S.; Loh, I. Botolinum toxin in rhinitis: Literature review and posterior nasal injection in allergic rhinitis. *Laryngoscope* **2017**, *127*, 2447–2454. [CrossRef] [PubMed]
124. Ozcan, C.; Ismi, O. Botulinum toxin for rhinitis. *Curr. Allergy Asthma Rep.* **2016**, *16*, 58. [CrossRef] [PubMed]
125. Braun, T.; Gurkov, R.; Kramer, M.F.; Krause, E. Septal injection of botulinum neurotoxin a for idiopathic rhinitis: A pilot study. *Am. J. Otolaryngol.* **2012**, *33*, 64–67. [CrossRef] [PubMed]

126. Hashemi, S.M.; Okhovat, A.; Amini, S.; Pourghasemian, M. Comparing the effects of botulinum toxin-a and cetirizine on the treatment of allergic rhinitis. *Allergol. Int.* **2013**, *62*, 245–249. [CrossRef] [PubMed]
127. Mozafarinia, K.; Abna, M.; Khanjani, N. Effect of botulinum neurotoxin a injection into the submucoperichondrium of the nasal septum in reducing idiopathic non-allergic rhinitis and persistent allergic rhinitis. *Iran. J. Otorhinolaryngol.* **2015**, *27*, 253–259. [PubMed]
128. Rohrbach, S.; Junghans, K.; Kohler, S.; Laskawi, R. Minimally invasive application of botulinum toxin a in patients with idiopathic rhinitis. *Head Face Med.* **2009**, *5*, 18. [CrossRef] [PubMed]
129. Zhu, Z.; Stone, H.F.; Thach, T.Q.; Garcia, L.; Ruegg, C.L. A novel botulinum neurotoxin topical gel: Treatment of allergic rhinitis in rats and comparative safety profile. *Am. J. Rhinol. Allergy* **2012**, *26*, 450–454. [CrossRef] [PubMed]

toxins

MDPI

Article

A Study and Review of Effects of Botulinum Toxins on Mast Cell Dependent and Independent Pruritus

Roshni Ramachandran [1], Marc J. Marino [1], Snighdha Paul [1], Zhenping Wang [2], Nicholas L. Mascarenhas [2], Sabine Pellett [3], Eric A. Johnson [3], Anna DiNardo [2] and Tony L. Yaksh [1,*]

1 Department of Anesthesiology, University of California, San Diego, La Jolla, CA 92093, USA; roramachandran@ucsd.edu (R.R.); mjmarino@ad.ucsd.edu (M.J.M.); spaul@westernu.edu (S.P.)
2 Department of Medicine, Division of Dermatology, University of California, San Diego, La Jolla, CA 92093, USA; zhenping.w@gmail.com (Z.W.); nmascare@ucsd.edu (N.L.M.); adinardo@ucsd.edu (A.D.)
3 Department of Bacteriology, University of Wisconsin, Madison, WI 53706, USA; sabine.pellett@wisc.edu (S.P.); eric.johnson@wisc.edu (E.A.J.)
* Correspondence: tyaksh@ucsd.edu; Tel.: +1-619-543-3597

Received: 7 March 2018; Accepted: 21 March 2018; Published: 23 March 2018

Abstract: Pruriceptive itch originates following activation of peripheral sensory nerve terminals when pruritogens come in contact with the skin. The ability of botulinum neurotoxins (BoNTs) to attenuate transmitter release from afferent terminals provides a rationale for studying its effect on pruritus. This study investigated the effects of BoNT/A1 and BoNT/B1 on mast cell dependent (Compound 48/80:48/80) and independent (Chloroquine:CQ) scratching. C57Bl/6 male mice received intradermal injection of 1.5 U of BoNT/A1, BoNT/B1 or saline 2, 7, 14 and 21 days prior to ipsilateral 48/80 or CQ at the nape of the neck. Ipsilateral hind paw scratching was determined using an automated recording device. The effect of BoNTs on 48/80 mediated mast cell degranulation was analyzed in human and murine mast cells and the presence of SNAREs was determined using qPCR, immunostaining and Western blot. Pre-treatment with BoNT/A1 and BoNT/B1 reduced 48/80 and CQ induced scratching behavior starting on day 2 with reversal by day 21. Both serotypes inhibited 48/80 induced mast cell degranulation. qPCR and immunostaining detected SNAP-25 mRNA and protein, respectively, in mast cells, however, Western blots did not. This study demonstrates the long-lasting anti-pruritic effects of two BoNT serotypes, in a murine pruritus model using two different mechanistically driven pruritogens. These data also indicate that BoNTs may have a direct effect upon mast cell degranulation.

Keywords: botulinum toxin; itch; SNARE; VAMP; mast cells; compound 48/80; chloroquine

Key Contribution: BoNT serotypes show long lasting anti-pruritic effects and may have a direct effect on mast cells.

1. Introduction

Pruritus or itch is an unpleasant sensation that promotes scratching as a primary response. Chronic itch is a debilitating and dominating symptom accompanying several disorders including skin conditions such as atopic dermatitis (AD) as well as in systemic (renal and liver failure) [1–3] and neurological disorders (diabetic neuropathy and shingles) [4,5]. Pruriceptive itch, as seen in AD, originates following the activation of peripheral sensory nerve terminals associated with allergic reactions induced by insect bites or when pruritogens come in contact with the skin. Among the several subtypes of primary afferent nerve fibers, a role for C-fibers has been demonstrated in detecting and transmitting pruriceptive signals to the neuraxis [6,7].

Many forms of itch are mediated by histamine released from mast cells that activate a subset of neurons expressing TRPV1 receptors as evidenced by the effects of TRPV1 antagonism in histamine evoked activation of dorsal root ganglion (DRG) neurons [8] and reduced histamine evoked scratching behavior [9]. Pruritogens, such as chloroquine (CQ), induce itch via mast cell-independent pathways [10]. Mas-related G protein coupled receptor (Mrgpr) has emerged as a novel class of receptors in histamine independent itch pathways and MrgprA3 is the receptor for CQ. In contrast to histamine dependent pathways, where TRPV1 functions downstream of histamine receptors to promote itch, the histamine-independent pathway utilizes TRPA1 as a key transduction channel downstream of the MrgprA3 receptor [11,12].

Botulinum neurotoxins (BoNTs), including the A1 (Botox) and B1 (Myobloc) serotypes, attenuate neurotransmitter release in neurons by the cleavage of terminal soluble N-ethylmaleimide-sensitive-factor attachment protein receptors (SNAREs) [13–15]. Data indicate that when BoNT/A1 and B1 are given subcutaneously in the paw, the toxin is taken up in the peripheral terminal and transported back to the central terminal of the primary afferent [16,17]. Studies from our lab as well as from other groups have shown that both subcutaneous (sc) BoNT/A1 and BoNT/B1 reduce local intradermal capsaicin evoked flares in animal [17,18] and human models [19–22], reflecting the local inhibitory effect upon release of vasodilatory peptides (substance P (sP)/ calcitonin gene-related peptide (CGRP)) from the peripheral terminal evoked by TRPV1 receptor. In addition, following peripheral delivery of BoNTs, cleaved SNAREs are detected in the dorsal root ganglia and dorsal horn along with an associated block of sP release [17]. While BoNTs primarily seem to affect motor neurons in botulism, it is well known that BoNTs can efficiently enter and block neurotransmission in other neuronal subpopulations as well. However, entry and effects on non-neuronal secreting cells, such as mast cells, are less explored, in part because the vesicle release machinery utilizes different (non-neuronal) SNARE proteins that based on the literature are not the targets of medically employed BoNTs. However, an anti-pruritic effect of BoNT/A1 has been demonstrated clinically in several skin disorders, including dermatitis [23], burn induced itch [24], and lichen simplex [25], a localized variant of AD in which acetylcholine appears to be a dominant pruritic mediator. BoNT/A1 also reduced the itch intensity, blood flow and neurogenic inflammation in response to the histamine prick test in human skin [19]. These results jointly suggest the use of BoNTs in treating pruritus, although the mechanism of action remains unknown including whether observed effects are a result of direct action of the BoNT on mast cells or an indirect effect via neurons. The present study demonstrates anti-pruritic effects of BoNT/A1 and BoNT/B1 on histamine dependent compound 48/80 and histamine-independent CQ-induced scratching behavior in mice, and for the first time shows an effect of the BoNTs on cultured murine and human mast cells.

2. Results

2.1. *BoNT/A1 and BoNT/B1 Injection Reduced 48/80 and CQ Induced Scratching*

Behavioral responses were recorded for 40 min in the C57Bl/6 mice following intradermal injection of 48/80 and CQ at the nape of the neck. Both pruritogens injected unilaterally induced ipsilateral scratching behavior. The total number of scratches in the 40 min period increased significantly following intradermal injection of mast cell-dependent 48/80 and mast cell-independent CQ (Figure 1).

Bouts of scratching induced by 48/80 and CQ were reduced by 1.5 U of ipsilateral BoNT/A1 and BoNT/B1 given locally (intradermal) two days prior to the intradermal injections of pruritogens. Analysis of total scratching in the 40 min period showed that this reduction was statistically significant. Importantly, the 1.5 U of intradermal BoNT-A1 or BoNT-B1 did not produce detectable alterations in motor function or strength. Animals displayed normal grasping behavior as measured by a suspension test where the animals were required to grip onto the wire mesh for at least 1 min and showed normal hind limb placing and stepping reflexes [17].

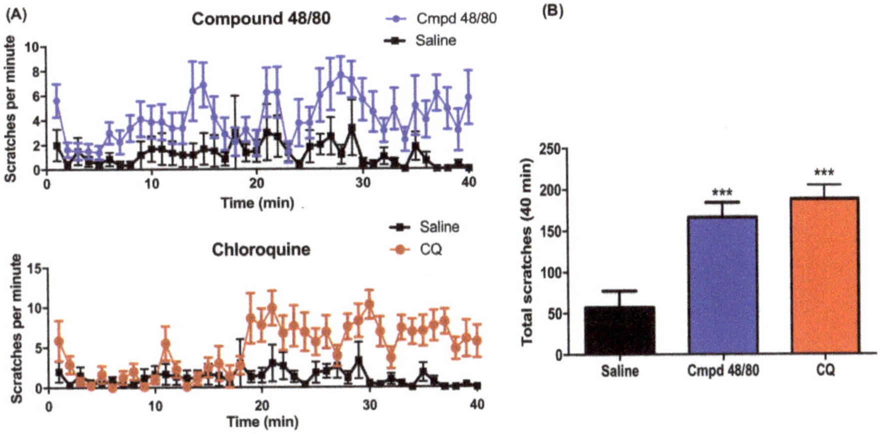

Figure 1. Compound 48/80 and chloroquine induced scratches: (**A**) time course of scratching induced by intradermal injection of compound 48/80 (50 µL of 1 mg/kg) (N = 8) or Chloroquine (50 µL of 2mg/mL) (N = 8) over a period of 40 min (CQ); (**B**) histogram showing cumulative scratch count following compound 48/80 and CQ in 40 min. All data are expressed as Mean ± SEM. *** $p < 0.001$ as compared to the saline treated group (N = 7).

2.2. BoNT/A1 and BoNT/B1 Have a Long Duration of Effect in Reducing Compound 48/80 and CQ Induced Scratching

One of the hallmarks of pharmaceutical BoNTs is their long duration of action, lasting 2–6 months in humans after intramuscular injection. Local intramuscular injection of BoNT/A1 in mice results in local paralysis that peaks at day 2 after injection and slowly decreases in effect over the following 2–3 weeks [26]. To determine whether effects of BoNT/A1 and B1 on 48/80 and CQ induced scratching have a similarly long-lasting duration, 1.5 U BoNT/A1 or BoNT/B1 or saline were given on days 2, 7, 14 and 21 days prior to administration of 48/80 and CQ treatment on the same side of the neck. BoNT/A1 and BoNT/B1 significantly reduced 48/80 induced scratching behavior on days 2, 7 and 14, but not on day 21 as compared to the saline treated group, suggesting a reversal of effect of BoNT by day 21 (Figure 2). A similar long-lasting effect of BoNT/A1 and B1 was observed on CQ induced scratching as well, where pretreatment with unilateral BoNT/A1 and B1 significantly reduced CQ induced scratching behavior on days 2, 7 and 14 with a complete reversal by day 21 (Figure 2). In both cases, a slow recovery to normal scratching behavior was observed over time, similarly as is seen with muscle paralysis after BoNT treatment. Interestingly, even though BoNT/A1 has a significantly longer duration of action than BoNT/B1 in causing muscle paralysis, in the pruritus assay, both toxins had a similar duration of action in suppressing 48/80 or CQ induced scratching behavior.

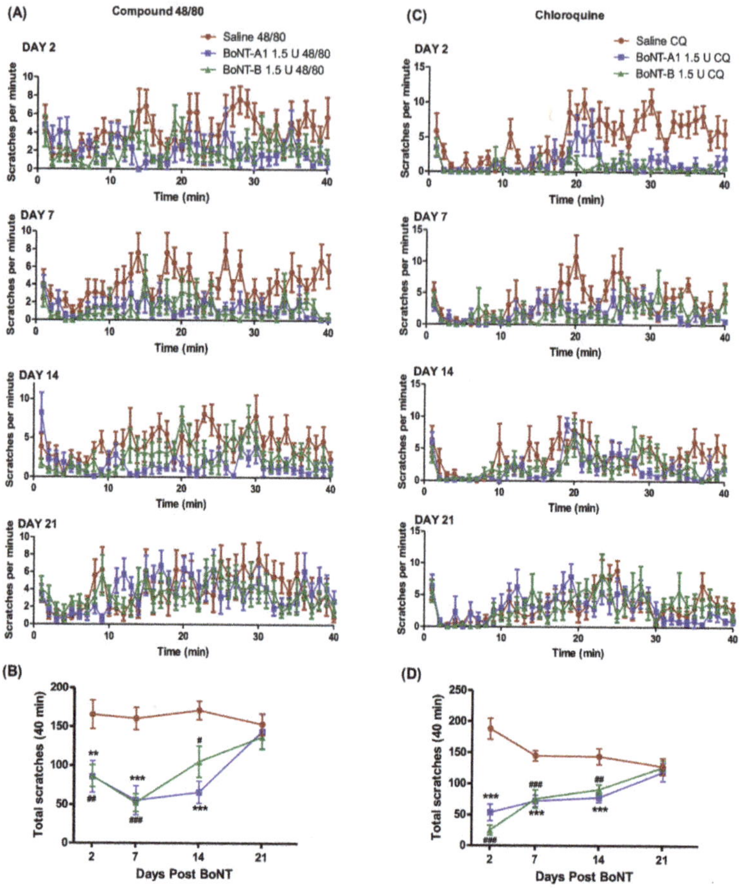

Figure 2. Duration of action of BoNT/A1 and BoNT/B1 in reducing compound 48/80 and chloroquine induced scratching: Mice were treated with intradermal saline (control), BoNT/A1 (1.5 U), or BoNT/B1 (1.5 U) at 2, 7, 14, or 21 days prior to intradermal administration of compound 48/80 (**A**,**B**) or Chloroquine (**C**,**D**). The total scratches per minute were observed over a 40 min time interval after administration of compound 48/80 or chloroquine. Plots indicate mean ± SEM for cumulative flinches observed at days 2, 7, 14 and 21. ** $p < 0.01$, *** $p < 0.001$ vs. saline; # $p < 0.05$, ## $p < 0.01$, ### $p < 0.001$ as compared to saline, $N = 8$ animals per group.

2.3. BoNT/A1 and BoNT/B1 Reduce Compound 48/80 Induced Murine and Human Mast Cell Degranulation

The inhibitory effects of BoNT/A1 and B1 on 48/80 induced scratching observed in the in vivo studies could be due to a direct effect of the BoNTs on mast cells or secondary to the inhibition of mediator release from primary afferents inhibited by BoNTs. In order to determine whether BoNT/A1 and B1 directly affected the functioning of mast cells, an in vitro assay using isolated murine and human iPSC derived mast cells was performed. The primary murine mast cells were treated with 48/80 for 20 min at 37 °C, leading to degranulation as evidenced by β-hexosaminidase release compared to untreated control cells. As expected, treatment with CQ did not induce mast cell degranulation. Interestingly, pre-treatment of both murine and human mast cells with 0.5 U of BoNT/A1 and /B1 for 24 h significantly reduced 48/80 mast cell degranulation (Figure 3). This indicates a direct effect of BoNT/A1 and B1 on mast cells.

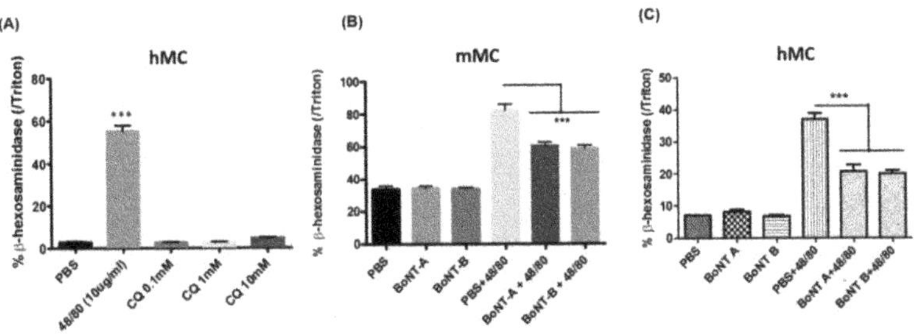

Figure 3. Effect of BoNT on compound 48/80 induced mast cell degranulation in human (hMC) and mouse mast cell culture (mMC): Mast cell β-hexosaminidase release (as index of mast cell degranulation) following compound 48/80 (48/80, 10 μg/mL) and chloroquine (CQ) (**A**); mast cell β-hexosaminidase release induced by 48/80 (1μg/mL) 24 h after treatment with 0.5 U of BoNT/A1 or BoNT/B1 in murine mast cell culture (**B**) and in human mast cell culture (**C**). *** $p < 0.001$ compared to other groups.

2.4. Western Blot Analysis of Expression and Effect of BoNT/A1 and BoNT/B1 on SNAP-25 and VAMP 1/2/3 in Human and Murine Mast Cells

The cellular target of BoNT/A1 is the neuronal SNAP-25 and for BoNT/B1 is VAMP-1 and 2, which are essential components in the neuronal vesicle release machinery. The BoNTs cleave their respective target SNARE proteins, which is the mode of action by which BoNTs block neurotransmitter release. While the degranulation machinery identified in mast cells utilizes SNAP-23 and VAMP-7/8, which are not cleaved by BoNT/A1 and /B1, the observed inhibition of degranulation of mast cells by BoNTs indicates a mechanism other than SNARE cleavage. In order to confirm this in our model, cultured murine and human mast cells were treated with BoNT/A1 and BoNT/B1 for 24 h and SNAP-25 and VAMP isoforms were analyzed using Western blot. Consistent with previous reports, Western blot analysis did not detect expression of SNAP-25 (Figure 4). It should be noted that spinal cord samples loaded as a positive control on the same immunoblot membrane clearly showed SNAP-25 expression, suggesting that mast cells do not express SNAP-25 at detectable levels. Though expression of VAMP-1/2/3 was observed in mast cells, BoNT/B1 surprisingly did not reduce full-length VAMP 1/2/3 levels in these BoNT treated mast cells, suggesting no cleavage of BoNT-B1 specific VAMP proteins.

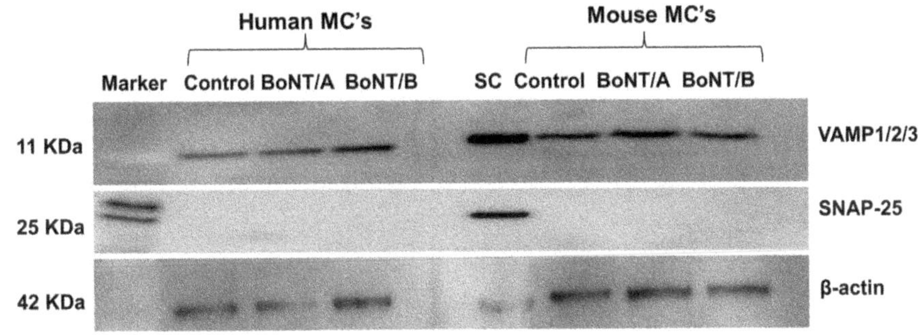

Figure 4. Expression of SNARE proteins in mast cells: Representative image of Western blots showing expression of SNAP-25 or VAMP-1/2/3 in the mast cells with or without BoNT/A1 or B1 treatment (0.5 U for 24 h). Spinal cord (SC) tissue was used as a positive control for SNAP-25 expression. Mast cells did not express SNAP-25 and hence no effect of BoNT/A1 on SNAP-25 was observed. VAMP 1/2/3 were expressed in mast cells; however, they were not affected by pre-treatment with BoNT/B1; this was repeated three times.

2.5. *Expression of SNAP-25 and VAMP 1/2/3 Cleavage with or without BoNT/A1 or B1 Treatment, Respectively, in Human and Murine Mast Cells*

Although Western blot did not detect any expression of SNAP-25 in human and mast cell culture, immunostaining was able to detect cleaved products of SNAP-25 following BoNT/A1 treatment on both human and murine mast cells. The SNAP-25 antibody used in the present study detects only the cleaved products (cSNAP-25). The control groups of murine and human MC did not show cSNAP-25 staining; however pre-treatment of the mast cells with BoNT/A1 for 4 h showed a dose-dependent increase in cSNAP-25 staining. DAPI was used to stain the nuclei of the mast cells (Figure 5A). RT-qPCR analysis on human and mouse mast cells showed expression of SNAP-25 mRNA, suggesting the presence of at least low levels of SNAP-25 in mast cells (Figure 5B). The VAMP antibody used recognizes the intact molecule. Therefore, reduction of VAMP protein expression was used as a measure of VAMP cleavage. In control animals, VAMP expression was observed in the control group along with the DAPI stained nuclei. Following pre-treatment with BoNT/B1, the cells showed a reduction in VAMP expression. Thus, VAMP cleavage was significantly greater in the BoNT/B1 treated group as compared to PBS control (Figure 5A).

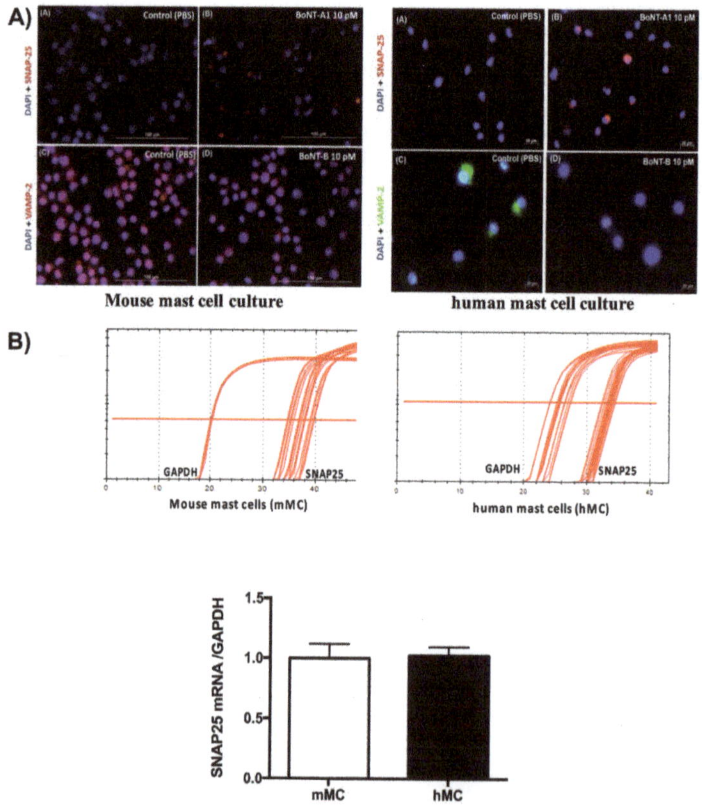

Figure 5. Detection of cSNAP-25 and VAMP-2, respectively, in mouse and human mast cell culture: (**A**) representative images of BoNT/A1-cleaved SNAP-25 and VAMP-2 immunostaining following treatment with BoNT/A1 and BoNT/B1 (10 pM); (**B**) RT-qPCR of SNAP-25 expression in mouse and human mast cell culture. $N = 3$.

3. Discussion

The present study demonstrated the anti-pruritic effects of two well characterized and clinically employed BoNT serotypes, Botulinum Toxin A1 (Botox©) and Botulinum Toxin B1 (MyoBloc©) over time in a murine pruritus model using two different mechanistically driven pruritogens. While involvement of SNARE proteins in release of pruritus stimulating mediators from mast cells has been demonstrated [27,28], effects of BoNT/A1 and BoNT/B1 on mast cell release has not been explored. The present study showed that BoNTs may have a direct effect on mast cells in altering its local degranulation, and that this effect may be independent of SNARE cleavage.

3.1. *Mast Cell Dependent and Independent Pruritogens*

Pruriceptive itch is induced peripherally due to the activation of nerve fibers located in the epidermis and is the type of itch observed in several dermatological conditions such as atopic dermatitis, psoriasis, etc. [29]. Pruriceptive itch can be experimentally triggered by several exogenous and endogenous substances. In the present study, we utilized two pruritogens, mast cell dependent, 48/80 and mast cell independent, CQ. Compound 48/80 degranulates mast cells to release histamine [30], which induces itch by binding to and activating C-fibers via gating the TRPV1 channel [8,9]. Other mediators released from mast cells such as serotonin, bradykinin, and prostaglandin can potentiate the effects of histamine induced itch sensation [31]. CQ, on the other hand, elicits itch in a mast cell independent pathway, presumably by activating Mrgpr /TRPA1 receptors [11,12]. A recent study shows that 48/80 may have a direct action on neurons in addition to degranulating mast cells [32] and the interpretation of the results in this study does consider this possibility. However, it should be noted that a previous study has reported mast cell mediated neuronal activity of 48/80 [33].

3.2. *Anti-Pruritic Effect of Botulinum Toxin*

BoNT/A1 and BoNT/B1 have been extensively used in clinical and pre-clinical studies for elucidating the mechanisms by which they can inhibit pain transduction in several pain related disorders. Ample evidence now suggests that BoNTs influence release of several neurotransmitters such as acetylcholine, glutamate, CGRP, sP, and serotonin [34–36]. The release of these neurotransmitters may play a contributing role in induced itch [37,38]. Patients with AD show an increase in density of nerve fibers containing CGRP and sP [39]. Furthermore, pre-clinical studies in pain models have shown that peripheral BoNT can block the release of neurotransmitters from the local afferents as well as from the central nerve terminals [17,18,40–43], suggesting a possible pathway in which BoNTs may influence the transmission of itch signals to higher brain centers. Our data from the present study suggests that both BoNT/A1 and BoNT/B1 significantly inhibited the scratching behavior induced by two mechanistically different pruritogens. These findings are in accordance with a clinical study showing that BoNT/A1 could reduce the histamine pin prick induced itch intensity in human skin along with diminished blood flow and neurogenic inflammation [19]. Further clinical studies have suggested anti-pruritic effects of BoNT/A1 on conditions accompanied with itch such as lichen simplex, rhinitis, inverse psoriasis, burn induced itch and dermatitis [23–25]. However, no studies have determined the effect of BoNT/B1 in pruritus so far.

3.3. *Duration of Action of BoNT*

Activity of BoNT is attributed to neuronal cell entry by the toxin, release of the light chain (LC) into the cells cytosol, and cleavage of terminal SNAREs by the LC, blocking vesicular transmitter release [13]. The duration of action of BoNT depends on the persistence of the catalytically active intracellular LC [44,45]. While in humans the duration of pharmaceutical BoNTs varies from two to six months, depending on the dose, mice usually recover from paralytic effects after local intramuscular injection within three weeks [26,46]. Similarly, the BoNT/A1 and B1 induced reduction in itch behavior in the murine model used in this study lasted for about two weeks, with mice showing gradual reversal that was complete by day 21 (Figure 3). This similarity in duration and gradual reversal indicates a possibly similar mechanism of action of BoNTs in mast cells as in neurons, or an indirect effect of BoNTs in pruritus due to neuronal release inhibition.

3.4. Possible Mechanism of Action of BoNT/A1 and BoNT/B1 in Reducing Induced Itch

Effects of both the pruritogens, 48/80 and CQ are believed to be mediated by the activation of C-fiber terminals in the epidermis. Compelling evidence suggests the role of TRPV1 and TRPA1 ion channels in these subsets of neurons downstream to histamine and CQ [11,12] to mediate calcium induced activation of SNAREs that mobilize synaptic vesicle release, thereby promoting itch sensation. Patients with AD show intense staining of CGRP and substance P-immunoreactive fibers, and uptake of BoNT has previously shown to inhibit the release of these neurotransmitters. Therefore, the reduction in induced itch behavior in mice by BoNT/A1 and B1 could be at least in part due to an effect of the toxins on the C-fibers, rather than a direct effect on mast cells.

Interestingly, we observed that pre-treatment with both BoNT/A1 and BoNT/B1 impaired 48/80 induced mast cell degranulation in cultured murine and human mast cells, indicating that BoNTs may also have a direct effect on mast cells. This is in agreement with previous experiments conducted by Park and colleagues that showed a decrease in mast cell activity seven days following BoNT/A1 treatment in rat skin tissue [47]. While the mast cell release machinery involves SNAREs, which are the target of BoNTs in neurons, the SNARE isoforms considered to be required for mast cell degranulation (SNAP-23 and VAMP-7 and 8) are insensitive to BoNT/A1 and /B1 [28,48,49]. In our study, very low levels of SNAP-25 mRNA expression were observed in both murine and human mast cells, with immunohistochemistry studies confirming the findings for both SNAP-25 and VAMP-1/2/3 and indicating cleavage of these SNARE isoforms by BoNT/A1 and B1. However, western blot data suggested absence or very low levels of SNAP-25 in mast cells, and levels of the BoNT/B1 sensitive VAMP-1/2/3 in mast cells appeared to be unaffected by BoNT/B1. Similar discrepancy in the SNAP-25 expression in mast cells using various detection methods has been previously reported [50]. This result, although confounding, is intriguing and leads to the speculation that BoNTs may utilize a non-canonical mechanism other than SNARE cleavage to inhibit release of secretory granules from mast cells. For example, one possibility could be hindrance in the trafficking of membrane proteins such as TRP receptor subunits to the plasma membrane of mast cells. The role of BoNT/A1 in inhibiting TRPV1 receptor function by affecting regulated endocytosis and reduction in TRPV1 receptor expression has been previously demonstrated in the trigeminal as well as in suburothelial nerve fibers [51,52] (Shimizu et al., Apostolidis et al.). Furthermore, studies have shown that 48/80 degranulation of mast cells employ calcium induced exocytosis in mast cells [53] and BoNTs primarily inhibit the normal depolarization- evoked calcium currents [54]. More studies are required to elucidate the inhibitory mechanism of botulinum toxins on mast cell degranulation and whether the observed in vivo effects are due to direct or indirect action of BoNTs on mast cells.

4. Materials and Methods

4.1. Animals

Adult male C57Bl/6 mice, 25–30 g (Harlan Sprague Dawley Inc., Indianapolis, IN, USA), were housed in the vivarium for a minimum of 2 days before use, maintained on a 12/12-h day-night cycle and given free access to food and water. All studies were carried out according to protocols approved by the Institutional Animal Care and Use Committee of the University of California, San Diego, CA, USA. Ethical approval code and date: S00137M and 26 March 2015 (IACUC).

4.2. Drugs

Drugs employed were compound 48/80 (48/80) (1 mg/mL) or CQ (2 mg/mL) (Sigma Aldrich, St Louis, MO, USA). BoNT/A1 (Botox©, onabotulinumtoxin A, Allergan Inc., Carlsbad, CA, USA) and

BoNT/B1 (Myobloc©, Rimabotulinumtoxin B, Solstice Neurosciences, Louisville, KY, USA) solutions were prepared from stock solutions of 50 U/mL and 5000 U/mL, respectively. These products were then serially diluted to the final concentration in 0.9% saline. All solutions were stored at 4 °C and brought to room temperature prior to use.

4.3. Drug Delivery

Mice were anesthetized (2.5% isoflurane, with 80% oxygen and 20% room air) and were shaven on the dorsolateral aspect of the neck and upper shoulder. Using a 29 G needle (insulin syringe) intradermal injection of 50 µL of BoNT/A1 or BoNT/B1 (1.5 U) or saline was administered. Intradermal injections of 48/80 or CQ (50 µL) were administered on the day of behavioral testing.

4.4. Behavior

On the day of testing, animals were placed in a plexiglass cylindrical chamber and a detection band was placed around the hind paw ipsilateral to the shaven area. To initiate scratching behavior, intradermal (ID) injection of 48/80 or CQ was administered in the middle of the shaven area of skin using a 29 G needle. The itch behavior is recorded over the period of 40 min using a paw motion detector (PMD). The PMD detects the movement of a non-ferrous metal band placed around one hind paw of the rodent (band weight = 0.1 g). The testing apparatus consists of cylindrical chambers (mouse: 8.5 cm diameter/22.5 cm tall). Under each cylinder is a pair of circular concentric electromagnetic coils, which serve respectively as antennae for transmission and reception. The transmitter coil assembly emits a 5–8 mW, 6–8 kHz, sinusoidal electromagnetic field. The detection principal is that Eddy currents created by the movements of the ferrous and nonferrous metals perturb the EM field. Such perturbations are detected and produce an output waveform [55,56]. Data were acquired electronically.

4.5. Mast Cell Culture

Primary murine MCs were generated from C57BL/6 mouse bone marrow and cultured in RPMI 1640 medium (Life Technologies, Carlsbad, CA, USA) supplemented with 10% heat-inactivated fetal bovine serum (Life Technologies, Carlsbad, CA, USA), 25 mM HEPES (pH 7.4), 4 mM L-glutamine, 0.1 mM nonessential amino acids, 1 mM sodium pyruvate, 50 µM 2-mercaptoethanol, 100 IU/mL penicillin, and 100 µg/mL streptomycin. Recombinant murine IL-3 (1 ng/mL, R&D Systems, Minneapolis, MN, USA) and recombinant murine stem cell factor (20 ng/mL, R&D Systems, Minneapolis, MN, USA) were also included to allow for in vitro differentiation. After 4 weeks, the MCs were fully differentiated, as confirmed by the expression of CD117 (c-Kit) and FcεRI. Cell maturation was confirmed by metachromatic staining with toluidine blue. The purity of MCs was greater than 98%. For the detailed procedure, see [57].

Primary human MCs were derived from human cord blood CD34+CD45+ cells from healthy donors (STEMCELL Technologies, Seattle, WA, USA) according to Kirshenbaum and Metcalfe [58]. They were cultured in Stemline II hematopoietic stem cell medium (Sigma Aldrich, St. Louis, MO, USA) with recombinant human SCF and IL-6 (100 ng/mL, Peprotech, Rock Hill, NJ, USA) for 9 weeks. MC differentiation was confirmed by CD117 (c-Kit) and FcεRI expression, and maturation was confirmed by metachromatic staining with toluidine blue. The purity of MCs was greater than 98%.

4.6. Mast Cell Degranulation Assay

Degranulation was assessed by measuring the activity of β hexosaminidase in the supernatants of 1×10^5 MCs in 200 µL Tyrode's buffer (0.1% BSA, 0.1% glucose, 2 mmol/L $MgCl_2$, 137.5 mmol/L NaCl, 12 mmol/L $NaHCO_3$, 2.6 mmol/L KCl, pH 7.4) incubated for 24 h with 0.5 U of BoNT-A1 or -B1 before the addition of 1 µg/mL 48/80 (Sigma Aldrich, St Louis, MO, USA). For comparison of mast cell degranulation by 48/80 to CQ, 10 µg/mL 48/80 was used. For each sample assayed, supernatant aliquots (20 µL) were mixed with substrate solution (100 µL) which consisted of 10 mM

4-methylumbelliferyl-2-acetamide-2-deoxy-b-D-glucopyranoside (EMD Millipore, Billerica, MA, USA) in 0.1 M sodium citrate buffer (pH 4.5) and were incubated for 2 h at 37 °C in the dark. The reaction mixtures were excited at 365 nm and measured at 460 nm in a fluorescence plate reader (Gemini EM microplate spectrofluorometer; Molecular Devices, Sunnyvale, CA, USA). To determine the total cellular content of this enzyme, an equivalent number of cells were lysed with 1% Triton X-100 (Sigma Aldrich, St Louis, MO, USA). Release of β-hexosaminidase was calculated as the percentage of the total enzyme content.

4.7. *Immunohistochemistry on Mast Cells*

Mast cells were attached to a glass slide by using Shandon Cytospin 2 cytocentrifuge (Thermo Fisher Scientific, Waltham, MC, USA). The cells were stained with 1 mg/mL anti BoNT/A1-cleaved-SNAP-25 Ab, which recognizes only the BoNT/A1cleavage product of SNAP-25 and not the full-length SNAP-25, and anti-VAMP-2 Ab (Synaptic Systems, Goettingen, Germany) according to the manufacturer's instructions. Slides were mounted in ProLong Anti-Fade reagent with DAPI (Molecular Probes, Eugene, OR, USA). We imaged the cells using the Bx51 research microscope (Olympus, Center Valley, PA, USA) and X-Cite 120 fluorescence illumination systems (EXFO Photonic Solutions, Mississauga, ON, Canada).

4.8. *mRNA Isolation and Real-Time Quantitative PCR*

Total RNA was isolated using Trizol Reagent (Invitrogen, Carlsbad, CA, USA) and 1 μg of total RNA was used for cDNA synthesis by using iScript cDNA Synthesis Kit (Bio-Rad Laboratories, Hercules, CA, USA) according to the manufacturer's instructions. cDNA was amplified using Real time-PCR in an ABI 7300 Real-Time PCR system (Applied Biosystems, Foster City, CA, USA). RNA analysis reagents (SYBR Green Master Mix) were from Bio-Rad, Hercules, CA, USA. We used the comparative ΔΔ cycle threshold method to quantify gene expression. Target gene expression levels in the test samples were normalized to the endogenous reference glyceraldehyde-3-phosphate dehydrogenase (GAPDH) (F: 5′-CCA ACC GCG AGA AGA TGA CC-3′ and R: 5′-GAT CTT CAT GAG GTA GTC AGT-3′) levels and reported as the fold difference relative to GAPDH gene expression in untreated baseline control. All assays were performed in triplicate and the experiments were repeated at least three times.

4.9. *Western Blot Analysis*

Following 24 h treatment with BoNT-A1 or BoNT-B1 on murine and human mast cells, cell lysates were prepared by solubilizing cells in RIPA buffer (Life Technologies, Carlsbad, CA, USA) with protease inhibitor cocktail (Sigma Aldrich, St Louis, MO, USA), at 1×10^7 cells/mL. Cells were incubated for 1 h on ice for complete lysis, and the lysates clarified by centrifugation at 4 °C, for 10 min at 12,000 RPM. Supernatants were collected and stored on ice for immediate use, or at –80 °C until needed. Total protein concentration of the clarified cell lysates was determined by BCA protein assay (Life Technologies, Carlsbad, CA, USA) prior to loading on a gel.

For the Western blot analysis, five micrograms of total cell lysate of each sample were separated on a 12% Bis-Tris NuPAGE gel with MES running buffer (all from Life Technologies). For the mouse spinal cord cell lysate (SC) controls, primary mouse spinal cord cell lysates were prepared as previously described [45], and 8 μl of untreated primary mouse spinal cord cell lysates were used. Proteins were transferred to a PVDF membrane (Millipore 0.45 micron for the SNAP-25 blots, and GE Healthcare (Little Chalfont, UK) 0.2 micron for the VAMP blots) by semi-dry transfer. The membranes were probed with antibodies to beta-actin (Abcam, Cambridge, UK) and VAMP-1/2/3 (Synaptic Systems) (top gel), a polyclonal anti-SNAP-25 antibody (Synaptic Systems) (middle gel), or a monoclonal anti-SNAP-25 antibody (Synaptic Systems) (bottom gel). Images were obtained using PhosphaGlo reagent (KPL, Gaithersburg, MD, USA) and a Fotodyne/FOTO/Analyst FX imaging system (Fotodyne, Hartland, WI, USA).

4.10. Statistical Analysis

The data for each variable was put in tabular form (i.e., Excel worksheet). Summary statistics were computed and include group means and standard deviations and numbers of animals per group. Statistical analysis was performed using GraphPad Prism 6, v6.0c (GraphPad Software, San Diego, CA, USA). For comparison of 48/80 and CQ induced scratching, results were compared using a one-way ANOVA across doses or time. Bonferroni post hoc tests were used to compare groups at similar doses or times. For all post hoc comparisons, multiplicity adjusted p-values were calculated. In each case, Bonferroni post hoc tests (e.g., t-tests with Bonferroni corrections) were undertaken and presented in the graphics and figure legends for values between $p < 0.01$ and $p < 0.0001$.

Acknowledgments: This work was supported by DA15353 (TY), 5R21AI113580-02 (RR) and DA02110 (SP).

Author Contributions: R.R. and T.L.Y. conceived and designed the experiments; R.R., M.J.M., S.P., Z.W., N.L.M. and S.P. performed the experiments; R.R., S.P. and Z.W. analyzed the data; A.D. and E.A.J. contributed to reagents/materials/analysis tools; R.R. wrote the paper.

Conflicts of Interest: The authors declare no conflict of interest.

References

1. Balaskas, E.V.; Chu, M.; Uldall, R.P.; Gupta, A.; Oreopoulos, D.G. Pruritus in continuous ambulatory peritoneal dialysis and hemodialysis patients. *Perit. Dial. Int.* **1993**, *13* (Suppl. 2), S527–S532. [PubMed]
2. Chia, S.C.; Bergasa, N.V.; Kleiner, D.E.; Goodman, Z.; Hoofnagle, J.H.; Di Bisceglie, A.M. Pruritus as a presenting symptom of chronic hepatitis C. *Dig. Dis. Sci.* **1998**, *43*, 2177–2183. [CrossRef] [PubMed]
3. Yosipovitch, G.; Greaves, M.W.; Schmelz, M. Itch. *Lancet* **2003**, *361*, 690–694. [CrossRef]
4. Oaklander, A.L.; Bowsher, D.; Galer, B.; Haanpää, M.; Jensen, M.P. Herpes zoster itch: Preliminary epidemiologic data. *J. Pain* **2003**, *4*, 338–343. [CrossRef]
5. Ikoma, A.; Steinhoff, M.; Ständer, S.; Yosipovitch, G.; Schmelz, M. The neurobiology of itch. *Nat. Rev. Neurosci.* **2006**, *7*, 535–547. [CrossRef] [PubMed]
6. Schmelz, M.; Schmidt, R.; Weidner, C.; Hilliges, M.; Torebjörk, H.E.; Handwerker, H.O. Chemical response pattern of different classes of C-nociceptors to pruritogens and algogens. *J. Neurophysiol.* **2003**, *89*, 2441–2448. [CrossRef] [PubMed]
7. Schmelz, M.; Schmidt, R.; Bickel, A.; Handwerker, H.O.; Torebjörk, H.E. Specific C-receptors for itch in human skin. *J. Neurosci.* **1997**, *17*, 8003–8008. [PubMed]
8. Shim, W.-S.; Tak, M.-H.; Lee, M.-H.; Kim, M.; Kim, M.; Koo, J.-Y.; Lee, C.-H.; Kim, M.; Oh, U. TRPV1 mediates histamine-induced itching via the activation of phospholipase A2 and 12-lipoxygenase. *J. Neurosci.* **2007**, *27*, 2331–2337. [CrossRef] [PubMed]
9. Imamachi, N.; Park, G.H.; Lee, H.; Anderson, D.J.; Simon, M.I.; Basbaum, A.I.; Han, S.-K. TRPV1-expressing primary afferents generate behavioral responses to pruritogens via multiple mechanisms. *Proc. Natl. Acad. Sci. USA* **2009**, *106*, 11330–11335. [CrossRef] [PubMed]
10. McNaughton, F.L.; Obianwu, H.O.; Isah, A.O.; Arhewoh, I.M. Chloroquine-induced Pruritus. *Indian J. Pharm. Sci.* **2010**, *72*, 283–289.
11. Liu, Q.; Tang, Z.; Surdenikova, L.; Kim, S.; Patel, K.N.; Kim, A.; Ru, F.; Guan, Y.; Weng, H.-J.; Geng, Y.; et al. Sensory neuron-specific GPCR Mrgprs are itch receptors mediating chloroquine-induced pruritus. *Cell* **2009**, *139*, 1353–1365. [CrossRef] [PubMed]
12. Wilson, S.R.; Gerhold, K.A.; Bifolck-Fisher, A.; Liu, Q.; Patel, K.N.; Dong, X.; Bautista, D.M. TRPA1 is required for histamine-independent, Mas-related G protein-coupled receptor-mediated itch. *Nat. Neurosci.* **2011**, *14*, 595–602. [CrossRef] [PubMed]
13. Schiavo, G.; Rossetto, O.; Santucci, A.; DasGupta, B.R.; Montecucco, C. Botulinum neurotoxins are zinc proteins. *J. Biol. Chem.* **1992**, *267*, 23479–23483. [PubMed]
14. Montecucco, C.; Schiavo, G. Mechanism of action of tetanus and botulinum neurotoxins. *Mol. Microbiol.* **1994**, *13*, 1–8. [CrossRef] [PubMed]
15. Schiavo, G.; Matteoli, M.; Montecucco, C. Neurotoxins affecting neuroexocytosis. *Physiol. Rev.* **2000**, *80*, 717–766. [CrossRef] [PubMed]

16. Bach-Rojecky, L.; Lacković, Z. Central origin of the antinociceptive action of botulinum toxin type A. *Pharmacol. Biochem. Behav.* **2009**, *94*, 234–238. [CrossRef] [PubMed]
17. Marino, M.J.; Terashima, T.; Steinauer, J.J.; Eddinger, K.A.; Yaksh, T.L.; Xu, Q. Botulinum toxin B in the sensory afferent: Transmitter release, spinal activation, and pain behavior. *Pain* **2014**, *155*, 674–684. [CrossRef] [PubMed]
18. Filipović, B.; Matak, I.; Bach-Rojecky, L.; Lacković, Z. Central action of peripherally applied botulinum toxin type A on pain and dural protein extravasation in rat model of trigeminal neuropathy. *PLoS ONE* **2012**, *7*, e29803. [CrossRef] [PubMed]
19. Gazerani, P.; Pedersen, N.S.; Drewes, A.M.; Arendt-Nielsen, L. Botulinum toxin type A reduces histamine-induced itch and vasomotor responses in human skin. *Br. J. Dermatol.* **2009**, *161*, 737–745. [CrossRef] [PubMed]
20. Krämer, H.H.; Angerer, C.; Erbguth, F.; Schmelz, M.; Birklein, F. Botulinum Toxin A reduces neurogenic flare but has almost no effect on pain and hyperalgesia in human skin. *J. Neurol.* **2003**, *250*, 188–193. [CrossRef] [PubMed]
21. Tugnoli, V.; Capone, J.G.; Eleopra, R.; Quatrale, R.; Sensi, M.; Gastaldo, E.; Tola, M.R.; Geppetti, P. Botulinum toxin type A reduces capsaicin-evoked pain and neurogenic vasodilatation in human skin. *Pain* **2007**, *130*, 76–83. [CrossRef] [PubMed]
22. Carmichael, N.M.E.; Dostrovsky, J.O.; Charlton, M.P. Peptide-mediated transdermal delivery of botulinum neurotoxin type A reduces neurogenic inflammation in the skin. *Pain* **2010**, *149*, 316–324. [CrossRef] [PubMed]
23. Wollina, U.; Karamfilov, T. Adjuvant botulinum toxin A in dyshidrotic hand eczema: A controlled prospective pilot study with left-right comparison. *J. Eur. Acad. Dermatol. Venereol.* **2002**, *16*, 40–42. [CrossRef] [PubMed]
24. Akhtar, N.; Brooks, P. The use of botulinum toxin in the management of burns itching: Preliminary results. *Burns* **2012**, *38*, 1119–1123. [CrossRef] [PubMed]
25. Heckmann, M.; Heyer, G.; Brunner, B.; Plewig, G. Botulinum toxin type A injection in the treatment of lichen simplex: An open pilot study. *J. Am. Acad. Dermatol.* **2002**, *46*, 617–619. [CrossRef] [PubMed]
26. Pellett, S.; Tepp, W.H.; Whitemarsh, R.C.M.; Bradshaw, M.; Johnson, E.A. In vivo onset and duration of action varies for botulinum neurotoxin A subtypes 1–5. *Toxicon* **2015**, *107*, 37–42. [CrossRef] [PubMed]
27. Moon, T.C.; Befus, A.D.; Kulka, M. Mast cell mediators: Their differential release and the secretory pathways involved. *Front. Immunol.* **2014**, *5*, 569. [CrossRef] [PubMed]
28. Lorentz, A.; Baumann, A.; Vitte, J.; Blank, U. The SNARE Machinery in Mast Cell Secretion. *Front. Immunol.* **2012**, *3*, 143. [CrossRef] [PubMed]
29. Potenzieri, C.; Undem, B.J. Basic mechanisms of itch. *Clin. Exp. Allergy* **2012**, *42*, 8–19. [CrossRef] [PubMed]
30. Kuraishi, Y.; Nagasawa, T.; Hayashi, K.; Satoh, M. Scratching behavior induced by pruritogenic but not algesiogenic agents in mice. *Eur. J. Pharmacol.* **1995**, *275*, 229–233. [CrossRef]
31. Wallengren, J. Neuroanatomy and neurophysiology of itch. *Dermatol. Ther.* **2005**, *18*, 292–303. [CrossRef] [PubMed]
32. Schemann, M.; Kugler, E.M.; Buhner, S.; Eastwood, C.; Donovan, J.; Jiang, W.; Grundy, D. The mast cell degranulator compound 48/80 directly activates neurons. *PLoS ONE* **2012**, *7*, e52104. [CrossRef] [PubMed]
33. De Jonge, F.; De Laet, A.; Van Nassauw, L.; Brown, J.K.; Miller, H.R.P.; van Bogaert, P.P.; Timmermans, J.P.; Kroese, A.B.A. In vitro activation of murine DRG neurons by CGRP-mediated mucosal mast cell degranulation. *Am. J. Physiol.-Gastrointest. Liver Physiol.* **2004**, *287*, G178–G191. [CrossRef] [PubMed]
34. Durham, P.L.; Cady, R.; Cady, R. Regulation of calcitonin gene-related peptide secretion from trigeminal nerve cells by botulinum toxin type A: Implications for migraine therapy. *Headache* **2004**, *44*, 35–42. [CrossRef] [PubMed]
35. Meng, J.; Ovsepian, S.V.; Wang, J.; Pickering, M.; Sasse, A.; Aoki, K.R.; Lawrence, G.W.; Dolly, J.O. Activation of TRPV1 mediates calcitonin gene-related peptide release, which excites trigeminal sensory neurons and is attenuated by a retargeted botulinum toxin with anti-nociceptive potential. *J. Neurosci.* **2009**, *29*, 4981–4992. [CrossRef] [PubMed]
36. Heyer, G.; Vogelgsang, M.; Hornstein, O.P. Acetylcholine is an inducer of itching in patients with atopic eczema. *J. Dermatol.* **1997**, *24*, 621–625. [CrossRef] [PubMed]
37. Hong, J.; Buddenkotte, J.; Berger, T.G.; Steinhoff, M. Management of itch in atopic dermatitis. *Semin. Cutan. Med. Surg.* **2011**, *30*, 71–86. [CrossRef] [PubMed]

38. Koga, K.; Chen, T.; Li, X.-Y.; Descalzi, G.; Ling, J.; Gu, J.; Zhuo, M. Glutamate acts as a neurotransmitter for gastrin releasing peptide-sensitive and insensitive itch-related synaptic transmission in mammalian spinal cord. *Mol. Pain* **2011**, *7*, 47. [CrossRef] [PubMed]
39. Tobin, D.; Nabarro, G.; Baart de la Faille, H.; van Vloten, W.A.; van der Putte, S.C.; Schuurman, H.J. Increased number of immunoreactive nerve fibers in atopic dermatitis. *J. Allergy Clin. Immunol.* **1992**, *90*, 613–622. [CrossRef]
40. Dolly, J.O.; Lawrence, G.W.; Meng, J.; Wang, J.; Ovsepian, S.V. Neuro-exocytosis: Botulinum toxins as inhibitory probes and versatile therapeutics. *Curr. Opin. Pharmacol.* **2009**, *9*, 326–335. [CrossRef] [PubMed]
41. Ramachandran, R.; Lam, C.; Yaksh, T.L. Botulinum toxin in migraine: Role of transport in trigemino-somatic and trigemino-vascular afferents. *Neurobiol. Dis.* **2015**, *79*, 111–122. [CrossRef] [PubMed]
42. Cui, M.; Khanijou, S.; Rubino, J.; Aoki, K.R. Subcutaneous administration of botulinum toxin A reduces formalin-induced pain. *Pain* **2004**, *107*, 125–133. [CrossRef] [PubMed]
43. Huang, P.P.; Khan, I.; Suhail, M.S.A.; Malkmus, S.; Yaksh, T.L. Spinal botulinum neurotoxin B: Effects on afferent transmitter release and nociceptive processing. *PLoS ONE* **2011**, *6*, e19126.
44. Keller, J.E.; Neale, E.A. The role of the synaptic protein SNAP-25 in the potency of botulinum neurotoxin type A. *J. Biol. Chem.* **2001**, *276*, 13476–13482. [CrossRef] [PubMed]
45. Whitemarsh, R.C.M.; Tepp, W.H.; Bradshaw, M.; Lin, G.; Pier, C.L.; Scherf, J.M.; Johnson, E.A.; Pellett, S. Characterization of botulinum neurotoxin A subtypes 1 through 5 by investigation of activities in mice, in neuronal cell cultures, and in vitro. *Infect. Immun.* **2013**, *81*, 3894–3902. [CrossRef] [PubMed]
46. Keller, J.E. Recovery from botulinum neurotoxin poisoning in vivo. *Neuroscience* **2006**, *139*, 629–637. [CrossRef] [PubMed]
47. Park, T.H. The effects of botulinum toxin A on mast cell activity: Preliminary results. *Burns* **2013**, *39*, 816–817. [CrossRef] [PubMed]
48. Guo, Z.; Turner, C.; Castle, D. Relocation of the t-SNARE SNAP-23 from lamellipodia-like cell surface projections regulates compound exocytosis in mast cells. *Cell* **1998**, *94*, 537–548. [CrossRef]
49. Vaidyanathan, V.V.; Puri, N.; Roche, P.A. The last exon of SNAP-23 regulates granule exocytosis from mast cells. *J. Biol. Chem.* **2001**, *276*, 25101–25106. [CrossRef] [PubMed]
50. Woska, J.R.; Gillespie, M.E. SNARE complex-mediated degranulation in mast cells. *J. Cell. Mol. Med.* **2012**, *16*, 649–656. [CrossRef] [PubMed]
51. Shimizu, T.; Shibata, M.; Toriumi, H.; Iwashita, T.; Funakubo, M.; Sato, H.; Kuroi, T.; Ebine, T.; Koizumi, K.; Suzuki, N. Reduction of TRPV1 expression in the trigeminal system by botulinum neurotoxin type-A. *Neurobiol. Dis.* **2012**, *48*, 367–378. [CrossRef] [PubMed]
52. Apostolidis, A.; Popat, R.; Yiangou, Y. Decreased sensory receptors P2X3 and TRPV1 in suburothelial nerve fibers following intradetrusor injections of Botulinum toxin for human detrusor overactivity. *J. Urol.* **2005**, *174*, 977–983. [CrossRef] [PubMed]
53. Cochrane, D.E.; Douglas, W.W. Calcium-induced extrusion of secretory granules (exocytosis) in mast cells exposed to 48-80 or the ionophores A-23187 and X-537A. *Proc. Natl. Acad. Sci. USA* **1974**, *71*, 408–412. [CrossRef] [PubMed]
54. Hirokawa, N.; Heuser, J.E. Structural evidence that botulinum toxin blocks neuromuscular transmission by impairing the calcium influx that normally accompanies nerve depolarization. *J. Cell Biol.* **1981**, *88*, 160–171. [CrossRef] [PubMed]
55. Yaksh, T.L.; Ozaki, G.; McCumber, D.; Rathbun, M.; Svensson, C.; Malkmus, S.; Yaksh, M.C. An automated flinch detecting system for use in the formalin nociceptive bioassay. *J. Appl. Physiol.* **2001**, *90*, 2386–2402. [CrossRef] [PubMed]
56. Marino, M.; Huang, P.; Malkmus, S.; Robertshaw, E.; Mac, E.A.; Shatterman, Y.; Yaksh, T.L. Development and validation of an automated system for detection and assessment of scratching in the rodent. *J. Neurosci. Methods* **2012**, *211*, 1–10. [CrossRef] [PubMed]
57. Wang, Z.; Lai, Y.; Bernard, J.J.; Macleod, D.T.; Cogen, A.L.; Moss, B.; Di Nardo, A. Skin mast cells protect mice against vaccinia virus by triggering mast cell receptor S1PR2 and releasing antimicrobial peptides. *J. Immunol.* **2012**, *188*, 345–357. [CrossRef] [PubMed]
58. Kirshenbaum, A.S.; Metcalfe, D.D. Growth of human mast cells from bone marrow and peripheral blood-derived CD34+ pluripotent progenitor cells. *Methods Mol. Biol.* **2006**, *315*, 105–112. [PubMed]

toxins

MDPI

Article

Monocentric Prospective Study into the Sustained Effect of Incobotulinumtoxin A (XEOMIN®) Botulinum Toxin in Chronic Refractory Migraine

Ioana Ion [1,*], Dimitri Renard [1], Anne Le Floch [1], Marie De Verdal [1], Stephane Bouly [1], Anne Wacongne [1], Alessandro Lozza [2] and Giovanni Castelnovo [1]

1 Department of Neurology, Nimes University Hospital, 30900 Nimes, France; dimitri.RENARD@chu-nimes.fr (D.R.); anne.LEFLOCH@chu-nimes.fr (A.L.F.); marie.DEVERDAL@chu-nimes.fr (M.D.V.); stephane.BOULY@chu-nimes.fr (S.B.); anne.WACONGNE@chu-nimes.fr (A.W.); giovanni.castelnovo@chu-nimes.fr (G.C.)

2 Neurological Institute, Foundation Casimiro Mondino, 27100 Pavia, Italy; alessandro.lozza@mondino.it

* Correspondence: IOANAMARIA.ION@chu-nimes.fr; Tel.: +33-064-316-8679

Received: 16 April 2018; Accepted: 28 May 2018; Published: 1 June 2018

Abstract: Refractory chronic migraine is a disabling disorder impacting quality of life. BOTOX® (Onabotulinumtoxin A) is approved as a prophylactic treatment of chronic migraine in patients unresponsive to at least three prior preventive treatments. The objective of this study was to determine the prophylactic effect of 145 U XEOMIN® (Incobotulinumtoxin A) injected at 31 specific sites in adult patients with refractory chronic migraine. Sixty-one patients (8 men and 53 women, mean age 50) with migraine were recruited, including 20 patients with isolated chronic migraine, 18 patients with chronic migraine associating tension-type headache, 12 patients with migraine associating medication *overuse headache*, and 11 patients with episodic disabling migraine. The mean number of injections and duration of treatment per patient was 3.5 (range 2–13) and 21 (6–68) months, respectively. From baseline to first injection, 44 patients (73%) had >50% reduction in frequency of migraine episodes, 29 patients (48%) showed >50% reduction in number of headache days, and 28 patients (46%) had a >50% reduction in drug intake. Stable response for all three parameters was observed after the last injection. XEOMIN® thus seems to represent an effective and sustained prophylactic treatment of chronic migraine.

Keywords: refractory chronic migraine; tension headache; medication *overuse headache*; prophylactic treatment; XEOMIN®

Key Contribution: In this study, XEOMIN® proved to be an effective prophylactic treatment with sustained efficacy in patients with a refractory CM and EDM.

1. Introduction

Between 2% and 15% of the world's population suffers from migraines, with a wide variation of frequency of attacks [1]. Refractory chronic migraine (CM) is a disabling illness causing significant interference with quality of life, despite promising results from trials of acute and prophylactic treatments. CM affects up to a fifth of migraine patients [1].

Despite the development of new pathophysiological hypotheses (and associated recent advancements on drug development), the benefit of the majority of conventional migraine preventive drugs does not exceed 50% over placebo [2]. A recent meta-analysis shows that only high dose topiramate and sodium valproate were more effective than placebo at reducing migraine by more than 50% [3].

The National Institute for Health and Clinical Excellence (NICE) and the US Food and Drug Administration have both recently approved BOTOX® (botulinum toxin type A—BoNT/A) for the prophylaxis of CM, specifically in refractory (i.e., not responding to at least three prior prophylactic treatments) CM patients [4,5]. In studies analyzing efficacy of BOTOX® in migraine patients, treatment also seemed to be effective in patients with migraine and associated medication *overuse headache* [MOH]) [6]. It was recently suggested that BOTOX® also represents an effective and safe intervention to target psychiatric comorbidities of migraine with improvements in depression and anxiety [7]. Double-blind, placebo-controlled trials of toxin A injections in patients with isolated episodic disabling migraine headaches (EDM) or tension-type headache (TTH) did not show significant effect of BoNT/A onabotulinum, even after controlling for a high placebo effect and after dose stratification [8–10]. However, patient numbers were low in these studies. Available clinical trials analyzing BONT/A efficacy in patients with isolated TTH show conflicting data, with a majority of studies showing no efficacy [11].

Botulinum toxin A efficacy has never been analyzed in patients with migraine and associated TTH.

XEOMIN® inhibits the release of acetylcholine from peripheral cholinergic nerve endings acting like a myorelaxant, but also like an analgesic by suppressing the peripheral and central sensitization [12]. Unlike other neurotoxins, XEOMIN® triggers minimal allergic reactions as it has no binding albumin protein [13].

To the best of our knowledge, XEOMIN® efficacy in migraine or other headache types has never been reported. The objective of our study was to assess the effect of XEOMIN® treatment in refractory CM (isolated or associated with TTH or MOH) and EDM patients.

2. Results

Demographic and clinical features of patients are shown in Table 1. Sixty-one patients (8 men and 53 women; mean age 50, range 22–73) were recruited, including 20 patients with isolated CM, 18 with CM-TTH, 12 with CM-MOH, and 11 with EDM. Before inclusion, nonsteroidal anti-inflammatory drugs, paracetamol, morphine, and triptans were used in 18, 20, 9, and 32 of the 61 patients, respectively. The mean number of injections and mean duration of treatment per patient was 3.5 (range 2–13) and 21 (range 6–68) months, respectively (Table 2).

Table 1. Demographic and clinical features.

Demographic Features	
Sex: men/women	8/53
Age: years, mean ± SD	50 ± 10
Headache type	
Isolated chronic migraine	20 (33%)
Chronic migraine + tension-type headache	18 (29%)
Chronic migraine + medication *overuse headache*	12 (20%)
Episodic disabling migraine	11 (18%)

Table 2. Treatment effect of XEOMIN®.

XEOMIN® responders	44 (73%)
Mean number of injections	3.5 (2–13)
Mean duration of treatment (months)	21 (6–68)
Mean duration of effect (weeks)	13.63

For the entire patient group, between baseline and the episode after the last injection, a >50% reduction in frequency of migraine episodes and headache days was observed in 44 (73%) and 29 patients (48%), respectively, whereas a >50% decrease in drug intake was observed in 28 patients (46%). In total, 44 patients (73%) were considered responders, including 18 CM, 16 CM-TTH, 6 CM-MOH, and 4 EDM patients. The 17 non-responders showed absence of therapeutic response in six patients and <50% response in 11 patients after two injections.

Compared to non-responders, responders showed >50% reduction of consumption of any acute medication after a mean of two years of treatment ($p < 0.001$). The mean number of pain-relief pills per month reduced from baseline to the episode after the last injection: 51 to 18 for morphine, 67 to 14 for paracetamol, 12 to 4 for triptan, and 12 to 5 for nonsteroidal anti-inflammatory drugs.

Median migraine episodes decreased from 8.5 (range 1–30) at baseline to 2 (range 0–16) after the first injection ($p < 0.001$) and to 2 (range 0–15) after the last injection ($p < 0.001$) (without difference in efficacy between the first and last injection, $p = 0.3$), corresponding to a 76% decrease from baseline to both later time points (Figure 1). Mean headache days decreased from 20.8 (SD 9.6) at baseline to 8.5 (SD 8.2) after the first injection ($p < 0.001$) and to 7.3 (SD 7.6) after the last injection ($p < 0.001$) (without difference in efficacy between the first and last injection, $p = 0.4$), corresponding to a 41% and 36% decrease from baseline to the first and last injection, respectively (Figure 1).

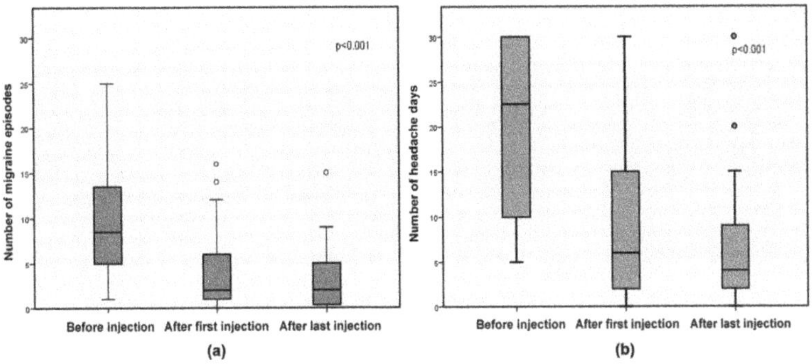

Figure 1. Responder group: box-and-whisker diagrams, presented as medians and interquartile ranges of (**a**) number of migraine episodes and (**b**) number of headache days. Circles represent outliers.

In the subgroup of patients with isolated CM (Figure 2), mean migraine episodes decreased from 9.83 (SD 6.23) at baseline to 4.06 (SD 4.04) and 4.26 (SD 3.98) after the first (59% reduction, $p < 0.001$) and last injection (57% reduction, $p < 0.001$), respectively (without difference in efficacy between first and last injection, $p = 0.8$); mean number of headache days was reduced from 13.11 (SD 7.71) at baseline to 4.40 (SD 4.27) (69% decrease, $p < 0.001$) after the first injection and to 4.66 (SD 4.21) after the last injection (67% decrease, $p < 0.001$) (without difference in efficacy between the first and last injection, $p = 0.9$).

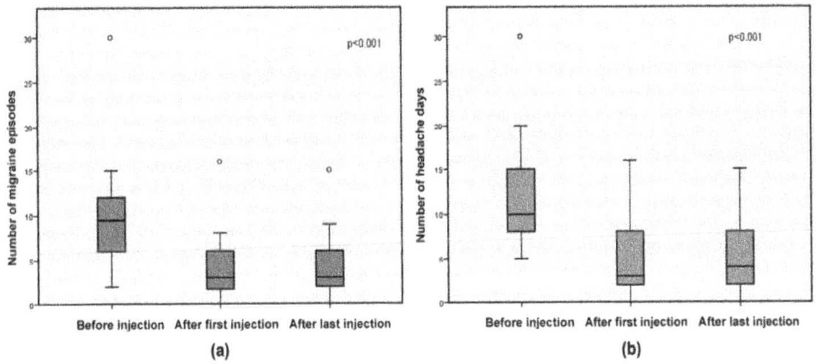

Figure 2. Isolated chronic migraine subgroup: box-and-whisker diagrams, presented as medians and interquartile ranges of (**a**) number of migraine episodes and (**b**) number of headache days. Circles represent outliers.

In the subgroup of patients with headache type other than isolated CM (Figure 3), the median number of migraine episodes decreased from 8 (range 1–30) at baseline to 2 (range 0–14) after the first injection (69% decrease, $p < 0.001$) and to 1 (range 0–9) (93% decrease, $p < 0.001$) after the last injection (without difference in efficacy between the first and last injection, $p = 0.1$), and median number of headache days from 27 (range 8–30) at baseline to 9 (range 0–30) after the first injection (57% decrease, $p < 0.001$), and to 4.5 (0–30) after the last injection (69% decrease, $p < 0.001$) (without difference in efficacy between the first and last injection, $p = 0.3$).

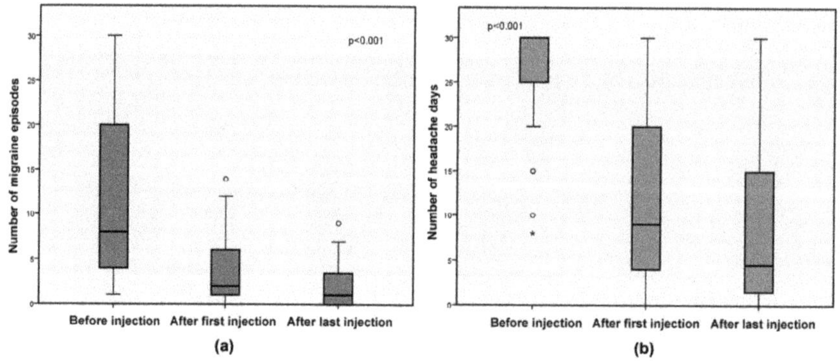

Figure 3. CM/TTH, CM-MOH and EDM subgroup: box-and-whisker diagrams, presented as medians and interquartile ranges of (**a**) number of migraine episodes and (**b**) number of headache days. Circles represent outliers.

When comparing both subgroups (isolated CM vs. non-isolated CM), non-isolated CM patients showed more frequent treatment response than isolated CM patients ($p < 0.001$ for both number of migraine episodes between baseline and first injection and between baseline and last injection; $p < 0.001$ for both the number of headache days between baseline and first injection and between baseline and last injection; $p < 0.001$ for both reduction in drug intake between baseline and first injection and between baseline and last injection).

The treatment was generally well tolerated. The most frequent adverse events reported were neck pain (7%) and flu-like syndrome (5%), but all these symptoms were transitory, disappearing after a maximum of 72 h, did not interfere with patient activity, and did not need further management. Overall, no patients discontinued treatment due to adverse events.

3. Discussion

In this study, XEOMIN® proved to be an effective prophylactic treatment with sustained efficacy in patients with a refractory CM and EDM. Treatment efficacy was observed both in patients with isolated migraine and in patients with migraine and associated TTH or MOH. XEOMIN® was well tolerated and no serious adverse events were observed.

To the best of our knowledge, this is the first prospective study analyzing the prophylactic efficacy of XEOMIN® in patients with refractory migraine and the efficacy of botulinum toxin in patients with migraine and associated TTH.

The PREEMPT 2 study has demonstrated that BOTOX® is effective for prophylaxis of adult CM patients [14]. BoNT/A treatment was also effective (significant reduction of headache days and triptan intake) in the subgroup of patients with CM and associated MOH in the PREEMT study [6].

One retrospective case series reporting on 21 Xeomin®-treated CM patients showed improvement in headache severity and frequency [15].

The treatment response we found in our XEOMIN® study corresponded to that observed in the earlier BOTOX® study [16]. However, in contrast with the PREEMPT 2 study where only the number of headache/migraine days was analyzed, we also assessed the number of migraine episodes and the reduction in drug intake. Our data support evidence that XEOMIN® treatment is effective on all three headache parameters.

In our study, the incobotulinum effect was sustained (lasting from the very first injection to the last) in all responders.

Study limitations included the lack of a control group (because of the known high placebo effect for headache treatment and especially for injectable therapies), the small sample size, and the non-inclusion of specific tools assessing depression, disability and quality of life. The long-term follow-up of the patients included in our study is ongoing.

A double-blind BOTOX® and XEOMIN® treatment study should be conducted in more patients (and compared with a placebo arm) with isolated migraine and with migraine associating other headache types in order to compare the efficacy of both BoNT/A treatments in the different patient groups.

4. Conclusions

These results suggest that IncobotulinumtoxinA toxin may be an effective and safe prophylactic treatment for a variety of refractory migraines. Its effect is sustained over time, reducing medication overuse, as suggested in the open-label phase of PREEMPT.

5. Materials and Methods

Between August 2009 and January 2016, we invited all adult patients with CM (isolated or associated with TTH or MOH) to a specialized headache consultation at our center (Nîmes University Hospital, France) or with EDM to be included in our study. The diagnosis of the different headache types analyzed in our study fulfilled the criteria of the International Classification of Headache Disorders ICHD-3 [17]. Pregnancy was an exclusion criterion. Signed written informed consent was obtained in all included patients.

Each patient was injected with a total of 145 UI of XEOMIN® at 31 specific points, topographically similar to the myogenic trigger points associated with referred pain locations (facial, pericranial and cervical muscles) [7]. The injections were scheduled at an interval between 3 and 6 months.

We prospectively evaluated the benefit of XEOMIN® by calculating the number of migraine episodes and headache days, and the drug intake (expressed in number of pills of nonsteroidal anti-inflammatory drugs, paracetamol, morphine, and triptans) during the six months preceding the first injection, during the 3 to 6 months after the first injection, and during the 3 to 6 months after the last injection.

Responders were defined as patients with at least 50% reduction in frequency of migraine episodes and/or headache days. Responder analyses were performed for the entire patient group and for 2 pre-specified patient subgroups (i.e., patients with isolated CM and patients with headache type other than isolated CM). Further injections were stopped in case of non-response after 2 injections.

The software used for statistical analysis was Statistical Package for Social Sciences (SPSS 20). Paired *t*-test was used to study differences between outcome variables (with $p < 0.05$ deemed as significant difference). Median was used for the groups with abnormal distribution, and mean for the rest of the analyses when permitted.

Author Contributions: Conceptualization, G.C. and I.I; Methodology, I.I.; Software, I.I.; Validation, A.L., M.D.V. and A.L.F.; Formal Analysis, I.I.; Investigation, G.C.; Resources, A.W.; Data Curation, S.B.; Writing-Original Draft Preparation, I.I.; Writing-Review & Editing, D.R.; Visualization, D.R.; Supervision, G.C.; Project Administration, G.C.

Funding: This research received no external funding.

Acknowledgments: We would like to thank Sarah Kabani (Department of Biostatistics, Epidemiology, Public Health and Innovation in Methodology (BESPIM), CHU de Nîmes, 4 Rue du Professeur Debré, 30029 Nîmes Cedex 09) for substantive editing of our manuscript.

Conflicts of Interest: The authors declare no conflicts of interest.

References

1. Stovner, L.; Hagen, K.; Jensen, R.; Katsarava, Z.; Lipton, R.; Scher, A.; Steiner, T.; Zwart, J.-A. The Global Burden of Headache: A Documentation of Headache Prevalence and Disability Worldwide. *Cephalalgia* **2007**, *27*, 193–210. [CrossRef] [PubMed]
2. Shamliyan, T.A.; Choi, J.-Y.; Ramakrishnan, R.; Miller, J.B.; Wang, S.-Y.; Taylor, F.R.; Kane, R.L. Preventive Pharmacologic Treatments for Episodic Migraine in Adults. *J. Gen. Intern. Med.* **2013**, *28*, 1225–1237. [CrossRef] [PubMed]
3. Jackson, J.L.; Cogbill, E.; Santana-Davila, R.; Eldredge, C.; Collier, W.; Gradall, A.; Sehgal, N.; Kuester, J. A Comparative Effectiveness Meta-Analysis of Drugs for the Prophylaxis of Migraine Headache. *PLoS ONE* **2015**, *10*, e0130733. [CrossRef] [PubMed]
4. Aurora, S.K.; Winner, P.; Freeman, M.C.; Spierings, E.L.; Heiring, J.O.; DeGryse, R.E.; VanDenburgh, A.M.; Nolan, M.E.; Turkel, C.C. OnabotulinumtoxinA for Treatment of Chronic Migraine: Pooled Analyses of the 56-Week PREEMPT Clinical Program. *Headache* **2011**, *51*, 1358–1373. [CrossRef] [PubMed]
5. Dodick, D.W.; Turkel, C.C.; DeGryse, R.E.; Aurora, S.K.; Silberstein, S.D.; Lipton, R.B.; Diener, H.-C.; Brin, M.F. OnabotulinumtoxinA for Treatment of Chronic Migraine: Pooled Results From the Double-Blind, Randomized, Placebo-Controlled Phases of the PREEMPT Clinical Program. *Headache* **2010**, *50*, 921–936. [CrossRef] [PubMed]
6. Silberstein, S.D.; Blumenfeld, A.M.; Cady, R.K.; Turner, I.M.; Lipton, R.B.; Diener, H.-C.; Aurora, S.K.; Sirimanne, M.; DeGryse, R.E.; Turkel, C.C.; et al. OnabotulinumtoxinA for treatment of chronic migraine: PREEMPT 24-week pooled subgroup analysis of patients who had acute headache medication overuse at baseline. *J. Neurol. Sci.* **2013**, *331*, 48–56. [CrossRef] [PubMed]
7. Zhang, H.; Zhang, H.; Wei, Y.; Lian, Y.; Chen, Y.; Zheng, Y. Treatment of chronic daily headache with comorbid anxiety and depression using botulinum toxin A: A prospective pilot study. *Int. J. Neurosci.* **2017**, *127*, 285–290. [CrossRef] [PubMed]
8. Ramachandran, R.; Yaksh, T.L. Therapeutic use of botulinum toxin in migraine: Mechanisms of action: Botulinum toxins as a prophylaxis for migraine. *Br. J. Pharmacol* **2014**, *171*, 4177–4192. [CrossRef] [PubMed]
9. Luvisetto, S.; Gazerani, P.; Cianchetti, C.; Pavone, F. Botulinum Toxin Type A as a Therapeutic Agent against Headache and Related Disorders. *Toxins* **2015**, *7*, 3818–3844. [CrossRef] [PubMed]
10. Shuhendler, A.J.; Lee, S.; Siu, M.; Ondovcik, S.; Lam, K.; Alabdullatif, A.; Zhang, X.; Machado, M.; Einarson, T.R. Efficacy of Botulinum Toxin Type A for the Prophylaxis of Episodic Migraine Headaches: A Meta-analysis of Randomized, Double-Blind, Placebo-Controlled Trials. *Pharmacotherapy* **2009**, *29*, 784–791. [CrossRef] [PubMed]
11. Silberstein, S.; Göbel, H.; Jensen, R.; Elkind, A.; DeGryse, R.; Walcott, J.; Turkel, C. Botulinum Toxin Type A in the Prophylactic Treatment of Chronic Tension-Type Headache: A Multicentre, Double-Blind, Randomized, Placebo-Controlled, Parallel-Group Study. *Cephalalgia* **2006**, *26*, 790–800. [CrossRef] [PubMed]
12. Durham, P.L.; Cady, R. Insights into the Mechanism of OnabotulinumtoxinA in Chronic Migraine: November/December 2011. *Headache* **2011**, *51*, 1573–1577. [CrossRef] [PubMed]
13. Frevert, J.; Dressler, D. Complexing proteins in botulinum toxin type A drugs: A help or a hindrance? *Biol. Targets Ther.* **2010**, 325. [CrossRef] [PubMed]
14. Diener, H.; Dodick, D.; Aurora, S.; Turkel, C.; DeGryse, R.; Lipton, R.; Silberstein, S.; Brin, M. OnabotulinumtoxinA for treatment of chronic migraine: Results from the double-blind, randomized, placebo-controlled phase of the PREEMPT 2 trial. *Cephalalgia* **2010**, *30*, 804–814. [CrossRef] [PubMed]
15. Kazerooni, R.; Lim, J.; Ashley Blake, P.; Lessig, S. IncobotulinumtoxinA for Migraine: A Retrospective Case Series. *Clin. Ther.* **2015**, *37*, 1860–1864. [CrossRef] [PubMed]

16. Ranoux, D.; Martiné, G.; Espagne-Dubreuilh, G.; Amilhaud-Bordier, M.; Caire, F.; Magy, L. OnabotulinumtoxinA injections in chronic migraine, targeted to sites of pericranial myofascial pain: An observational, open label, real-life cohort study. *J. Headache Pain* **2017**, *18*, 75. [CrossRef] [PubMed]
17. Headache Classification Committee of the International Headache Society (IHS). The International Classification of Headache Disorders, 3rd edition (beta version). *Cephalalgia* **2013**, *33*, 629–808. [CrossRef]

toxins

MDPI

Review

The Expanding Therapeutic Utility of Botulinum Neurotoxins

Elena Fonfria [1,*], Jacquie Maignel [2], Stephane Lezmi [2], Vincent Martin [2], Andrew Splevins [1], Saif Shubber [3], Mikhail Kalinichev [2], Keith Foster [1], Philippe Picaut [4] and Johannes Krupp [2]

1 Ipsen Bioinnovation, 102 Park Drive, Milton Park, Abingdon, Oxfordshire OX14 4RY, UK; andrew.splevins@ipsen.com (A.S.); keith.foster@ipsen.com (K.F.)
2 Ipsen Innovation, 5 Avenue du Canada, 91940 Les Ulis, France; jacquie.maignel@ipsen.com (J.M.); stephane.lezmi@ipsen.com (S.L.); vincent.martin@ipsen.com (V.M.); mikhail.kalinichev@ipsen.com (M.K.); johannes.krupp@ipsen.com (J.K.)
3 Ipsen Biopharm Ltd., Wrexham Industrial Estate, 9 Ash Road, Wrexham LL13 9UF, UK; saif.shubber@ipsen.com
4 Ipsen Bioscience, 650 Kendall Street, Cambridge, MA 02142, USA; philippe.picaut@ipsen.com
* Correspondence: elena.fonfria@ipsen.com; Tel.: +44-(0)1235-44-88-79

Received: 13 April 2018; Accepted: 16 May 2018; Published: 18 May 2018

Abstract: Botulinum neurotoxin (BoNT) is a major therapeutic agent that is licensed in neurological indications, such as dystonia and spasticity. The BoNT family, which is produced in nature by clostridial bacteria, comprises several pharmacologically distinct proteins with distinct properties. In this review, we present an overview of the current therapeutic landscape and explore the diversity of BoNT proteins as future therapeutics. In recent years, novel indications have emerged in the fields of pain, migraine, overactive bladder, osteoarthritis, and wound healing. The study of biological effects distal to the injection site could provide future opportunities for disease-tailored BoNT therapies. However, there are some challenges in the pharmaceutical development of BoNTs, such as liquid and slow-release BoNT formulations; and, transdermal, transurothelial, and transepithelial delivery. Innovative approaches in the areas of formulation and delivery, together with highly sensitive analytical tools, will be key for the success of next generation BoNT clinical products.

Keywords: new indications; formulation; delivery

Key Contribution: Review presenting the current therapeutic landscape of BoNTs, their biological effects distal to the site of injection, and the challenges faced in their pharmaceutical development.

---

1. Current Therapeutic Landscape

Based upon the use of neutralising antibodies, there are currently seven different serotypes of botulinum neurotoxin (BoNT) that have been reported, from BoNT A through to G. More recently, an eighth serotype has been identified at the protein sequence level, BoNT/X, although this has not yet been produced or characterised as a protein [1]. Over the last 15 years, it has also been recognised that within each serotype there are multiple sub-types, each with a unique protein sequence and a distinct molecular entity [2]. All BoNT serotypes and their subtypes inhibit the neurotransmitter release from nerve terminals through the prevention of acetylcholine release at the neuromuscular junction, which results in flaccid paralysis. Despite this, the intracellular target proteins, receptors, pharmacodynamic properties, and potencies vary substantially between BoNT serotypes.

Despite the great diversity of natural BoNTs and the fact that there are several manufacturers of BoNT for both aesthetic and therapeutic applications, to date, all of the commercially available BoNT products are serotype BoNT/A1, except for a single serotype BoNT/B product, Myobloc®/Neurobloc®.

However, BoNT/B showed to be less potent in the clinic than had been anticipated based on its efficacy during animal studies. The reason for this has recently been identified as a residue difference within human synaptotagmin II, which is the protein receptor for BoNT/B [3,4]. The residue difference is within the binding recognition sequence of synaptotagmin II and renders human synaptotagmin II a lower affinity receptor for BoNT/B than in other species. The low affinity for human synaptotagmin II requires higher doses of toxin to be injected in order to achieve efficacy that is similar to BoNT/A, and this results in a different safety profile and a high rate (up to 18%) of neutralizing antibodies as compared to BoNT/A (0 to 5%) ([5]; FDA label). For this reason, the BoNT/B product is not widely used. The identification of the molecular explanation for BoNT/B having lower efficacy in humans has enabled the design of modified BoNT/B sequences that are able to bind human synaptotagmin II with higher affinity, and so to potentially have improved therapeutic characteristics [6].

The three most widely used and commercially available BoNT/A products are Dysport® (abobotulinumtoxinA, Ipsen, Paris, France), Botox® (onabotulinumtoxinA, Allergan, Dublin, Ireland), and Xeomin® (incobotulinumtoxinA, Merz, Frankfurt am Main, Germany). While the mechanism of action of these three products is the same, there are differences between them, since the BoNT/A that is produced and purified is specific to each toxin manufacturer, and the final formulation is different for each product. For example, the potency units are different for each product, and they are not interchangeable [7]. The unit is defined as the mouse LD50 by the intraperitoneal route, and each company assesses these in its own proprietary assay. This means that a "Dysport® unit" is not the same as a "Botox® unit", or yet again, a "Xeomin® unit". The clinically approved doses, which are measured in the respective units, are again, therefore, different between the products. The amount of human serum albumin also differs (highest in Xeomin® [1 mg], when compared to Botox® [500 μg], and lowest in Dysport® [125 μg]), and most importantly, the amount of neurotoxin is different in each individual product (3.24 ng per 500 U vial for Dysport®; 0.73 ng per 100 U vial for Botox®; 0.44 ng per 100 U vial for Xeomin® [8]), leading to potentially different efficacy profiles in humans.

An excellent review of commercially available BoNT products and their manufacture is provided in Pickett, 2014 [9]. The key aspects of the major BoNT products that are available in the United States and Europe are given in Table 1. Currently, all of the commercially available BoNT products are manufactured using native *Clostridium botulinum* as the production organism, although some companies are exploring the use of recombinant expression using *Escherichia coli*. This would allow a standardised and safer manufacturing process for BoNT/A and for other serotypes and genetically modified versions of the neurotoxin.

Table 1. Characteristics of current major botulinum neurotoxin (BoNT) products.

	AboA [1]	**IncoA** [2]	**OnaA** [3]	**RimaB** [4]
1st Approval	1991	2005	1989	2000
Serotype	A1	A1	A1	B
Strain	Hall	Hall	Hall	Bean
Purification Method s	Chromatography	Unpublished	Crystallization	Chromatography
Complex Size	>500 kD	150 kD	900 kD	700 kD
Excipients	HSA (125 μg) Lactose	HSA (1 mg) Sucrose	HSA (500 μg) Sodium chloride	HSA (500 μg/mL) Sodium succinate Sodium chloride
Stabilization	Lyophilization	Lyophilization	Vacuum drying	Solution
Solubilization	Normal saline	Normal saline	Normal saline	N/A
pH	~7	~7	~7	5.6
Unitage (U/vial)	300, 500	100, 200	100, 200	2500, 5000, 10,000
Shelf Life (months)	24	36	36	24
Neurotoxin Protein (ng/vial) †	4.35	0.6	5	~25, 50, 100

† Protein (ng/vial) is for entire neurotoxin complex, the total protein load being dominated by albumin. HSA = human serum albumin. [1] AboA = abobotulinumtoxinA (Dysport®). Dysport® PI, Ipsen, 2015. [2] IncoA = incobotulinumtoxinA (Xeomin®). Xeomin® PI, Merz, 2015. [3] OnaA = onabotulinumtoxinA (Botox®). Botox® PI, Allergan, 2015. [4] RimaB = rimabotulinumtoxinB (Myobloc®/Neurobloc®). Myobloc® PI, Worldwide Meds, 2010.

In the United States of America (USA) and Europe, both Dysport® and Botox® are approved for use in adult upper and lower limb spasticity, while Xeomin® is only approved for use in adult upper limb spasticity (the Xeomin adult lower limb Phase 3 pivotal study did not meet its primary endpoint at the 400 U dose [NCT01464307, https://clinicaltrials.gov/]). Dysport® is the only BoNT/A product approved in the USA for the use in children with lower limb spasticity. The Botox® study is still ongoing, (NCT01603628), while the Xeomin® pivotal Phase 3 study did not meet its primary endpoint (NCT01893411).

Over the last two decades, the localized efficacy of BoNT/A, and its well tolerated safety profile, has resulted in significant growth of on-label use across multiple therapeutic and aesthetic indications. BoNT/As are well tolerated, which has also favoured significant growth in its empirical/off-label use in a variety of movement, ophthalmologic, gastrointestinal, urologic, orthopedic, dermatologic, secretory, and pain disorders.

BoNT is injected locally in skeletal muscles (on-label such as cervical dystonia, hemifascial spasm, blepharospasm, spasticity in adult and children; or, off-label such as writer cramp, tremors, spasmodic dysphonia), smooth muscles (on-label neurogenic detrusor overactivity, idiopathic bladder overactivity; or, off label such as bladder pain syndrome, detrusor sphincter dyssynergia) or exocrine gland hyperfunction (on-label sialorrhea, axillary hyperhidrosis; or, off-label, such as Frey's syndrome, plantar/palmar hyperhidrosis). More recently, BoNT has been used in pain related disorders (on-label chronic migraine or off-label, such as osteoarthritis, neuropathic pain, lower back pain). In aesthetic, BoNT is used to treat multiple facial hyperkinetic lines that are related to striated muscles spasm (on-label glabellar lines, lateral canthal lines, front lines; or, off-label such as lateral eyebrow lift, nasal lines, mid and lower face, neck).

Currently available BoNT products have certain limitations. As the injection is local, there is the risk, although very low, for the toxin to diffuse locally in the vicinity of the tissue injected and induce unwanted effects, or more importantly, to spread far from the original injection site. These unwanted side effects are influenced by the injection technique, the dose, and the volume. The injection procedure can also be a limitation, as it necessitates the specific training for injectors and can be painful for patients, hence there is a need to develop novel formulations and delivery techniques, such as transdermal delivery or products with a longer duration of response (BoNT/A products are reinjected every three to four months in most indications, while an injection interval of six to nine months duration would be of clinical interest). Limitations of the current toxin products may also relate to vial size (3 to 10 mL) relative to some therapeutic indications where the injection volume can be 15 to 30 mL. In addition to these limitations, when seeking to expand the approved clinical indications for BoNT products, there is a strong need to assess the risk-benefit profile through well-designed research clinical trials.

2. Alternative Serotypes, Broadening the Therapeutic Landscape

Although only BoNT/A or BoNT/B serotype products are currently available as licenced clinical products, several other serotypes of BoNT have been explored as potential therapeutic agents in humans. The use of BoNT/F as an alternative serotype in patients who had become resistant to BoNT/A through antibody formation was first reported in 1992 [10]. Subsequent studies confirmed the clinical benefit of BoNT/F in dystonic patients, and revealed that it had a significantly shorter duration of response [11–17].

Another BoNT serotype, with an even shorter duration of response, is BoNT/E. A comparison of BoNT/E and BoNT/A in the *extensor digitorum brevis* muscle of human volunteers using compound muscle action potential (CMAP) to assess the efficacy that was demonstrated a much faster recovery following BoNT/E administration [18]. Surprisingly, in this study, when the *extensor digitorum brevis* was injected with a combination of both BoNT/A and E, recovery was similar to that observed with BoNT/E alone; this is not consistent with the findings in a number of animal experiments, nor with the understanding that BoNT/A light chain survives in the neuronal cytosol and results in ongoing paralysis, even after the BoNT/E has worn off [19–21]. Short acting BoNTs, such as E and F, have potential clinical applications in therapeutic areas where a significantly shorter duration of response (3–6 weeks) when compared to that of BoNT/A (3–4 months) is required, for example, in orthopedics and rehabilitation medicine [22]. Recently, a biotechnology company, Bonti, announced that it is developing a BoNT/E product, EB-001, in aesthetic and therapeutic indications. The first phase 2 study, with EB-001 in glabellar frown lines, demonstrated the safety and clinical efficacy for this indication. Bonti have also initiated a phase 2 clinical study to evaluate the safety and efficacy of EB-001 by intramuscular injection in reducing musculoskeletal pain in patients undergoing elective augmentation mammoplasty. Ipsen also have a recombinant BoNT/E in phase 1 clinical studies; this is the first recombinant botulinum neurotoxin ever to have entered clinical trials in humans.

In addition to its shorter duration of response, which offers therapeutic differentiation from existing BoNT products, preclinical studies also indicate that BoNT/E has additional properties that may open up novel therapeutic applications. Experimental studies in rats showed that BoNT/E that was injected into the hippocampus inhibited glutamate release and reduced both focal and generalised kainic acid-induced seizures [23]. BoNT/E also prevented neuronal loss and long term cognitive defects that were associated with kainic acid seizures, and reduced sensitivity to electrical stimulation of kindling, indicating an antiepileptogenic activity. The authors suggested that this activity is a result of selective inhibition of excitatory glutaminergic versus GABAergic transmission by BoNT/E attributable to preferential localisation of SNAP-25 in excitatory hippocampal neurons.

A third alternative to BoNT/A, which was explored for its potential therapeutic utility, is serotype BoNT/C. A comparison of the neuromuscular blockade induced by BoNT/C, assessed electrophysiologically in the *extensor digitorum brevis* muscle of human volunteers, showed an efficacy and duration of action that was very similar to BoNT/A [24]. The same authors reported that it was used to treat two patients with idiopathic facial hemispasm and one patient with blepharospasm with long lasting beneficial effects. BoNT/C injections, like BoNT/A injections, did not affect the motor neuron count in human volunteers, showing it to be well tolerated [25]. BoNT/C was successfully tested in a pilot series of BoNT/A non-responsive patients with focal dystonia (four with torticollis and two with blepharospasm) [26]. Patients did not develop secondary resistance to BoNT/C after chronic use. The activity of BoNT/C in BoNT/A-resistant patients was further confirmed in patients with cervical dystonia [27]. Despite this early clinical interest, as of yet, no commercial product based upon BoNT/C has been produced, possibly reflecting that it is not sufficiently differentiated from BoNT/A in its clinical characteristics.

In addition to the BoNT serotypes that are described above, potential differences between BoNT/A subtypes have also been explored. Comparison of BoNT/A subtypes 1 to 5 revealed distinct characteristics both in vitro and in vivo [28,29]. BoNT/A2 was more potent in vitro and in vivo compared to BoNT/A1 [28,30–32]. As BoNT/A2 was reported to enter neuronal cells faster than BoNT/A1, this was proposed to be responsible for the difference in potency [30]. It has also been suggested that a higher occupancy of the cellular receptors by BoNT/A2 as compared to BoNT/A1 is the underlying mechanism [33]. The crystal structure of BoNT/A2 bound to the luminal domain of its cognate protein receptor SV2C, has been recently resolved, showing that the mode of binding of BoNT/A2 to SV2C does not substantially differ from that of BoNT/A1 [34]. The intoxication symptoms in mice that were injected i.v. with 10^4 units/mL of BoNT/A2 have been reported to differ from those in mice injected i.v. with 10^5 units/mL of BoNT/A1 [29,35]. Using a twitch tension assay in mouse hemi-diaphragm and rat grip strength model it was proposed that BoNT/A2 was a more potent neuromuscular blocker and spread less to the contralateral limb than BoNT/A1 [32]. For further discussion of the differences in spread between BoNT/A1 and BoNT/A2, see Section 4.4. It has also been reported that BoNT/A2 is less immunogenic than BoNT/A1 [36], but the comparison compared a complexed form in the case of BoNT/A1 with purified BoNT/A2, so there is the potential that the differential presence of complexing proteins influenced the measured immunogenicity. The authors also claimed that BoNT/A2 was less susceptible to neutralisation by human antisera raised to BoNT/A1 complex toxoid vaccine. In healthy volunteers, BoNT/A2 caused a reduction in CMAP with a comparable onset and duration as onabotulinumtoxin A [37]. Subsequently, BoNT/A2 was compared to onabotulinumtoxin A in post-stroke spasticity. BoNT/A2 was reported to show higher efficacy and less spread, as measured by the hand grip of the unaffected side, than the A1 toxin [38]. Animal models have also shown that BoNT/A2 could be a promising therapeutic in Parkinson's disease and inflammatory and neuropathic pain [39–41]. In 2016, Shionogi & Co. Ltd. (Osaka, Japan) announced a licence agreement with Tokoshima University for BoNT/A2, and is undertaking its global development as a novel BoNT therapeutic.

3. Novel Indications

3.1. Pain and Migraine

Pain is the most common reason for a patient to seek medical help, and it is seen by physicians as a symptom of an underlying medical condition [42]. While acute pain typically measures in days to weeks, chronic pain can persist from months to years, thus representing a major health-care issue with a serious impact on quality of life and significant socio-economic cost [43,44]. Chronic pain is classified as inflammatory (such as osteoarthritis, rheumatoid arthritis), neuropathic (such as diabetic, post-herpetic neuralgia), or dysfunctional (such as tension type headache, migraine, interstitial cystitis, irritable bowel syndrome) [45]. Current medication for acute and chronic pain includes opioids, cyclooxygenase inhibitors, acetaminophen, as well as several repositioned drugs, such as the antidepressant drug duloxetine and the antiepileptic drug pregabalin. While these drugs offer some pain relief, they are not consistently effective, often result in tolerance when being taken over a prolonged period and cause serious side-effects that hinder their use [46]. Therefore, there is a need for new pain therapeutics that can offer improved efficacy, reduced propensity to cause tolerance, and fewer side-effects. There is rapidly growing evidence that BoNT can offer an effective, long-lasting pain relief, and very few side-effects in a wide range of medical conditions.

The initial evidence of pain relief in response to BoNT treatment is linked to several serendipitous observations in clinical studies involving muscle hyperactivity and muscle pain in patients with spasticity, dystonia, and related conditions. While muscle relaxant effects may play a role in some of these conditions, there is growing evidence that they cannot account for all mechanisms mediating pain relief following BoNT treatment across a growing range of medical conditions. For example, even in conditions involving intramuscular-administered BoNT, effects in pain can precede and/or last longer in comparison to the muscle-relaxant effects [47,48]. Also, it is now well-accepted that, in addition to local uptake in the synaptic terminal, a distinct secondary uptake pathway results in retrograde transport of BoNT and its activity at distal sites [49]. The retrograde transport of BoNT from the site of uptake at the sensory neuron ending into the dorsal root ganglion and the spinal cord is believed to play a pivotal role for the activity of BoNT in pain [50,51]. In addition to neurons, BoNT can impact the functional activity of glial cells, such as Schwann cells and astrocytes, which suggests the presence of yet another mechanism of pain modulation by BoNT [52–54].

Since the initial discovery several decades ago, the field of therapeutic application of BoNT in pain has been growing rapidly, which was predominately led by observations and studies performed in clinical settings. Despite the rapid growth of the field, prophylactic treatment of chronic migraine is the only pain indication currently approved based on the outcome of two multi-center phase 3 studies [55] and their combined *post hoc* analysis [56]. Reflecting the recent grade A recommendation of the American Academy of Neurology, BoNT/A should be used in chronic migraine and should not be used (as ineffective) in episodic migraine [57]. Apart from these two migraine indications with clear recommendations on the use of BoNT/A, there are a number of other types of headaches where the evidence is not as clear, as both positive and negative clinical results have been obtained. For example, the effects of BoNT/A in tension-type headache, which is the most common primary headache and pain condition, have been evaluated in several open-label and randomized, placebo-controlled studies. BoNT/A injected into the pericranial muscles every three months during 18 months (in an open-label study) or only once (in a double-blind study), reduced the severity of headache, reduced pericranial muscle tenderness, and increased the number of headache-free days [58]. In contrast, BoNT/A failed to improve any measures of tension-type headache in two other placebo-controlled, double-blind clinical studies [59,60]. Interestingly, in another double-blind placebo-controlled study, no difference was seen between the BoNT/A and the placebo group on Day 60, but a significant number of patients reported a 50% decrease in headache days at Day 90 [61]. This suggests that, at least with tension-type headache, longer post-treatment periods need to be evaluated in order to see the effect. Similar discrepancies in the efficacy of BoNT in pain across clinical studies have been seen in other indications, such as osteopathic pain [62].

What makes it difficult for a given pain indication to interpret and to compare the results across clinical studies, is the fact that there is no consistency in the experimental variables used, such as sites and routes of injection, number of injections needed, doses, administration regimens (single vs. repeated), etc. Back-translating the human findings into an appropriate animal model with the objective to perform a systematic evaluation of the experimental variables can greatly benefit the field. Furthermore, performing clinical studies in large animals, which show pain conditions that are closer to humans in etiology, can provide additional value. For example, in a placebo-controlled, randomized, double-blind clinical study, intra-articular injection of BoNT/A reduced the joint pain in osteoarthritic dogs [63]. In another randomized, placebo-controlled study in dogs, sub-cutaneous administration of BoNT into the mammary glands 24 h before bilateral, radical, cancer-related mastectomy significantly decreased the post-operative need for rescue morphine analgesia [64]. These findings are well aligned with those showing BoNT/A-mediated pain relief in cancer patients after surgery and/or radiation [65].

Overall, while the diverse pool of clinical studies assessing the efficacy of BoNT in pain is an important source of potential new indications, the questions of where, when, and how to inject require systematic assessment in pre-clinical studies. In addition, pre-clinical studies have been essential in building our understanding of potential mechanisms of BoNT-induced pain relief [28,66,67]. Testing BoNT in disease-relevant animal models, including those in rodents and in larger species, combined with a better understanding of the mechanisms that are involved, can build a solid case for initiation of clinical studies in a new pain or headache indication.

3.2. *Osteoarthritis*

Osteoarthritis (OA) is the most common form of arthritis in humans and OA-related joint pain is a major health concern [68]. Since no disease modifying agents for OA exist, the clinical focus is on pain management and minimizing the functional impairment of the joint.

In OA, changes to the joint articular cartilage surfaces and underlying cartilage matrix lead to the loss of joint space and joint misalignment, as well as inflammation of the joint synovium [69,70]. Fissures and fractures in the cartilage surface appear. Changes at the interface between cartilage and bone, the osteochondral junction, allow for the penetration of sensory and sympathetic nerves from the richly innervated bone marrow [70]. The inflammation eventually causes both the peripheral and central sensitization of neurons, leading to spontaneous joint pain at rest and hyperalgesia. Despite progress on the exact mechanism leading to the pain sensation [71], our detailed mechanistic understanding remains sketchy. However, it seems reasonable to assume that release of sensory neuropeptides such as substance P, calcitonin gene-related peptide (CGRP), and neurokinin A, contributes to the pain sensation in OA [62,72]. Since BoNTs can inhibit the release of these peptides, intra-articular BoNT administration may be able to directly reduce peripheral sensitization, and indirectly reduce central sensitization.

From clinical studies, there is however limited evidence that intra-articular BoNT injections have beneficial effects. Hsieh and colleagues [73] studied 46 patients with symptomatic OA knee who were randomly assigned to a BoNT/A treatment group (100 U Botox®) into the affected knee) or a control group. The pain visual analogue scale score in the treatment group significantly decreased from the pretreatment value early after treatment (one week) and was still decreased at the six-month post-treatment follow-up, resulting in a significant difference to the control group at both timepoints. Similar findings were obtained with two other evaluation scales, thus showing that intra-articular injection of BoNT/A provided pain relief and improved functional abilities for the patients with OA knee in this study. However, in a recent double-blind, randomized, placebo-controlled, 12-week trial using a single ultrasound-guided intra-articular injection of BoNT/A in 121 patients no significant differences in clinical efficacy parameters were found between Botox® and placebo in the entire population [74]. In another study recently completed in 176 patients with OA knee with Botox®, no statistically significant difference was observed on any of the parameter assessing pain between the onabotulinum toxin and placebo (NCT02230956). Both of the studies add to earlier clinical studies using intra-articular BoNT injections in various rheumatic conditions that were recently reviewed by Khenioui and colleagues [62]. Although the 16 reviewed studies were heterogeneous and had various shortcomings that prohibited the reaching of a generalized conclusion with a satisfactory level of confidence, the reviewing authors did notice that they provided some trend towards the anti-nociceptive effect of intra-articular BoNT/A. Such results show that more research is necessary to understand the mechanism of action and the behaviour of the botulinum toxin when being injected intra-articular. Furthermore, the potential analgesic effects of intra-articular BoNT injections in clinical studies could be explained based on the results of preclinical studies [63,75–78]. New botulinum toxins that are engineered to specifically target some pain receptors and act on some biomarkers could be developed in future as novel therapeutics.

3.3. Overactive Bladder and Neurogenic Detrusor Overactivity

The bladder is a densely innervated organ, and its functions (storing and discarding urine) are under the synergistic control of the sensory, parasympathetic, and somatic nervous system [79]. Overactive bladder (OAB) is a syndrome where urinary urgency is often accompanied by frequency and nocturia. The mechanisms underlying OAB are still a matter of debate. A 'myogenic' hypothesis proposes that OAB results primarily from detrusor myocyte overexcitability, whereas a more recent, 'urothelium-based', hypothesis highlights the action of the mucosa on afferences sensitization and overactivity. Interestingly, specific cell types, such as urothelial cells [80], and, more recently, telocytes [81], have emerged as pivotal in the development of pathological conditions. Neurogenic detrusor overactivity (NDO) is described in patients with neurologic lesions (e.g., multiple sclerosis, spinal cord injury) where a sacral spinal micturition reflex develops through the activation and the remodelling of C fibres.

Oral antimuscarinic agents are the first line pharmacological therapy for urine storage dysfunction. BoNT started being used off-label in the early 2000s as a second line therapy in OAB [82]. Soon, it became clear that BoNTs action was not limited to its action on parasympathetic structures and acetylcholine release controlling detrusor contractility, but that it was also targeting sensory afferents. Animal models showed that BoNT/A was able to decrease the release of ATP and increase the level of NO [83,84], thus reducing the bladder afferences sensitization, and also decrease CGRP and substance P release, acting on the inflammatory component that may accumulate in bladder dysfunction [85]. Furthermore, clinical evidence highlighted the effect of BoNT/A on nerve growth factor (NGF) release, as well as TRPV1 expression, which are involved in the development of detrusor overactivity [86,87].

Moreover, clinical data suggest that BoNT/B may be efficacious at lower doses in the autonomic nervous system of the human bladder when compared to the somatic nervous system, and this was also shown by experiments in rodents [88,89], see also Figure 1. Therefore, there may be a therapeutic opportunity for treating patients with different serotypes [3], within the limits of species sensitivity, as discussed earlier, in Section 2. SV2/SNAP25 are more abundant in cholinergic as compared to sensory fibres in the human bladder [90], which may explain some cases of urinary retention in patients being treated by intradetrusor injections of BoNT/A. Intrathecal administration of BoNT/A in spinal cord-injured rats, the prototypical animal model of neurogenic detrusor overactivity, resulted in normalization of pathological bladder contractions and bladder basal pressure [91]. This may open research opportunities for natural or engineered neurotoxins that are targeting the afferent and pivotal component of the disease with a different therapeutic profile compared to BoNT/A.

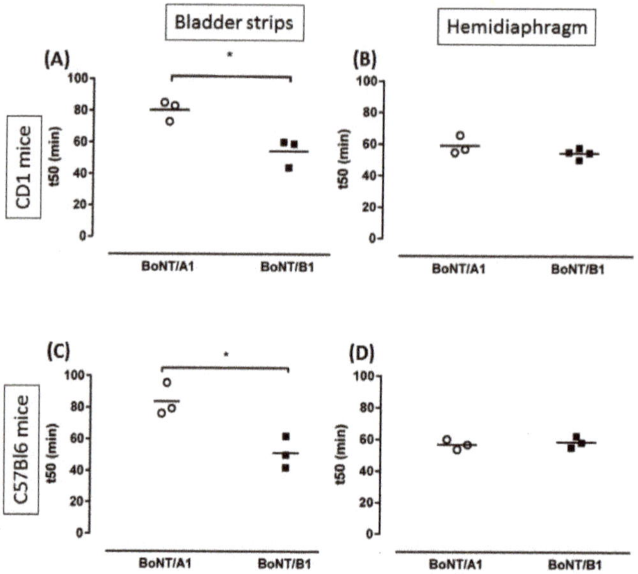

Figure 1. Whatever the mouse strain, BoNT/B1 is significantly more potent than BoNT/A1 in a model of detrusor contractions (**A**,**C**), while the potencies of BoNT/A1 and BoNT/B1 were equal in the phrenic nerve-hemidiaphragm preparation (**B**,**D**).* $p < 0.05$ (unpaired Student's t test) [89].

3.4. Wound Healing

The healing of a wound comprises four overlapping phases: haemostasis, inflammation, tissue proliferation, and remodeling (for review see [92]). Increased metabolic activity and inflammation during healing can induce muscle contractions around the edges of the wound, which in turn, creates repetitive tension on the wound [93]. This has the potential to not only delay the healing of the wound, but also to increase fibrosis and induce or aggravate hypertrophic scarring. Chemoimmobilisation of the musculature adjacent and under a surgical wound through injection of BoNT could thus be beneficial for the overall wound healing process and the cosmetic appearance of the healed wound.

Indeed, there is clinical evidence that BoNT/A may have beneficial effects in wound healing. For example, using a visual analogue scale in patients who had undergone surgery for facial wounds, Ziade and colleagues [94] found a statistically significant improvement in scarring of the tissue in those patients who had been injected with BoNT within three days post-surgery, compared to patients not injected with BoNT. However, no statistically significant differences were found between the two groups in this study when using other assessment methods. Similarly, a systematic review of the literature for the use of BoNTs for the prevention of hypertrophic scars that included ten clinical studies, found improved cosmetic outcomes among certain studies. However, due to the heterogeneity of the studies, as well as other factors, the authors concluded that the data were not supportive of the clinical usage of BoNT for this indication at this time, but recommended randomized controlled trials to reach a firm conclusion [95]. At the time of writing, April 2018, two randomized controlled clinical trials are currently ongoing (NCT02623829 and NCT02886988).

While the clinical data are thus suggestive, but presently are not yet conclusive, preclinical experimental work has provided evidence that BoNTs do have beneficial effects in wound healing. For example, using a study design that allowed for each animal to be its own control, Lee and colleagues [96] showed significant differences in wound size between BoNT-treated and untreated control wounds. The treated wounds also showed less infiltration of inflammatory cells, a smaller number of fibroblasts, less fibrosis, and a lower expression of transforming growth factor (TGF)-β1, as compared to the control wounds. TGF-β1 is a fibrotic cytokine that has pleiotropic actions in wound healing [97], and it is involved in the formation of hypertrophic scars. The finding by Lee and colleagues [96] that BoNT-treated wounds show a lower expression of TGF-β1 may be the result of the chemoimmobilisation of the muscle. However, BoNTs may also directly interfere with the expression of TGF-β1 in fibroblasts and fibroblast proliferation [98,99].

4. BoNT Effects Remote from the Site of Injection

4.1. Neuronal Retrograde Transport and Central Effects

The vast majority of clinical effects that are exhibited by BoNTs are attributed to their well-established actions at the site of injection [100–105]. However, in some instance, the in situ activity of BoNT seems insufficient to fully explain its clinical efficacy, thus raising the idea that other "non-classical" actions on the central nervous system might also be involved [51,106,107]. Indeed, some data have shown that peripherally injected BoNT triggers distant changes at various central levels.

For example, the involvement of cortical networks after BoNT/A administration has been reported. Patients suffering from cervical dystonia were shown to display a higher neuronal excitability (measurement of P22/N30 cortical component of median nerve somatosensory evoked potentials) and reduced gray matter volume that was assessed by magnetic resonance imaging (MRI) in discrete cortex areas [108,109]. Local injections of BoNT/A in cervical muscles had long-lasting beneficial effects on these central alterations.

Some studies also assessed the effect of BoNT/A peripheral muscular injections on brainstem activity in patients with blepharospasm [110] or dysphonia [111]. In the first study, unilateral BoNT/A injections in the *orbicularis oculi* decreased in a strong and similar fashion the blink reflex after the stimulation of supra-orbital nerve in both ipsilateral and contralateral muscles. On the other hand, the activity of injected muscle measured by electromyography was not inhibited in the same proportion as the latter parameter. According to the authors, the beneficial action of BoNT/A in blepharospasm is thus more likely due to changes in brainstem interneuronal pathways than local muscular action [110]. The same conclusions were reached by Bielamowicz and Ludlow [111], who observed after unilateral BoNT/A administration in *thyroaritenoid* muscles decreased activation levels and spasmodic bursts that were measured by electromyography in both injected and contralateral muscles.

Central changes at the spinal cord level were also demonstrated. Marchand-Pauvert, Aymard [112] investigated, in patients exhibiting lower limb spasticity, the recurrent inhibition from a BoNT/A-injected muscle (*soleus*) to a distant untreated muscle (*quadriceps femoris*). After stimulation of the tibialis nerve that contains motoneurons innervating the *soleus*, the recurrent inhibition was found to be decreased in comparison with measurements that were recorded before treatment. The authors hypothesized that this effect was unlikely due to the local action of the neurotoxin in the injected muscle or on spindle afferent input, but is more likely due to a modification of spinal synaptic transmission. Indeed, they suggested that BoNT/A underwent retrograde neuronal transport from the injected muscle to the spinal cord and locally reduced the stimulation of motoneuron terminals on Renshaw cells, inhibitory interneurons projecting to motoneurons innervating the *quadriceps* muscle. This probably led to the decreased recurrent inhibition of the latter muscle [112]. A similar study obtained comparable findings [113], providing more evidence for a central action of BoNT in humans as a result of a putative neuronal retrograde transport.

Cellular and electrophysiological alterations in Renshaw cells were also found in rats that were injected peripherally with neurotoxins [114,115], indicating that such a phenomenon could also exist in animals. Antonucci, Rossi [21] demonstrated that BoNT/A injections in the hippocampus, whisker pads, or optic tectum led to the appearance of cleaved SNAP25 in the contralateral hippocampus, in the neuropil surrounding facial neurons soma, and in the retina, respectively. Interestingly, in the latter pathway, pretreatment with colchicine (which inhibits microtubule-dependent retrograde transport) abolished the appearance of cleaved SNAP25 in the retina. These first sets of data suggest that either an active form of BoNT/A or cleaved SNAP25 itself could have been transported from nerve terminals to neuron soma. The authors tried to answer that question by injecting BoNT/A in the optic tectum of rats, and, three days later, concomitantly sectioning the optic nerve and injecting BoNT/E in the eye vitreous. As expected, BoNT/E rapidly eliminated SNAP25 cleaved by BoNT/A from the eye. However, 25 days later, the appearance of SNAP25 cleaved by BoNT/A was observed, suggesting the presence of active BoNT/A in the same region [21].

Similar results were found in various in vivo studies, with the appearance of cleaved SNAP25 at the spinal cord level following peripheral BoNT/A injections in rat or mice hindlimb (Figure 2) [52,116–118], and in the brainstem after BoNT/A administration in the whisker pad [119–121] or in the optic tectum [122]. However, direct evidence for a retrograde transport of BoNT would be to detect an active form (either holotoxin or light chain) in central regions after peripheral administration. To our knowledge, this has never been demonstrated, although a work from Wang, Martin [123] showed the presence of fluorescently tagged BoNT/A heavy chain (thus not active) in mice spinal cord after hindlimb injection.

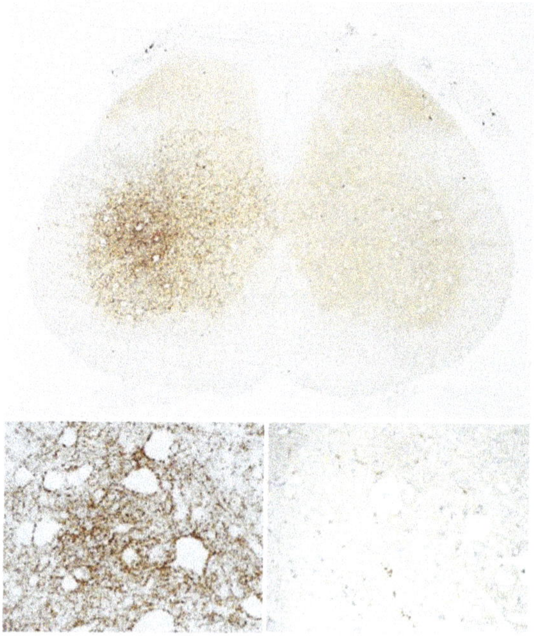

Figure 2. Immunohistochemistry staining of cleaved SNAP25 in rat lumbar spinal cord after BoNT/A injection in the left gastrocnemius muscle. Intense staining was found in the ipsilateral ventral horn neuropil, and only traces were found in the contralateral side (SL, VM, unpublished data).

Data from in vitro experiments shed some light on this question. Indeed, numerous works were able to demonstrate, in motoneuron or hippocampal neuron cultures, retrograde transport of either BoNT/A holotoxin or its heavy chain domain [49,120,123–125]. Interesting to note, heavy chains of both BoNT/A and tetanus toxin were found to share the same retrograde carriers when being retrogradely transported [120]. More precisely, BoNT/A heavy chain is thought to be internalized in nerve terminals within a specific pool of non-recycling synaptic vesicles [124], and undergo axonal retrograde transport in autophagosomes that finally fuse to lysosomes at the soma level [123]. In an elegant study, Bomba-Warczak, Vevea [49] used microfluidic chambers to demonstrate that application at the soma side of anti-BoNT/A antibodies or heavy chain competing with holotoxin prevents the appearance of cleaved SNAP25 in this compartment following BoNT/A application at the axon side. These data are thus in favor of a retrograde transport of BoNT/A holotoxin to the soma of the primary neuron, which is then exposed to the extracellular medium before entering the secondary neuron, leading to distal effects [49].

In vitro data are thus suggestive of retrograde transport of BoNT/A besides its classical mechanism of action, underlining some clinical observations. However, the axonal transport of a functional form of the toxin still needs to be clearly demonstrated in vivo. Apart from BoNT/A, little is known about the potential retrograde transport of other BoNT serotypes. Some data support the existence of such phenomenon for BoNT/E, but apparently, to a lesser extent than for BoNT/A [21,120,125]. BoNT/B [126] and BoNT/D [49] were also shown to undergo retrograde transport.

4.2. Diffusion within the Injected Muscle, Local Spread and Contributing Factors

When injected in a tissue, BoNTs present with a remarkable safety profile, mostly remaining within the injected organ, allowing for their use for various medical applications, as indicated in various reviews and meta-analyses [127–129]. While the diffusion of the injected toxin is somehow expected within the injected muscle or in very close neighboring muscles, local spread can be observed beyond the site of injection leading to different unexpected effects, depending of the targeted area. Local adverse effects that are associated with the intramuscular use of BoNT are thus due to excessive local muscle weakness and leakage to nearby muscles, and are reported as leading potentially to severe adverse events [130]. When used for the treatment of blepharospasm the most frequently reported adverse reactions were eyelid ptosis (21%), superficial punctate keratitis (6%), and dry eye (6%) for Botox® and eyelid ptosis (19%), dry eye (16%), and dry mouth (16%) for Xeomin® (for further details see prescribing information for both products, FDA). When used for the treatment of cervical dystonia, the most frequently reported adverse reactions were dysphagia (19%), upper respiratory infection (12%), neck pain (11%), and headache (11%) for Botox®; muscular weakness (16%), dysphagia (15%), dry mouth (13%), and injection site discomfort (13%) for Dysport®; and, dysphagia (18%), neck pain (15%), and muscle weakness (11%) for Xeomin® (for further details see prescribing information, FDA). Theses adverse effects suggest that unbound toxin moves away from the muscle, most likely through the extracellular space and determined by a concentration gradient. The dose, volume, and injection techniques that are used to target the different muscles are important to limit the occurrence of such adverse reactions.

The evaluation of local spread has been conducted in humans and animal models using electrophysiology and/or tissue markers, such as cleaved SNAP25 or other surrogate markers (for example, see Figure 3). Using electrophysiology and periodic acid-Schiff stain to identify glycogen content in muscle fibers, it was estimated that BoNT/A can pass through the *tibialis* muscle fascia (thick fibrous tissue covering the muscle), and the presence of the *tibialis* fascia can reduce the local spread by 20% in the rat [131]. This local spread was also confirmed in larger species, such as in the cat [132], and primates [133]. In rabbits that were injected with 2.5 U/kg of BoNT/A (unknown origin) by i.m. route in the *longissimus dorsalis* muscle, the intra-muscular diffusion of the toxin from the injection site was reported over a distance of 3 to 4.5 cm, and local spread across facial planes identified over a distance of 1.5 to 2.5 cm with the same intensity as within the injected muscle [134]. In the mouse, N-CAM (a marker that is expressed in denervated muscles) was strongly expressed in the myofiber of the injected *tibialis* muscle, but limited expression was detected in the ipsilateral *gastrocnemius* and *quadriceps femoris* muscles of the injected leg, suggesting a limited local spread in this model using three different BoNT/A formulations (Dysport®, Botox®, and Xeomin®) [135].

Regarding the effect of injection volume, little is known and the literature does not support a substantial influence on local spread. In humans treated for dynamic forehead lines at relatively low doses of BoNT/A (5 U Botox® /injection site) the area affected was slightly greater with an injected volume of 250 μL when compared to a volume of 50 μL; the increase in local diffusion was estimated to be around 1.5 times higher (+50%) for a five times larger injection volume [136]. Similarly, in humans, doubling the concentration (same dose in half the injection volume) resulted in significantly greater effects on the injected muscle, as assessed by CMAP amplitude evaluation (effect on the intra-muscular diffusion). However, effects in nearby muscles were only slightly dependent on the injected volume, with limited differences between the groups [137].

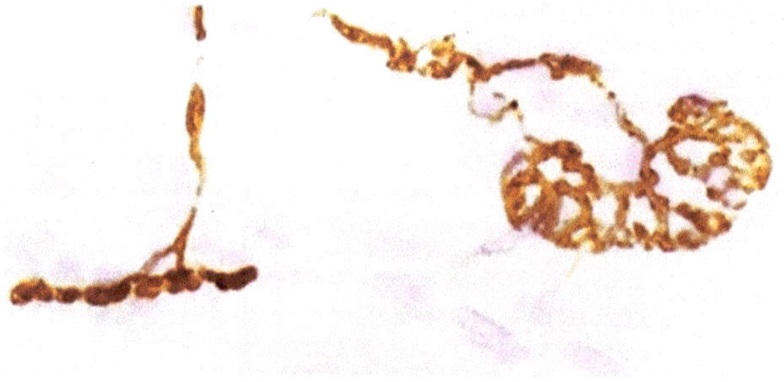

Figure 3. Immunohistochemistry staining of cleaved SNAP25 in rat muscle injected with BoNT/A (SL, VM, unpublished data).

4.3. *Systemic Spread and Contributing Factors*

Beyond local spread, leakage from the injection site may occur, resulting in a hematogenous spread and systemic exposure, leading to symptoms that are consistent with the mechanism of action of botulinum toxin [138]. Hematogenous spread may result in signs of asthenia, generalized muscle weakness, diplopia, blurred vision, ptosis, dysphagia, dysphonia, dysarthria, urinary incontinence, and breathing difficulties. These symptoms have been reported hours to weeks after injection. Extremely rare cases of swallowing and breathing difficulties have been reported [138–140], as indicated in all the commercially available BoNT labels. These observations are extremely rare and BoNTs present with a very good benefit/risk balance [128,129].

Various factors may affect the fate the injected toxin and its effect in the body, such as volume/concentration, amount of toxin, formulation, needle size, number of injections, precision of injection, and the biologic properties of the injected toxin (mechanism of action, duration of action, half-life in tissues), as well as the anatomy of the target area and tissue type [138,141].

BoNT serotype is also an important contributing factor affecting systemic spread. There was potentially greater spread to nearby and remote non-injected muscles that are associated with BoNT/A when compared to BoNT/B at equivalent efficacious doses in the mouse and primate using the CMAP test [134]. Similar observations were reported in the mouse, in which i.m. LD_{50} was 13.9 U/kg for BoNT/A (Botox®) and 104.6 U/kg for BoNT/B (Myobloc®), while safety margins (LD_{50}/ED_{50}) were lower for BoNT/B (5.4) than BoNT/A (13.9) [142], suggesting that BoNT/B is less safe. Other factors probably influence spread and its clinical consequences (e.g., toxin half-life in tissues and blood, distribution of receptors, co-receptors, and SNARE proteins in the targeted physiological system [muscular or autonomic], etc.). This was confirmed by a Japanese group using the CMAP test in the injected and contralateral limb muscle in the rat to compare toxins at equivalent efficacious doses [143]. They determined that BoNT/CD is the most prone to spread remotely, and that BoNT/D is least prone to spread. The rank order of BoNT serotypes based upon spread in this study in rats was CD > A > E > C > B > F > D. Interestingly, when ranked based upon safety index a different order was obtained: F > C > D > E > A > CD > B, with BoNT/F being the safest. Recent data obtained using CMAP amplitude and/or cleaved SNAP25 immunohistochemistry in remote muscles, also support the dose dependent systemic spread effect in rats that were injected with BoNT/A [116,117].

4.4. New BoNT Therapeutics with Decreased Spread

Spread could be an important differentiating factor in the BoNT therapeutic landscape. BoNT/A3 [144] and BoNT/A2 [38] are two subtypes that may offer reduced spread. BoNT/A2 has been reported as showing less spread to neighbouring muscles than BoNT/A1 [38]. In a study with healthy volunteers, the effect of 6.5 U BoNT/A2 and 10 U BoNT/A1 that is injected into the *extensor digitorum brevis* muscle on either side of the same subject were compared [37]. Although a similar onset, duration, and magnitude of the effect was seen for the two toxins, there was less spread of the effect to the neighbouring *abductor hallucis* muscle for BoNT/A2 compared to BoNT/A1. In a randomized double-blinded controlled phase 2/3 study in post-stroke spasticity, hand grip strength on the unaffected side was significantly reduced after BoNT/A1 treatment, but not after BoNT/A2, which is again consistent with less spread of A2 when compared to A1. In a later study, BoNT/A2 was reported to have reduced systemic toxicity, which is in agreement with the reduced spread that was reported in the clinical studies above [145], and also reduced anterograde transport compared to BoNT/A1, as measured by muscle contraction and immunocytochemical analysis [31,117]. However, despite these encouraging results, there is much lower number of safety data in humans for BoNT/A2 as compared to BoNT/A1, and as such, more human exposure to BoNT/A2 will be needed prior to establishing BoNT/A2 as a differentiated therapeutic. The biological properties and potential clinical utility of BoNT/A2 are discussed more fully in Section 2 above.

5. Novel Formulations

5.1. Current Products and Challenges Associated with Formulation of BoNTs

The BoNT formulations for the main commercially available products have existed for over 20 years. The formulation of BoNTs is challenging, owing to their structural complexities, the analytical tools that are available, and the low product concentrations used. The extremely high potency and selectivity of BoNT for cholinergic neurons, with a human lethal dose of parenteral injection estimated as between 0.1–1 ng/kg [146], requires that pharmaceutical preparations of BoNT comprise vanishingly small quantities of the toxin itself. Drug products have been shown to contain between 0.44 and 3.24 ng of the 150 kDa toxin per vial [8], and as such, present unique challenges for the formulation and the analytical strategy employed to assess stability. BoNTs in this respect differ from conventional biologics where much of the focus of formulation is on controlling protein aggregation [147]. One of the primary challenges in the formulation of BoNTs is minimising loss during manufacture and storage. BoNTs are also very susceptible to denaturation due to surface denaturation, heat, and alkaline conditions. Due to these contributing factors, the lyophilisation or freeze-drying of the toxin complex or the neurotoxin is the favoured method of distributing the product in a form that is stable and readily used by the clinician [9]. All BoNT/A clinical products currently available, apart from in Japan, Korea and Taipei, are dried powder products that need to be reconstituted for use. The BoNT/B product has been provided as a liquid, which is ready for use, since its license approval in December 2000. This product may be painful when injected, however, due to the acidic pH of the solution. Medytox was the first BoNT/A liquid product launched, Innotox®, but limited to Korea, Taipei, and Japan, as of today. Allergan licenced worldwide rights to Innotox outside Korea from Medytox. Most of the major clinical BoNT/A manufacturers are working to develop liquid formulations. Liquid formulation is considered the next generation of toxin products because of its convenience and ease of administration. Recently, Ipsen has reported a phase 2 clinical trial of a ready-to-use liquid formulation of abobotulinumtoxinA (abobotulinumtoxinA solution for injection, ASI). This formulation was shown to be efficacious, with comparable results to reconstituted abobotulinumtoxinA, and to have a favorable safety profile in subjects with severe to moderate glabellar lines [148]. Another feature of all the existing product formulations is the presence of human serum albumin (HSA) as a stabilising agent. This is not desirable due to the theoretical risk of contamination with pathogens. As part of the development of next generation liquid formulations, companies are exploring formulations that have different stabilisers and components, including the omission of excipients from animal origin and HSA.

5.2. Slow-Release Formulations

Advanced formulations for BoNT include the slow or sustained release formulations, which aim to release BoNTs over a defined period in a controlled manner. This may be through colloidal carrier technology and/or exploiting the thermo-responsive nature of polymeric solutions. Depending on the clinical application, such formulations may provide a benefit to the existing delivery methods that are used. The clinical use of a slow-release formulation or depot requires careful consideration. In many indications, the accuracy of injection is a critical factor during treatment, with skilled injectors depositing the BoNT at the neuromuscular junctions to minimise the spread to adjacent muscles. In many treatments, this is performed in multiple locations within a muscle to achieve the desired outcome. A successful slow-release depot would, therefore, have to remain in situ without migration for the period of release. The duration of BoNT therapeutic benefit in movement disorders is typically 3–4 months [149]. Currently, the sustained release profile for most clinically applicable depot formulations is no more than approximately seven days, which would not produce a significant improvement in duration for BoNTs. For a significant improvement in the duration of BoNT effects, release over 3–4 weeks is likely to be necessary. The challenge of formulating to achieve the desired release profile is therefore much greater and further compounded by the additional complexity of needing to stabilise a large and complex protein at 37 °C for this duration. Also, any depot would need to be sufficiently small that the lasting presence is not uncomfortable for the patient.

5.3. Analytical Challenges

If a slow-release formulation were to be developed, it would be desirable to demonstrate the release profile of the drug over time, both in vitro and in vivo. The concentration at the point of administration, however, is already in the picomolar range, a level at which most pharmacokinetic studies are performed. It seems likely that the released material from a slow-release depot would be at even lower concentration, and over a greater time. Accurate determination of this profile is important for a product possessing such high potency as BoNT [146]. This increases the analytical challenge in preparing such a formulation, ensuring the accuracy of the final dose, and developing a consistent release profile. The absence of circulating biomarkers for the intoxication of neurons by the toxin further increases the complexity, as the pharmacological measure is only obtained from measurement of the local paralysis, electrophysiology, or other functional responses. With recent advances in analytical sensitivities [150,151], the accurate detection of BoNT at the required concentrations is beginning to become achievable, but the technologies are still not in routine use. This analytical improvement will be vital for development of slow-release formulations of BoNTs.

6. Novel Delivery Methods

Currently clinical BoNT products are delivered by local injection into the target tissue. This can be a painful process and requires clinical expertise on the part of the administrating physician to ensure the correct local delivery and avoid the application to adjacent tissues resulting in a lack of therapeutic efficacy and/or off-target effects. For conditions such as hyperhidrosis, application can require multiple subcutaneous injections in sensitive locations, such as the palm or axilla, resulting in discomfort or even pain for the patient. Injection in such situations can require local analgesia or pain block. In bladder applications, where multiple injections via cystoscopy are required, this can require local or even general anaesthesia. Other limitations to the injection of BoNT products include erythema, swelling, and potential for infection. In aesthetic use in facial areas, there is also the risk of bruising and/or bleeding. Bleeding can also be an issue for injections of BoNT into the bladder urothelium. Development of needle-free delivery would therefore be of great benefit in such circumstances, requiring less specialised clinician input, increased convenience, and reduced discomfort/pain for the patient. Non-invasive delivery of BoNTs is challenging owing to the biological barriers limiting successful access to the intended tissue and the large size of the protein. Approaches under development involve either a physical or chemical approach to transiently permeabilise the barrier and enable entry of the BoNT. To date, all of the needle-free approaches in development are aimed at the relatively superficial delivery and not replacing intramuscular injection to deeper muscles involved in many of the movement disorders where BoNT is used therapeutically.

6.1. *Transdermal Delivery*

Development of transdermal drug delivery methods has a long history and has already made a significant contribution to medical practice [152], although largely for small molecule drugs to date. A number of investigators have studied the ability of enhancers to increase skin permeability and enable the transdermal entry of BoNT. One approach that has received a lot of attention is the use of Cell Penetrating Peptides (CPP), and particularly ones that are derived from the transactivator of transcription (TAT) protein of human immunodeficiency virus. Revance Therapeutics Inc. have progressed this approach for transdermal delivery of BoNT/A to the clinic for both lateral canthal lines and axillary hyperhidrosis. The neurotoxin construct that was progressed by Revance, RT001, consists of a purified 150 kDa BoNT/A protein formulated in a poloxamer gel containing a CPP, RTP004, a single chain peptide consisting of 35 L-amino acids. RTP004 has two domains, a core sequence of 15 lysines that confer positive charge to the peptide, and a protein transduction domain that is derived from residues 49–57 of the TAT protein [153]. The CPP associates with the neurotoxin protein non-covalently via ionic interactions between cationic regions within the CPP and the negatively charged surface of the neurotoxin protein. The resulting complex enables transcutaneous flux of the neurotoxin via cell to cell micropinocytosis. Varying the CPP was found to vary the delivery characteristics of the payload, enabling the delivery to different depths of penetration; the longer the peptide the deeper the penetration. In RT001, the CPP is formulated to deliver the BoNT/A to the mid-dermis appropriate for treatment of lateral canthal lines and hyperhidrosis. Phase 1 studies with RT001 showed it to be safe and tolerable [154]. Subsequently, a number of phase 2 studies demonstrated RT001 to be safe and effective in the treatment of moderate to severe lateral canthal lines or hyperhidrosis [155–157]. While in 2015, Revance announced that it had commenced dosing patients in a Phase 3 pivotal study to evaluate the safety and efficacy of RT001 for the treatment of lateral canthal lines the study did not achieve its co-primary endpoints, and was discontinued. Revance is now focused on developing an injectable form of BoNT/A combined with its proprietary peptide technology, RT002, which is claimed to spread less from the site of injection and to give a greater safety margin and enable the enhanced duration of therapeutic benefit.

Another approach to transdermal delivery of BoNT/A, which was developed by Anterios Inc., was the use of liposomes of a controlled size range to deliver BoNT/A for hyperhidrosis. Anterios was acquired by Allergan plc in 2016. In 2015, the lead Anterios formulation, ANT-1207, entered a phase 2 trial (NCT02479139) for axillary hyperhidrosis. Allergan have yet to report on the outcome of this study.

Chajchir and colleagues reported on the use of a microcrystal and nanoparticle formulation, InParT (Transdermal Corp), reconstituted with Botox® at 2 U/mL for transdermal delivery in the treatment of upper facial lines [158]. The formulation was found to be effective versus placebo based on patient reported Facial Line Outcome scores. The formulation was applied daily for a period of 4 to 7 weeks, with a 12 week follow up period. The improved outcome scores were maintained during the whole study period. Given the very low dose of BoNT/A that was employed, this result is surprising, but may reflect the frequent initial dosing regimen.

Transdermal delivery of BoNT/A using a short synthetic peptide, TD-1, as an enhancing agent has been reported to reduce plasma extravasation and blood flow changes that are evoked by electrical stimulation of the hind-paw in a rat model of neurogenic inflammation [159]. Peptide-mediated transdermal delivery of BoNT/A was proposed to offer an easy and non-invasive route of administration for the treatment of neurogenic inflammation.

Perhaps the most unusual and potentially risky uses of CPP to achieve transdermal delivery of BoNT was the direct fusion of the TAT peptide to the light chain of BoNT/A [160,161]. This was reported to enable the direct application and delivery of the light chain into cells without the need for any of the other domains of BoNT that mediate neuronal specific binding and the translocation of the light chain into the cytosol [160]. Transcutaneous delivery through mouse skin was also evaluated by immunohistochemistry. The authors discuss the therapeutic potential of such an approach, but it did not consider the lack of selective targeting or the potential for non-specific entry into any cell that was exposed to the fusion protein. Such a lack of cell selectivity must significantly increase the risk of non-specific toxicity and represent a significant safety barrier to therapeutic application of such a fusion protein.

The requirement for an enhancer to enable the transdermal delivery of BoNT is demonstrated by the inability of BoNT/A applied directly to the skin to impact palmar hyperhidrosis [162]. Without any enhancer to allow for the entry of the neurotoxin across the dermal barrier no effect above control was observed, clearly showing the inability of a large multi-domain protein, like BoNT, to cross the dermal layer unaided.

In addition to chemical enhancing agents, the use of physical approaches to disrupt the permeability barrier of the skin and enable entry of BoNT has been explored. Kavanagh and Shams reported the use of iontophoresis to deliver BoNT/A for the treatment of palmar hyperhidrosis, with an improvement in the sweat rate of 66%, which is a similar result to that obtained with intradermal BoNT/A [163]. Subsequently, Pacini and colleagues confirmed in rats that pulsed current iontophoresis delivered BoNT/A through living skin [164]. Following iontophoresis, BoNT/A was clearly detected in association with cutaneous striated skeletal muscle fibres in the deep dermis of the rat skin. Transdermal delivery by jet nebulization of BoNT/A in combination with lidocaine has been reported to be an effective and painless method for the successful treatment of palmar, plantar, and axillary hyperhidrosis [165]. An emerging technology for transdermal drug delivery is the use of microneedles [166], and the use of microneedles for the delivery of BoNT/A into the skin has been reported [167]. As yet, however, there are surprisingly few publications on this route of transdermal delivery for neurotoxin.

6.2. *Transurothelial Delivery*

The other major application of BoNT to have received considerable attention in regards to needle-free delivery is the use in the bladder for treatment of OAB and NDO. The current procedure is invasive, requiring cystoscopic guidance and multiple injections into the bladder, and often necessitating intravenous sedation or anaesthesia. If a less invasive, needle-free method of administration could be demonstrated to be effective, this would be preferable. There is also evidence that whilst injection of BoNT into the bladder wall impacts both the afferent and efferent nerves, approaches that avoid injection impact only afferent nerves, which may be therapeutically advantageous [168].

Intraluminal instillation of BoNT/A without injection failed to deliver toxin into the bladder wall due to the impermeability of the bladder urothelium to large macromolecules and degradation of the toxin by urine proteases [169,170]. In order to enable the entry of BoNT into the bladder wall, it is necessary to use chemical agents to denude the urothelium. One such approach is the use of the organic solvent dimethyl sulphoxide (DMSO) [170]. The safety and the efficacy of co-administration of BoNT/A with DMSO has been demonstrated in a clinical trial in women with refractory OAB [171]. Protamine sulphate has also been employed to denude the bladder urothelium and aid access of BoNT/A to the bladder wall [169,172]. Protamine sulphate pre-treatment of bladder prior to the instillation of BoNT/A has been reported to be safe and potentially effective in patients with refractory OAB [173]. Instillation of BoNT/A was reported to reduce the inflammatory effects that are caused by the prior injection of cyclophosphamide in a rat model of cystitis [174]. In this case, it was proposed that the permeability barrier of the bladder urothelium had been impaired by the cyclophosphamide-induced inflammation enabling access of the instilled BoNT/A. Hyaluronan-phosphatidylethanolamine (HA-PE) has been reported to be another potential chemical agent allowing for bladder instillation of BoNT/A to be effective [175]. Based upon SNAP25 cleavage, the instillation of BoNT/A with HA-PE was as effective as intra-detrusor injection in enabling BoNT/A delivery into the bladder.

Inert heat sensitive hydrogel preparations that increase the residence time of neurotoxin adjacent to the urothelium and allow for slow release exposure has been used to enhance the effectiveness of instilled BoNT/A. OnabotulinumtoxinA embedded in the hydrogel TC-3 has shown efficacy in the treatment of OAB [176]. TC-3 is produced by an Israeli company UroGen Pharma Ltd. (Ra'anana, Israel) as RTGel^{TM}. In 2016, UroGen licensed the worldwide rights to develop RTGel^{TM} in combination with BoNT/A to Allergan Inc. (Dublin, Ireland), who are currently conducting phase 2 studies in OAB. Liposomes are being developed as a delivery vehicle enabling intravesical BoNT/A delivery in the bladder by the US biotech Lipella Pharmaceuticals [177]. Bladder instillation of liposome encapsulated BoNT/A was effective at treating the symptoms of OAB in patients [178].

As with transdermal delivery, in the bladder, physical methods to enhance the permeability of the urothelium have been employed as well as chemical. Low energy shock waves have been reported to enable delivery of intravesical BoNT/A into the bladder wall and block acetic acid-induced hyperactivity in a rat model of bladder hyperactivity [179]. The use of intravesical electromotive BoNT/A delivery in the bladder has been widely studied, both in animal models [180] and clinical application [180–183]. Intravesical electromotive BoNT/A has been reported to be effective in women with OAB [181] and in NDO in children [182,184]. In children, a long-term follow-up study has shown it to be a safe and effective method of treating NDO resulting from myelomeningocele [183].

6.3. Transepithelial Delivery

One other area where needle-free delivery of BoNT/A has been explored is topical intranasal delivery. Successful intranasal delivery of BoNT/A and the relief of symptoms of allergic rhinitis in rats was achieved using the proprietary CPP RT001 formulation [185]. Effective relief of idiopathic rhinitis in some patients has been reported following simple intranasal application of a sponge soaked in BoNT/A solution [186].

7. Conclusions

BoNTs have proved to be highly effective therapeutic proteins offering symptomatic relief across a wide spectrum of neurological and muscular conditions that are characterized by neuronal hyperactivity. The increasing understanding of the biology of the neurotoxins and the availability of highly differentiated toxin serotypes and subtypes offers the prospect in coming years of expanding this therapeutic benefit and extending it to a greater range of clinical conditions, offering the benefit of being more specific and the efficacy of these unique therapeutic proteins to a much greater number of patients. Whilst botulinum toxins have the advantage of being extremely potent with an extended duration of biological activity, properties that are key to their clinical success, these very characteristics present significant challenges to the scientific field of pharmaceutical development. Furthermore, in the coming years, modified and recombinant toxins would expand even more the future therapeutic utility of BoNTs.

Author Contributions: All authors contributed to the writing of one or more sections of the review. E.F. and J.K. co-design the review. E.F. and K.F. coordinated the production of the review.

Conflicts of Interest: All authors are Ipsen employees.

References

1. Zhang, S.; Masuyer, G.; Zhang, J.; Shen, Y.; Lundin, D.; Henriksson, L.; Miyashita, S.-I.; Martínez-Carranza, M.; Dong, M.; Stenmark, P. Identification and characterization of a novel botulinum neurotoxin. *Nat. Commun.* **2017**, *8*, 14130. [CrossRef] [PubMed]
2. Hill, K.K.; Smith, T.J. Genetic diversity within Clostridium botulinum serotypes, botulinum neurotoxin gene clusters and toxin subtypes. In *Botulinum Neurotoxins*; Springer: Berlin, Germany, 2012; pp. 1–20.
3. Peng, L.; Berntsson, R.P.-A.; Tepp, W.H.; Pitkin, R.M.; Johnson, E.A.; Stenmark, P.; Dong, M. Botulinum neurotoxin DC uses synaptotagmin I and II as receptors, and human synaptotagmin II is not an effective receptor for type B, DC and G toxins. *J. Cell Sci.* **2012**, *125*, 3233–3242. [CrossRef] [PubMed]
4. Strotmeier, J.; Willjes, G.; Binz, T.; Rummel, A. Human synaptotagmin-II is not a high affinity receptor for botulinum neurotoxin B and G: Increased therapeutic dosage and immunogenicity. *FEBS Lett.* **2012**, *586*, 310–313. [CrossRef] [PubMed]
5. Dressler, D.; Bigalke, H.; Benecke, R. Botulinum toxin type B in antibody-induced botulinum toxin type A therapy failure. *J. Neurol.* **2003**, *250*, 967–969. [CrossRef] [PubMed]
6. Tao, L.; Peng, L.; Berntsson, R.P.-A.; Liu, S.M.; Park, S.; Yu, F.; Boone, C.; Palan, S.; Beard, M.; Chabrier, P.-E. Engineered botulinum neurotoxin B with improved efficacy for targeting human receptors. *Nat. Commun.* **2017**, *8*, 53. [CrossRef] [PubMed]
7. Brin, M.F.; James, C.; Maltman, J. Botulinum toxin type A products are not interchangeable: A review of the evidence. *Biol. Targets Ther.* **2014**, *8*, 227. [CrossRef] [PubMed]
8. Frevert, J. Content of botulinum neurotoxin in botox®/vistabel®, dysport®/azzalure®, and xeomin®/bocouture®. *Drugs R D* **2010**, *10*, 67–73. [CrossRef] [PubMed]
9. Pickett, A. Botulinum toxin as a clinical product: Manufacture and pharmacology. In *Clinical Applications of Botulinum Neurotoxin*; Foster, K., Ed.; Springer: Berlin, Germany, 2014; pp. 7–49.
10. Ludlow, C.; Hallett, M.; Rhew, K.; Cole, R.; Shimizu, T.; Bagley, J.; Schulz, G.; Yin, S.; Koda, J. Therapeutic use of type F botulinum toxin. *N. Engl. J. Med.* **1992**, *326*, 349–350. [PubMed]
11. Greene, P.E.; Fahn, S. Use of botulinum toxin type F injections to treat torticollis in patients with immunity to botulinum toxin type A. *Mov. Disord.* **1993**, *8*, 479–483. [CrossRef] [PubMed]
12. Greene, P.E.; Fahn, S. Response to botulinum toxin F in seronegative botulinum toxin A—Resistant patients. *Mov. Disord.* **1996**, *11*, 181–184. [CrossRef] [PubMed]
13. Mezaki, T.; Kaji, R.; Kohara, N.; Fujii, H.; Katayama, M.; Shimizu, T.; Kimura, J.; Brin, M. Comparison of Therapeutic Efficacies of Type A and F Botulinum Toxins for Blepharospasm A double-blind, controlled study. *Neurology* **1995**, *45*, 506–508. [CrossRef] [PubMed]
14. Houser, M.; Sheean, G.; Lees, A. Further studies using higher doses of botulinum toxin type F for torticollis resistant to botulinum toxin type A. *J. Neurol. Neurosurg. Psychiatry* **1998**, *64*, 577–580. [CrossRef] [PubMed]
15. Sheean, G.; Lees, A. Botulinum toxin F in the treatment of torticollis clinically resistant to botulinum toxin A. *J. Neurol. Neurosurg. Psychiatry* **1995**, *59*, 601–607. [CrossRef] [PubMed]
16. Chen, R.; Karp, B.I.; Hallett, M. Botulinum toxin type F for treatment of dystonia Long-term experience. *Neurology* **1998**, *51*, 1494–1496. [CrossRef] [PubMed]
17. Billante, C.R.; Zealear, D.L.; Billante, M.; Reyes, J.H.; Sant'Anna, G.; Rodriguez, R.; Stone, R. Comparison of neuromuscular blockade and recovery with botulinum toxins A and F. *Muscle Nerve* **2002**, *26*, 395–403. [CrossRef] [PubMed]
18. Eleopra, R.; Tugnoli, V.; Rossetto, O.; De Grandis, D.; Montecucco, C. Different time courses of recovery after poisoning with botulinum neurotoxin serotypes A and E in humans. *Neurosci. Lett.* **1998**, *256*, 135–138. [CrossRef]
19. Adler, M.; Keller, J.E.; Sheridan, R.E.; Deshpande, S.S. Persistence of botulinum neurotoxin A demonstrated by sequential administration of serotypes A and E in rat EDL muscle. *Toxicon* **2001**, *39*, 233–243. [CrossRef]
20. Whitemarsh, R.C.M.; Tepp, W.H.; Johnson, E.A.; Pellett, S. Persistence of botulinum neurotoxin a subtypes 1–5 in primary rat spinal cord cells. *PLoS ONE* **2014**, *9*, e90252. [CrossRef] [PubMed]
21. Antonucci, F.; Rossi, C.; Gianfranceschi, L.; Rossetto, O.; Caleo, M. Long-distance retrograde effects of botulinum neurotoxin A. *J. Neurosci.* **2008**, *28*, 3689–3696. [CrossRef] [PubMed]

22. Scheps, D.; de la Paz, M.L.; Jurk, M.; Hofmann, F.; Frevert, J. Design of modified botulinum neurotoxin A1 variants with a shorter persistence of paralysis and duration of action. *Toxicon* **2017**, *139*, 101–108. [CrossRef] [PubMed]
23. Costantin, L.; Bozzi, Y.; Richichi, C.; Viegi, A.; Antonucci, F.; Funicello, M.; Gobbi, M.; Mennini, T.; Rossetto, O.; Montecucco, C. Antiepileptic effects of botulinum neurotoxin E. *J. Neurosci.* **2005**, *25*, 1943–1951. [CrossRef] [PubMed]
24. Eleopra, R.; Tugnoli, V.; Rossetto, O.; Montecucco, C.; De Grandis, D. Botulinum neurotoxin serotype C: A novel effective botulinum toxin therapy in human. *Neurosci. Lett.* **1997**, *224*, 91–94. [CrossRef]
25. Eleopra, R.; Tugnoli, V.; Quatrale, R.; Gastaldo, E.; Rossetto, O.; De Grandis, D.; Montecucco, C. Botulinum neurotoxin serotypes A and C do not affect motor units survival in humans: An electrophysiological study by motor units counting. *Clin. Neurophysiol.* **2002**, *113*, 1258–1264. [CrossRef]
26. Eleopra, R.; Tugnoli, V.; De Grandis, D.; Montecucco, C. Botulinum toxin serotype C treatment in subjects affected by focal dystonia and resistant to botulinum toxin serotype A. *Neurology* **1998**, *50*, A72.
27. Eleopra, R.; Tugnoli, V.; Quatrale, R.; Rossetto, O.; Montecucco, C.; Dressler, D. Clinical use of non-A botulinum toxins: Botulinum toxin type C and botulinum toxin type F. *Neurotox. Res.* **2006**, *9*, 127–131. [CrossRef] [PubMed]
28. Pellett, S.; Tepp, W.H.; Whitemarsh, R.C.; Bradshaw, M.; Johnson, E.A. In vivo onset and duration of action varies for botulinum neurotoxin A subtypes 1–5. *Toxicon* **2015**, *107*, 37–42. [CrossRef] [PubMed]
29. Whitemarsh, R.C.; Tepp, W.H.; Bradshaw, M.; Lin, G.; Pier, C.L.; Scherf, J.M.; Johnson, E.A.; Pellett, S. Characterization of botulinum neurotoxin A subtypes 1 through 5 by investigation of activities in mice, in neuronal cell cultures, and in vitro. *Infect. Immun.* **2013**, *81*, 3894–3902. [CrossRef] [PubMed]
30. Pier, C.L.; Chen, C.; Tepp, W.H.; Lin, G.; Janda, K.D.; Barbieri, J.T.; Pellett, S.; Johnson, E.A. Botulinum neurotoxin subtype A2 enters neuronal cells faster than subtype A1. *FEBS Lett.* **2011**, *585*, 199–206. [CrossRef] [PubMed]
31. Akaike, N.; Shin, M.C.; Wakita, M.; Torii, Y.; Harakawa, T.; Ginnaga, A.; Kato, K.; Kaji, R.; Kozaki, S. Transsynaptic inhibition of spinal transmission by A2 botulinum toxin. *J. Physiol.* **2013**, *591*, 1031–1043. [CrossRef] [PubMed]
32. Torii, Y.; Kiyota, N.; Sugimoto, N.; Mori, Y.; Goto, Y.; Harakawa, T.; Nakahira, S.; Kaji, R.; Kozaki, S.; Ginnaga, A. Comparison of effects of botulinum toxin subtype A1 and A2 using twitch tension assay and rat grip strength test. *Toxicon* **2011**, *57*, 93–99. [CrossRef] [PubMed]
33. Kroken, A.R.; Blum, F.C.; Zuverink, M.; Barbieri, J.T. Entry of Botulinum neurotoxin subtypes A1 and A2 into neurons. *Infect. Immun.* **2017**, *85*, e00795-16. [CrossRef] [PubMed]
34. Benoit, R.M.; Schärer, M.A.; Wieser, M.M.; Li, X.; Frey, D.; Kammerer, R.A. Crystal structure of the BoNT/A2 receptor-binding domain in complex with the luminal domain of its neuronal receptor SV2C. *Sci. Rep.* **2017**, *7*, 43588. [CrossRef] [PubMed]
35. Tepp, W.H.; Lin, G.; Johnson, E.A. Purification and characterization of a novel subtype A3 botulinum neurotoxin. *Appl. Environ. Microbiol.* **2012**, *78*, 3108–3113. [CrossRef] [PubMed]
36. Torii, Y.; Goto, Y.; Nakahira, S.; Kozaki, S.; Ginnaga, A. Comparison of the immunogenicity of botulinum toxin type A and the efficacy of A1 and A2 neurotoxins in animals with A1 toxin antibodies. *Toxicon* **2014**, *77*, 114–120. [CrossRef] [PubMed]
37. Mukai, Y.; Shimatani, Y.; Sako, W.; Asanuma, K.; Nodera, H.; Sakamoto, T.; Izumi, Y.; Kohda, T.; Kozaki, S.; Kaji, R. Comparison between botulinum neurotoxin type A2 and type A1 by electrophysiological study in healthy individuals. *Toxicon* **2014**, *81*, 32–36. [CrossRef] [PubMed]
38. Kaji, R. Clinical differences between A1 and A2 botulinum toxin subtypes. *Toxicon* **2015**, *107*, 85–88. [CrossRef] [PubMed]
39. Itakura, M.; Kohda, T.; Kubo, T.; Semi, Y.; Azuma, Y.-T.; Nakajima, H.; Kozaki, S.; Takeuchi, T. Botulinum neurotoxin A subtype 2 reduces pathological behaviors more effectively than subtype 1 in a rat Parkinson's disease model. *Biochem. Biophys. Res. Commun.* **2014**, *447*, 311–314. [CrossRef] [PubMed]
40. Shin, M.-C.; Yukihira, T.; Ito, Y.; Akaike, N. Antinociceptive effects of A1 and A2 type botulinum toxins on carrageenan-induced hyperalgesia in rat. *Toxicon* **2013**, *64*, 12–19. [CrossRef] [PubMed]
41. Ma, L.; Nagai, J.; Sekino, Y.; Goto, Y.; Nakahira, S.; Ueda, H. Single Application of A2 NTX, a Botulinum Toxin A2 Subunit, Prevents Chronic Pain Over Long Periods in Both Diabetic and Spinal Cord Injury–Induced Neuropathic Pain Models. *J. Pharmacol. Sci.* **2012**, *119*, 282–286. [CrossRef] [PubMed]

42. Debono, D.J.; Hoeksema, L.J.; Hobbs, R.D. Caring for patients with chronic pain: Pearls and pitfalls. *J. Am. Osteopath. Assoc.* **2013**, *113*, 620–627. [CrossRef] [PubMed]
43. Van Hecke, O.; Torrance, N.; Smith, B.H. Chronic pain epidemiology—Where do lifestyle factors fit in? *Br. J. Pain* **2013**, *7*, 209–217. [CrossRef] [PubMed]
44. Reid, K.J.; Harker, J.; Bala, M.M.; Truyers, C.; Kellen, E.; Bekkering, G.E.; Kleijnen, J. Epidemiology of chronic non-cancer pain in Europe: Narrative review of prevalence, pain treatments and pain impact. *Curr. Med. Res. Opin.* **2011**, *27*, 449–462. [CrossRef] [PubMed]
45. Woolf, C.J. Overcoming obstacles to developing new analgesics. *Nat. Med.* **2010**, *16*, 1241–1247. [CrossRef] [PubMed]
46. Kissin, I. The development of new analgesics over the past 50 years: A lack of real breakthrough drugs. *Anesth. Analg.* **2010**, *110*, 780–789. [CrossRef] [PubMed]
47. Tarsy, D.; First, E.R. Painful cervical dystonia: Clinical features and response to treatment with botulinum toxin. *Mov. Disord.* **1999**, *14*, 1043–1045. [CrossRef]
48. Freund, B.; Schwartz, M. Temporal relationship of muscle weakness and pain reduction in subjects treated with botulinum toxin A. *J. Pain* **2003**, *4*, 159–165. [CrossRef] [PubMed]
49. Bomba-Warczak, E.; Vevea, J.D.; Brittain, J.M.; Figueroa-Bernier, A.; Tepp, W.H.; Johnson, E.A.; Yeh, F.L.; Chapman, E.R. Interneuronal Transfer and Distal Action of Tetanus Toxin and Botulinum Neurotoxins A and D in Central Neurons. *Cell Rep.* **2016**, *16*, 1974–1987. [CrossRef] [PubMed]
50. Cocco, A.; Albanese, A. Recent developments in clinical trials of bont. *Toxicon* **2017**, *123*, S89.
51. Caleo, M.; Restani, L. Direct central nervous system effects of botulinum neurotoxin. *Toxicon* **2017**, *147*, 68–72. [CrossRef] [PubMed]
52. Marinelli, S.; Vacca, V.; Ricordy, R.; Uggenti, C.; Tata, A.M.; Luvisetto, S.; Pavone, F. The analgesic effect on neuropathic pain of retrogradely transported botulinum neurotoxin A involves Schwann cells and astrocytes. *PLoS ONE* **2012**, *7*, e47977. [CrossRef] [PubMed]
53. Silva, L.B.D.; Poulsen, J.N.; Arendt-Nielsen, L.; Gazerani, P. Botulinum neurotoxin type A modulates vesicular release of glutamate from satellite glial cells. *J. Cell. Mol. Med.* **2015**, *19*, 1900–1909. [CrossRef] [PubMed]
54. Zychowska, M.; Rojewska, E.; Makuch, W.; Luvisetto, S.; Pavone, F.; Marinelli, S.; Przewlocka, B.; Mika, J. Participation of pro-and anti-nociceptive interleukins in botulinum toxin A-induced analgesia in a rat model of neuropathic pain. *Eur. J. Pharmacol.* **2016**, *791*, 377–388. [CrossRef] [PubMed]
55. Aurora, S.; Dodick, D.W.; Turkel, C.; DeGryse, R.; Silberstein, S.; Lipton, R.; Diener, H.; Brin, M. OnabotulinumtoxinA for treatment of chronic migraine: Results from the double-blind, randomized, placebo-controlled phase of the PREEMPT 1 trial. *Cephalalgia* **2010**, *30*, 793–803. [CrossRef] [PubMed]
56. Silberstein, S.D.; Dodick, D.W.; Aurora, S.K.; Diener, H.-C.; DeGryse, R.E.; Lipton, R.B.; Turkel, C.C. Per cent of patients with chronic migraine who responded per onabotulinumtoxinA treatment cycle: PREEMPT. *J. Neurol. Neurosurg. Psychiatry* **2015**, *86*, 996–1001. [CrossRef] [PubMed]
57. Simpson, D.M.; Hallett, M.; Ashman, E.J.; Comella, C.L.; Green, M.W.; Gronseth, G.S.; Armstrong, M.J.; Gloss, D.; Potrebic, S.; Jankovic, J. Practice guideline update summary: Botulinum neurotoxin for the treatment of blepharospasm, cervical dystonia, adult spasticity, and headache Report of the Guideline Development Subcommittee of the American Academy of Neurology. *Neurology* **2016**, *86*, 1818–1826. [CrossRef] [PubMed]
58. Relja, M.; Telarović, S. Botulinum toxin in tension-type headache. *J. Neurol.* **2004**, *251*, i12–i14. [CrossRef] [PubMed]
59. Padberg, M.; De Bruijn, S.; De Haan, R.; Tavy, D. Treatment of chronic tension-type headache with botulinum toxin: A double-blind, placebo-controlled clinical trial. *Cephalalgia* **2004**, *24*, 675–680. [CrossRef] [PubMed]
60. Schulte-Mattler, W.J.; Krack, P.; Group, B.S. Treatment of chronic tension-type headache with botulinum toxin A: A randomized, double-blind, placebo-controlled multicenter study. *Pain* **2004**, *109*, 110–114. [CrossRef] [PubMed]
61. Silberstein, S.D.; Göbel, H.; Jensen, R.; Elkind, A.H.; Degryse, R.; Walcott, J.M.; Turkel, C. Botulinum toxin type A in the prophylactic treatment of chronic tension-type headache: A multicentre, double-blind, randomized, placebo-controlled, parallel-group study. *Cephalalgia* **2006**, *26*, 790–800. [CrossRef] [PubMed]

62. Khenioui, H.; Houvenagel, E.; Catanzariti, J.F.; Guyot, M.A.; Agnani, O.; Donze, C. Usefulness of intra-articular botulinum toxin injections. A systematic review. *Jt. Bone Spine* **2016**, *83*, 149–154. [CrossRef] [PubMed]
63. Heikkilä, H.; Hielm-Björkman, A.; Morelius, M.; Larsen, S.; Honkavaara, J.; Innes, J.; Laitinen-Vapaavuori, O. Intra-articular botulinum toxin A for the treatment of osteoarthritic joint pain in dogs: A randomized, double-blinded, placebo-controlled clinical trial. *Vet. J.* **2014**, *200*, 162–169. [CrossRef] [PubMed]
64. Vilhegas, S.; Cassu, R.; Barbero, R.; Crociolli, G.; Rocha, T.; Gomes, D. Botulinum toxin type A as an adjunct in postoperative pain management in dogs undergoing radical mastectomy. *Vet. Rec.* **2015**, *177*, 391. [CrossRef] [PubMed]
65. Mittal, S.; Machado, D.G.; Jabbari, B. OnabotulinumtoxinA for treatment of focal cancer pain after surgery and/or radiation. *Pain Med.* **2012**, *13*, 1029–1033. [CrossRef] [PubMed]
66. Lacković, Z.; Filipović, B.; Matak, I.; Helyes, Z. Activity of botulinum toxin type A in cranial dura: Implications for treatment of migraine and other headaches. *Br. J. Pharmacol.* **2016**, *173*, 279–291. [CrossRef] [PubMed]
67. Drinovac Vlah, V.; Filipović, B.; Bach-Rojecky, L.; Lacković, Z. Role of central versus peripheral opioid system in antinociceptive and anti-inflammatory effect of botulinum toxin type A in trigeminal region. *Eur. J. Pain* **2017**, *22*, 583–591. [CrossRef] [PubMed]
68. Nelson, A.E. Osteoarthritis year in review 2017: Clinical. *Osteoarthr. Cartil.* **2018**, *26*, 319–325. [CrossRef] [PubMed]
69. Kidd, B.L. Osteoarthritis and joint pain. *Pain* **2006**, *123*, 6–9. [CrossRef] [PubMed]
70. Martell-Pelletier, J.; Barr, A.J.; Cicuttini, F.M.; Conaghan, P.G.; Cooper, C.; Goldring, M.B.; Goldring, S.R.; Jones, G.; Teichthal, A.J.; Pelletier, J. Osteoarthritis. *Nat. Rev. Dis. Prim.* **2016**, *2*, 16072. [CrossRef] [PubMed]
71. Ivanusic, J.J. Molecular Mechanisms That Contribute to Bone Marrow Pain. *Front. Neurol.* **2017**, *8*, 458. [CrossRef] [PubMed]
72. Schaible, H.-G.; Ebersberger, A.; Von Banchet, G.S. Mechanisms of Pain in Arthritis. *Ann. N. Y. Acad. Sci.* **2002**, *966*, 343–354. [CrossRef] [PubMed]
73. Hsieh, L.-F.; Wu, C.-W.; Chou, C.-C.; Yang, S.-W.; Wu, S.-H.; Lin, Y.-J.; Hsu, W.-C. Effects of botulinum toxin landmark-guided intra-articular injection in subjects with knee osteoarthritis. *PM&R* **2016**, *8*, 1127–1135.
74. Arendt-Nielsen, L.; Jiang, G.; DeGryse, R.; Turkel, C. Intra-articular onabotulinumtoxinA in osteoarthritis knee pain: Effect on human mechanistic pain biomarkers and clinical pain. *Scand. J. Rheumatol.* **2017**, *46*, 303–316. [CrossRef] [PubMed]
75. Krug, H.E.; Frizelle, S.; McGarraugh, P.; Mahowald, M.L. Pain behavior measures to quantitate joint pain and response to neurotoxin treatment in murine models of arthritis. *Pain Med.* **2009**, *10*, 1218–1228. [CrossRef] [PubMed]
76. Anderson, S.; Krug, H.; Dorman, C.; McGarraugh, P.; Frizelle, S.; Mahowald, M. Analgesic effects of intra-articular botulinum toxin Type B in a murine model of chronic degenerative knee arthritis pain. *J. Pain Res.* **2010**, *3*, 161. [CrossRef] [PubMed]
77. Wang, L.; Wang, K.; Chu, X.; Li, T.; Shen, N.; Fan, C.; Niu, Z.; Zhang, X.; Hu, L. Intra-articular injection of Botulinum toxin A reduces neurogenic inflammation in CFA-induced arthritic rat model. *Toxicon* **2017**, *126*, 70–78. [CrossRef] [PubMed]
78. Yoo, K.Y.; Lee, H.S.; Cho, Y.K.; Lim, Y.S.; Kim, Y.S.; Koo, J.H.; Yoon, S.J.; Lee, J.H.; Jang, K.H.; Song, S.H. Anti-inflammatory Effects of Botulinum Toxin Type A in a Complete Freund's Adjuvant-Induced Arthritic Knee Joint of Hind Leg on Rat Model. *Neurotox. Res.* **2014**, *26*, 32–39. [CrossRef] [PubMed]
79. Chapple, C. Chapter 2: Pathophysiology of neurogenic detrusor overactivity and the symptom complex of "overactive bladder". *Neurourol. Urodyn.* **2014**, *33* (Suppl. S3), S6–S13. [CrossRef] [PubMed]
80. Merrill, L.; Gonzalez, E.J.; Girard, B.M.; Vizzard, M.A. Receptors, channels, and signalling in the urothelial sensory system in the bladder. *Nat. Rev. Urol.* **2016**, *13*, 193–204. [CrossRef] [PubMed]
81. Traini, C.; Fausssone-Pellegrini, M.S.; Guasti, D.; Del Popolo, G.; Frizzi, J.; Serni, S.; Vannucchi, M.G. Adaptive changes of telocytes in the urinary bladder of patients affected by neurogenic detrusor overactivity. *J. Cell. Mol. Med.* **2018**, *22*, 195–206. [CrossRef] [PubMed]
82. Schurch, B.; Stohrer, M.; Kramer, G.; Schmid, D.M.; Gaul, G.; Hauri, D. Botulinum-A toxin for treating detrusor hyperreflexia in spinal cord injured patients: A new alternative to anticholinergic drugs? Preliminary results. *J. Urol.* **2000**, *164*, 692–697. [CrossRef]

83. Khera, M.; Somogyi, G.T.; Kiss, S.; Boone, T.B.; Smith, C.P. Botulinum toxin A inhibits ATP release from bladder urothelium after chronic spinal cord injury. *Neurochem. Int.* **2004**, *45*, 987–993. [CrossRef] [PubMed]
84. Collins, V.M.; Daly, D.M.; Liaskos, M.; McKay, N.G.; Sellers, D.; Chapple, C.; Grundy, D. OnabotulinumtoxinA significantly attenuates bladder afferent nerve firing and inhibits ATP release from the urothelium. *BJU Int.* **2013**, *112*, 1018–1026. [CrossRef] [PubMed]
85. Lucioni, A.; Bales, G.T.; Lotan, T.L.; McGehee, D.S.; Cook, S.P.; Rapp, D.E. Botulinum toxin type A inhibits sensory neuropeptide release in rat bladder models of acute injury and chronic inflammation. *BJU Int.* **2008**, *101*, 366–370. [CrossRef] [PubMed]
86. Jhang, J.F.; Kuo, H.C. Botulinum Toxin A and Lower Urinary Tract Dysfunction: Pathophysiology and Mechanisms of Action. *Toxins (Basel)* **2016**, *8*, 120. [CrossRef] [PubMed]
87. Giannantoni, A.; Conte, A.; Farfariello, V.; Proietti, S.; Vianello, A.; Nardicchi, V.; Santoni, G.; Amantini, C. Onabotulinumtoxin-A intradetrusorial injections modulate bladder expression of NGF, TrkA, p75 and TRPV1 in patients with detrusor overactivity. *Pharmacol. Res.* **2013**, *68*, 118–124. [CrossRef] [PubMed]
88. Loiseau, C.; Iezhova, T.; Valkiunas, G.; Chasar, A.; Hutchinson, A.; Buermann, W.; Smith, T.B.; Sehgal, R.N. Spatial variation of haemosporidian parasite infection in African rainforest bird species. *J. Parasitol.* **2010**, *96*, 21–29. [CrossRef] [PubMed]
89. Maignel-Ludop, J.; Huchet, M.; Krupp, J. Botulinum Neurotoxins Serotypes A and B induce paralysis of mouse striated and smooth muscles with different potencies. *Pharmacol. Res. Perspect.* **2017**, *5*, e00289. [CrossRef] [PubMed]
90. Coelho, A.; Dinis, P.; Pinto, R.; Gorgal, T.; Silva, C.; Silva, A.; Silva, J.; Cruz, C.D.; Cruz, F.; Avelino, A. Distribution of the high-affinity binding site and intracellular target of botulinum toxin type A in the human bladder. *Eur. Urol.* **2010**, *57*, 884–890. [CrossRef] [PubMed]
91. Coelho, A.; Oliveira, R.; Cruz, F.; Cruz, C.D. Impairment of sensory afferents by intrathecal administration of botulinum toxin A improves neurogenic detrusor overactivity in chronic spinal cord injured rats. *Exp. Neurol.* **2016**, *285*, 159–166. [CrossRef] [PubMed]
92. Eming, S.A.; Martin, P.; Tomic-Canic, M. Wound repair and regeneration: Mechanisms, signaling, and translation. *Sci. Transl. Med.* **2014**, *6*, 265sr266. [CrossRef] [PubMed]
93. Lebeda, F.J.; Dembek, Z.F.; Adler, M. Kinetic and reaction pathway analysis in the application of botulinum toxin A for wound healing. *J. Toxicol.* **2012**, *2012*, 159726. [CrossRef] [PubMed]
94. Ziade, M.; Domergue, S.; Batifol, D.; Jreige, R.; Sebbane, M.; Goudot, P.; Yachouh, J. Use of botulinum toxin type A to improve treatment of facial wounds: A prospective randomised study. *JPRAS* **2013**, *66*, 209–214. [CrossRef] [PubMed]
95. Prodromidou, A.; Frountzas, M.; Vlachos, D.-E.G.; Vlachos, G.D.; Bakoyiannis, I.; Perrea, D.; Pergialiotis, V. Botulinum toxin for the prevention and healing of wound scars: A systematic review of the literature. *Plast. Surg.* **2015**, *23*, 260–264. [CrossRef]
96. Lee, B.-J.; Jeong, J.-H.; Wang, S.-G.; Lee, J.-C.; Goh, E.-K.; Kim, H.-W. Effect of botulinum toxin type a on a rat surgical wound model. *Clin. Exp. Otorhinolaryngol.* **2009**, *2*, 20. [CrossRef] [PubMed]
97. Kiritsi, D.; Nyström, A. The role of TGFβ in wound healing pathologies. *Mech. Ageing Dev.* **2017**. [CrossRef] [PubMed]
98. Xiao, Z.; Zhang, F.; Lin, W.; Zhang, M.; Liu, Y. Effect of botulinum toxin type A on transforming growth factor beta1 in fibroblasts derived from hypertrophic scar: A preliminary report. *Aesth. Plast. Surg.* **2010**, *34*, 424–427. [CrossRef] [PubMed]
99. Xiao, Z.; Zhang, M.; Liu, Y.; Ren, L. Botulinum toxin type a inhibits connective tissue growth factor expression in fibroblasts derived from hypertrophic scar. *Aesth. Plast. Surg.* **2011**, *35*, 802–807. [CrossRef] [PubMed]
100. Pirazzini, M.; Rossetto, O.; Eleopra, R.; Montecucco, C. Botulinum Neurotoxins: Biology, Pharmacology, and Toxicology. *Pharmacol. Rev.* **2017**, *69*, 200–235. [CrossRef] [PubMed]
101. Popoff, M.R.; Poulain, B. Bacterial toxins and the nervous system: Neurotoxins and multipotential toxins interacting with neuronal cells. *Toxins (Basel)* **2010**, *2*, 683–737. [CrossRef] [PubMed]
102. Poulain, B. How do the Botulinum Neurotoxins block neurotransmitter release: From botulism to the molecular mechanism of action. *Botulinum J.* **2008**, *1*, 14–87. [CrossRef]
103. Rossetto, O. Botulinum Toxins: Molecular Structures and Synaptic Physiology. *Botulinum Toxin Treat. Clin. Med.* **2018**, 1–12. [CrossRef]

104. Rossetto, O.; Pirazzini, M.; Montecucco, C. Botulinum neurotoxins: Genetic, structural and mechanistic insights. *Nat. Rev. Microbiol.* **2014**, *12*, 535–549. [CrossRef] [PubMed]
105. Rummel, A. The long journey of botulinum neurotoxins into the synapse. *Toxicon* **2015**, *107*, 9–24. [CrossRef] [PubMed]
106. Matak, I.; Lackovic, Z.; Relja, M. Botulinum toxin type A in motor nervous system: Unexplained observations and new challenges. *J. Neural Transm. (Vienna)* **2016**, *123*, 1415–1421. [CrossRef] [PubMed]
107. Mazzocchio, R.; Caleo, M. More than at the neuromuscular synapse: Actions of botulinum neurotoxin A in the central nervous system. *Neuroscientist* **2015**, *21*, 44–61. [CrossRef] [PubMed]
108. Kanovsky, P.; Streitova, H.; Dufek, J.; Znojil, V.; Daniel, P.; Rektor, I. Change in lateralization of the P22/N30 cortical component of median nerve somatosensory evoked potentials in patients with cervical dystonia after successful treatment with botulinum toxin A. *Mov. Disord.* **1998**, *13*, 108–117. [CrossRef] [PubMed]
109. Delnooz, C.C.; Pasman, J.W.; van de Warrenburg, B.P. Dynamic cortical gray matter volume changes after botulinum toxin in cervical dystonia. *Neurobiol. Dis.* **2015**, *73*, 327–333. [CrossRef] [PubMed]
110. Behari, M.; Raju, G.B. Electrophysiological studies in patients with blepharospasm before and after botulinum toxin A therapy. *J. Neurol. Sci.* **1996**, *135*, 74–77. [CrossRef]
111. Bielamowicz, S.; Ludlow, C.L. Effects of botulinum toxin on pathophysiology in spasmodic dysphonia. *Ann. Otol. Rhinol. Laryngol.* **2000**, *109*, 194–203. [CrossRef] [PubMed]
112. Marchand-Pauvert, V.; Aymard, C.; Giboin, L.S.; Dominici, F.; Rossi, A.; Mazzocchio, R. Beyond muscular effects: Depression of spinal recurrent inhibition after botulinum neurotoxin A. *J. Physiol.* **2013**, *591*, 1017–1029. [CrossRef] [PubMed]
113. Aymard, C.; Giboin, L.S.; Lackmy-Vallee, A.; Marchand-Pauvert, V. Spinal plasticity in stroke patients after botulinum neurotoxin A injection in ankle plantar flexors. *Physiol. Rep.* **2013**, *1*, e00173. [CrossRef] [PubMed]
114. Clowry, G.J.; Walker, L.; Davies, P. The effects of botulinum neurotoxin A induced muscle paresis during a critical period upon muscle and spinal cord development in the rat. *Exp. Neurol.* **2006**, *202*, 456–469. [CrossRef] [PubMed]
115. Gonzalez-Forero, D.; Pastor, A.M.; Geiman, E.J.; Benitez-Temino, B.; Alvarez, F.J. Regulation of gephyrin cluster size and inhibitory synaptic currents on Renshaw cells by motor axon excitatory inputs. *J. Neurosci.* **2005**, *25*, 417–429. [CrossRef] [PubMed]
116. Cai, B.B.; Francis, J.; Brin, M.F.; Broide, R.S. Botulinum neurotoxin type A-cleaved SNAP25 is confined to primary motor neurons and localized on the plasma membrane following intramuscular toxin injection. *Neuroscience* **2017**, *352*, 155–169. [CrossRef] [PubMed]
117. Koizumi, H.; Goto, S.; Okita, S.; Morigaki, R.; Akaike, N.; Torii, Y.; Harakawa, T.; Ginnaga, A.; Kaji, R. Spinal Central Effects of Peripherally Applied Botulinum Neurotoxin A in Comparison between Its Subtypes A1 and A2. *Front. Neurol.* **2014**, *5*, 98. [CrossRef] [PubMed]
118. Matak, I.; Riederer, P.; Lackovic, Z. Botulinum toxin's axonal transport from periphery to the spinal cord. *Neurochem. Int.* **2012**, *61*, 236–239. [CrossRef] [PubMed]
119. Filipovic, B.; Matak, I.; Bach-Rojecky, L.; Lackovic, Z. Central action of peripherally applied botulinum toxin type A on pain and dural protein extravasation in rat model of trigeminal neuropathy. *PLoS ONE* **2012**, *7*, e29803. [CrossRef] [PubMed]
120. Restani, L.; Giribaldi, F.; Manich, M.; Bercsenyi, K.; Menendez, G.; Rossetto, O.; Caleo, M.; Schiavo, G. Botulinum neurotoxins A and E undergo retrograde axonal transport in primary motor neurons. *PLoS Pathog.* **2012**, *8*, e1003087. [CrossRef] [PubMed]
121. Wu, C.; Xie, N.; Lian, Y.; Xu, H.; Chen, C.; Zheng, Y.; Chen, Y.; Zhang, H. Central antinociceptive activity of peripherally applied botulinum toxin type A in lab rat model of trigeminal neuralgia. *Springerplus* **2016**, *5*, 431. [CrossRef] [PubMed]
122. Restani, L.; Novelli, E.; Bottari, D.; Leone, P.; Barone, I.; Galli-Resta, L.; Strettoi, E.; Caleo, M. Botulinum neurotoxin A impairs neurotransmission following retrograde transynaptic transport. *Traffic* **2012**, *13*, 1083–1089. [CrossRef] [PubMed]
123. Wang, T.; Martin, S.; Papadopulos, A.; Harper, C.B.; Mavlyutov, T.A.; Niranjan, D.; Glass, N.R.; Cooper-White, J.J.; Sibarita, J.B.; Choquet, D.; et al. Control of autophagosome axonal retrograde flux by presynaptic activity unveiled using botulinum neurotoxin type A. *J. Neurosci.* **2015**, *35*, 6179–6194. [CrossRef] [PubMed]

124. Harper, C.B.; Papadopulos, A.; Martin, S.; Matthews, D.R.; Morgan, G.P.; Nguyen, T.H.; Wang, T.; Nair, D.; Choquet, D.; Meunier, F.A. Botulinum neurotoxin type-A enters a non-recycling pool of synaptic vesicles. *Sci. Rep.* **2016**, *6*, 19654. [CrossRef] [PubMed]
125. Lawrence, G.W.; Ovsepian, S.V.; Wang, J.; Aoki, K.R.; Dolly, J.O. Extravesicular intraneuronal migration of internalized botulinum neurotoxins without detectable inhibition of distal neurotransmission. *Biochem. J.* **2012**, *441*, 443–452. [CrossRef] [PubMed]
126. Ramachandran, R.; Lam, C.; Yaksh, T.L. Botulinum toxin in migraine: Role of transport in trigemino-somatic and trigemino-vascular afferents. *Neurobiol. Dis.* **2015**, *79*, 111–122. [CrossRef] [PubMed]
127. Bentivoglio, A.R.; Fasano, A.; Ialongo, T.; Soleti, F.; Lo Fermo, S.; Albanese, A. Fifteen-year experience in treating blepharospasm with Botox or Dysport: Same toxin, two drugs. *Neurotox. Res.* **2009**, *15*, 224–231. [CrossRef] [PubMed]
128. Dong, Y.; Wu, T.; Hu, X.; Wang, T. Efficacy and safety of botulinum toxin type A for upper limb spasticity after stroke or traumatic brain injury: A systematic review with meta-analysis and trial sequential analysis. *Eur. J. Phys. Rehabil. Med.* **2017**, *53*, 256–267. [PubMed]
129. Gu, H.Y.; Song, J.K.; Zhang, W.J.; Xie, J.; Yao, Q.S.; Zeng, W.J.; Zhang, C.; Niu, Y.M. A systematic review and meta-analysis of effectiveness and safety of therapy for overactive bladder using botulinum toxin A at different dosages. *Oncotarget* **2017**, *8*, 90338–90350. [CrossRef] [PubMed]
130. Naumann, M.; Jankovic, J. Safety of botulinum toxin type A: A systematic review and meta-analysis. *Curr. Med. Res. Opin.* **2004**, *20*, 981–990. [CrossRef] [PubMed]
131. Shaari, C.M.; George, E.; Wu, B.L.; Biller, H.F.; Sanders, I. Quantifying the spread of botulinum toxin through muscle fascia. *Laryngoscope* **1991**, *101*, 960–964. [CrossRef] [PubMed]
132. Yaraskavitch, M.; Leonard, T.; Herzog, W. Botox produces functional weakness in non-injected muscles adjacent to the target muscle. *J. Biomech.* **2008**, *41*, 897–902. [CrossRef] [PubMed]
133. Arezzo, J.C. NeuroBloc/Myobloc: Unique features and findings. *Toxicon* **2009**, *54*, 690–696. [CrossRef] [PubMed]
134. Borodic, G.E.; Joseph, M.; Fay, L.; Cozzolino, D.; Ferrante, R.J. Botulinum A toxin for the treatment of spasmodic torticollis: Dysphagia and regional toxin spread. *Head Neck* **1990**, *12*, 392–399. [CrossRef] [PubMed]
135. Carli, L.; Montecucco, C.; Rossetto, O. Assay of diffusion of different botulinum neurotoxin type a formulations injected in the mouse leg. *Muscle Nerve* **2009**, *40*, 374–380. [CrossRef] [PubMed]
136. Hsu, T.S.; Dover, J.S.; Arndt, K.A. Effect of volume and concentration on the diffusion of botulinum exotoxin A. *Arch. Dermatol.* **2004**, *140*, 1351–1354. [CrossRef] [PubMed]
137. Wohlfarth, K.; Schwandt, I.; Wegner, F.; Jurgens, T.; Gelbrich, G.; Wagner, A.; Bogdahn, U.; Schulte-Mattler, W. Biological activity of two botulinum toxin type A complexes (Dysport and Botox) in volunteers: A double-blind, randomized, dose-ranging study. *J. Neurol.* **2008**, *255*, 1932–1939. [CrossRef] [PubMed]
138. Brodsky, M.A.; Swope, D.M.; Grimes, D. Diffusion of botulinum toxins. *Tremor Other Hyperkinet. Mov.* **2012**, *2*. [CrossRef]
139. Bakheit, A.M.; Ward, C.D.; McLellan, D.L. Generalised botulism-like syndrome after intramuscular injections of botulinum toxin type A: A report of two cases. *J. Neurol. Neurosurg. Psychiatry* **1997**, *62*, 198. [CrossRef] [PubMed]
140. Bhatia, K.P.; Munchau, A.; Thompson, P.D.; Houser, M.; Chauhan, V.S.; Hutchinson, M.; Shapira, A.H.; Marsden, C.D. Generalised muscular weakness after botulinum toxin injections for dystonia: A report of three cases. *J. Neurol. Neurosurg. Psychiatry* **1999**, *67*, 90–93. [CrossRef] [PubMed]
141. Ramirez-Castaneda, J.; Jankovic, J.; Comella, C.; Dashtipour, K.; Fernandez, H.H.; Mari, Z. Diffusion, spread, and migration of botulinum toxin. *Mov. Disord.* **2013**, *28*, 1775–1783. [CrossRef] [PubMed]
142. Aoki, R.K. Botulinum neurotoxin serotypes A and B preparations have different safety margins in preclinical models of muscle weakening efficacy and systemic safety. *Toxicon* **2002**, *40*, 923–928. [CrossRef]
143. Torii, Y.; Goto, Y.; Takahashi, M.; Ishida, S.; Harakawa, T.; Sakamoto, T.; Kaji, R.; Kozaki, S.; Ginnaga, A. Quantitative determination of biological activity of botulinum toxins utilizing compound muscle action potentials (CMAP), and comparison of neuromuscular transmission blockage and muscle flaccidity among toxins. *Toxicon* **2010**, *55*, 407–414. [CrossRef] [PubMed]
144. Johnson, E.A.; Tepp, W.H.; Lin, G. Purification, Characterization, and Use of Clostridium Botulinum Neurotoxin BoNT/A3. Patent WO2013049139, 4 April 2013.

145. Torii, Y.; Goto, Y.; Nakahira, S.; Kozaki, S.; Kaji, R.; Ginnaga, A. Comparison of systemic toxicity between botulinum toxin subtypes A1 and A2 in mice and rats. *Basic Clin. Pharmacol. Toxicol.* **2015**, *116*, 524–528. [CrossRef] [PubMed]
146. Schantz, E.J.; Johnson, E.A. Properties and Use of Botulinum Toxin and Other Microbial Neurotoxins in Medicine. *Microbiol. Rev.* **1992**, *56*, 80–99. [PubMed]
147. Frokjaer, S.; Otzen, D.E. Protein drug stability: A formulation challenge. *Nature* **2005**, 298–306. [CrossRef] [PubMed]
148. Ascher, B.; Kestemont, P.; Boineau, D.; Bodokh, I.; Stein, A.; Heckmann, M.; Dendorfer, M.; Pavicic, T.; Volteau, M.; Tse, A.; et al. Liquid Formulation of AbobotulinumtoxinA Exhibits a Favorable Efficacy and Safety Profile in Moderate to Severe Glabellar Lines: A Randomized, Double-Blind, Placebo- and Active Comparator-Controlled Trial. *Aesthet. Surg. J.* **2018**, *38*, 183–191. [CrossRef] [PubMed]
149. Jankovic, J. Botulinum toxin in clinical practice. *J. Neurol. Neurosurg. Psychiatry* **2004**, *75*, 951–957. [CrossRef] [PubMed]
150. Bagramyan, K.; Barash, J.R.; Arnon, S.S.; Kalkum, M. Attomolar Detection of Botulinum Toxin Type A in Complex Biological Matrices. *PLoS ONE* **2008**. [CrossRef] [PubMed]
151. Mason, J.T.; Xu, L.; Sheng, Z.-M.; He, J.; O'Leary, T.J. Liposome polymerase chain reaction assay for the sub-attomolar detection of cholera toxin and botulinum toxin type A. *Nat. Protocol.* **2006**, *1*, 2003–2011. [CrossRef] [PubMed]
152. Prausnitz, M.R.; Langer, R. Transdermal drug delivery. *Nat. Biotechnol.* **2008**, *26*, 1261–1268. [CrossRef] [PubMed]
153. Waugh, J.M.; Lee, J.; Dake, M.D.; Browne, D. Nonclinical and clinical experiences with CPP-based self-assembling peptide systems in topical drug development. *Cell Penetr. Pept. Methods Protocol.* **2011**, 553–572.
154. Jones, T.; Jeremy Scott, C.; Tranowski, D.; Joshi, T. Safety and Tolerability of Topical Botulinum Toxin Type A in Healthy Adults. In Proceedings of the 69th Annual Meeting of the Society for Investigative Dermatology, Montreal, QC, Canada, 6–9 May 2009.
155. Brandt, F.; O'connell, C.; Cazzaniga, A.; Waugh, J.M. Efficacy and safety evaluation of a novel botulinum toxin topical gel for the treatment of moderate to severe lateral canthal lines. *Dermatol. Surg.* **2010**, *36*, 2111–2118. [CrossRef] [PubMed]
156. Glogau, R.; Brandt, F.; Kane, M.; Monheit, G.D.; Waugh, J.M. Results of a randomized, double-blind, placebo-controlled study to evaluate the efficacy and safety of a botulinum toxin type A topical gel for the treatment of moderate-to-severe lateral canthal lines. *J. Drugs Dermatol.* **2012**, *11*, 38–45. [PubMed]
157. Glogau, R.G. Topically applied botulinum toxin type A for the treatment of primary axillary hyperhidrosis: Results of a randomized, blinded, vehicle-controlled study. *Dermatol. Surg.* **2007**, *33*, S76–S80. [CrossRef] [PubMed]
158. Chajchir, I.; Modi, P.; Chajchir, A. Novel topical BoNTA (CosmeTox, toxin type A) cream used to treat hyperfunctional wrinkles of the face, mouth, and neck. *Aesthet. Plast. Surg.* **2008**, *32*, 715–722. [CrossRef] [PubMed]
159. Carmichael, N.M.; Dostrovsky, J.O.; Charlton, M.P. Peptide-mediated transdermal delivery of botulinum neurotoxin type A reduces neurogenic inflammation in the skin. *Pain* **2010**, *149*, 316–324. [CrossRef] [PubMed]
160. Saffarian, P.; Peerayeh, S.N.; Amani, J.; Ebrahimi, F.; Sedighian, H.; Halabian, R.; Fooladi, A.A.I. TAT-BoNT/A (1–448), a novel fusion protein as a therapeutic agent: Analysis of transcutaneous delivery and enzyme activity. *Appl. Microbiol. Biotechnol.* **2016**, *100*, 2785–2795. [CrossRef] [PubMed]
161. Saffarian, P.; Peerayeh, S.N.; Amani, J.; Ebrahimi, F.; Sedighianrad, H.; Halabian, R.; Imani Fooladi, A.A. Expression and purification of recombinant TAT-BoNT/A (1–448) under denaturing and native conditions. *Bioengineered* **2016**, *7*, 478–483. [CrossRef] [PubMed]
162. Chow, A.; Wilder-Smith, E. Effect of transdermal botulinum toxin on sweat secretion in subjects with idiopathic palmar hyperhidrosis. *Br. J. Dermatol.* **2009**, *160*, 721–722. [CrossRef] [PubMed]
163. Kavanagh, G.M.; Shams, K. Botulinum toxin type A by iontophoresis for primary palmar hyperhidrosis. *J. Am. Acad. Dermatol.* **2006**, *55*, S115–S117. [CrossRef] [PubMed]
164. Pacini, S.; Gulisano, M.; Punzi, T.; Ruggiero, M. Transdermal delivery of Clostridium botulinum toxin type A by pulsed current iontophoresis. *J. Am. Acad. Dermatol.* **2007**, *57*, 1097–1099. [CrossRef] [PubMed]

165. Iannitti, T.; Palmieri, B.; Aspiro, A.; Di Cerbo, A. A preliminary study of painless and effective transdermal botulinum toxin A delivery by jet nebulization for treatment of primary hyperhidrosis. *Drug Des. Dev. Ther.* **2014**, *8*, 931. [CrossRef] [PubMed]
166. Bariya, S.H.; Gohel, M.C.; Mehta, T.A.; Sharma, O.P. Microneedles: An emerging transdermal drug delivery system. *J. Pharm. Pharmacol.* **2012**, *64*, 11–29. [CrossRef] [PubMed]
167. Torrisi, B.M.; Zarnitsyn, V.; Prausnitz, M.; Anstey, A.; Gateley, C.; Birchall, J.C.; Coulman, S. Pocketed microneedles for rapid delivery of a liquid-state botulinum toxin A formulation into human skin. *J. Control. Release* **2013**, *165*, 146–152. [CrossRef] [PubMed]
168. Tyagi, P.; Kashyap, M.; Yoshimura, N.; Chancellor, M.; Chermansky, C.J. Past, Present and Future of Chemodenervation with Botulinum Toxin in the Treatment of Overactive Bladder. *J. Urol.* **2017**, *197*, 982–990. [CrossRef] [PubMed]
169. Khera, M.; Somogyi, G.T.; Salas, N.A.; Kiss, S.; Boone, T.B.; Smith, C.P. In vivo effects of botulinum toxin A on visceral sensory function in chronic spinal cord-injured rats. *Urology* **2005**, *66*, 208–212. [CrossRef] [PubMed]
170. Shimizu, S.; Wheeler, M.; Saito, M.; Weiss, R.; Hittelman, A. 907 Effect of intravesical botulinum toxin a delivery (using dmso) in rat overactive bladder model. *J. Urol.* **2012**, *187*, e370. [CrossRef]
171. Petrou, S.P.; Parker, A.S.; Crook, J.E.; Rogers, A.; Metz-Kudashick, D.; Thiel, D.D. Botulinum a toxin/dimethyl sulfoxide bladder instillations for women with refractory idiopathic detrusor overactivity: A phase 1/2 study. *Mayo Clin. Proc.* **2009**, *84*, 702–706. [CrossRef] [PubMed]
172. Vemulakonda, V.M.; Somogyi, G.T.; Kiss, S.; Salas, N.A.; Boone, T.B.; Smith, C.P. Inhibitory effect of intravesically applied botulinum toxin A in chronic bladder inflammation. *J. Urol.* **2005**, *173*, 621–624. [CrossRef] [PubMed]
173. Sweeney, D.; O'Leary, M.; Erickson, J.; Marx, S.; Chancellor, M. Safety and efficacy with bladder botulinum toxin in elderly patients. In Proceedings of the International Continence Society Annual Meeting, Montreal, QC, Canada, 28 August–2 September 2005.
174. Chuang, Y.-C.; Yoshimura, N.; Huang, C.-C.; Wu, M.; Chiang, P.-H.; Chancellor, M.B. Intravesical botulinum toxin A administration inhibits COX-2 and EP4 expression and suppresses bladder hyperactivity in cyclophosphamide-induced cystitis in rats. *Eur. Urol.* **2009**, *56*, 159–167. [CrossRef] [PubMed]
175. El Shatoury, M.; Di Young, L.; Turley, E.; Yazdani, A.; Dave, S. Early experimental results of using a novel delivery carrier, hyaluronan-phosphatidylethanolamine (HA-PE), which may allow simple bladder instillation of botulinum toxin A as effectively as direct detrusor muscle injection. *J. Pediatr. Urol.* **2017**. [CrossRef] [PubMed]
176. Krhut, J.; Navratilova, M.; Sykora, R.; Jurakova, M.; Gärtner, M.; Mika, D.; Pavliska, L.; Zvara, P. Intravesical instillation of onabotulinum toxin A embedded in inert hydrogel in the treatment of idiopathic overactive bladder: A double-blind randomized pilot study. *Scand. J. Urol.* **2016**, *50*, 200–205. [CrossRef] [PubMed]
177. Chuang, Y.-C.; Tyagi, P.; Huang, C.-C.; Yoshimura, N.; Wu, M.; Kaufman, J.; Chancellor, M.B. Urodynamic and immunohistochemical evaluation of intravesical botulinum toxin A delivery using liposomes. *J. Urol.* **2009**, *182*, 786–792. [CrossRef] [PubMed]
178. Chuang, Y.-C.; Kaufmann, J.H.; Chancellor, D.D.; Chancellor, M.B.; Kuo, H.-C. Bladder instillation of liposome encapsulated onabotulinumtoxina improves overactive bladder symptoms: A prospective, multicenter, double-blind, randomized trial. *J. Urol.* **2014**, *192*, 1743–1749. [CrossRef] [PubMed]
179. Chuang, Y.-C.; Huang, T.-L.; Tyagi, P.; Huang, C.-C. Urodynamic and immunohistochemical evaluation of intravesical botulinum toxin A delivery using low energy shock waves. *J. Urol.* **2016**, *196*, 599–608. [CrossRef] [PubMed]
180. Kajbafzadeh, A.-M.; Montaser-Kouhsari, L.; Ahmadi, H.; Sotoudeh, M. Intravesical electromotive botulinum toxin type A administration: Part I—Experimental study. *Urology* **2011**, *77*, 1460–1464. [CrossRef] [PubMed]
181. Schiotz, H.A.; Mai, H.T.; Zabielska, R. Intravesical Electromotive Botulinum Toxin in Women with Overactive Bladder—A Pilot Study. *ARC J. Gynecol. Obs.* **2017**, *2*, 4–10.
182. Kajbafzadeh, A.-M.; Ahmadi, H.; Montaser-Kouhsari, L.; Sharifi-Rad, L.; Nejat, F.; Bazargan-Hejazi, S. Intravesical electromotive botulinum toxin type A administration—Part II: Clinical application. *Urology* **2011**, *77*, 439–445. [CrossRef] [PubMed]

183. Ladi-Seyedian, S.-S.; Sharifi-Rad, L.; Kajbafzadeh, A.-M. Intravesical Electromotive Botulinum Toxin Type "A" Administration for Management of Urinary Incontinence Secondary to Neuropathic Detrusor Overactivity in Children: Long-Term Follow-up. *Urology* **2017**, in press. [CrossRef] [PubMed]
184. Kajbafzadeh, A.-M.; Sharifi-Rad, L.; Ladi-Seyedian, S.-S. Intravesical electromotive botulinum toxin type A administration for management of concomitant neuropathic bowel and bladder dysfunction in children. *Int. J. Colorectal Dis.* **2016**, *31*, 1397–1399. [CrossRef] [PubMed]
185. Zhu, Z.; Stone, H.F.; Thach, T.Q.; Garcia, L.; Ruegg, C.L. A novel botulinum neurotoxin topical gel: Treatment of allergic rhinitis in rats and comparative safety profile. *Am. J. Rhinol. Allergy* **2012**, *26*, 450–454. [CrossRef] [PubMed]
186. Rohrbach, S.; Junghans, K.; Köhler, S.; Laskawi, R. Minimally invasive application of botulinum toxin A in patients with idiopathic rhinitis. *Head Face Med.* **2009**, *5*, 18. [CrossRef] [PubMed]

toxins

MDPI

Review

Analgesic Effects of Botulinum Toxin in Children with CP

Josephine Sandahl Michelsen, Gitte Normann and Christian Wong *

Department of Orthopedics, Hvidovre Hospital, Hvidovre 2650, Denmark;
Josephine.sandahl.michelsen@regionh.dk (J.S.M.); gittenormann@gmail.com (G.N.)
* Correspondence: Christian.nai.en.tierp-wong@regionh.dk; Tel.: +45-38626966

Received: 30 March 2018; Accepted: 13 April 2018; Published: 19 April 2018

Abstract: Experiencing pain is the greatest contributor to a reduced quality of life in children with cerebral palsy (CP). The presence of pain is quite common (~60%) and increases with age. This leads to missed school days, less participation, and reduced ambulation. Despite these alarming consequences, strategies to relieve the pain are absent and poorly studied. Moreover, it is difficult to evaluate pain in this group of children, especially in cases of children with cognitive deficits, and tools for pain evaluation are often inadequate. Botulinum toxin has been shown to alleviate pain in a variety of disorders and could potentially have an analgesic effect in children with CP as well. Even though most of the studies presented here show promising results, many also have limitations in their methodology as it is unlikely to capture all dimensions of pain in this heterogeneous group using only one assessment tool. In this review, we present a new way of examining the analgesic effect of botulinum toxin in children with CP using a variety of pain scores.

Keywords: pain; cerebral palsy; botulinum toxin A

Key Contribution: This review describes the causes of pain in children with cerebral palsy; how to evaluate this and the analgesic effect of botulinum toxin; including a description of a prospective study protocol examining the effect of botulinum toxin on muscle-related pain.

---

1. Pain in Children with Cerebral Palsy

1.1. Introduction

Cerebral palsy (CP) is a heterogeneous group of non-progressive neurological disorders caused by damage to either the fetal or the infant brain, affecting the development of posture and movement. CP is the most common cause of physical disability in children, affecting 2.5 children for every 1000 children being born. CP causes variances in the level of motor function, from ambulatory children to nonambulatory children that depend on full-time assistance. Motor function is classified using the Gross Motor Function Classification System (GMFCS), where level 1 describes the most functional group and level 5 describes the least function group. Secondary musculoskeletal problems such as spasticity, muscle deformities, hip dislocation, or scoliosis often occur and can contribute to the pain experienced by this population. Cognitive, perceptional, or communicative disturbances are often present, which can make pain scoring difficult [1].

The pain these children experience includes both chronic pain and pain related to procedures such as physiotherapy (assisted stretching), passive joint movement, botulinum toxin injections, and surgery, with physiotherapy being reported as the cause of the most intense and most frequent pain [2,3]. Recurrent nonprocedural musculoskeletal pain is also a serious and disabling problem and has been reported in 62% of children with CP [4].

Pain is reported to be the most important factor affecting the quality of life and the participation of children with CP, and it is reported to be an even stronger contributor than GMFCS levels [4–11].

In this review, we describe the characteristics of pain in children with CP and the problems with recognizing and grading pain. We also discuss if botulinum toxin can be used to treat pain in this group of patients. As this review focuses on botulinum toxin as a treatment for general musculoskeletal pain, studies on procedural pain will not be discussed in detail.

1.2. Prevalence and Intensifiers

A European multicenter project (SPARCLE) involving seven European countries began in 2004 to study the prevalence of pain in 818 eight to twelve year old children with CP (SPACLE 1) [4–11]. Of these children, 60% had experienced pain in the last week according to self-reports and 73% according to parental reports. A follow-up study was conducted in 2009 (SPARCLE2) including 594 of the children who had participated in the first study and were now considered adolescents. During the five years of the study, the frequency of pain had increased to 74% and 77%, respectively. The prevalence reported in this study seems consistent with other studies reporting 48–67% [2,3,12–19]. In contrast, Alriksson-Schmidt and Hägglund (2016) included 2777 children and assessed pain among all GMFCS groups, but reported only a prevalence of 32.4% [20]. In contrast to many of the other studies, only children aged 0–14 were included, which easily could have lowered the prevalence as increasing age has been shown to be a contributing factor [2,4,14]. The SPACLE studies actually found that an age of more than 14 years was the only significant predictor for recurrent musculoskeletal pain [4]. Findlay et al. (2015) also showed that an increasing age, together with a presence of pain, negatively affected the quality of life of children [14]. Compared to the general population where approximately every fifth child experiences chronic pain [21,22], there is no doubt that children with CP experience pain more often.

The presence of pain in children with CP has been correlated with missed school days, less participation in activities, and reduced ambulation [23,24], which, combined with the negative impact on their quality of life, make the high prevalence of pain even more alarming.

Despite the high prevalence of pain, strategies to reduce it are inadequate or absent [12,13,25–27]. This indicates that there is a need for more knowledge and awareness, and strategies to reduce the pain need to be optimized.

1.3. Pain Characteristic, Location, and Frequency

The location, intensity, frequency, and origins (neuropathic, nociceptive) of the pain seem to vary across this heterogeneous population, which contributes to its complexity. Even the factors triggering the pain can vary. Inactivity, physical activity, stress, weather, and sleep have all been described as intensifiers [10,15,28].

The pain that children with CP experience can be both neuropathic and nociceptive in origin. A recent study [27] used quantitative sensory testing (QST) to determine the sensory detection and the pain thresholds in 30 children and adolescents with CP. When compared with the reference values from healthy controls, the children with CP were less sensitive to mechanical and thermal stimuli, but were more sensitive to mechanic pain. This might explain the high prevalence of musculoskeletal pain and pain during assisted stretching. The study proposed that the alternation in sensory detection is caused by a dysfunction in the sensory tract neurons, which makes neuropathic pain possible. This study proposes that an increased sensitivity to mechanic pain could be a contributing factor to the general experience of pain. As a consequence, the treatment of pain must involve strategies aimed to reduce the causes or effects of the (mechanic) pain.

Several secondary problems related to the diagnosis of cerebral palsy have been described by physicians as contributing factors to the pain. This includes hip dislocation, dystonia, muscle spasms, spasticity, deformities, constipation, and abnormal joint compression due to an abnormal gait pattern [12]. Pain seems to be most commonly located in the lower extremities [12,14,15]. The cause and the location of the pain seem to vary across GMFCS levels. The most functional children (GMFCS 1) complain of pain in the lower extremities, especially in the feet as a result of spasticity and muscular deformities, whereas the least functional children (GMFCS V) seem to have more pain in the hip and the abdominal region as a result of hip dislocation and constipation [12,20].

The pain intensity ranges from mild to severe, with most children reporting mild–moderate pain that occurs once or twice a week and does not affect their ability to perform activities [2,10–14]. Approximately one-quarter experience moderate–severe pain on a daily basis and report that the pain affects their ability to perform activities [2,12,14].

Pain intensity and frequency have been shown to correlate with increasing age [2,4,14] and GMFCS level [10,13,16,22] However, the correlation with the GFMCS levels is not consistent throughout all studies [2,14,17,19]. A gender difference has also been found as a trend, where girls experience more pain than boys [12,17], but only one study has shown significant results [20].

1.4. Pain is Unrecognized and Undertreated

A study from Penner et al. in 2013, where caregivers and a physician independently evaluated the presence of pain, suggested that musculoskeletal pain in particular is missed by physicians, and as a consequence, might be undertreated [13]. The presence of cognitive deficits can make it difficult for these children to report the pain and for the physician to recognize it. This observation is supported by a study from Stallard et al. (2001), where parental pain diaries were used to follow 34 non-communicative and cognitively impaired children during a two-day observation [29]. Even though 25 of the 34 children had pain on at least one of the two days, no-one received active pain management.

Literature describing the degree of pain management in children with CP is sparse, which could reflect an unrecognized and undertreated problem. A recently published study showed that only half of children with CP used specific pain strategies (medication, massage, activity, rest, and coping strategies) to relieve their pain [27], and Russo et al. (2008) have shown that only 16% used analgesia to relieve their pain [15]. The same is seen in the adult population [25,26]. Engel et al. showed in 2002 that even though many pain interventions such as ibuprofen, stretching, exercise, acetaminophen, and massage were perceived as moderately helpful, only a small group of patients were using them [25]. Moreover, a large variation in the efficacy of the interventions has been demonstrated [26], which seems plausible due to the heterogeneity of this patient group. As a consequence, an individual and multilevel pain management seems of great importance.

1.5. Pain Scoring

Recommendations in pain scoring have pointed out the use of self-reports to score the pain [30,31], and the most common tool used at the hospitals seems to be numeric intensity scales, which are usually the visual analogue scale (VAS) or the faces pain rate scales for smaller children (e.g., Wong–Baker FACES scale, faces pain scale). However, children with neurological deficits might also show atypical pain behavior such as drooling and laughing [3,32,33], which can make it difficult for physicians, caregivers, and parents to recognize the pain. Moreover, some of these children are not able to communicate due to cognitive deficits, which make pain scoring even more difficult. In recent years, several behavioral-based tools for pain scoring (NCCPC, pediatric pain profile and FLACC) have been developed for children with neurological and communitive deficits [30,31,33,34]. Most of these behavioral scoring tools have been modified in a revised edition, making it possible to add individual pain behavior to the scale and thus ensure that the level of pain is captured and correctly scored. Russo et al. (2008) proposed another problem in that some children and parents might see the pain as part of the underlying condition and as something that they have to live with. They might be unaware that the pain can be relieved, which may prevent them from seeking help [15].

Even if proper pain-scoring tools are available in the clinic, physicians have to be aware of the problem, be able to recognize pain behaviors, and to have knowledge of possible strategies to relieve the pain.

One reason for this issue of undertreated pain could be the difficulties in assessing the pain due the heterogeneity of the cognitive impairments related to CP, which makes it impossible to use a single standardized test [30,31].

In conclusion, there is no doubt that pain is an important and neglected issue in children with CP, which, when undertreated, has significant consequences such as missed school days, reduced participation, and a lower quality of life. Part of the problem seems to be the heterogeneity of the pain in its location, intensity, and cause. Pain is perhaps one of the most subjective feelings in the world, and as a consequence, there is a need for sufficient pain-scoring tools that are able to capture all dimensions of the pain independent of any potential cognitive deficits. Sufficient strategies in pain management might be difficult to find due to the complexity of the pain, and therefore, pain warrants individual assessment and treatment.

2. Existing Literature on the Analgesic Effect of Botulinum Toxin

2.1. The Mechanism of Botulinum Toxin

The mechanism of botulinum toxin on a cellular level is believed to be the blockage of the release of acetylcholine to the motor endplates, thereby preventing muscular contraction. Acetylcholine is transported in small vesicles and is released from the neuron through exocytosis. Large proteins called snares are connected to the outside of the vesicle and to the membrane of the neuron. Upon exocytosis, the snares perform a complex which enables the fusion and the release of the neurotransmitter. Botulinum toxin prevents the release of acetylcholine by cleaving one or more of the three snares (SNAP-25, Syntaxin, and VAMP) that form the complex. The snares involved in the docking of the vesicle are not specific to the neurotransmitter being transported [35]. Nonclinical studies have shown that botulinum toxin also blocks the release of neurotransmitters (e.g., glutamate, CGRP and substance P) that are involved in pain and inflammatory pathways [35,36]. The analgesic effect of botulinum toxin seems to be multifactorial. Botulinum toxin seems to have the ability to reduce pain indirectly as a muscle relaxant or by blocking local nociceptive neuropeptides involved in the peripheral sensitization caused by inflammation or injury. Besides its local effect, nonclinical studies have also suggested that botulinum toxin can be transported by retrograde axonal transport to the dorsal root, where it can exert a more central analgesic effect [35,36]. This is supported by studies showing bilateral analgesic effects following an ipsilateral injection of botulinum toxin [35]. By preventing the release of these neurotransmitters in the central nervous system, botulinum toxin may relieve neuropathic pain.

This analgesic effect of botulinum toxin is also supported by clinical studies where a pain-relieving effect has been observed in various pain disorders [36,37]. An excessive review from Safarpour et al. (2018) found level A evidence (effective) for post-herpetic neuralgia, trigeminal neuralgia, and post-traumatic neuralgia. Level B evidence (probably effective) was found for diabetic neuropathy, plantar fasciitis, piriformis syndrome, pain caused by knee arthroplasty, male pelvic pain syndrome, chronic back pain, and neuropathic pain secondary to traumatic spinal cord injury. Only level C evidence (possibly effective) was observed for female pelvic pain, knee osteoarthritis, and postoperative pain in children with CP [37]. In conclusion, the various ways by which botulinum toxin can exert its effects may support the theory that it has a pain-relieving effect for all causes of pain and not only those related to muscular hyperactivity.

2.2. Botulinum Toxin A for Spasticity-Related Pain

Studies on other populations with spasticity have shown promising results for botulinum toxin A as a treatment for spasticity-related pain. This has been described thoroughly by B. Jabbari et al. (2015), who examined several studies [38]. Five out of nine studies on upper limb spasticity showed positive results, and in four of the studies, the pain-relieving effect was shown in approximately 90% of the patients. Jabbari et al. proposed the use of invalidated pain scores as the reason for the lack of a measurable effect in the other studies. Lower limb spasticity was also examined by Jabbari, but the literature was sparse. Only three studies were examined but a reduction in limb pain or the number of painful spasms was seen in each of the studies as a result of the treatment.

Similar positive results were shown by Wissel et al. (2000). They studied the management of spasticity-associated pain with botulinum toxin A injections in a heterogeneous population of 60 patients with spasticity (including nine children with CP), and they reported a pain reduction in 90% of the patients [39]. Recently, they published an even larger double-blinded, randomized study, including 273 stroke patients who confirmed the result, and the reduction was sustained through to week 52 [40]. This suggests a long-lasting analgesic effect on spasticity-related pain, and the same effect may be seen in children with CP.

2.3. Botulinum Toxin A as a Treatment for Pain in Children with CP

The aforementioned mechanisms for botulinum toxin suggest that botulinum toxin could be a possible treatment for all kinds of pain that children with CP experience. However, the existing literature is sparse.

Botulinum toxin injections have, since the early 1990s, been used to reduce spasticity in children with cerebral palsy, to improve motor function, and to delay the need for surgery [41]. A Norwegian registry-based study (2012) examined the characteristics of children treated with botulinum toxin [42] and found that approximately two-thirds of all children with spastic CP were treated with botulinum toxin to improve their motor function. Pain relief and ease of care were less common indications for treatment. Interestingly, the study also showed that children with severe cognitive deficits were less commonly treated.

Pin et al. (2013) reviewed the evidence for the efficacy of botulinum toxin in children with CP (GMFCS IV and V) [43]. The study examined different parameters (pain reduction, motor function, ease of care, and comfort) and found that the level of methodological quality was weak to moderate in many of the studies. Out of 19 studies, only six studies included pain as an endpoint, with one measuring postoperative pain and five measuring general pain. Two studies [44,45] showed that the treatment had a significant effect, while one study showed a trend towards an analgesic effect, but the result was not significant [46]. These studies will be described in detail later in this review. The last three studies [47–49] were case studies and therefore, no statistical analyses were conducted. A total of six patients with pain were examined in the three case studies, and a positive effect was reported in all of them. The type of pain was painful shoulder luxation, hip pain, and pain during nursing and physiotherapy. A long-lasting effect of 6 and 7 months was reported in two patients [47,49]. Pin et al. concluded that only weak to moderate evidence exists for the effect of botulinum toxin in relieving spasticity-related (general) pain.

The analgesic effect of botulinum toxin in children with cerebral palsy has often only been investigated as a secondary or exploratory endpoint, sometimes only as part of a quality-of-life questionnaire or as an individual treatment goal [46,50,51]. Vles et al. (2008) used the VAS score to study the effect of botulinum toxin injection in regards to individual therapeutic goals [46]. The VAS score ranges from 0–10, where a score of 0 reflects a very satisfactory treatment, while a score of 10 reflects a very dissatisfactory treatment. Pain reduction was set as a treatment goal for four out of 55 children, and three of them reported individual scores of 9.4 to 0, 5.5 to 2.7, and 4.0 to 2.0 pre- and post-treatment. The last one did not find any change after the treatment and had the same score of 7.4 before and after the injection. Despite the positive effect seen in three of the children, no significant effect was found.

The effect on pain after botulinum toxin injections in children with cerebral palsy has, to our knowledge, only been measured as a primary endpoint in three studies [44,45,52]. Barwood et al. (2000) used an observational pain score and the level of analgesic requirements to study the effect of botulinum toxin on postoperative pain after hip adductor release [44]. A 74% reduction in the mean pain score was observed in children receiving botulinum toxin injections as compared to placebo. The group receiving treatment also needed 50% less analgesics than the children receiving a placebo treatment.

Rivard et al. (2009) used parent-proxy ratings to evaluate the analgesic effect of botulinum toxin injections on general pain in children with cerebral palsy [52]. Of the children with CP, 62% did not experience any pain one month post-injection. The assessment was done solely as a telephone interview, and therefore, the results have to be seen with caution. Lundy et al. (2009) used a validated behavioral pain score (the pediatric pain profile) to measure the effect of botulinum toxin in relieving hip pain in nonambulant children with CP [45]. The study showed promising results, with a reduction in hip pain in all participants from baseline to three months post-injection. Out of a maximum score of 60, the mean pain score fell from 42.2 (SD 8.6, range 20–59) at the baseline measurements to 9.5 (SD 5.2, range 1–23) at three months post-injection. The response to the treatment varied with individual reductions in the range of 12–58 points.

Another promising and long-lasting result was reported in a multicentered observational study by Chaléat-Valayer et al. (2011), which examined 282 children. Each child received injections with botulinum toxin based on self-selected therapeutic objectives. Those having an objective related to comfort and pain showed improvements of 80 percent at the end of the study, one year post-injection. Overall, the study also found that significantly fewer children experienced daily and intermittent pain as a result of the treatment [50].

Copeland et al. (2014) found in a double-blinded, randomized control study (RCT) that a significant pain reduction occurred between baseline and follow-up measurements, which was only evident in the group receiving the treatment [51]. However, the pain reduction was not significantly different from the group receiving the placebo treatment. Pain is, as described, an important factor for quality for life. An improvement in quality of life was also evident between the baseline and the follow-up measurements in the treatment group, which was significantly different from the placebo group at 16 weeks post-treatment.

Other RCT studies investigating pain have shown the same conflicting results, where patients respond positively to both the placebo and the treatment with botulinum toxin [38]. This may reflect a high placebo effect, which plausibly could be interrelated to the use of only one, highly subjective pain tool. This warrants a more strenuous methodological approach to evaluating pain in future studies.

Even though most of the studies presented here show promising results for botulinum toxin as a treatment for pain, many of the studies has limitations in regards to their methodology. This includes the absence of a control group, the exclusion of some GMFCS levels, the use of proxy reports, and the measurement of the effect of pain through the use of only one subjective measurement or as an individual therapeutic goal.

The absence of sufficient evidence for the efficacy of botulinum toxin as a treatment for pain in children with CP could also be caused by a lack of a proper evaluation of the pain as a result of the use of different pain-scoring tools. For such a heterogeneous group as these children, it is unlikely that all dimensions of pain will be captured using only one assessment tool.

In conclusion, further investigation into this matter is needed to establish a pain-relieving effect of botulinum toxin. This should include a detailed description of the type, the location, the intensity, and the frequency of pain, as well as the degree of cognitive deficits in this heterogeneous population, a more thorough examination of the pain, and the inclusion of a broader spectrum of this patient population.

3. Botulinum Toxin A as a Treatment for Spasticity-Related Pain

3.1. *A Novel Approach—The Use of a Variety of Pain Scores*

We are commencing a prospective multicenter study investigating the effect of a single injection of abobotulinumtoxinA (Dysport) on the pain and the quality of life in children with CP. Based on the parents' and patients' feedback after botulinum toxin treatment, we are hopeful that botulinum toxin could be a possible pain treatment for children with cerebral palsy. The process by which botulinum toxin alleviates pain and whether botulinum toxin injected locally in the muscles could have more direct effect on pain and inflammatory pathways is still not fully understood. Only children suffering from spasticity-related pain in the lower extremities will therefore be included in this study. This will be measured by the presence of a pain response (r-FLACC) and increased muscle tone during passive joint movement. If a painful reaction in a muscle is being detected, the muscle will be a target for treatment. However, the children must experience at least moderate pain (4 on the r-FLACC) to be considered for this study. In contrast to the previous studies already mentioned in this review, we will focus on a more thorough methodological approach to investigate the effect of the botulinum toxin on pain. The level of pain will be measured pre-injection and 4, 12, and 28 weeks post-injection, which will enable us to measure a possible long-lasting effect. To capture as many dimensions of the children's pain experiences, we will use a variety of pain scores. The revised FLACC during passive range of motion will also be used to measure localized pain in the muscles. The pain scoring will be done blinded using a video recording of the session. The pediatric pain profile previous used by Lundy et al. (2009) [45] will be used to investigate both the characteristics of the pain and to evaluate the level of daily pain. All communicative children will be asked to evaluate the pain on an intensity scale using VAS or Wong-Baker, since a self-reported rating is the gold standard for pain evaluation, but as mentioned, it not always applicable in this patient population. For the non-communicative children, proxy reports by the parents will therefore be utilized in the pediatric pain profile. In general, one observer will perform all pain scoring measurements to ensure a uniform and standardized evaluation. In this study, we will include children with CP belonging to all GMFCS levels for a comprehensive analysis of this heterogeneous group of disabled children.

Pain has a negative impact on quality of life as previously described. We will therefore monitor the quality of life with questionnaires (CPchild and CPQOL) throughout the study period. Recommendations state that it is essential to define a realistic, therapeutic, and measurable goal for the treatment [41]. A goal will therefore be set for each child describing a desirable pain-related effect of the treatment. It could be fewer awakenings during the night or to be able to perform activities previously described as painful. The goal attainment scale will be used to monitor the progress at each follow-up (4, 12, 28 weeks post-treatment).

It is still not clear whether a decrease in spasticity will relieve the pain or if other mechanisms are involved. Spasticity measurements (Modified Ashworth Scale and Tardieu scale) will therefore be performed throughout the study period by the same rater. This might enable us to correlate the pain with the presence of spasticity even though some criticism has been reported regarding the reliability of these measurements [53].

In conclusion, we hope to be able to perform a comprehensive study where we examine the possible effects of muscular botulinum toxin injections in children with cerebral palsy, with a focus on spasticity-related pain. It would have been preferable but ultimately not feasible to include a placebo treatment due to ethical considerations which prevent the use of sham injections, which (in principle) are without effect and painful to perform.

3.2. *Botulinum Toxin Injection—Limitations and Safety*

Botulinum toxin injections seem to have a pain-relieving effect but have limitations, as with all other treatments. Botulinum toxin injections have been considered as a safe treatment for spasticity in children with CP, but minor side effects like pain at the injection site, urinary incontinence, and influenza-like symptoms have been observed [54]. The injections are considered painful for many of the children and some children will thus be offered general or local anesthesia before the injection. Even though general and local anesthetics are generally considered safe, they are associated with an elevated risk of adverse events. In addition, the development of antibodies against the toxin can occur in some children, thereby preventing an effective response to the treatment [55], and there is always a chance that the toxin will spread and cause a partial, unintended paralysis and weakness in the muscles. Another limitation is the duration of the treatment. Nonclinical studies have shown that the motor endplate recovers after approximately three months [56], and even though the therapeutic effect has been observed to persist for up to several months [40,47,49,50], a strategy involving repeated injections is necessary for a sustained effect. Delgado et al. examined in 2017 the safety and efficacy of repeated injections in 216 children with cerebral palsy, and they did not find any reason to suspect a high risk for adverse events, and the clinical improvements were also sustained through repeated treatment cycles [57]. The study confirmed a long-lasting therapeutic effect as one out of five patients showed an effect duration of at least 28 weeks. The main indication for treating with botulinum toxin has been the presence of spasticity, but as spasticity can develop into structural contractures over time, some children will be unfit for the treatment with increasing age. Botulinum toxin has been considered useful for other pain conditions, and hypotheses have been made regarding the direct effects of botulinum toxin on pain and the inflammatory effect, as mentioned previously. Pain due to contractures, deformities, simple muscle overload or other causes unrelated to spasticity in children with CP might therefore be alleviated with botulinum toxin, but it should only be considered in moderate and severe pain if less invasive pharmacological and nonpharmacological strategies are ineffective [58].As injection treatment requires accurate skills and is time-consuming, expensive, invasive, and has possible side effects, it is important to weigh these limitations and concerns against the possible beneficial effects of the treatment prior to commencing the treatment.

Acknowledgments: Funds to cover the costs to publish in this open access comes from a pending study sponsored by Ipsen A/B.

Conflicts of Interest: First author is conducting the above described study and last author is supervising the study. Second author has no conflict of interest. Ipsen A/B is sponsoring this study, but has not been taking part in the creation of this article. The founding sponsors commented on the above described pending study in the design of the study, and will be allowed to comment on manuscripts coming from this study before submission. The founding sponsors will have no role in the collection, analyses, or interpretation of data; in the writing of the manuscript, and in the decision to publish the results.

References

1. Rosenbaum, P.; Paneth, N.; Leviton, A.; Goldstein, M.; Bax, M.; Damiano, D.; Dan, B.; Jacobsson, B. A report: The definition and classification of cerebral palsy April 2006. *Dev. Med. Child Neurol.* **2007**, *109* (Suppl. 109), 8–14.
2. Jayanath, S.; Ong, L.C.; Marret, M.J.; Fauzi, A.A. Parent-reported pain in non-verbal children and adolescents with cerebral palsy. *Dev. Med. Child Neurol.* **2016**, *58*, 395–401. [CrossRef] [PubMed]
3. Hadden, K.L.; Von Baeyer, C.L. Pain in children with cerebral palsy: Common triggers and expressive behaviors. *Pain* **2002**, *99*, 281–288. [CrossRef]
4. Ramstad, K.; Jahnsen, R.; Skjeldal, O.H.; Diseth, T.H. Characteristics of recurrent musculoskeletal pain in children with cerebral palsy aged 8 to 18 years. *Dev. Med. Child Neurol.* **2011**, *53*, 1013–1018. [CrossRef] [PubMed]
5. Colver, A.; Rapp, M.; Eisemann, N.; Ehlinger, V.; Thyen, U.; Dickinson, H.O.; Parkes, J.; Parkinson, K.; Nystrand, M.; Fauconnier, J.; et al. Self-reported quality of life of adolescents with cerebral palsy: A cross-sectional and longitudinal analysis. *Lancet* **2015**, *385*, 705–716. [CrossRef]
6. Colver, A.; Thyen, U.; Arnaud, C.; Beckung, E.; Fauconnier, J.; Marcelli, M.; FMcManus, V.; Michelsen, S.I.; Parkes, J.; Parkinson, K.; et al. Association between participation in life situations of children with cerebral palsy and their physical, social, and attitudinal environment: A cross-sectional multicenter European study. *Arch. Phys. Med. Rehabil.* **2012**, *93*, 2154–2164. [CrossRef] [PubMed]
7. Fauconnier, J.; Dickinson, H.O.; Beckung, E.; Marcelli, M.; McManus, V.; Michelsen, S.I.; Parkes, J.; Parkinson, K.N.; Thyen, U.; Arnaud, C.; et al. Participation in life situations of 8–12 year old children with cerebral palsy: Cross sectional European study. *BMJ* **2009**, *338*, b1458. [CrossRef] [PubMed]
8. Dang, V.M.; Colver, A.; Dickinson, H.O.; Marcelli, M.; Michelsen, S.I.; Parkes, J.; Parkinson, K.; Rapp, M.; Arnaud, C.; Nystrand, M.; et al. Predictors of participation of adolescents with cerebral palsy: A European multi-centre longitudinal study. *Res. Dev. Disabil.* **2015**, *36*, 551–564. [CrossRef] [PubMed]
9. Ramstad, K.; Jahnsen, R.; Skjeldal, O.H.; Diseth, T.H. Mental health, Health related quality of life and recurrent musculoskeletal pain in children with cerebral palsy aged 8 to 18 years. *Disabil. Rehabil.* **2012**, *34*, 1589–1595. [CrossRef] [PubMed]

10. Parkinson, K.N.; Dickinson, H.O.; Arnaud, C.; Lyons, A.; Colver, A.; Beckung, E.; Thyen, U. Pain in young people aged 13 to 17 years with cerebral palsy: Cross-sectional, multicentre European study. *Arch. Dis. Child.* **2013**, *98*, 434–440. [CrossRef] [PubMed]
11. Parkinson, K.N.; Gibson, L.; Dickinson, H.O.; Colver, A.F. Pain in children with cerebral palsy: A cross-sectional multicentre European study. *Acta Paediatr.* **2010**, *99*, 446–451. [CrossRef] [PubMed]
12. Penner, M.; Xie, W.Y.; Binepal, N.; Switzer, L.; Fehlings, D. Characteristics of pain in children and youth with cerebral palsy. *Pediatrics* **2013**, *132*, e407–e413. [CrossRef] [PubMed]
13. Houlihan, C.M.; Hanson, A.; Quinlan, N.; Puryear, C.; Stevenson, R.D. Intensity, perception, and descriptive characteristics of chronic pain in children with cerebral palsy. *J. Pediatr. Rehabil. Med.* **2008**, *1*, 145–153. [PubMed]
14. Findlay, B.; Switzer, L.; Narayanan, U.; Chen, S.; Fehlings, D. Investigating the impact of pain, age, Gross Motor Function Classification System, and sex on health-related quality of life in children with cerebral palsy. *Dev. Med. Child Neurol.* **2016**, *58*, 292–297. [CrossRef] [PubMed]
15. Russo, R.; Miller, M.; Haan, E.; Cameron, I.D.; Crotty, M. Pain Characteristics and Their Association with Quality of Life and Self-concept in Children with Hemiplegic Cerebral Palsy Identified from a Population Register. *Clin. J. Pain* **2008**, *24*, 335–342. [CrossRef] [PubMed]
16. Barney, C.C.; Krach, L.E.; Rivard, P.F.; Belew, J.L.; Symons, F.J. Motor function predicts parent-reported musculoskeletal pain in children with cerebral palsy. *Pain Res. Manag.* **2013**, *18*, 323–327. [CrossRef] [PubMed]
17. Doralp, S.; Bartlett, D.J. The Prevalence, Distribution, and Effect of Pain among Adolescents with Cerebral Palsy. *Pediatr. Phys. Ther.* **2010**, *22*, 26–33. [CrossRef] [PubMed]
18. Yamaguchi, R.; Perry, K.N.; Hines, M. Pain, pain anxiety and emotional and behavioural problems in children with cerebral palsy. *Disabil. Rehabil.* **2013**, *36*, 125–130. [CrossRef] [PubMed]
19. Kennes, J.; Rosenbaum, P.; Hanna, S.E.; Walter, S.; Russell, D.; Raina, P.; Bartlett, D.; Galuppi, B. Health status of school-aged children with cerebral palsy: Information from a population-based sample. *Dev. Med. Child Neurol.* **2002**, *44*, 240–247. [CrossRef] [PubMed]
20. Alriksson-Schmidt, A.; Hagglund, G. Pain in children and adolescents with cerebral palsy: A population-based registry study. *Acta Paediatr.* **2016**, *105*, 665–670. [CrossRef] [PubMed]
21. Rustøen, T.; Wahl, A.K.; Hanestad, B.R.; Lerdal, A.; Paul, S.; Miaskowski, C. Prevalence and characteristics of chronic pain in the general Norwegian population. *Eur. J. Pain* **2004**, *8*, 555–565. [CrossRef] [PubMed]
22. Perquin, C.W.; Hazebroek-Kampschreur, A.A.J.M.; Hunfeld, J.A.M.; Bohnen, A.M.; van Suijlekom-Smit, L.W.A.; Passchier, J.; van der Wouden, J.C. Pain in children and adolescents: A common experience. *Pain* **2000**, *87*, 51–58. [CrossRef]
23. Houlihan, C.M.; O'Donnell, M.; Conaway, M.; Stevenson, R.D. Bodily pain and health-related quality of life in children with cerebral palsy. *Dev. Med. Child Neurol.* **2004**, *46*, 305–310. [CrossRef] [PubMed]
24. Tervo, R.C.; Symons, F.; Stout, J.; Novacheck, T. Parental report of pain and associated limitations in ambulatory children with cerebral palsy. *Arch. Phys. Med. Rehabil.* **2006**, *87*, 928–934. [CrossRef] [PubMed]
25. Engel, J.M.; Kartin, D.; Jensen, M.P. Pain treatment in persons with cerebral palsy: Frequency and helpfulness. *Am. J. Phys. Med. Rehabil.* **2002**, *81*, 291–296. [CrossRef] [PubMed]
26. Jensen, M.P.; Engel, J.M.; Hoffman, A.J.; Schwartz, L. Natural history of chronic pain and pain treatment in adults with cerebral palsy. *Am. J. Phys. Med. Rehabil.* **2004**, *83*, 439–445. [CrossRef] [PubMed]
27. Blankenburg, M.; Junker, J.; Hirschfeld, G.; Michel, E.; Aksu, F.; Wager, J.; Zernikow, B. Quantitative sensory testing profiles in children, adolescents and young adults (6–20 years) with cerebral palsy: Hints for a neuropathic genesis of pain syndromes. *Eur. J. Paediatr. Neurol.* **2017**. [CrossRef] [PubMed]
28. Jahnsen, R.; Villien, L.; Aamodt, G.; Stanghelle, J.K.; Holm, I. Musculoskeletal pain in adults with cerebral palsy compared with the general population. *J. Rehabil. Med.* **2004**, *36*, 78–84. [CrossRef] [PubMed]
29. Stallard, P.; Williams, L.; Lenton, S.; Velleman, R. Pain in cognitively impaired, non-communicating children. *Arch. Dis. Child.* **2001**, *85*, 460–462. [CrossRef] [PubMed]
30. Kingsnorth, S.; Orava, T.; Provvidenza, C.; Adler, E.; Ami, N.; Gresley-Jones, T.; Mankad, D.; Slonim, N.; Fay, L.; Joachimides, N.; et al. Chronic Pain Assessment Tools for Cerebral Palsy: A Systematic Review. *Pediatrics* **2015**, *136*, e947–e960. [CrossRef] [PubMed]
31. Warlow, T.A.; Hain, R.D.W. 'Total Pain' in Children with Severe Neurological Impairment. *Children* **2018**, *5*, 13. [CrossRef] [PubMed]

32. Swiggum, M.; Hamilton, M.L.; Gleeson, P.; Roddey, T. Pain in Children with Cerebral Palsy: Implications for Pediatric Physical Therapy. *Pediatr. Phys. Ther.* **2010**, *22*, 86–92. [CrossRef] [PubMed]
33. Pedersen, L.K.; Rahbek, O.; Nikolajsen, L.; Møller-Madsen, B. Assessment of pain in children with cerebral palsy focused on translation and clinical feasibility of the revised FLACC score. *Scand. J. Pain* **2015**, *9*, 49–54. [CrossRef]
34. Maliviya, S.; Voepel-Lewis, T.; Burke, C.; Merkel, S.; Tait, A.R. The revised FLACC observational pain tool: Improved reliability and validity for pain assessment in children with cognitive impairment. *Pediatr. Anesth.* **2006**, *16*, 258–265. [CrossRef] [PubMed]
35. Pellett, S.; Yaksh, T.L.; Ramachandran, R. Current Status and Future Directions of Botulinum Neurotoxins for Targeting Pain Processing. *Toxins* **2015**, *7*, 4519–4563. [CrossRef] [PubMed]
36. Oh, H.M.; Chung, M.E. Botulinum Toxin for Neuropathic Pain: A Review of the Literature. *Toxins* **2015**, *7*, 3127–3154. [CrossRef] [PubMed]
37. Safarpour, Y.; Jabbari, B. Botulinum toxin Treatment of Pain Syndromes—An evidence based review. *Toxincon* **2018**, accepted. [CrossRef] [PubMed]
38. Jabbari, B. Botulinum Neurotoxins for Relief of Pain Associated with Spasticity. In *Botulinum Toxin Treatment of Pain Disorders*; Springer: New York, NY, USA, 2015; pp. 153–166. ISBN 978-1-4939-2501-8.
39. Wissel, J.; Müller, J.; Dressnandt, J.; Heinen, F.; Naumann, M.; Topka, H.; Poewe, W. Management of spasticity associated pain with botulinum toxin A. *J. Pain Symptom Manag.* **2000**, *20*, 44–49. [CrossRef]
40. Wissel, J.; Ganapathy, V.; Ward, A.B.; Borg, J.; Ertzgaard, P.; Herrmann, C.; Haggstrom, A.; Sakel, M.; Ma, J.; Dimitrova, R.; et al. OnabotulinumtoxinA Improves Pain in Patients with Post-stroke Spasticity: Findings from a Randomized, Double-Blind, Placebo-Controlled Trial. *J. Pain Symptom Manag.* **2016**, *52*, 17–26. [CrossRef] [PubMed]
41. Strobl, W.; Theologis, T.; Brunner, R.; Kocer, S.; Viehweger, E.; Pascual-Pascual, I.; Placzek, R. Best Clinical Practice in Botulinum Toxin Treatment for Children with Cerebral Palsy. *Toxins* **2015**, *7*, 1629–1648. [CrossRef] [PubMed]
42. Elkamil, A.I.; Skranes, J.; Lamvik, T.; Vik, T. Botulinum neurotoxin treatment in children with cerebral palsy: A population-based study in Norway. *Eur. J. Paediatr. Neurol.* **2012**, *16*, 522–527. [CrossRef] [PubMed]
43. Pin, T.W.; Elmasry, J.; Lewis, J. Efficacy of botulinum toxin A in children with cerebral palsy in Gross Motor Function Classification System levels IV and V: A systematic review. *Dev. Med. Child Neurol.* **2013**, *55*, 304–313. [CrossRef] [PubMed]
44. Barwood, S.; Baillieu, C.; Boyd, R.; Brereton, K.; Low, J.; Nattrass, G.; Graham, H.K. Analgesic effects of botulinum toxin A: A randomized, placebo-controlled clinical trial. *Dev. Med. Child Neurol.* **2000**, *42*, 116–121. [CrossRef] [PubMed]
45. Lundy, C.T.; Doherty, G.M.; Fairhurst, C.B. Botulinum toxin type A injections can be an effective treatment for pain in children with hip spasms and cerebral palsy. *Dev. Med. Child Neurol.* **2009**, *51*, 705–710. [CrossRef] [PubMed]
46. Vles, G.F.; de Louw, A.J.; Speth, L.A.; van Rhijn, L.V.; Janssen-Potten, Y.J.M.; Hendriksen, J.G.; Vles, J.S.H. Visual Analogue Scale to score the effects of Botulinum Toxin A treatment in children with cerebral palsy in daily clinical practice. *Eur. J. Paediatr. Neurol.* **2008**, *12*, 231–238. [CrossRef] [PubMed]
47. Gooch, J.L.; Sandell, T.V. Botulinum toxin for spasticity and athetosis in children with cerebral palsy. *Arch. Phys. Med. Rehabil.* **1996**, *77*, 508–511. [CrossRef]
48. Koman, L.A.; Mooney, J.F., 3rd; Smith, B.; Goodman, A.; Mulvaney, T. Management of cerebral palsy with botulinum-A toxin: Preliminary investigation. *J. Pediatr. Orthop.* **1993**, *13*, 489–495. [CrossRef] [PubMed]
49. Mall, V.; Heinen, F.; Linder, M.; Philipsen, A.; Korinthenberg, R. Treatment of cerebral palsy with botulinum toxin A: Functional benefit and reduction of disability. Three case reports. *Pediatr. Rehabil.* **1997**, *1*, 235–237. [CrossRef] [PubMed]
50. Cheléat-Valayer, E.; Parraette, B.; Colin, C.; Denis, A.; Oudin, S.; Bérard, C.; Bernard, J.C.; Bourg, V.; Deleplanque, B.; Dulieu, I.; et al. A French observational study of botulinum toxin use in the management of children with cerebral palsy: BOTULOSCOPE. *Eur. J. Paediatr. Neurol. Soc.* **2011**, *15*, 439–449. [CrossRef] [PubMed]
51. Copeland, L.; Edwards, P.; Thorley, M.; Donaghey, S.; Gascoigne-Pees, L.; Kentish, M.; Cert, G.; Lindsley, J.; McLennan, K.; Sakzewski, L. Botulinim toxin A for nonambulatory children with cerebral palsy: A double blind randomized controlled trial. *J. Pediatr.* **2014**, *165*, 140–146. [CrossRef] [PubMed]

52. Rivard, P.F.; Nugent, A.C.; Symons, F.J. Parent-proxy ratings of pain before and after botulinum toxin type A treatment for children with spasticity and cerebral palsy. *Clin. J. Pain* **2009**, *25*, 412–417. [CrossRef] [PubMed]
53. Mutlu, A.; Livanelioglu, A.; Gunel, M.K. Reliability of Ashworth and Modified Ashworth Scales in Children with Spastic Cerebral Palsy. *BMC Musculoskelet. Disord.* **2008**, *9*, 44. [CrossRef] [PubMed]
54. Bakheit, A.M.O.; Severa, S.; Cosgrove, A.; Morton, B.; Roussounis, S.H.; Doderlein, L.; Lin, J.P. Safety profile and efficacy of botulinum toxin A (Dysport) in children with muscle spasticity. *Dev. Med. Child Neurol.* **2001**, *23*, 234–238. [CrossRef]
55. Jakovic, J.; Schwartz, K. Response and immunoresistance to botulinum toxin injections. *Neurology* **1995**, *45*, 1743–1746. [CrossRef]
56. De Paiva, A.; Meunier, F.A.; Molgó, J.; Aoki, K.R.; Dolly, J.O. Functional repair of motor endplates after botulinum neurotoxin type A poisoning: Biphasic switch of synaptic activity between nerve sprouts and their parent terminals. *Proc. Natl. Acad. Sci. USA* **1999**, *96*, 3200–3205. [CrossRef] [PubMed]
57. Delgado, M.R.; Bonikowski, M.; Carranza, J.; Dabrowski, E.; Matthews, D.; Russman, B.; Tilton, A.; Velez, J.C.; Grandoulier, A.-S.; Picaut, P. Safety and efficiaty of repeat open-label abobotulinumtoxinA treatment in pediatric cerebral palsy. *J. Child Neurol.* **2017**, *32*, 1058–1064. [CrossRef] [PubMed]
58. Tamburin, S.; Lacerenza, M.R.; Castelnuovo, G.; Agostini, M.; Paolucci, S.; Bartolo, M.; Bonazza, S.; Federico, A.; Formaglio, F.; Giusti, E.M.; et al. Pharmacological and non-pharmacological strategies in the integrated treatment of pain in neurorehabilitation. Evidence and recommendations from the Italian Consensus Conference on Pain in Neurorehabilitation. *Eur. J. Phys. Rehabil. Med.* **2016**, *52*, 741–752. [PubMed]

toxins

MDPI

Article

Lumbar Sympathetic Block with Botulinum Toxin Type A and Type B for the Complex Regional Pain Syndrome

Yongki Lee [1], Chul Joong Lee [2], Eunjoo Choi [1], Pyung Bok Lee [1], Ho-Jin Lee [1] and Francis Sahngun Nahm [1,*]

[1] Department of Anesthesiology and Pain Medicine, Seoul National University Bundang Hospital, Seongnam 13620, Korea; yongkilee.md@gmail.com (Y.L.); ejchoi@snubh.org (E.C.); painfree@snubh.org (P.B.L.); zenerdiode03@gmail.com (H.-J.L.)
[2] Zeropain Clinic, Seoul 02830, Korea; may97lee@yahoo.com
* Correspondence: hiitsme@hanmail.net; Tel.: +82-31-787-7499

Received: 8 March 2018; Accepted: 16 April 2018; Published: 19 April 2018

Abstract: A lumbar sympathetic ganglion block (LSB) is a therapeutic method for complex regional pain syndrome (CRPS) affecting the lower limbs. Recently, LSB with botulinum toxin type A and B was introduced as a novel method to achieve longer duration of analgesia. In this study, we compared the botulinum toxin type A (BTA) with botulinum toxin type B (BTB) in performing LSB on patients with CRPS. LSB was performed with either BTA or BTB on patients with CRPS in their lower extremities. The length of time taken for patients to return to the pre-LSB pain score and the adverse effect of LSB with BTA/BTB were investigated. The median length of time taken for the patients to return to the pre-LSB pain score was 15 days for the BTA group and 69 days for the BTB group ($P = 0.002$). Scores on a visual analogue scale decreased in the patients of both groups, and no significant adverse effects were experienced. In conclusion, the administration of either BTA or BTB for LSB is a safe method to prolong the sympathetic blocking effect in patients with CRPS. BTB is more effective than BTA to prolong the sympathetic blocking effect in CRPS patients.

Keywords: botulinum toxin; complex regional pain syndrome; lumbar sympathetic ganglion block; pain

Key Contribution: The administration of either BTA or BTB for LSB is a safe method to prolong the sympathetic blocking effect in patients with CRPS. BTB is more effective than BTA to prolong the sympathetic blocking effect in CRPS patients.

1. Introduction

Complex regional pain syndrome (CRPS) is a rare chronic pain syndrome that causes sensory symptoms such as spontaneous pain and allodynia, as well as motor and autonomic nervous system symptoms [1]. It is an intractable pain disorder that requires a multimodal treatment approach, and there is currently no single treatment method that is specific to CRPS [2]. Of the existing methods, sympathetic blocks are known to reduce pain as well as improve motor and autonomic nervous system functions [3]. Despite the small body of research on the effectiveness of sympathetic blocks, the procedure is widely used for the treatment of CRPS [3,4].

A nerve block using local anesthetics is generally administered to the lumbar sympathetic chain in patients with CRPS in their lower extremities. The blocking effect is temporary in most patients, and therefore, achieving a more long-term effect necessitates one or more of the following additional procedures: repeated sympathetic blocks with local anesthetics, radiofrequency thermocoagulation or neurodestructive procedures that use alcohol or phenol. The merits of a chemical neurolysis of the sympathetic nerve using alcohol or phenol include that it is a simple, economical procedure that can elicit a relatively long-term treatment effect. However, complications can occur, such as genitofemoral neuralgia, which has a prevalence of about 4–10% [5,6]. Moreover, post-sympathectomy neuralgia can occur after chemical sympathetic neurolysis with alcohol or phenol [7]. Radiofrequency thermocoagulation is reported to have similar long-term effects to those of neurodestructive procedures that use phenol [6]. Due to the anatomical location of the lumbar sympathetic chain, however, difficulties have been associated with the procedural method in terms of needle positioning during radiofrequency lesioning [8]. Additionally, radiofrequency lumbar sympatholysis is related to post-sympathectomy neuralgia [9], similar to the chemical sympatholysis.

Botulinum toxin (BT) inhibits the release of acetylcholine from cholinergic nerve endings and is typically used in the treatment of dystonia [10]. The sympathetic blocking effect can be obtained by injecting BT at the sympathetic ganglion, because presynaptic fibers of sympathetic ganglia are also cholinergic. There have been several reports on the prolonged sympathetic blocking effect of BT. When botulinum toxin type A (BTA) was injected into the superior cervical ganglion of a rabbit, the sympathetic blocking effect lasted for a minimum of 1 month and no pathological changes occurred [11]. Another study reported on BT use for a ganglion impar block in patients with chronic perineal pain; a ganglion impar block that used BTA was performed and resulted in pain relief for 3 months and longer [12]. Moreover, Carroll et al. [13] reported that a sympathetic block that used BTA in patients with CRPS in their lower extremities yielded a blocking effect (without any serious complications) for approximately 2 months longer than a block that only used local anesthetics.

Differences exist between BT type A and type B (BTB) with regard to their mechanism of action and target proteins, and moreover BTB can block the release of acetylcholine in the cholinergic nerve fiber [10,14]. Based on this mechanism of action, BTB has been used in clinical practice for treating cervical dystonia [15], adductor muscle spasms [16], piriformis syndrome [17], subacromial bursitis [18], overactive bladder [19] and hyperhidrosis [20]. However, only a few studies have compared the effects of BTA and BTB. When BT was used in patients with cervical dystonia, type A had a longer duration of action than type B [21], but there is no clear conclusion regarding the clinical effect of this difference. Additionally, BTB has been reported to spread into the surrounding tissue less than BTA [14]. With these background studies in mind, we searched the literature for the use of BTB for a lumbar sympathetic block (LSB), but only one case report was found [22]. Furthermore, there has been no published research comparing the effect of the two types of BT when used for LSB. Therefore, the purpose of this retrospective observational study was to compare the effect of BTA and BTB when performing LSB in patients with CRPS in the lower extremities.

2. Results

A total of 18 patients were included in this study. The demographic data of the patients are shown in Table 1.

Table 1. Demographic data.

Variables	BTA Group (n = 5)	BTB Group (n = 13)
Gender (M/F)	5/0	10/3
Age (median, range) years	26 (21–43)	23 (20–47) M 23 (20–39)/F 36 (23–47)
10-cm VAS score (median, range)		
Pre-LSB	7.5 (3.5–8.5)	6.0 (2.0–10.0) M 5.5 (3.5–10.0)/F 6.0 (2.0–10.0)
Post-LSB	3.0 (2.0–5.0)	3.0 (1.0–7.0) M 3.0 (2.0–6.0)/F 5.0 (1.0–7.0)

Values represent the number of patients. M: male, F: female, BTA: botulinum toxin A, BTB: botulinum toxin B, VAS: visual analogue scale, LSB: lumbar sympathetic block.

One patient in group A and one patient in group B complained of dizziness after the procedure, but the symptoms improved within a week without any particular treatment.

There were no significant differences among the demographic characteristics between the groups. The median duration of observation was 56 days (range 14–570 days). The time taken to return to the pre-procedure VAS score was significantly longer in group B than group A (Figure 1). The median time to return to baseline pain was 69 days in group B (95% CI, 45.5–92.5 days) compared to 15 days for group A (95% CI, 12.9–17.2 days) ($P = 0.002$). The VAS scores that were recorded 1 week after the procedure were found to be significantly lower in both groups compared to those which were recorded prior to the procedure. The median VAS score change that occurred between these time points was 2.5 (range 1.0–6.0) ($P = 0.043$) in group A and 3.0 (range 0.5–5.0) ($P = 0.001$) in group B. However, there was no significant difference in the delta-VAS score before and after treatment in both groups 1 week after the procedure ($P = 0.633$).

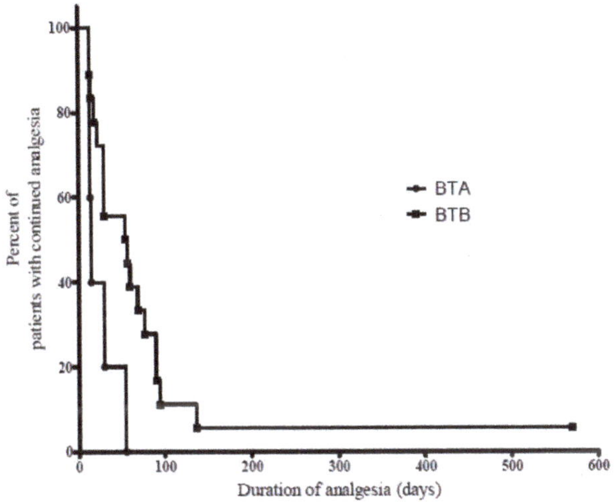

Figure 1. Log-rank analysis of the duration of analgesia. The median duration of analgesia was 15 (95% CI, 12.9–17.1) days for the BTA group, and 69 (95% CI, 45.5–92.5) days for the BTB group. There was a significant difference in the duration of analgesia between the two groups ($P = 0.002$).

3. Discussion

In our study, the sympathetic blocking effect of BTB was longer than that of BTA in the patients with CRPS in the lower limbs. Chemical sympathectomy is used widely: it is economical, easy to perform and anticipated long-term effects. In patients with neuropathic pain or CRPS, however, there is no high-quality evidence for the use of chemical sympathectomy, and it is only recommended for use with caution only in clinically selected patients [4,23]. When sympathetic nerves are destroyed through chemical, surgical, or radiofrequency methods, further neuropathic pain can occur due to nerve destruction [24]. Post-sympathectomy neuralgia is a syndrome of pain with a burning nature, which can last 2–3 months [25]. This syndrome can be more severe and debilitating than the initial pain complaint [24], which is thought to be a result of the sensitization of the viscerosomatic nociceptive spinal neuron caused by the sympathectomy. An additional contributing factor may be differentiation hyperactivity in the sensitized neurons as a result of the axotomy [4,26]. Due to the anatomical location, genitofemoral neuralgia can also occur after chemical lumbar sympathectomy [5,6]. Additionally, surgical sympathectomy has been found to produce postsympathectomy neuralgia in up to 39% of patients [27].

BT has seven serotypes, and among these, types A and B are used for the treatment of various conditions. The target site of the toxin is the neuromuscular junction, and the toxin works by dissolving the SNARE [soluble N-ethylmaleimide sensitive factor attachment protein (SNAP) receptor] complex which functions in exocytosis. Type A works on SNAP25, and type B works on synaptobrevin. As a result, BT blocks the release of acetylcholine and exocytosis, causing flaccid paralysis [10]. Therefore, BT is used in the treatment of pain that occurs from dystonia and excessive muscle contraction [28].

BT is also reported to be effective in neuropathic pain syndromes, such as trigeminal neuralgia, postherpetic neuralgia, and CRPS, as well as pain caused by dystonia [13,29–31]. The effectiveness of BT is due not only to the repression of the secretion of acetylcholine, but also to the blocking of the exocytosis of various pain-related neurotransmitters such as substance P and calcitonin gene-related peptide [32–34]. Therefore, there can be additional benefit in using BT for sympathetic block, not only prolonging the duration of sympathetic block but also interrupting the cascade of pain-related neurotransmitters in CRPS.

Few studies have directly injected BT near the nerve, especially near the sympathetic ganglion [35]. In the first study to report on the action and effect of BT on the sympathetic ganglion, BTA was injected into the surgically exposed superior cervical ganglion of a rabbit [11]. The effect of BTA was compared through miosis to a control group that received normal saline, and there was a dose-dependent sympathetic blocking effect of BTA. However, there was no significant change in the number or shape of the nerve cells as compared to the control group. In rabbits in which miosis was observed, the mean time of duration was 5.3 weeks. These findings suggest that BT causes a sympathetic block without causing any histological changes, and this blocking effect reflects the largest difference when compared to chemical sympathectomy using alcohol or phenol.

There was a crossover study that compared the duration of pain relief when using only local anesthetics versus using both local anesthetics and BTA together in performing a lumbar sympathetic ganglion block in nine patients with CRPS in the lower extremities [13]. When BTA was used, the median time taken to return to the level of pain prior to the procedure was 69 days, whereas only 8 days were required when only local anesthetics were used. In addition, with the exception of one patient who complained of nausea and vomiting, which improved without any particular treatment, there were no incidents of adverse effects. This shows that a long-term blocking effect can be safely attained by injecting BTA near the sympathetic ganglion in humans.

A few studies have compared the duration of the blocking effect when using BTA or BTB in a sympathetic block. In a randomized double-blind study that compared the duration of the effect using BTA or BTB in patients with cervical dystonia, similar durations of 14.0 weeks and 12.1 weeks were found, respectively, and this small difference was statistically significant [21]. Similar results were observed in preclinical research [36]. In another study that compared the effect of BTA and BTB in toxin-naïve cervical dystonia patients, no significant difference in the duration of action was found, and the durations were 13.1 weeks and 13.7 weeks, respectively [37].

In our study, BTB resulted in a 4-fold longer duration compared to BTA. These results are contrary to preceding studies; however, the disease and the treatment areas are different. Previous researches that compared the two types of BT have been limited to cervical dystonia and aesthetic treatments. Both of these procedures can involve injecting BT directly into the muscle, and the results may differ when injecting BT closer to the sympathetic ganglia. When BT was injected into the paws of the monkeys, the spreading of toxin was smaller with BTB than with BTA [14]. This result implies that the BTB can be more focused than BTA at the targeted tissue. However, this result conflicts with clinical data that has reported more side effects, such as dry mouth and dysphagia, when BTB was used [38]. Nevertheless, these adverse effects were mostly light to moderate and tended to decrease when injections were repeated, which suggest that rather than occurring from the toxin spreading from the injected area, the side effects likely occurred because of the high sensitivity of BTB to cholinergic autonomic neurons, particularly postganglionic neurons, e.g., the M3 receptor [39]. The results of the present study, including longer duration of action in BTB can be explained in light of the fact that BTB spreads less to surrounding tissues than BTA and that BTB works more specifically on cholinergic autonomic neurons in the sympathetic ganglia.

Our result that LSB with BTA showed only 15 days (95% CI, 12.9–17.2 days) of median time to return of baseline pain was quite short compared to the previous study result. The previous study by Carroll et al. reported that the 95% confidence interval of the median duration of LSB with BTA was 12–253 days [13], which was very wide. Only three of the eight patients in the study of Carroll et al. showed significantly prolonged effect of BTA. Another possible reason is that the study design of the previous manuscript was 'cross-over design'. According to the article by Nordmann et al. "the successive LSB provided increasing duration of completely pain free period" [40]. Therefore, the repetitive LSB with local bupivacaine only and bupivacaine with BTA in the study by Carroll et al. resulted in the prolonged effect of LSB.

There are limitations to our study. First, this was a retrospective study. Due to the lack of information on BTB use for LSB, there were difficulties in designing and performing a prospective double-blinded study. We used BTA 100 IU and BTB 5000 IU for LSB. In the previous studies which compared the BTA with BTB in the patients with cervical dystonia, the dose ratio of 1 U BTA was comparable to 40–67 U BTB [21,37]. From this, we set the equivalent dose ratio of 1 U BTA to 50 U BTB (BTA 100 = BTB 5000 U) in our study. We think our study can provide a foundation for future well-designed studies on BT use for LSB. Second, because of the retrospective design, we could not measure various changes in symptoms and signs (e.g., oedema, cold sensation and mechanical allodynia), but could measure only the VAS scores, in each patient. Third, the sample size was quite small; however, CRPS is a rare, intractable disorder; therefore, it was not easy to recruit many CRPS patients for a 3-year study period. A multi-center study is necessary to recruit many patients.

4. Conclusions

In this study, the authors confirmed that both BTA and BTB can be used with no serious side effects when used for an LSB in patients with CRPS type 1 in their lower extremities. In terms of the duration of pain relief, BTB was found to be more effective than BTA. However, this research is limited in that it was a retrospective study and did not include many patients in the BTA group. A well-designed, randomized prospective study is needed to compare the effects of the two types of BT in LSB.

5. Materials and Methods

5.1. Study Participants

This retrospective observational study was approved by the institutional review board of our hospital (IRB No. B-1311/228-102), and written consent was obtained from the patients and their guardians after they received an explanation of the methods and the purpose of the procedure as well as recent research results.

The inclusion criteria for patients consisted of the following: (1) patients who visited the pain center at our university hospital and were diagnosed with CRPS type 1 in the unilateral lower extremities from March 2010 to June 2013 and (2) patients who received LSB with either BTA or BTB. The diagnosis of CRPS was made according to the criteria known as the 'Budapest research criteria' [41], which is a revised version of the criteria that were originally proposed by the International Association for the Study of Pain (IASP) [42]. According to the criteria, the patients should meet at least one symptom in all four categories (sensory, vasomotor, sudomotor/edema, and motor/trophic change) and at least one sign in two or more categories. Furthermore, LSB with BT was performed on patients who had previously shown significant pain reduction (50% or more) after LSB with 5 mL of 0.25% ropivacaine. The exclusion criteria consist of the following: (1) patients who had received any neuro-destructive procedure on the lumbar sympathetic ganglia using radiofrequency thermocoagulation or chemicals (alcohol or phenol) or (2) patients who had received a sympathetic block within 6 months.

5.2. LSB Procedure

Percutaneous LSB was performed in the operating room with fluoroscopic guidance (Figure 2). The patient was placed in a prone position on a radiographic table with a 15-cm-high pillow underneath the patient's abdomen to reduce lumbar lordosis. The patient was given an intravenous infusion of lactated Ringer's solution and was monitored by pulse oximetry, electrocardiogram and blood pressure readings during each procedure. For the LSB procedure, a 21-gauge 15 cm Chiba needle (Cook Inc., Bloomington, IN, USA) was advanced under the oblique projection of a C-arm fluoroscopy. When the Chiba needle was inserted properly at the anterolateral side of the L3 vertebral body, 1–2 mL of contrast agent (Omnipaque®, Nycomed Ireland Ltd., Cork, Ireland) was injected to confirm adequate spread around the target site (anterolateral border of the vertebral body) and to identify any intramuscular or intravascular spreading. When the contrast agent did not spread adequately, the same procedure was repeated by inserting another needle at the L2 vertebral level. In group A, BTA 100 IU (Botox®, Allergan Inc., Irvine, CA, USA) combined with 0.25% ropivacaine (2.5 cc) was injected; in group B, 5000 IU BTB (Myobloc™, Solstice Neurosciences Inc., Louisville, KY, USA) combined with 0.25% ropivacaine (2.5 cc) was injected. When the needle was inserted only at the L3 level, the entire dosage of the medication was injected. Furthermore, when the needle was inserted at the L2 and L3 level, the dosage of BTA or BTB was divided in half and combined with 0.25% ropivacaine (2.5 cc) for injection at each level. After LSB, Skin temperature was measured 30 min after the LSB. The sympathetic block was considered successful when the skin temperature of the affected side increased by $\geq$2 °C.

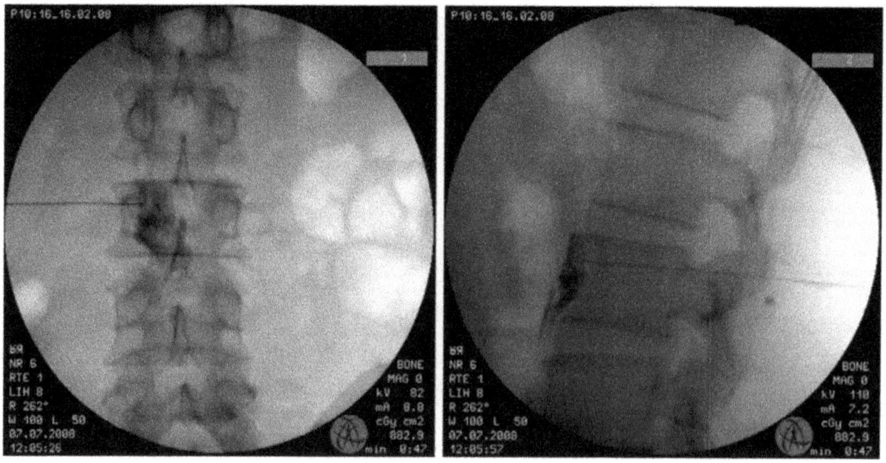

Figure 2. Spread of the contrast agent during the lumbar sympathetic block. The contrast agent was confined to the anterolateral border of the vertebral body without any psoas spread laterally or intravascularly. (**1**) Antero-posterior view. (**2**) lateral view of the fluoroscopy.

5.3. Data Collection and Statistical Analyses

From the patients' medical records and demographic data, the VAS scores prior to and 1 week after the procedure were examined, and the number of elapsed days until the VAS score returned to the pre-LSB state was recorded. The occurrence of any adverse effects or complications was also examined. The primary endpoint—the time taken to return to the baseline VAS score—was analyzed using Kaplan–Meier analysis. The difference between the two groups was analyzed by the log-rank test.

The secondary endpoint—the VAS score change from before to after the procedure—was expressed as the median with a range and was tested using the Wilcoxon signed rank test. PASW® software version 18.0 (Chicago, IL, USA, 2009) was used for the statistical analysis, and *P*-values < 0.05 were considered statistically significant.

Author Contributions: Y.L. drafted this article. C.J.L. contributed the idea of this study. E.C. analyzed the data. P.B.L. provided the critical revision of this article. H.-J.L. contributed the data collection. F.S.N. Conceived and designed this study.

Conflicts of Interest: The authors declare no conflict of interest.

References

1. Birklein, F. Complex regional pain syndrome. *J. Neurol.* **2005**, *252*, 131–138. [CrossRef] [PubMed]
2. Harden, R.N.; Oaklander, A.L.; Burton, A.W.; Perez, R.S.; Richardson, K.; Swan, M.; Barthel, J.; Costa, B.; Graciosa, J.R.; Bruehl, S. Complex regional pain syndrome: Practical diagnostic and treatment guidelines, 4th edition. *Pain Med.* **2013**, *14*, 180–229. [CrossRef] [PubMed]
3. Sharma, A.; Williams, K.; Raja, S.N. Advances in treatment of complex regional pain syndrome: Recent insights on a perplexing disease. *Curr. Opin. Anaesthesiol.* **2006**, *19*, 566–572. [CrossRef] [PubMed]
4. Straube, S.; Derry, S.; Moore, R.A.; McQuay, H.J. Cervico-thoracic or lumbar sympathectomy for neuropathic pain and complex regional pain syndrome. *Cochrane Database Syst. Rev.* **2010**, *7*, Cd002918.
5. Kim, W.O.; Yoon, K.B.; Kil, H.K.; Yoon, D.M. Chemical lumbar sympathetic block in the treatment of plantar hyperhidrosis: A study of 69 patients. *Dermatol. Surg.* **2008**, *34*, 1340–1345. [CrossRef] [PubMed]
6. Manjunath, P.S.; Jayalakshmi, T.S.; Dureja, G.P.; Prevost, A.T. Management of lower limb complex regional pain syndrome type 1: An evaluation of percutaneous radiofrequency thermal lumbar sympathectomy versus phenol lumbar sympathetic neurolysis -a pilot study. *Anesth. Analg.* **2008**, *106*, 647–649. [CrossRef] [PubMed]
7. Schott, G.D. Interrupting the sympathetic outflow in causalgia and reflex sympathetic dystrophy. *BMJ* **1998**, *316*, 792–793. [CrossRef] [PubMed]
8. Haynsworth, R.F., Jr.; Noe, C.E. Percutaneous lumbar sympathectomy: A comparison of radiofrequency denervation versus phenol neurolysis. *Anesthesiology* **1991**, *74*, 459–463. [CrossRef] [PubMed]
9. Rocco, A.G. Radiofrequency lumbar sympatholysis. The evolution of a technique for managing sympathetically maintained pain. *Reg. Anesth.* **1995**, *20*, 3–12. [PubMed]
10. Chen, S. Clinical uses of botulinum neurotoxins: Current indications, limitations and future developments. *Toxins* **2012**, *4*, 913–939. [CrossRef] [PubMed]
11. Kim, H.J.; Seo, K.; Yum, K.W.; Oh, Y.S.; Yoon, T.G.; Yoon, S.M. Effects of botulinum toxin type a on the superior cervical ganglia in rabbits. *Auton. Neurosci.* **2002**, *102*, 8–12. [CrossRef]
12. Lim, S.J.; Park, H.J.; Lee, S.H.; Moon, D.E. Ganglion impar block with botulinum toxin type a for chronic perineal pain—A case report. *Korean J. Pain* **2010**, *23*, 65–69. [CrossRef] [PubMed]
13. Carroll, I.; Clark, J.D.; Mackey, S. Sympathetic block with botulinum toxin to treat complex regional pain syndrome. *Ann. Neurol.* **2009**, *65*, 348–351. [CrossRef] [PubMed]
14. Callaway, J.E.; Arezzo, J.C.; Grethlein, A.J. Botulinum toxin type b: An overview of its biochemistry and preclinical pharmacology. *Dis. Mon.* **2002**, *48*, 367–383. [CrossRef] [PubMed]
15. Chinnapongse, R.B.; Lew, M.F.; Ferreira, J.J.; Gullo, K.L.; Nemeth, P.R.; Zhang, Y. Immunogenicity and long-term efficacy of botulinum toxin type b in the treatment of cervical dystonia: Report of 4 prospective, multicenter trials. *Clin. Neuropharmacol.* **2012**, *35*, 215–223. [CrossRef] [PubMed]
16. Choi, E.J.; Byun, J.M.; Nahm, F.S.; Lee, P.B. Obturator nerve block with botulinum toxin type b for patient with adductor thigh muscle spasm—A case report. *Korean J. Pain* **2011**, *24*, 164–168. [CrossRef] [PubMed]
17. Lang, A.M. Botulinum toxin type B in piriformis syndrome. *Am. J. Phys. Med. Rehabil.* **2004**, *83*, 198–202. [CrossRef] [PubMed]
18. Lee, J.H.; Lee, S.H.; Song, S.H. Clinical effectiveness of botulinum toxin type b in the treatment of subacromial bursitis or shoulder impingement syndrome. *Clin. J. Pain* **2011**, *27*, 523–528. [CrossRef] [PubMed]
19. Dykstra, D.; Enriquez, A.; Valley, M. Treatment of overactive bladder with botulinum toxin type B: A pilot study. *Int. Urogynecol. J. Pelvic Floor Dysfunct.* **2003**, *14*, 424–426. [CrossRef] [PubMed]

20. Baumann, L.; Slezinger, A.; Halem, M.; Vujevich, J.; Mallin, K.; Charles, C.; Martin, L.K.; Black, L.; Bryde, J. Double-blind, randomized, placebo-controlled pilot study of the safety and efficacy of myobloc (botulinum toxin type B) for the treatment of palmar hyperhidrosis. *Dermatol. Surg.* **2005**, *31*, 263–270. [CrossRef] [PubMed]
21. Comella, C.L.; Jankovic, J.; Shannon, K.M.; Tsui, J.; Swenson, M.; Leurgans, S.; Fan, W. Comparison of botulinum toxin serotypes A and B for the treatment of cervical dystonia. *Neurology* **2005**, *65*, 1423–1429. [CrossRef] [PubMed]
22. Choi, E.; Cho, C.W.; Kim, H.Y.; Lee, P.B.; Nahm, F.S. Lumbar sympathetic block with botulinum toxin type B for complex regional pain syndrome: A case study. *Pain Physician* **2015**, *18*, E911–E916. [PubMed]
23. Furlan, A.D.; Lui, P.W.; Mailis, A. Chemical sympathectomy for neuropathic pain: Does it work? Case report and systematic literature review. *Clin. J. Pain* **2001**, *17*, 327–336. [CrossRef] [PubMed]
24. Kapetanos, A.T.; Furlan, A.D.; Mailis-Gagnon, A. Characteristics and associated features of persistent post-sympathectomy pain. *Clin. J. Pain* **2003**, *19*, 192–199. [CrossRef] [PubMed]
25. Macrae, W.A. Chronic pain after surgery. *Br. J. Anaesth.* **2001**, *87*, 88–98. [CrossRef] [PubMed]
26. Kramis, R.C.; Roberts, W.J.; Gillette, R.G. Post-sympathectomy neuralgia: Hypotheses on peripheral and central neuronal mechanisms. *Pain* **1996**, *64*, 1–9. [CrossRef]
27. Rieger, R. Video-assisted retroperitoneoscopic lumbar sympathectomy. *Eur. Surg.* **2012**, *44*, 10–13. [CrossRef]
28. Wissel, J.; Muller, J.; Dressnandt, J.; Heinen, F.; Naumann, M.; Topka, H.; Poewe, W. Management of spasticity associated pain with botulinum toxin a. *J. Pain Symptom. Manag.* **2000**, *20*, 44–49. [CrossRef]
29. Shehata, H.S.; El-Tamawy, M.S.; Shalaby, N.M.; Ramzy, G. Botulinum toxin-type A: Could it be an effective treatment option in intractable trigeminal neuralgia? *J. Headache Pain* **2013**, *14*, 92. [CrossRef] [PubMed]
30. Xiao, L.; Mackey, S.; Hui, H.; Xong, D.; Zhang, Q.; Zhang, D. Subcutaneous injection of botulinum toxin a is beneficial in postherpetic neuralgia. *Pain Med.* **2010**, *11*, 1827–1833. [CrossRef] [PubMed]
31. Park, J.; Park, H.J. Botulinum toxin for the treatment of neuropathic pain. *Toxins* **2017**, *9*, 260. [CrossRef] [PubMed]
32. Cui, M.; Khanijou, S.; Rubino, J.; Aoki, K.R. Subcutaneous administration of botulinum toxin a reduces formalin-induced pain. *Pain* **2004**, *107*, 125–133. [CrossRef] [PubMed]
33. Jeynes, L.C.; Gauci, C.A. Evidence for the use of botulinum toxin in the chronic pain setting—A review of the literature. *Pain Pract.* **2008**, *8*, 269–276. [CrossRef] [PubMed]
34. Aoki, K.R. Review of a proposed mechanism for the antinociceptive action of botulinum toxin type A. *Neurotoxicology* **2005**, *26*, 785–793. [CrossRef] [PubMed]
35. Fabregat, G.; De Andres, J.; Villanueva-Perez, V.L.; Asensio-Samper, J.M. Subcutaneous and perineural botulinum toxin type A for neuropathic pain: A descriptive review. *Clin. J. Pain* **2013**, *29*, 1006–1012. [CrossRef] [PubMed]
36. Roger Aoki, K. Botulinum neurotoxin serotypes A and B preparations have different safety margins in preclinical models of muscle weakening efficacy and systemic safety. *Toxicon* **2002**, *40*, 923–928. [CrossRef]
37. Pappert, E.J.; Germanson, T. Botulinum toxin type B vs. Type A in toxin-naive patients with cervical dystonia: Randomized, double-blind, noninferiority trial. *Mov. Disord.* **2008**, *23*, 510–517. [CrossRef] [PubMed]
38. Dressler, D.; Benecke, R. Autonomic side effects of botulinum toxin type b treatment of cervical dystonia and hyperhidrosis. *Eur. Neurol.* **2003**, *49*, 34–38. [CrossRef] [PubMed]
39. Arezzo, J.C. Neurobloc/myobloc: Unique features and findings. *Toxicon* **2009**, *54*, 690–696. [CrossRef] [PubMed]
40. Nordmann, G.R.; Lauder, G.R.; Grier, D.J. Computed tomography guided lumbar sympathetic block for complex regional pain syndrome in a child: A case report and review. *Eur. J. Pain* **2006**, *10*, 409–412. [CrossRef] [PubMed]
41. Harden, R.N.; Bruehl, S.; Stanton-Hicks, M.; Wilson, P.R. Proposed new diagnostic criteria for complex regional pain syndrome. *Pain Med.* **2007**, *8*, 326–331. [CrossRef] [PubMed]
42. Stanton-Hicks, M.; Janig, W.; Hassenbusch, S.; Haddox, J.D.; Boas, R.; Wilson, P. Reflex sympathetic dystrophy: Changing concepts and taxonomy. *Pain* **1995**, *63*, 127–133. [CrossRef]

toxins

MDPI

Review

Botulinum Toxin for Central Neuropathic Pain

Jihye Park [1] and Myung Eun Chung [2,*]

[1] Department of Rehabilitation Medicine, Seoul St. Mary's Hospital, College of Medicine, The Catholic University of Korea, 222, Banpo-daero, Seocho-gu, Seoul 06591, Korea; sophia@catholic.ac.kr

[2] Department of Rehabilitation Medicine, St. Paul's Hospital, College of Medicine, The Catholic University of Korea, Wangsan-ro 180, Dongdaemoon-Gu, Seoul 02559, Korea

* Correspondence: coltrane@catholic.ac.kr; Tel.: +82-2-958-2307; Fax: +82-2-968-2307

Received: 30 April 2018; Accepted: 28 May 2018; Published: 1 June 2018

Abstract: Botulinum toxin (BTX) is widely used to treat muscle spasticity by acting on motor neurons. Recently, studies of the effects of BTX on sensory nerves have been reported and several studies have been conducted to evaluate its effects on peripheral and central neuropathic pain. Central neuropathic pain includes spinal cord injury-related neuropathic pain, post-stroke shoulder pain, multiple sclerosis-related pain, and complex regional pain syndrome. This article reviews the mechanism of central neuropathic pain and assesses the effect of BTX on central neuropathic pain.

Keywords: botulinum toxin; BTX; central neuropathic pain; spinal cord injury; post-stroke shoulder pain; complex regional pain syndrome

Key Contribution: This review summarizes the mechanism of central neuropathic pain and botulinum toxin action against it based on preclinical and clinical studies.

1. Introduction

Botulinum toxins (BTXs) are neurotoxic substances produced by *Clostridium botulinum*, a gram-positive anaerobic bacterium. In botulism poisoning, flaccid paralysis occurs by inhibiting the release of neurotransmitters from the peripheral cholinergic nerve terminals of the skeletal and autonomic nervous system. Paralysis begins at the ocular muscles and then spreads to the muscles of the face, before reaching the respiratory muscles and causing respiratory failure.

BTX has traditionally been found in seven serotypes: A, B, C1, D, E, F, and G [1]. They have similar molecular weights and common subunit structures, but differ in their reaction mechanisms, durations of effect, and side effects.

In recent years, using molecular genetic analysis, many genes have been discovered that encode new BTXs. Thus, subtypes, such as BTX/A1, BTX/A2, BTX/B1, and BTX/B2, and chimeric types, such as BTX/DC, BTX/CD and BTX/FA, have been found.

Clinical use of BTX began in 1973, when Scott demonstrated that injecting the toxin into orbicularis oculi muscles was effective in treating strabismus. Over the next several decades, its application expanded to a variety of diseases.

BTX has a molecular weight of 150 kDa, consists of an inactive single-chain polypeptide, and folds into a 3-domain structure. The light chain (50 kDa) is a zinc-dependent protease that constitutes an active toxin and cleaves the soluble *N*-ethyl-maleimide-sensitive factor attachment receptor (SNARE) complex [2,3]. The heavy chain (100 kDa) consists of an N-terminal translocation domain and a C-terminal receptor binding domain, and it acts in neuron-specific binding. The light and heavy chains are linked by disulfide bonds, which partially obscure the active sites of the toxin. When the single-chain disulfide bond is reduced, the light chain metalloprotease can be released to act as a toxin.

The main functional effect of BTX occurs in the neuromuscular junction, where it inhibits the release of acetylcholine from the presynaptic nerve ending, resulting in muscular and autonomic paralysis [4]. The toxin-mediated muscle relaxation process proceeds in three phases: Binding, internalization, and the inhibition of neurotransmitter release. Specific binding to neurons is mediated by heavy chains [5] and internalization is mediated by receptor-mediated endocytosis [6,7]. Once BTX is internalized, the light chains within the vesicles are translocated across the vesicle membrane and released into the neuronal cytoplasm. SNARE is involved in the exocytosis of acetylcholine vesicles, located at the nerve endings, by attaching acetylcholine vesicles to the cell membrane, thus, allowing acetylcholine exocytosis to occur [8]. BTX causes degradation of the SNARE protein, resulting in paralysis. Based on these mechanisms, BTX is clinically used to treat muscle spasticity associated with central nervous system (CNS) disorders, such as stroke, brain injury, spinal cord injury (SCI), cerebral palsy, and multiple sclerosis (MS).

However, two other functional effects of BTXs exist: The effects on the afferent limb of the motor nervous system and the analgesic effect on the sensory nerve system. Several preclinical studies have shown that BTX inhibits neuromodulator and transmitter secretion, which is important for neurotransmission in the sensory pathway, and, thus, BTX may reduce neuropathic pain.

Preclinical and clinical studies have reported the effects of BTX on peripheral neuropathic pain and, generally, demonstrated a high level of evidence for some diseases [9]. However, few studies have reported its therapeutic effects on central neuropathic pain, and its effects have not been proven. The aim of this article is to review the mechanism of central neuropathic pain and to investigate the effect of BTX on central neuropathic pain.

A PubMed and EMBASE search (1980~March 2018) was performed as follows: 'Botulinum toxins', 'neuropathic pain', 'neuropathy', 'pain', 'allodynia', 'hyperalgesia' and 'spinal cord injury', 'post-stroke pain', 'multiple sclerosis', and 'complex regional pain syndrome'. The results included animal studies, randomized controlled trials (RCTs), observational studies, case reports, and reviews. Editorials, guidelines, and trial protocols were excluded. Two reviewers individually assessed the abstracts to determine the eligibility of the studies. Articles not available in English and studies conducted in children ($\leq$18 years of age) were also excluded.

2. Mechanism of Central Neuropathic Pain

The International Association for the Study of Pain (IASP) defines neuropathic pain as pain caused by a lesion or disease of the somatosensory nervous system [10]. Neuropathic pain is a clinical description that requires a demonstrable lesion or a disease that satisfies the established neurological diagnostic criteria. It has two typical symptoms, allodynia and hyperalgesia. Allodynia describes a pain due to a stimulus that does not normally provoke pain and hyperalgesia refers to increased pain from a stimulus that normally provokes pain [10].

Several molecular mechanisms are involved in the development of allodynia and hyperalgesia. After nerve injury, changes in the expression of sodium and calcium channels cause spontaneous activity in nerve endings, resulting in spontaneous pain. This is an important factor that causes sensitization. In addition, various cytokines, including glutamate, substance P, and proinflammatory cytokines, are involved in sensitization. Inflamed or ischemic tissues become acidified and this cellular environment causes pain by stimulating the release of neuropeptides from the primary afferent nerve tissue [11]. When neuropeptides, such as calcitonin gene-related protein (CGRP) and substance P, are secreted into the endoneurium, they cause local blood flow and blood vessel leakage, leading to edema and pain.

Because central neuropathic pain is defined by IASP as a pain caused by a lesion or disease of the central somatosensory nervous system [10], central neuropathic pain is a heterogenous group of neuropathic pain conditions. Major diagnostic conditions include: (1) Central pain associated with SCI; (2) central post-stroke pain; and (3) central pain associated with MS.

The mechanisms of neuropathic pain, following SCI, in various animal models have been published (Figure 1). Cellular and molecular responses to SCI occur at various levels, from the distal terminals of primary afferent neurons to the cortical area along the nervous system, leading to neuropathic pain.

Several changes in the primary afferent neuron have been suggested. A definite factor that mediates SCI-related pain is an increased excitability of dorsal root ganglion (DRG) neurons. The spontaneous activity of nociceptive DRG neurons has been shown to increase after SCI [12], and some authors have demonstrated that the expression of the capsaicin-sensitive cation channel transient receptor potential vanilloid type 1 (TRPV1) in DRG neurons increases after SCI, which is enhanced by capsaicin-evoked ion currents and calcium responses in DRG neurons [13].

Neuronal hyperexcitability in the spinal dorsal horn is also associated with SCI-related neuropathic pain [14,15]. This phenomenon might occur through chronic glial cell activation [16,17], dendritic spine remodeling [18,19], dysregulation of glutamate homeostasis [16], glutamate receptor activation [20], loss of GABAergic inhibitory interneurons [21,22], interruption of descending inhibitory modulation by serotonin [23,24], or upregulation of voltage-gated calcium channel alpha-2-delta-1 subunit proteins [25].

In patients with central pain following SCI, neurons in the somatosensory thalamus fire in bursts of action potentials more frequently than do similar neurons in patients without pain [26]. In rats with contusive SCI, thalamic ventralis postero-lateralis neurons exhibited a dysrhythmia in that a significantly higher proportion fired spontaneously when compared with neurons in uninjured rats [27]. Based on these results, abnormal thalamic processes following SCI may mediate neuropathic pain. Additionally, in rats with SCI, neurons in the primary somatosensory cortex had significantly higher spontaneous firing rates, greater evoked responses to noxious mechanical stimulation, and a greater tendency to fire bursts of action potentials [28]. Another study also revealed that phosphorylation of AMPA-type glutamate receptors in the primary somatosensory cortex play an important role in the development of hypersensitivity after SCI [29].

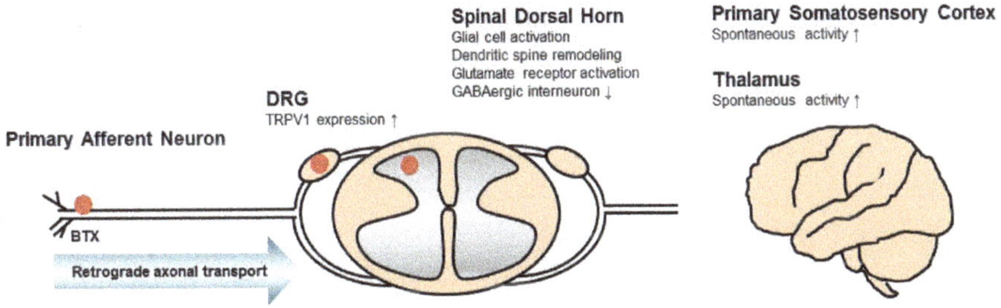

Figure 1. Illustrated mechanism of central neuropathic pain associated with spinal cord injury (SCI). These mechanisms include transient receptor potential vanilloid type 1 (TRPV1) overexpression in dorsal root ganglion (DRG) neurons, glial cell activation, dendritic spine remodeling, glutamate receptor activation and loss of GABAergic interneuron in the spinal dorsal horn, and spontaneous firing of neurons in the thalamus and primary somatosensory cortex. It has been suggested that the antinociceptive mechanism of botulinum toxins (BTXs) applied to the nerve endings not only affects the primary afferent neurons but also acts on the DRG and spinal dorsal horn through retrograde axonal transport.

The pathophysiology of central post-stroke pain, another important disease constituting central neuropathic pain, remains uncertain. Recent advances in brain imaging technology have increased the understanding of the role of specific anatomic locations. Several reports have suggested that central post-stroke pain commonly occurs in lesions affecting the thalamus, parietal cortex, dorsal putamen, posterior internal capsule, dorsal basal ganglia, brainstem, and lateral medulla [30–33]. Particularly, spinothalamic tracts terminated with the ventral posterolateral thalamus and lesions of the ventral posteromedial thalamus and medial lemniscal thalamocortical pathway were found to be the major factors causing central post-stroke pain [34,35]. These results have also been demonstrated in animal model experiments. Thermal hypersensitivity was observed in a rat model of the ventral posterior thalamic infarction [36], with thermal and mechanical hyperalgesia developing in rats with a thalamic hemorrhagic lesion [37].

In the middle cerebral artery occlusion rat model, increased *N*-methyl-D-aspartate (NMDA) and AMPA receptor mediated excitatory transmission of the dorsal horn, decreases in GABA and glycine receptor mediated inhibitory transmission, and an increase in descending facilitation was proposed to be involved in the development of central post-stroke pain [38]. In the ventral posterior thalamic lesion rat model, P2X7 expression in the medial thalamus was directly involved in nociceptive transmission, and short-term P2X7 inhibition led to a reduction of glutamatergic facilitation and neuronal hyperexcitability [39].

3. Mechanism of BTX for Central Neuropathic Pain

The initial analgesic effect of BTX is caused by a decrease in muscle spasms. However, many preclinical and clinical studies suggest that a different mechanism underlies the analgesic effect of BTX. The hypothesis is that BTX inhibits the secretion of neuropeptides and suppresses inflammation and pain.

Several preclinical studies have shown that BTX-A inhibits the release of neurotransmitters that regulate pain and inflammation. McMahon et al. showed that BTX preferentially attenuates the slow phase of KCl-evoked glutamate release, which may be associated with synaptic vesicle mobilization according to a study that utilized a guinea pig formalin-induced pain model [40]. Welch et al. reported that BTX inhibits potassium-evoked substance P secretion from cultured embryonic rat DRG neurons [41], and Durham et al. demonstrated that BTX-A can directly decrease the release of CGRP from cultured rat trigeminal ganglion neurons [42].

Xiao et al. demonstrated that BTX significantly reduces TRPV1 expression [43]. A neuropathic pain model was induced by transection of the lumbar 5 ventral root in male rats. BTX-A or normal saline was administered to the plantar surface by subcutaneous injection. TRPV1 expression increased significantly in the lumbar 4–5 DRG after the transection of the lumbar 5 ventral root, and this increase persisted for at least 21 days. Subcutaneous injection of BTX-A significantly, and dose-dependently, reduced the expression of TRPV1 in the DRG neuron and significantly reduced hyperalgesia. A similar effect occurred on the expression of P2X3, one of the purinergic receptors associated with nociceptors, in a study that evaluated the effect of BTX on P_2X_3 expression, with the same method. Subcutaneous administration of BTX-A significantly, and bilaterally, reduced mechanical allodynia and inhibited the P_2X_3 overexpression induced by the transection of the lumbar 5 ventral root [44].

One possible interpretation of these findings is that BTX reduces peripheral sensitization and afferent input to the spinal cord by inhibiting the release of neurotransmitters from peripheral nerve endings, thereby, indirectly a decreasing central sensitization. However, it has been hypothesized that the central effect may be direct by retrograde axonal transport of BTX along the branches of nociceptive neurons.

Immunohistochemical experiments have revealed that cleaved SNAP-25, a product of BTX-A action, is found not only in the peripheral region but also in the facial nucleus in the brain stem [45], superior colliculus [46], and motor region of the spinal cord [47,48]. Antonucci et al. found cleaved SNAP-25 in the ipsilateral facial nucleus after a BTX-A injection into rat whisker muscles [45]. Matak et al. found that cleaved SNAP-25 fragments were present in the ventral horn and dorsal horn of the spinal cord after low-dose toxin injections into the gastrocnemius muscle and sciatic nerve [47]. These authors also identified that cleaved SNAP-25 was not detected in the spinal cord when they injected BTX-A into a sciatic nerve pretreated with colchicine, an axonal transport blocker. Therefore, they suggested that BTX-A showed a central effect by microtubule-dependent retrograde axonal transport [49]. Wang et al., however, cited the possibility that disassociated cleaved SNAP-25 might have migrated from the terminal to the cell body, suggesting that the discovery of cleaved SNAP-25 in the CNS does not necessarily reflect the activity of BTX-A in the CNS [50].

Retrograde axonal transport is well known as a transport pathway for various substances, such as tetanus toxin, and this fact suggests that BTX may also use the same pathway. Several studies have reported that the heavy chain, or the entire toxin, undergoes retrograde transport after a peripheral injection of BTX-A. Restani et al. directly monitored the endocytosis and axonal transport of BTX-A, and they showed that BTX-A was internalized by spinal cord motor neurons and underwent fast axonal retrograde transport [51]. Wang et al. reported that fluorescently labeled BTX heavy chains were detected in spinal cord motor neurons after injection into the mouse hindlimb, which demonstrated retrograde transport of BTX [50].

Several studies of the behavioral effects of BTX-A have demonstrated the central antinociceptive effect of BTX-A. Bilateral pain associated with experimental diabetes [52], carrageenan-induced hyperalgesia, and paclitaxel-induced peripheral neuropathy [53] or acidic saline-induced mirror pain, [54] can be bilaterally reduced by the unilateral injection of BTX-A in rats. Bach-Rojecky et al. reported that mechanical and thermal hypersensitivity of the ipsilateral side, as well as the contralateral side, were decreased after subcutaneous unilateral BTX injection into the plantar surface of the hindlimb [52]. In addition, Favre-Guilmard et al. reported a significant anti-hyperalgesic effect in the uninjected contralateral hindpaw after subcutaneous administration of BTX-A to the plantar surface in carrageenan-induced hyperalgesia and paclitaxel-induced peripheral neuropathy models. These results suggest that the antinociceptive effect of BTX-A cannot be explained by the peripheral action and it is possible that BTX-A has a central action through the retrograde axonal transport [53]. This process is also expected to be a major mechanism in the BTX-A action on central neuropathic pain.

4. Clinical Studies of BTX for Central Neuropathic Pain

4.1. Neuropathic Pain after Spinal Cord Injury

Two case series of clinical reports with very small sample sizes have evaluated the effect of BTX-A on neuropathic pain in patients with SCI. Jabbari et al. [55] reported cases of two patients with burning pain in a dermatome due to spinal cord lesion at the cervical level (tumor or stroke). BTX-A (OnabotulinumtoxinA) was injected subcutaneously at multiple points in the area of the burning pain and allodynia. The effect was assessed by the visual analogue scale (VAS) and clinical changes. One patient received 100 units of BTX-A. One week after the injection, the VAS score decreased from 8–10 to 2–3 points, and the frequency of severe spontaneous pain was reduced by 80%. The second patient received 80 units; skin sensitivity and spontaneous burning pain were significantly reduced after approximately 10 days, and this effect lasted approximately three months. Han et al. [56] reported a case of a patient with allodynia and dysesthesia of the lower limb. BTX-A was injected subcutaneously at ~10 units into the painful foot area and the effect was evaluated by the change in VAS score. After four weeks, the pain severity and burst frequency were reduced.

A recent study has been reported on the effect of BTX-A on SCI-associated neuropathic pain. Han et al. [57] reported the effects of BTX-A in a randomized, double-blind, and placebo-controlled study in 40 patients with SCI-associated neuropathic pain. Patients were treated with subcutaneous injections of BTX-A (200 units) or normal saline and the VAS score, the Korean version of the short-form McGill Pain Questionnaire, and the WHOQoL-BREF quality of life assessment were assessed at four and eight weeks. Thus, BTX-A has been shown to be effective in treating intractable chronic neuropathic pain in patients with SCI. The above studies are summarized in Table 1.

Table 1. Summary of studies of botulinum toxin (BTX) for central neuropathic pain.

Author, Year	Study Design	Sample Size (*N*)	Diagnosis	Injection Site/Dose	Follow up	Pain Measure	Results
Jabbari, 2003 [55]	Case series	2	SCI	Subcutaneous injection at the site of allodynia/BTX-A 16–20 U/site		VAS	Pain was decreased; frequency of severe spontaneous pain was reduced
Han, 2014 [56]	Case report	1	SCI	Subcutaneous injection in the painful foot/BTX-A	Week 4	VAS	Pain severity and the frequency of burst was reduced
Han, 2016 [57]	Double-blind, randomized controlled study	40	SCI	Subcutaneous injection/BTX-A 200 U	Week 4, 8	VAS (100 mm), McGill Pain Questionnaire	Pain was reduced significantly in BTX-A treated group
Yelnik, 2007 [58]	Double-blind, randomized controlled study	20	stroke	Subscapularis muscle/BTX-A 500 U/injection + physical therapy	Week 1, 2, 4	verbal scale (10 point)	Pain improvement with BTX-A from first week
Marco, 2007 [59]	Double-blind, randomized controlled study	31	stroke	Pectoralis major muscle/BTX-A 500 U/injection + TENS for 6 weeks	Week 1, 4, 12, 24	VAS (100 mm)	Significantly greater pain improvement from the first week in BTX group
Kong, 2007 [60]	Double-blind, randomized controlled study	17	stroke	Pectoralis major, biceps brachii muscles/BTX-A 500 U	Week 4, 8, 12	VAS (0–10)	No difference in shoulder pain
Lim, 2008 [61]	Double-blind, randomized controlled study	29	stroke	Infraspinatus, pectoralis and subscapularis muscles + IA saline injection; IA triamcinolone (40 mg) injection + saline to the same muscles/BTX-A 100 U	Week 2, 6, 12	NRS	Significantly greater pain improvement in the BTX-A–treated at 12 weeks
Boer, 2008 [62]	Double-blind, randomized controlled study	22	stroke	Subscapular muscle/BTX-A 50 U, twice	Week 6, 12	VAS (vertical 100 mm)	No significant changes in pain
Shaw, 2011 [63]	Double-blind, randomized controlled study	333	stroke	Elbow, wrist and finger flexor muscles/ BTX-A, 4 times/injection + physical therapy 4 weeks	Week 4, 12, 48	verbal scale, NRS	Significant decrease at 12 months in the BTX group
Castiglione, 2011 [8]	Pilot study	5	stroke	IA shoulder joint/BTX-A 500 or 100 units	Week 2, 8	VAS	Decreased pain at 2 and 8 weeks after BTX-A injection

Table 1. *Cont.*

Author, Year	Study Design	Sample Size (*N*)	Diagnosis	Injection Site/Dose	Follow up	Pain Measure	Results
Marciniak, 2012 [64]	Double-blind, randomized controlled study	21	stroke	Pectoralis major ± teres major muscles/BTX-A 140–200 units	Week 2, 4, 12	VAS	Decreased pain scores at 4 weeks
Choi, 2016 [65]	Retrospective, unblinded, uncontrolled study	6	stroke	Subscapularis muscle/BTX-A	Week 1, 2, 4, 8	PI-NRS	Pain improvement with BTX-A injection
Carroll, 2009 [66]	Double-blind, randomized controlled study	18	CRPS	LSB/Bupivacaine 0.5% + 75 units of BTX-A	Week 4	VAS (10 cm)	The rate of pain return was significantly lower after LSB with BTA
Safarpour, 2010 [67]	Double-blind, randomized controlled study Uncontrolled, unblinded, open-label study	14 (6 control)	CRPS	Intradermally and subcutaneously into the allodynic area / 5 units per site (total 40–200 units)	Week 3, 8	Brief pain inventory, PIQ, McGill pain questionnaire, QST, patients satisfaction scale	No significant response after injection; study terminated prematurely because of intolerance
Kharkar, 2011 [68]	Retrospective, unblinded, uncontolled study	37	CRPS	Upper limb girdle muscles/BTX-A 10–20 units per muscle (total 100 units)	Week 4	Likert scale (11 point)	43% decrease in local pain scores
Safarpour, 2010 [69]	Case series	2	CRPS	Trigger point in the proximal muscle/BTX-A 20 units per site	□	VAS (1–10)	Alleviate both myofascial pain syndrome and the distal allodynia, discoloration and, tissue swelling
Birthi, 2012 [70]	Case report	1	CRPS	Subcutaneous injection on the dorsum of the hand/BTX-A 5 units per site (total 100 units)	weekly, 12 weeks	McGill Pain Questionnaire	Able to decrease daily opioid medication by 20% at 8th week; pain returned to baseline at 12th week
Choi, 2015 [71]	Case series	2	CRPS	Lumbar sympathetic block/levovupivacaine 0.25% + 5000 units of BTX-B	Week 8	VAS, LANSS	Pain intensity and LANSS score were significantly reduced
Buonocore, 2017 [72]	Case report	1	CRPS	TP, FDL, FHL muscles, tibial nerve around the tarsal tunnel/BTX-A 120 units per muscle, twice	Week 36	□	Significant decrease in the frequency of acute dysesthesias

SCI: Spinal cord injury; CRPS: Complex regional pain syndrome; VAS: Visual analog scale; NRS: Numeric rating scale; IA: Intra-articular; LANSS: Leeds assessment of neuropathic symptoms and signs; LSB: Lumbar sympathetic block; TP: Tibialis posterior; FDL: Flexor digitorum longus; FHL: Flexor hallucis longus.

4.2. Post-Stroke Shoulder Pain

Central post-stroke pain occurs after a cerebrovascular event, including lesion of the brainstem, thalamus, and cerebral cortex, and may affect half of the body [73]. Several authors have described central post-stroke pain as a central neuropathic pain syndrome that can occur after a stroke in the body part that corresponds to the cerebrovascular lesion and is characterized by pain and sensory abnormalities, where other causes of obvious nociceptive, psychogenic, or peripheral neuropathic origin have been ruled out [74,75].

Post-stroke shoulder pain is a common disease with an incidence rate ranging from 21–72% [76,77]. Many studies have examined the effects of BTX on the treatment of post-stroke shoulder pain, but the results are conflicting, and, thus, drawing conclusions remains difficult.

Yelnik et al. [58] conducted a double-blind RCT of the effect of BTX on post-stroke shoulder pain in 20 patients. Ten patients were injected with 500 units of BTX-A (AbobotulinumtoxinA) in the subscapularis muscle, and 10 patients in the control group underwent a placebo injection in the same muscle. All participants underwent rehabilitation, including stretching exercises. Pain was improved in the BTX injection group at one week, and pain scores using a 10-point verbal scale at four weeks showed a significant difference between the two groups. Marco et al. [59] reported a double-blind RCT for evaluating the effect of BTX. In 14 patients, 500 units of BTX-A (AbobotulinumtoxinA) was injected into the pectoralis major muscles, and 15 patients in the control group were injected with a placebo. Transcutaneous electrical nerve stimulation was applied for six weeks. After one week, pain during shoulder movement decreased in both groups, but the VAS score in the BTX injection group decreased more significantly, and this trend continued until six months. However, no significant difference in the shoulder range of motion or spasticity was found between the two groups. Kong et al. [60] conducted a double-blind RCT of 17 patients. Five hundred units of BTX-A (AbobotulinumtoxinA) was injected into the pectoralis major and biceps brachii muscles in the experimental group and normal saline was injected into the same region in the control group. The VAS scores at 4, 8, and 12 weeks after injection were not significantly different between the two groups. The median baseline VAS score of the patients was 6, and the scores decreased by 2–3 points in both groups.

Lim et al. [61] reported a double-blind RCT of 29 patients. In the experimental group, 100 units of BTX-A (OnabotulinumtoxinA) was injected into the infraspinatus, pectoralis, and subscapularis muscles, along with intra-articular saline. In contrast, the control group received an intra-articular triamcinolone (40 mg) injection and saline was injected into the muscles described above. The numeric rating scale at 12 weeks was reduced by 4.2 ± 0.4 points in the BTX-A intramuscular injection group and by 2.5 ± 0.8 points in the intra-articular triamcinolone injection group. Intramuscular injection of BTX-A was superior to intra-articular injection of triamcinolone ($p = 0.051$). Boer et al. [62] conducted a double-blind RCT of 22 patients. They injected 100 units of BTX-A (OnabotulinumtoxinA) into the subscapularis muscle in the experimental group and injected saline in the control group. Vertical VAS scores were not significantly different between the two groups at 6 weeks and 12 weeks. Shaw et al. [63] reported the effects of BTX-A (AbobotulinumtoxinA) on spasticity, function, and pain in patients with spasticity of the upper limb after stroke. This study was a multicenter RCT called BoTULS. The pain rating and pain scale evaluated at one and three months showed no significant difference between the two groups, but the pain rating evaluated at 12 months showed a significant decrease in the injection group. Marciniak et al. [64] evaluated the effects of BTX by injecting 140–200 units of BTX-A (OnabotulinumtoxinA) or saline into a pectoralis major muscle, with or without a teres major muscle. At four weeks, worst pain ratings decreased in both groups, but no significant difference was found between the two groups. The above studies are summarized in Table 1.

Post-stroke shoulder pain is thought to be caused by multiple factors, including both the nervous system and mechanical factors. Post-stroke shoulder pain may be associated with spasticity, but it is difficult to determine whether spasticity acts as a mechanism to cause post-stroke shoulder pain, whether it is increased by the shoulder pain, or both. It is well known that the improvement of spasticity may be associated with an improvement of pain, but the correlation between spasticity and pain is not linear, and multiple factors may be involved [78]. Several studies have suggested a musculoskeletal origin for post-stroke shoulder pain. Musculoskeletal conditions, such as subluxation, tendinitis, adhesive capsulitis, rotator cuff tear, and subacromial bursitis, may contribute to post-stroke shoulder pain. Whether these diseases can cause post-stroke shoulder pain is controversial, because these conditions may result from stroke.

In a study by Zeilig [79], those with post-stroke shoulder pain had higher heat-pain thresholds and exhibited higher rates of hyperpathia, allodynia, and dysesthesia in the affected shoulder and leg than those without post-stroke shoulder pain. The authors suggested that the finding of altered thermal sensitivity, which indicates damage to the spinothalamic-thalamocortical tract, was not restricted to the shoulder, but rather characterized the affected side. An additional support to this central neuropathic pain proposition was the higher rate of damage to the parietal cortex in the post-stroke shoulder pain group. From these results, various factors appear to cause post-stroke shoulder pain, but it seems to be attributable to central neuropathic pain.

Two systematic reviews of the effects of BTX on shoulder pain, including post-stroke shoulder pain, have been reported. In a Cochrane report that focused on BTX-A for shoulder pain, the authors included six RCTs comparing BTX with a placebo or active treatment. Five RCTs in participants with post-stroke shoulder pain indicated that, compared with placebo, a single intramuscular injection of BTX-A significantly reduced pain at three to six months postinjection, but not at one month [80]. Another systematic review included nine RCTs of BTX injections in patients with shoulder pain. The shoulder pain was due to hemiplegia in six studies, adhesive capsulitis in one study, subacromial bursitis or shoulder impingement syndrome in one study, and arthritis in one study [81]. They concluded that BTX injection resulted in minor to moderate pain relief and an increase in shoulder abduction in patients with chronic shoulder pain. Based on these two reviews, BTX injection in post-stroke shoulder pain is expected to be effective in reducing pain.

4.3. Multiple Sclerosis

MS is a chronic disease in which focal demyelinating lesions of the CNS occur at multiple sites due to autoimmune inflammatory processes. The plaques, located in the subcortical, brainstem, or spinal cord, cause neurological symptoms and signs, including abnormal coordination, motor, sensory, and cognitive function. According to one report, approximately 65% of MS patients with spasticity are known to suffer from pain [82]. Pain appears in the form of central dysesthetic pain, trigeminal neuralgia, Lhermitte's phenomenon, and tonic spasm. In a review published in 2013, the authors classified MS-related pain into nine categories and described each possible mechanism [82]. According to the authors, ongoing extremity pain is caused by thalamic or cortical deafferentation by multiple lesions along the spinothalamocortical pathways. In addition, Lhermitte's phenomenon and painful tonic spasm are caused by demyelination of the dorsal column primary afferents and the corticospinal pathway, respectively, providing a possible mechanism for central neuropathic pain.

Various double-blind RCTs of BTX effects on MS-associated detrusor overactivity and spasticity are available. A preliminary report on the effects of BTX on spastic dysphagia, myokymia, tonic spasm, and internuclear ophthalmoplegia also exists. However, no RCT has been performed to evaluate whether BTX is effective for MS-related pain. In a recent prospective, open-label study of 131 patients with spasticity, 19% were patients with MS, and 60% reported a significant reduction in spasticity-related pain after BTX-A treatment [83]. MS-related pain has the characteristics of central neuropathic pain and conducting well-designed research on whether BTX is effective for MS-related pain will be necessary in the future.

4.4. Complex Regional Pain Syndrome

Complex regional pain syndrome (CRPS) is a painful disease that can result from an imbalance due to trauma. Unlike other neuropathic pain syndromes, CRPS is accompanied by additional signs, such as abnormal blood flow control, sweating, and active and passive motor impairment. Not all CRPS signs can be fully explained by the peripheral mechanism and several studies suggest there might be a central mechanism [84]. The CNS undergoes functional and structural changes in people with chronic pain and these changes are thought to be particularly important in CRPS because they cause central sensitization [85,86]. CRPS is often spread beyond the original injury and in many cases, it has been reported to spread to the contralateral extremity in a mirror pattern [87,88]. Regarding the bilateral spreading of CRPS signs, it was suggested that trans-synaptic changes in the spinal cord dorsal horn, contralateral to the affected side, may underlie this spreading [89]. It is unclear whether CNS alterations are a primary abnormality in the disease or a secondary change due to pain, but changes in the CNS play an important role in CRPS, thus, this review addresses the disease.

Carroll et al. prospectively investigated 18 subjects with CRPS [66]. Lumbar sympathetic blocks were accomplished with bupivacaine alone or an additional 75 units of BTX-A. The rate of pain return was significantly lower and the duration of pain reduction was longer in the group with BTX-A injection compared to that with local anesthetic alone. Safarpour et al. conducted a double-blind, randomized, controlled, and open-label extension study [67]. BTX-A was injected intradermally and subcutaneously into the allodynic area, but no significant response occurred after treatment. Kharkar et al. injected 10–20 units of BTX-A per muscle in 37 patients with CRPS-related spasm or dystonia in the neck and/or upper limb girdle [68] and found a statistically significant decrease in local pain scores compared with baseline. Several additional case reports and case series with very small sample sizes are listed in Table 1.

Although no systematic review of the effect of BTX on CRPS is available, most studies have shown BTX to be effective in reducing pain. CRPS also has a multifactorial mechanism, but as central sensitization is reported as a major mechanism, BTX is expected to effectively reduce the pain.

5. Conclusions

The mechanism of central neuropathic pain has been examined according to various hypotheses, including neuronal hyperexcitability and dysfunction of the spinothalamic tract. To date, various preclinical and clinical studies have been published on whether BTX may be effective for central neuropathic pain. BTX inhibits the secretion of substance P and CGRP from DRG, inhibits the expression of TRPV1 and P_2X_3, and induces a central effect through retrograde axonal transport. In addition, several studies have demonstrated its effect on central neuropathic pain associated with SCI, stroke, MS, and CRPS. Effects of BTX on neuropathic pain after SCI, post-stroke shoulder pain, and CRPS has been shown; therefore, it can be considered as one of the treatment options. In the future, well-designed studies will be necessary to assess the effects of BTX on central neuropathic pain, and, furthermore, effective injection sites, injection techniques, and adequate doses should be considered.

Acknowledgments: This study was funded by Ministry of Science, ICT and Future Planning, Republic of Korea (NRF-2016R1C1B1016489).

Conflicts of Interest: The authors declare no conflicts of interest.

References

1. Simpson, L.L. The origin, structure, and pharmacological activity of botulinum toxin. *Pharmacol. Rev.* **1981**, *33*, 155–188. [PubMed]
2. Tian, J.H.; Wu, Z.X.; Unzicker, M.; Lu, L.; Cai, Q.; Li, C.; Schirra, C.; Matti, U.; Stevens, D.; Deng, C.; et al. The role of Snapin in neurosecretion: Snapin knock-out mice exhibit impaired calcium-dependent exocytosis of large dense-core vesicles in chromaffin cells. *J. Neurosci.* **2005**, *25*, 10546–10555. [CrossRef] [PubMed]
3. Ilardi, J.M.; Mochida, S.; Sheng, Z.H. Snapin: A SNARE-associated protein implicated in synaptic transmission. *Nat. Neurosci.* **1999**, *2*, 119–124. [CrossRef] [PubMed]

4. Matak, I.; Lacković, Z. Botulinum toxin A, brain and pain. *Prog. Neurobiol.* **2014**, *119–120*, 39–59. [CrossRef] [PubMed]
5. Evans, D.M.; Williams, R.S.; Shone, C.C.; Hambleton, P.; Melling, J.; Dolly, J.O. Botulinum neurotoxin type B. Its purification, radioiodination and interaction with rat-brain synaptosomal membranes. *Eur. J. Biochem.* **1986**, *154*, 409–416. [CrossRef] [PubMed]
6. Black, J.D. Interaction of 125I-labeled botulinum neurotoxins with nerve terminals. II. Autoradiographic evidence for its uptake into motor nerves by acceptor-mediated endocytosis. *J. Cell Biol.* **1986**, *103*, 535–544. [CrossRef] [PubMed]
7. Simpson, L.L. The binding fragment from tetanus toxin antagonizes the neuromuscular blocking actions of botulinum toxin. *J. Pharmacol. Exp. Ther.* **1984**, *229*, 182–187. [PubMed]
8. Castiglione, A.; Bagnato, S.; Boccagni, C.; Romano, M.C.; Galardi, G. Efficacy of intra-articular injection of botulinum toxin type A in refractory hemiplegic shoulder pain. *Arch. Phys. Med. Rehabil.* **2011**, *92*, 1034–1037. [CrossRef] [PubMed]
9. Safarpour, Y.; Jabbari, B. Botulinum toxin treatment of pain syndromes -an evidence based review. *Toxicon* **2018**. [CrossRef] [PubMed]
10. Merskey, H.B.N. (Ed.) *Classification of Chronic Pain: Descriptions of Chronic Pain Syndromes and Definitions of Pain Terms*, 2nd ed.; IASP Press: Seattle, WA, USA, 1994.
11. Reeh, P.W.; Kress, M. Molecular physiology of proton transduction in nociceptors. *Curr. Opin. Pharmacol.* **2001**, *1*, 45–51. [CrossRef]
12. Bedi, S.S.; Yang, Q.; Crook, R.J.; Du, J.; Wu, Z.; Fishman, H.M.; Grill, R.J.; Carlton, S.M.; Walters, E.T. Chronic spontaneous activity generated in the somata of primary nociceptors is associated with pain-related behavior after spinal cord injury. *J. Neurosci.* **2010**, *30*, 14870–14882. [CrossRef] [PubMed]
13. Ramer, L.M.; van Stolk, A.P.; Inskip, J.A.; Ramer, M.S.; Krassioukov, A.V. Plasticity of TRPV1-Expressing Sensory Neurons Mediating Autonomic Dysreflexia Following Spinal Cord Injury. *Front. Physiol.* **2012**, *3*, 257. [CrossRef] [PubMed]
14. Zhang, H.; Xie, W.; Xie, Y. Spinal cord injury triggers sensitization of wide dynamic range dorsal horn neurons in segments rostral to the injury. *Brain Res.* **2005**, *1055*, 103–110. [CrossRef] [PubMed]
15. Gwak, Y.S.; Kang, J.; Leem, J.W.; Hulsebosch, C.E. Spinal AMPA receptor inhibition attenuates mechanical allodynia and neuronal hyperexcitability following spinal cord injury in rats. *J. Neurosci. Res.* **2007**, *85*, 2352–2359. [CrossRef] [PubMed]
16. Putatunda, R.; Hala, T.J.; Chin, J.; Lepore, A.C. Chronic at-level thermal hyperalgesia following rat cervical contusion spinal cord injury is accompanied by neuronal and astrocyte activation and loss of the astrocyte glutamate transporter, GLT1, in superficial dorsal horn. *Brain Res.* **2014**, *1581*, 64–79. [CrossRef] [PubMed]
17. Gwak, Y.S.; Kang, J.; Unabia, G.C.; Hulsebosch, C.E. Spatial and temporal activation of spinal glial cells: Role of gliopathy in central neuropathic pain following spinal cord injury in rats. *Exp. Neurol.* **2012**, *234*, 362–372. [CrossRef] [PubMed]
18. Tan, A.M.; Stamboulian, S.; Chang, Y.W.; Zhao, P.; Hains, A.B.; Waxman, S.G.; Hains, B.C. Neuropathic pain memory is maintained by Rac1-regulated dendritic spine remodeling after spinal cord injury. *J. Neurosci.* **2008**, *28*, 13173–13183. [CrossRef] [PubMed]
19. Zhao, P.; Hill, M.; Liu, S.; Chen, L.; Bangalore, L.; Waxman, S.G.; Tan, A.M. Dendritic spine remodeling following early and late Rac1 inhibition after spinal cord injury: Evidence for a pain biomarker. *J. Neurophysiol.* **2016**, *115*, 2893–2910. [CrossRef] [PubMed]
20. Leem, J.W.; Kim, H.K.; Hulsebosch, C.E.; Gwak, Y.S. Ionotropic glutamate receptors contribute to maintained neuronal hyperexcitability following spinal cord injury in rats. *Exp. Neurol.* **2010**, *224*, 321–324. [CrossRef] [PubMed]
21. Meisner, J.G.; Marsh, A.D.; Marsh, D.R. Loss of GABAergic interneurons in laminae I-III of the spinal cord dorsal horn contributes to reduced GABAergic tone and neuropathic pain after spinal cord injury. *J. Neurotrauma* **2010**, *27*, 729–737. [CrossRef] [PubMed]
22. Berrocal, Y.A.; Almeida, V.W.; Puentes, R.; Knott, E.P.; Hechtman, J.F.; Garland, M.; Pearse, D.D. Loss of central inhibition: Implications for behavioral hypersensitivity after contusive spinal cord injury in rats. *Pain Res. Treat.* **2014**, *2014*, 178278. [CrossRef] [PubMed]
23. Hains, B.C.; Johnson, K.M.; Eaton, M.J.; Willis, W.D.; Hulsebosch, C.E. Serotonergic neural precursor cell grafts attenuate bilateral hyperexcitability of dorsal horn neurons after spinal hemisection in rat. *Neuroscience* **2003**, *116*, 1097–1110. [CrossRef]

24. Lin, C.Y.; Lee, Y.S.; Lin, V.W.; Silver, J. Fibronectin inhibits chronic pain development after spinal cord injury. *J. Neurotrauma.* **2012**, *29*, 589–599. [CrossRef] [PubMed]
25. Boroujerdi, A.; Zeng, J.; Sharp, K.; Kim, D.; Steward, O.; Luo, Z.D. Calcium channel alpha-2-delta-1 protein upregulation in dorsal spinal cord mediates spinal cord injury-induced neuropathic pain states. *Pain* **2011**, *152*, 649–655. [CrossRef] [PubMed]
26. Lenz, F.A.; Kwan, H.C.; Dostrovsky, J.O.; Tasker, R.R. Characteristics of the bursting pattern of action potentials that occurs in the thalamus of patients with central pain. *Brain Res.* **1989**, *496*, 357–360. [CrossRef]
27. Gerke, M.B.; Duggan, A.W.; Xu, L.; Siddall, P.J. Thalamic neuronal activity in rats with mechanical allodynia following contusive spinal cord injury. *Neuroscience* **2003**, *117*, 715–722. [CrossRef]
28. Quiton, R.L.; Masri, R.; Thompson, S.M.; Keller, A. Abnormal activity of primary somatosensory cortex in central pain syndrome. *J. Neurophysiol.* **2010**, *104*, 1717–1725. [CrossRef] [PubMed]
29. Jiang, L.; Voulalas, P.; Ji, Y.; Masri, R. Post-translational modification of cortical GluA receptors in rodents following spinal cord lesion. *Neuroscience* **2016**, *316*, 122–129. [CrossRef] [PubMed]
30. De Oliveira, R.A.; de Andrade, D.C.; Machado, A.G.; Teixeira, M.J. Central poststroke pain: Somatosensory abnormalities and the presence of associated myofascial pain syndrome. *BMC Neurol.* **2012**, *12*, 89. [CrossRef] [PubMed]
31. Kalita, J.; Kumar, B.; Misra, U.K.; Pradhan, P.K. Central post stroke pain: Clinical, MRI, and SPECT correlation. *Pain Med.* **2011**, *12*, 282–288. [CrossRef] [PubMed]
32. Landerholm, A.H.; Hansson, P.T. Mechanisms of dynamic mechanical allodynia and dysesthesia in patients with peripheral and central neuropathic pain. *Eur. J. Pain (Lond. Engl.)* **2011**, *15*, 498–503. [CrossRef] [PubMed]
33. Sprenger, T.; Seifert, C.L.; Valet, M.; Andreou, A.P.; Foerschler, A.; Zimmer, C.; Collins, D.L.; Goadsby, P.J.; Tolle, T.R.; Chakravarty, M.M. Assessing the risk of central post-stroke pain of thalamic origin by lesion mapping. *Brain J. Neurol.* **2012**, *135*, 2536–2545. [CrossRef] [PubMed]
34. Hong, J.H.; Bai, D.S.; Jeong, J.Y.; Choi, B.Y.; Chang, C.H.; Kim, S.H.; Ahn, S.H.; Jang, S.H. Injury of the spino-thalamo-cortical pathway is necessary for central post-stroke pain. *Eur. Neurol.* **2010**, *64*, 163–168. [CrossRef] [PubMed]
35. Krause, T.; Brunecker, P.; Pittl, S.; Taskin, B.; Laubisch, D.; Winter, B.; Lentza, M.E.; Malzahn, U.; Villringer, K.; Villringer, A.; et al. Thalamic sensory strokes with and without pain: Differences in lesion patterns in the ventral posterior thalamus. *J. Neurol. Neurosurg. Psychiatry* **2012**, *83*, 776–784. [CrossRef] [PubMed]
36. Blasi, F.; Herisson, F.; Wang, S.; Mao, J.; Ayata, C. Late-onset thermal hypersensitivity after focal ischemic thalamic infarcts as a model for central post-stroke pain in rats. *J. Cereb. Blood Flow Metab.* **2015**, *35*, 1100–1103. [CrossRef] [PubMed]
37. Lu, H.C.; Chang, W.J.; Kuan, Y.H.; Huang, A.C.; Shyu, B.C. A [14C]iodoantipyrine study of inter-regional correlations of neural substrates following central post-stroke pain in rats. *Mol. Pain* **2015**, *11*, 9. [CrossRef] [PubMed]
38. Takami, K.; Fujita-Hamabe, W.; Harada, S.; Tokuyama, S. Abeta and Adelta but not C-fibres are involved in stroke related pain and allodynia: An experimental study in mice. *J. Pharmacy Pharmacol.* **2011**, *63*, 452–456. [CrossRef] [PubMed]
39. Kuan, Y.H.; Shih, H.C.; Tang, S.C.; Jeng, J.S.; Shyu, B.C. Targeting P(2)X(7) receptor for the treatment of central post-stroke pain in a rodent model. *Neurobiol. Dis.* **2015**, *78*, 134–145. [CrossRef] [PubMed]
40. McMahon, H.T.; Foran, P.; Dolly, J.O.; Verhage, M.; Wiegant, V.M.; Nicholls, D.G. Tetanus toxin and botulinum toxins type A and B inhibit glutamate, gamma-aminobutyric acid, aspartate, and met-enkephalin release from synaptosomes. Clues to the locus of action. *J. Biol. Chem.* **1992**, *267*, 21338–21343. [PubMed]
41. Welch, M.J.; Purkiss, J.R.; Foster, K.A. Sensitivity of embryonic rat dorsal root ganglia neurons to Clostridium botulinum neurotoxins. *Toxicon* **2000**, *38*, 245–258. [CrossRef]
42. Durham, P.L.; Cady, R.; Cady, R. Regulation of calcitonin gene-related peptide secretion from trigeminal nerve cells by botulinum toxin type A: Implications for migraine therapy. *Headache* **2004**, *44*, 35–42; discussion 33–42. [CrossRef] [PubMed]
43. Xiao, L.; Cheng, J.; Zhuang, Y.; Qu, W.; Muir, J.; Liang, H.; Zhang, D. Botulinum toxin type A reduces hyperalgesia and TRPV1 expression in rats with neuropathic pain. *Pain Med.* **2013**, *14*, 276–286. [CrossRef] [PubMed]
44. Xiao, L.; Cheng, J.; Dai, J.; Zhang, D. Botulinum toxin decreases hyperalgesia and inhibits P2X3 receptor over-expression in sensory neurons induced by ventral root transection in rats. *Pain Med.* **2011**, *12*, 1385–1394. [CrossRef] [PubMed]
45. Antonucci, F.; Rossi, C.; Gianfranceschi, L.; Rossetto, O.; Caleo, M. Long-distance retrograde effects of botulinum neurotoxin A. *J. Neurosci.* **2008**, *28*, 3689–3696. [CrossRef] [PubMed]

46. Restani, L.; Antonucci, F.; Gianfranceschi, L.; Rossi, C.; Rossetto, O.; Caleo, M. Evidence for anterograde transport and transcytosis of botulinum neurotoxin A (BoNT/A). *J. Neurosci.* **2011**, *31*, 15650–15659. [CrossRef] [PubMed]
47. Matak, I.; Riederer, P.; Lackovic, Z. Botulinum toxin's axonal transport from periphery to the spinal cord. *Neurochem. Int.* **2012**, *61*, 236–239. [CrossRef] [PubMed]
48. Koizumi, H.; Goto, S.; Okita, S.; Morigaki, R.; Akaike, N.; Torii, Y.; Harakawa, T.; Ginnaga, A.; Kaji, R. Spinal Central Effects of Peripherally Applied Botulinum Neurotoxin A in Comparison between Its Subtypes A1 and A2. *Front. Neurol.* **2014**, *5*, 98. [CrossRef] [PubMed]
49. Matak, I.; Bach-Rojecky, L.; Filipovic, B.; Lackovic, Z. Behavioral and immunohistochemical evidence for central antinociceptive activity of botulinum toxin A. *Neuroscience* **2011**, *186*, 201–207. [CrossRef] [PubMed]
50. Wang, T.; Martin, S.; Papadopulos, A.; Harper, C.B.; Mavlyutov, T.A.; Niranjan, D.; Glass, N.R.; Cooper-White, J.J.; Sibarita, J.B.; Choquet, D.; et al. Control of autophagosome axonal retrograde flux by presynaptic activity unveiled using botulinum neurotoxin type A. *J. Neurosci.* **2015**, *35*, 6179–6194. [CrossRef] [PubMed]
51. Restani, L.; Giribaldi, F.; Manich, M.; Bercsenyi, K.; Menendez, G.; Rossetto, O.; Caleo, M.; Schiavo, G. Botulinum neurotoxins A and E undergo retrograde axonal transport in primary motor neurons. *PLoS Pathog.* **2012**, *8*, e1003087. [CrossRef] [PubMed]
52. Bach-Rojecky, L.; Salkovic-Petrisic, M.; Lackovic, Z. Botulinum toxin type A reduces pain supersensitivity in experimental diabetic neuropathy: Bilateral effect after unilateral injection. *Eur. J. Pharmacol.* **2010**, *633*, 10–14. [CrossRef] [PubMed]
53. Favre-Guilmard, C.; Auguet, M.; Chabrier, P.E. Different antinociceptive effects of botulinum toxin type A in inflammatory and peripheral polyneuropathic rat models. *Eur. J. Pharmacol.* **2009**, *617*, 48–53. [CrossRef] [PubMed]
54. Bach-Rojecky, L.; Lackovic, Z. Central origin of the antinociceptive action of botulinum toxin type A. *Pharmacol. Biochem. Behav.* **2009**, *94*, 234–238. [CrossRef] [PubMed]
55. Jabbari, B.; Maher, N.; Difazio, M.P. Botulinum toxin a improved burning pain and allodynia in two patients with spinal cord pathology. *Pain Med.* **2003**, *4*, 206–210. [CrossRef] [PubMed]
56. Han, Z.A.; Song, D.H.; Chung, M.E. Effect of subcutaneous injection of botulinum toxin A on spinal cord injury-associated neuropathic pain. *Spinal Cord.* **2014**, *52* (Suppl. 1), S5–S6. [CrossRef] [PubMed]
57. Han, Z.A.; Song, D.H.; Oh, H.M.; Chung, M.E. Botulinum toxin type A for neuropathic pain in patients with spinal cord injury. *Ann Neurol.* **2016**, *79*, 569–578. [CrossRef] [PubMed]
58. Yelnik, A.P.; Colle, F.M.; Bonan, I.V.; Vicaut, E. Treatment of shoulder pain in spastic hemiplegia by reducing spasticity of the subscapular muscle: A randomised, double blind, placebo controlled study of botulinum toxin A. *J. Neurol. Neurosurg. Psychiatry* **2007**, *78*, 845–848. [CrossRef] [PubMed]
59. Marco, E.; Duarte, E.; Vila, J.; Tejero, M.; Guillen, A.; Boza, R.; Escalada, F.; Espadaler, J.M. Is botulinum toxin type A effective in the treatment of spastic shoulder pain in patients after stroke? A double-blind randomized clinical trial. *J. Rehabil. Med.* **2007**, *39*, 440–447. [CrossRef] [PubMed]
60. Kong, K.H.; Neo, J.J.; Chua, K.S. A randomized controlled study of botulinum toxin A in the treatment of hemiplegic shoulder pain associated with spasticity. *Clin. Rehabil.* **2007**, *21*, 28–35. [CrossRef] [PubMed]
61. Lim, J.Y.; Koh, J.H.; Paik, N.J. Intramuscular botulinum toxin-A reduces hemiplegic shoulder pain: A randomized, double-blind, comparative study versus intraarticular triamcinolone acetonide. *Stroke* **2008**, *39*, 126–131. [CrossRef] [PubMed]
62. De Boer, K.S.; Arwert, H.J.; de Groot, J.H.; Meskers, C.G.; Mishre, A.D.; Arendzen, J.H. Shoulder pain and external rotation in spastic hemiplegia do not improve by injection of botulinum toxin A into the subscapular muscle. *J. Neurol. Neurosurg. Psychiatry* **2008**, *79*, 581–583. [CrossRef] [PubMed]
63. Shaw, L.C.; Price, C.I.; van Wijck, F.M.; Shackley, P.; Steen, N.; Barnes, M.P.; Ford, G.A.; Graham, L.A.; Rodgers, H.; Bo, T.I. Botulinum Toxin for the Upper Limb after Stroke (BoTULS) Trial: Effect on impairment, activity limitation, and pain. *Stroke* **2011**, *42*, 1371–1379. [CrossRef] [PubMed]
64. Marciniak, C.M.; Harvey, R.L.; Gagnon, C.M.; Duraski, S.A.; Denby, F.A.; McCarty, S.; Bravi, L.A.; Polo, K.M.; Fierstein, K.M. Does botulinum toxin type A decrease pain and lessen disability in hemiplegic survivors of stroke with shoulder pain and spasticity?: A randomized, double-blind, placebo-controlled trial. *Am. J. Phys. Med. Rehabil.* **2012**, *91*, 1007–1019. [CrossRef] [PubMed]
65. Choi, J.G.; Shin, J.H.; Kim, B.R. Botulinum Toxin A Injection into the Subscapularis Muscle to Treat Intractable Hemiplegic Shoulder Pain. *Ann. Rehabil. Med.* **2016**, *40*, 592–599. [CrossRef] [PubMed]
66. Carroll, I.; Clark, J.D.; Mackey, S. Sympathetic block with botulinum toxin to treat complex regional pain syndrome. *Ann. Neurol.* **2009**, *65*, 348–351. [CrossRef] [PubMed]

67. Safarpour, D.; Salardini, A.; Richardson, D.; Jabbari, B. Botulinum toxin A for treatment of allodynia of complex regional pain syndrome: A pilot study. *Pain Med.* **2010**, *11*, 1411–1414. [CrossRef] [PubMed]
68. Kharkar, S.; Ambady, P.; Venkatesh, Y.; Schwartzman, R.J. Intramuscular botulinum toxin in complex regional pain syndrome: Case series and literature review. *Pain Phys.* **2011**, *14*, 419–424.
69. Safarpour, D.; Jabbari, B. Botulinum toxin A (Botox) for treatment of proximal myofascial pain in complex regional pain syndrome: Two cases. *Pain Med.* **2010**, *11*, 1415–1418. [CrossRef] [PubMed]
70. Birthi, P.; Sloan, P.; Salles, S. Subcutaneous botulinum toxin A for the treatment of refractory complex regional pain syndrome. *PM R J. Inj. Funct. Rehabil.* **2012**, *4*, 446–449. [CrossRef] [PubMed]
71. Choi, E.; Cho, C.W.; Kim, H.Y.; Lee, P.B.; Nahm, F.S. Lumbar Sympathetic Block with Botulinum Toxin Type B for Complex Regional Pain Syndrome: A Case Study. *Pain Phys.* **2015**, *18*, E911–E916.
72. Buonocore, M.; Demartini, L.; Mandrini, S.; Dall'Angelo, A.; Dalla Toffola, E. Effect of Botulinum Toxin on Disabling Neuropathic Pain: A Case Presentation Suggesting a New Therapeutic Strategy. *PM R J. Inj. Funct. Rehabil.* **2017**, *9*, 200–203. [CrossRef] [PubMed]
73. Klit, H.; Finnerup, N.B.; Andersen, G.; Jensen, T.S. Central poststroke pain: A population-based study. *Pain* **2011**, *152*, 818–824. [CrossRef] [PubMed]
74. Andersen, G.; Vestergaard, K.; Ingeman-Nielsen, M.; Jensen, T.S. Incidence of central post-stroke pain. *Pain* **1995**, *61*, 187–193. [CrossRef]
75. Leijon, G.; Boivie, J.; Johansson, I. Central post-stroke pain–neurological symptoms and pain characteristics. *Pain* **1989**, *36*, 13–25. [CrossRef]
76. Dromerick, A.W.; Edwards, D.F.; Kumar, A. Hemiplegic shoulder pain syndrome: Frequency and characteristics during inpatient stroke rehabilitation. *Arch. Phys. Med. Rehabil.* **2008**, *89*, 1589–1593. [CrossRef] [PubMed]
77. Kalichman, L.; Ratmansky, M. Underlying pathology and associated factors of hemiplegic shoulder pain. *Am. J. Phys. Med. Rehabil.* **2011**, *90*, 768–780. [CrossRef] [PubMed]
78. Sheean, D.G. Is spasticity painful? *Eur. J. Neurol.* **2009**, *16*, 157–158. [CrossRef] [PubMed]
79. Zeilig, G.; Rivel, M.; Weingarden, H.; Gaidoukov, E.; Defrin, R. Hemiplegic shoulder pain: Evidence of a neuropathic origin. *Pain* **2013**, *154*, 263–271. [CrossRef] [PubMed]
80. Singh, J.A.; Fitzgerald, P.M. Botulinum toxin for shoulder pain. *Cochrane Database Syst. Rev.* **2010**. [CrossRef]
81. Wu, T.; Fu, Y.; Song, H.X.; Ye, Y.; Dong, Y.; Li, J.H. Effectiveness of Botulinum Toxin for Shoulder Pain Treatment: A Systematic Review and Meta-Analysis. *Arch. Phys. Med. Rehabil.* **2015**, *96*, 2214–2220. [CrossRef] [PubMed]
82. Truini, A.; Barbanti, P.; Pozzilli, C.; Cruccu, G. A mechanism-based classification of pain in multiple sclerosis. *J. Neurol.* **2013**, *260*, 351–367. [CrossRef] [PubMed]
83. Shaikh, A.; Phadke, C.P.; Ismail, F.; Boulias, C. Relationship Between Botulinum Toxin, Spasticity, and Pain: A Survey of Patient Perception. *Can. J. Neurol. Sci.* **2016**, *43*, 311–315. [CrossRef] [PubMed]
84. Jänig, W.; Baron, R. Complex regional pain syndrome: Mystery explained? *Lancet Neurol.* **2003**, *2*, 687–697. [CrossRef]
85. Woolf, C.J.; Thompson, S.W. The induction and maintenance of central sensitization is dependent on *N*-methyl-D-aspartic acid receptor activation; implications for the treatment of post-injury pain hypersensitivity states. *Pain* **1991**, *44*, 293–299. [CrossRef]
86. Del Valle, L.; Schwartzman, R.J.; Alexander, G. Spinal cord histopathological alterations in a patient with longstanding complex regional pain syndrome. *Brain Behav. Immun.* **2009**, *23*, 85–91. [CrossRef] [PubMed]
87. Forss, N.; Kirveskari, E.; Gockel, M. Mirror-like spread of chronic pain. *Neurology* **2005**, *65*, 748–750. [CrossRef] [PubMed]
88. Van Rijn, M.A.; Marinus, J.; Putter, H.; Bosselaar, S.R.; Moseley, G.L.; van Hilten, J.J. Spreading of complex regional pain syndrome: Not a random process. *J. Neural Transm.* **2011**, *118*, 1301–1309. [CrossRef] [PubMed]
89. Aira, Z.; Buesa, I.; Gallego, M.; Garcia del Cano, G.; Mendiable, N.; Mingo, J.; Rada, D.; Bilbao, J.; Zimmermann, M.; Azkue, J.J. Time-dependent cross talk between spinal serotonin 5-HT2A receptor and mGluR1 subserves spinal hyperexcitability and neuropathic pain after nerve injury. *J. Neurosci.* **2012**, *32*, 13568–13581. [CrossRef] [PubMed]

toxins MDPI

Article

Botulinum Toxin B Affects Neuropathic Pain but Not Functional Recovery after Peripheral Nerve Injury in a Mouse Model

Alba Finocchiaro [1,2], Sara Marinelli [1,3], Federica De Angelis [3], Valentina Vacca [1,3], Siro Luvisetto [1,3,*] and Flaminia Pavone [1,3,*]

1 National Research Council of Italy-CNR, Institute of Cell Biology and Neurobiology-IBCN, 00143 Roma, Italy; alba.finocchiaro@hotmail.it (A.F.); sara.marinelli@cnr.it (S.M.); valentina.vacca@ibcn.cnr.it (V.V.)
2 Department of Psycology, PhD School of Behavioural Neuroscience, Sapienza University, 00185 Roma, Italy
3 IRCCS Santa Lucia Foundation, 00143-Roma, Italy; federica.deangelis@uniroma1.it
* Correspondence: siro.luvisetto@cnr.it (S.L.); flaminia.pavone@cnr.it (F.P.); Tel.: +39-06-501-703-271 (S.L. & F.P.)

Received: 12 February 2018; Accepted: 15 March 2018; Published: 18 March 2018

Abstract: Clinical use of neurotoxins from *Clostridium botulinum* is well established and is continuously expanding, including in treatment of pain conditions. *Background*: The serotype A (BoNT/A) has been widely investigated, and current data demonstrate that it induces analgesia and modulates nociceptive processing initiated by inflammation or nerve injury. Given that data concerning the serotype B (BoNT/B) are limited, the aim of the present study was to verify if also BoNT/B is able not only to counteract neuropathic pain, but also to interfere with inflammatory and regenerative processes associated with the nerve injury. *Methods*: As model of neuropathic pain, chronic constriction injury (CCI) of the sciatic nerve was performed in CD1 male mice. Mice were intraplantarly injected with saline (control) or BoNT/B (5 or 7.5 pg/mouse) into the injured hindpaw. For comparison, another mouse group was injected with BoNT/A (15 pg/mouse). Mechanical allodynia and functional recovery of the injured paw was followed for 101 days. Spinal cords and sciatic nerves were collected at day 7 for immunohistochemistry. *Results and Conclusions:* The results of this study show that BoNT/B is a powerful biological molecule that, similarly to BoNT/A, can reduce neuropathic pain over a long period of time. However, the analgesic effects are not associated with an improvement in functional recovery, clearly highlighting an important difference between the two serotypes for the treatment of this chronic pain state.

Keywords: nerve regeneration; Schwann cells; glia; spinal cord; immunohistochemistry; allodynia; weight bearing; sciatic static index; walking track analysis

Key Contribution: Intraplantar injection of botulinum serotype B counteracts pain, but not functional deficits induced by chronic constriction of sciatic nerve in mice.

1. Introduction

The interest in botulinum neurotoxins (BoNTs) has been growing in the last years because they have become important therapeutic agents for many pathological conditions, including pain [1–4]. This was allowed by better comprehension of the mechanism of action of BoNTs [5,6].

Seven BoNT serotypes (A–G) have been recognized up until now, with a growing number of subtypes continuously identified [7]. All BoNTs are zinc endopeptidases that selectively cleave one of the SNARE (soluble *N*-ethylmaleimide-sensitive factor attachment protein receptor) proteins essential for the formation of SNARE complex, the core component of the eukaryotic neuroexocytosis [8]. Owing to their zinc endopeptidase activity, BoNT/A and /E cleave SNAP25 (synaptosomal-associated protein of 25 kDa), BoNT/B, /D, /F, and /G cleave VAMP (vesicle-associated membrane protein), while BoNT/C cleaves both SNAP25 and syntaxin [9].

Most of preclinical data on the analgesic effects of BoNTs derive from experiments with BoNT/A, which is also the serotype with the long-lasting action duration and lower toxicity. In the past years, we demonstrated the antiallodynic efficacy of BoNT/A in the mouse model of chronic constriction injury (CCI) of the sciatic nerve [10–14]. Antiallodynia was accompanied by structural changes in injured nerve and improvements in functional recovery of the injured hindlimb. In details, a single intraplantar (ipl) injection of BoNT/A in the injured hindpaw was sufficient to (i) inhibit glial cell activation; (ii) modulate pro- and anti-nociceptive interleukins; (iii) accelerate processes related to sciatic nerve regeneration; and (iv) improve functional recovery from CCI-induced atrophy of the injured hindpaw.

From a clinical view, BoNT/A has been approved by FDA for treatment of a wide variety of clinical conditions [2,15], but a downside may limit its use. As a matter of fact, the action of BoNTs is reversible, and after repeated treatment, BoNT/A can induce the phenomenon of tolerance, generating the need to continue therapy using other serotypes. Nowadays, the only serotype commercially available in replacement of BoNT/A is BoNT/B, but in view of the relevant clinical differences of the two serotypes [16], BoNT/B has been approved only for cervical dystonia.

As for basic science, only few studies focused on the use of BoNT/B in chronic pain. Peripheral administration of BoNT/B reduced peripheral inflammation and spinal nociceptive processing in inflammatory pain models, such as carrageenan [17], capsaicin [18], and formalin [18,19], and yields a long-lasting attenuation of allodynia in mice subjected either to spinal nerve ligation [20,21] or to cisplatin administration [21].

As suggested by the commentary of Pavone and Ueda [22], it is extremely important to understand the mechanisms underlying the action of BoNT serotypes other than serotype A. We decided to verify not only if BoNT/B could counteract CCI-induced neuropathic pain for a long time interval, but also if it could affect, as occurs for BoNT/A, the regenerative processes of the peripheral injured nerve, as well as the functional recovery of the injured hindlimb. In addition, we performed, in BoNT/B-treated CCI mice, immunohistochemistry analysis of spinal cord, looking for the expression of markers of activation of glial cells.

2. Results

2.1. *Effects of BoNT/B on Mechanical Nociceptive Threshold in CCI Mice*

To verify the analgesic properties of BoNT/B, we analyzed its effect on mechanical nociceptive threshold in CCI mice (Figure 1A). In CCI-saline mice, the mechanical nociceptive threshold in the ipsilateral hindpaw was around 50% lower compared to contralateral hindpaw. Since mice withdrew their ipsilateral hindpaw after very low stimuli (5–6 g), which did not evoke any reaction in contralateral hindpaw, we considered this response as allodynia. The ipsilateral allodynia was maintained for at least 3 weeks and, even if reduced, was still present after 3 months. On the contrary, a single ipl injection of BoNT/B (5 or 7.5 pg/paw at D5) in CCI mice (CCI-B5 and CCI-B7.5) clearly antagonizes allodynia, as indicated by the clear-cut enhancement of the ipsilateral withdrawal threshold, at values corresponding to 80% of the contralateral withdrawal threshold. Both in CCI-B5 and CCI-B7.5 mice, the antiallodynic effect was observed already at D6 (the day after the injection) and the significant difference with CCI-saline mice persisted for a very long time. Two-way ANOVA for repeated measures carried out for ipsilateral allodynia showed a significant main effect for treatment ($F_{2,27} = 10.941$; $p < 0.0003$), days ($F_{17,459} = 68.739$; $p < 0.0001$) and treatment x days interaction ($F_{34,459} = 7.031$; $p < 0.0001$). Post hoc comparisons vs. CCI-saline mice confirmed a significant difference (Tukey–Kramer, $p < 0.05$) from D6 to D31 for CCI-B5, and from D6 to D41 for CCI-B7.5 mice.

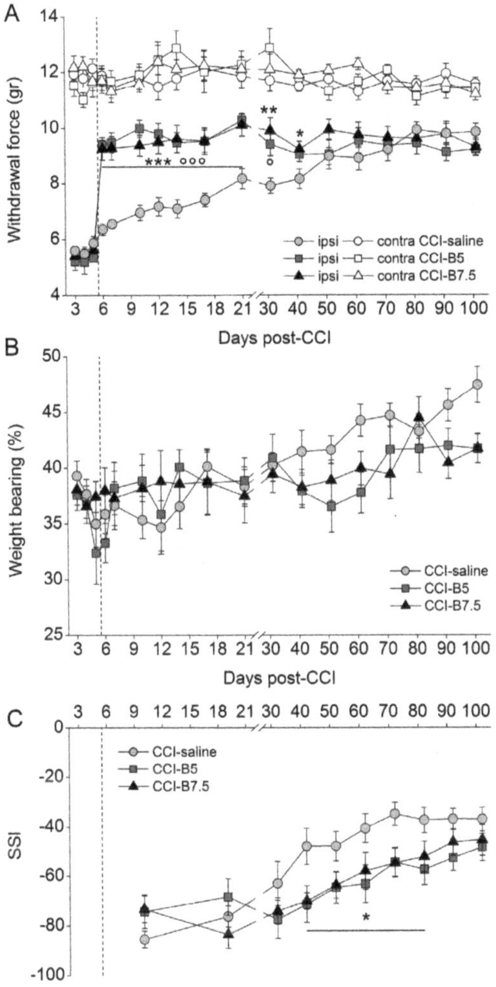

Figure 1. Mechanical allodynia and functional recovery in chronic constriction injury (CCI)-mice. (**A**) Mechanical allodynia measured on ipsilateral (closed symbols) and contralateral (open symbols) hindpaw of CCI-mice after a single ipsilateral injection of saline (CCI-saline: ○,●), BoNT/B 5 pg/paw (CCI-B5: □,■) and BoNT/B 7.5 pg/paw (CCI-B7.5: △,▲). Dotted line indicates the day of injection. In CCI-BoNT/B mice groups the strong antiallodynic effect was observed starting from the day after the injection and persisted for a very long time. Statistical symbols: (ooo) $p < 0.001$, (o) $p < 0.05$ for CCI-B5 vs. CCI-saline; (***) $p < 0.001$, (**) $p < 0.01$, (*) $p < 0.05$ for CCI-B7.5 vs. CCI-saline. (**B**) Weight bearing calculated as ratio of the weight distribution between the hindpaws, in CCI-saline (●), CCI-B5 (■) and CCI-B7.5 (▲) mice. In all mice groups there was a slow but incomplete functional recovery over time. The CCI-BoNT/B mice did not show difference compared to CCI-saline mice. (**C**) Walking track analysis: sciatic static index, SSI, calculated from hindpaws' footprints in CCI-saline (●), CCI-B5 (■) and CCI-B7.5 (▲) mice. BoNT/B slowed down the functional recovery of mice: CCI-BoNT/B mice expressed more negative values in respect to the CCI-saline mice. Statistical symbols: (*) $p < 0.05$ both for CCI-B5 and CCI-B7.5 vs. CCI-saline.

2.2. Effects of BoNT/B on Functional Recovery after CCI

Functional recovery was examined by (i) measuring the weight bearing between the two hindlimbs (incapacitance test); and, (ii) walking track analysis (footprint test), followed by calculation of the sciatic static index (SSI).

Figure 1B shows the reduction of the weight bearing to value <50% in CCI-mice, indicating a displacement of weight distribution toward the contralateral hindlimb. The graph indicates that, independently from the treatment, there was a slow recovery over time. Two-way ANOVA for repeated measures showed not significant effects for treatment ($F_{2,27} = 1.013$, $p = 0.3765$), days ($F_{17,459} = 5.341$, $p < 0.0001$), and treatment x days interactions ($F_{34,459} = 1.226$, $p = 0.1824$).

Figure 1C shows the SSI for CCI-saline, CCI-B5, and CCI-B7.5 mice calculated with the walking track analysis. All CCI mice manifested a severe impairment of motor function, as revealed by SSI values (around 80) until D32; then they showed a slow, but incomplete, functional recovery. In particular, in CCI-saline mice, the SSI values were slowly increased during the overall time course but, 2 months after CCI, impairments in functional recovery were still observed. Both CCI-B5 and CCI-B7.5 mice did not show improvement, indeed, their SSI values worsened in comparison to CCI-saline mice. At D101, CCI-B5 and CCI-B7.5 mice expressed SSI values similar to those of CCI-saline mice. Two-way ANOVA for repeated measures showed a significant main effect for days ($F_{9,243} = 32.786$; $p < 0.0001$) and for treatment x days ($F_{9,243} = 2.867$; $p = 0.0001$). Post hoc comparisons vs. CCI-saline showed a significant difference ($p < 0.05$) from D42 to D82, for both CCI-B5 and CCI-B7.5 mice.

2.3. Effect of BoNTs on Cytoskeleton and Myelin Sheath of Injured Sciatic Nerve

The axonal injury caused by CCI induces structural changes in damaged nerves, which begin almost immediately and determine a progressive degradation of cytoskeletal proteins. Ipsilateral sections of sciatic nerves were incubated with rabbit polyclonal antibody anti-neurofilament-200 (NF200), a marker of large-diameter axons. As evidenced by representative examples in Figure 2A, both CCI-saline and CCI-B7.5 mice showed disjointed and broken up tissue, with loss of axonal integrity and neurofilaments not equally distributed along the fibers. Conversely, in CCI-A15 mice, neurofilaments appeared almost uniform, with a tissue presenting a compact regular structure, more similar to naïve mice than to saline CCI mice.

Figure 2B shows IF of GFAP in ipsilateral sciatic nerve sections taken from CCI-saline, CCI-B7.5, and CCI-A15 mice. GFAP is a cytoskeleton constituent of Schwann cells (SCs) expressed both by immature dedifferentiate and mature non-myelinating cells. After peripheral nerve injury, SCs lose contact with axons, increase their GFAP expression, and acquire an immature dedifferentiated phenotype resembling non-myelin forming SCs. As previously reported [11], the expression of GFAP in injured sciatic nerves of all CCI mice groups was evaluated by means of RGB pixel analysis of IF images (Figure 2C). One-way ANOVA evidenced a significantly ($F_{2,38} = 11.913$; $p < 0.0001$) different expression of GFAP among groups. In respect to CCI-saline mice, post hoc comparisons showed that GFAP expression was significantly increased in CCI-A15 mice (Fisher's PLSD analysis, $p = 0.0274$) and significantly reduced in CCI-B7.5 mice ($p = 0.0397$), respectively. The expression of GFAP was also significantly different ($p < 0.0001$) between CCI-B7.5 and CCI-A15 mice.

Figure 2D shows IF of S100β marker of SCs, in ipsilateral sciatic nerve sections taken from CCI-saline, CCI-B7.5, and CCI-A15 mice. S100β is a glial-specific protein localized in the cytoplasm and nucleus of a wide range of cells, derived from neural crest, including SCs. In SCs, S100β is expressed both by immature dedifferentiating and mature myelinating cells. Differently from the expression of GFAP, the expression of S100β was not significantly different among the different CCI mice groups (quantification in Figure 2E).

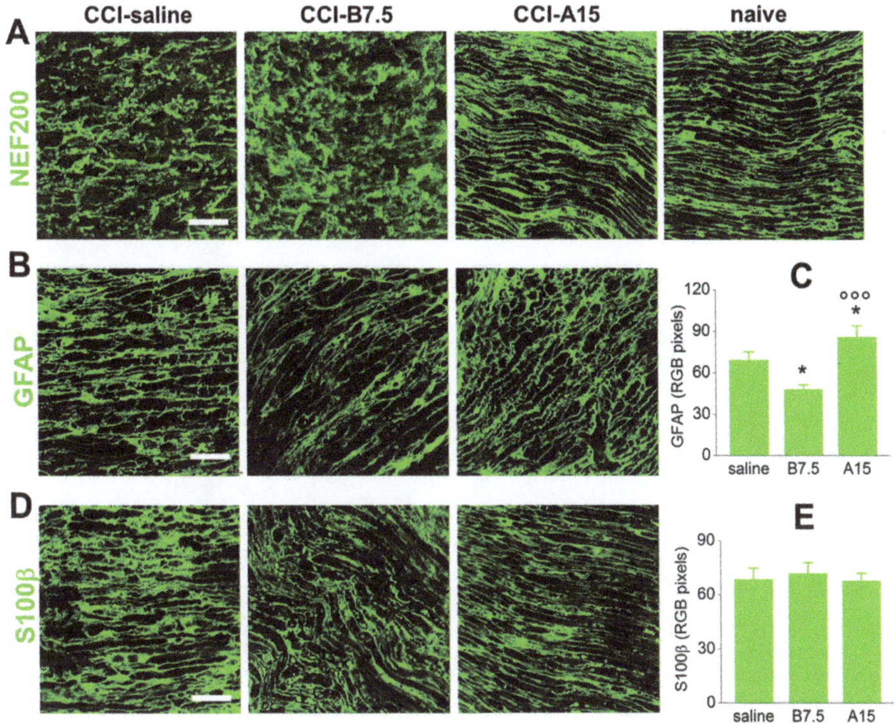

Figure 2. IF analysis of NF200, GFAP, and S100β in injured sciatic nerve. (**A**) Representative examples of confocal images at high magnification (63×) showing IF expression of NF200 in sciatic nerve sections, proximal to the lesion, from CCI-saline, CCI-B7.5, and CCI-A15 compared to naïve mice. As evidenced by morphological staining with NF200, CCI-saline and CCI-B7.5 showed similar tissue morphology with disjoined fibers, while CCI-A15 was similar to naïve mice, with almost regular tissue morphology and uniform and compact structure. Scale bar: 50 μm. (**B**) Representative examples of confocal images at high magnification (63×) showing IF expression of GFAP (green) and its quantification by RGB analysis (**C**), in sciatic nerve sections from CCI-saline, CCI-B7.5, and CCI-A15 mice. Scale bar: 50 μm. RGB analysis reveals an increased expression of GFAP in CCI-A15 mice and a decreased expression of GFAP in CCI-B7.5 mice, with respect to CCI-saline. (**D**) Representative examples of confocal images at high magnification (63×) showing IF expression of S100β (green) and its quantification by RGB analysis (**E**), in sciatic nerve sections from CCI-saline, CCI-B7.5, and CCI-A15 mice. Scale bar: 50 μm. RGB analysis reveals no different expression of S100β in all CCI mice groups. Statistical symbols: (*) $p < 0.05$ vs. CCI-saline; (ooo) $p < 0.001$ vs. CCI-B7.5.

2.4. Effects of BoNTs on Myelin-Associated Protein Expressed by SCs

Schwann cells play a key role in the clearance of myelin debris from damaged nerve. The loss of axon–SC contact is a signal that causes SC proliferation, an important event that promotes axon regeneration. During proliferation, myelinating and non-myelinating SCs change their phenotype from differentiated to dedifferentiated cells, and this switch is associated with expression of regeneration- and myelin-associated proteins (e.g., P0, PMP22).

To avoid enhancement of pro-inflammatory status associated with myelin debris and aggregates, SCs begin demyelination with fragmentation of the myelin sheath into small ovoid-like structures that occur near the Schmidt–Lanterman incisures [23,24].

Figure 3 shows IF for either P0 (marker of a major peripheral myelin protein; Figure 3A) or PMP22 (marker of peripheral myelin protein 22; Figure 3B), alone or co-stained with GFAP for SCs (green) and DAPI for nuclei (blue) in ipsilateral sciatic nerve sections taken from CCI-saline, CCI-B7.5, and CCI-A15 mice. As evidenced by the zoomed images in Figure 3A,B, both P0 and PMP22 were found aggregated and accumulated in characteristic ovoids in CCI-saline mice. Different results were observed in samples from CCI-B7.5 and CCI-A15 mice, where the presence of myelin aggregates in ovoids was less evident, and staining of P0 and PMP22 was reduced in respect to CCI-saline.

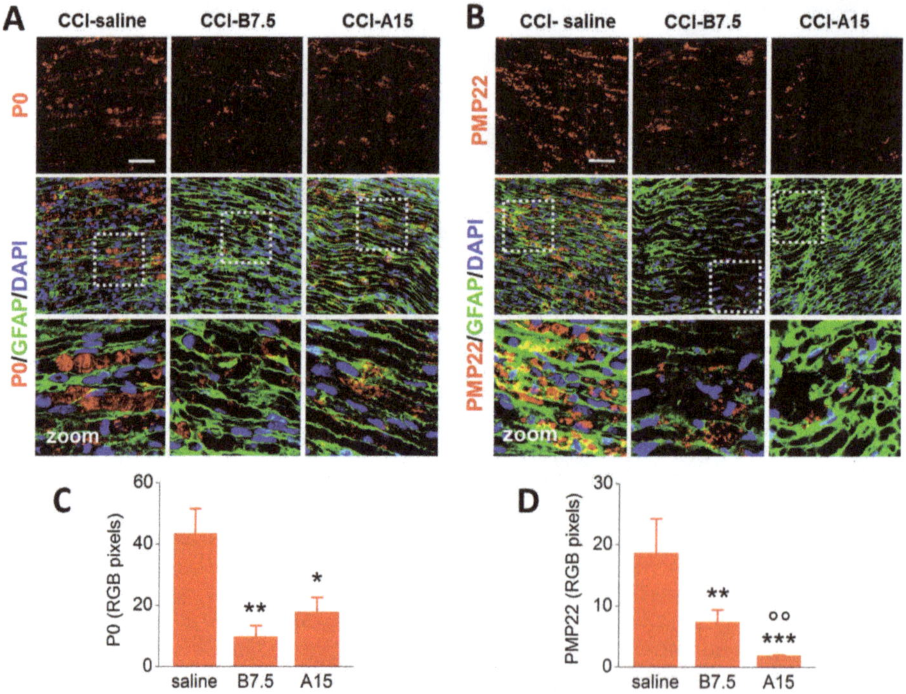

Figure 3. IF analysis of P0 and PMP22 in injured sciatic nerve. (**A**,**B**) Representative examples of confocal images at high magnification (63×) showing single IF expression of P0 or PMP22 (red), or double IF with GFAP (green), and their quantification by RGB analysis (**C**,**D**), in sciatic nerve sections from CCI-saline, CCI-B7.5, and CCI-A15 mice. White dotted squares in panels with double IF indicate the zone of the section where zooming (×2) was taken. Zoomed images: typical examples of myelin ovoids, which are more expressed in CCI-saline mice. Scale bar: 50 μm. RGB analyses reveal lower expression of P0 and PMP22 in CCI-A15 and CCI-B7.5 with respect to CCI-saline mice. Statistical symbols: (*) $p < 0.05$, (**) $p < 0.01$ vs. CCI-saline; (oo) $p < 0.01$ vs. CCI-B7.5.

RGB analysis and one-way ANOVA confirmed the different expression of P0 (Figure 3C) and PMP22 (Figure 3D) in the different CCI mice groups. As for P0, ANOVA indicated a significant main effect for treatment ($F_{2,17} = 5.468$; $p = 0.0147$); post hoc comparisons showed significantly reduced expression of P0 in both CCI-B7.5 ($p = 0.0052$) and CCI-A15 ($p = 0.0197$) vs. CCI-saline mice. Instead, CCI-B7.5 and CCI-A15 did not show any differences between them. As for PMP22, ANOVA indicated a significant main effect for treatment ($F_{2,18} = 7.952$; $p = 0.0034$); post hoc comparisons showed a significant reduced expression of PMP22 in both CCI-B7.5 ($p = 0.0019$) and CCI-A15 ($p = 0.0009$) vs. CCI-saline, and, differently from P0, in CCI-A15 vs. CCI-B7.5 ($p = 0.0029$).

2.5. Effect of BoNTs on the Immune Cells after CCI

After peripheral nerve damage, resident mast cells are the first immune cells to be activated. Activated mast cells degranulate and release a variety of proinflammatory mediators, which contribute to recruitment of neutrophils and, as a consequence, of infiltrating activated hematogenous macrophages [25], facilitating a rapid elimination of myelin debris and nerve regeneration.

Figure 4A shows the IF of CC1 (green), marker of chymase 1, a protein expressed by activated mast cells, in sciatic nerve sections from CCI mice. Compared to saline mice, the expression of mast cells was enhanced in both CCI-B7.5 and CCI-A15 mice groups. RGB analysis and one-way ANOVA (Figure 4B) for CC1 indicated a significant main effect for treatment ($F_{2,24} = 38.224$; $p < 0.0001$). Post hoc comparisons confirmed a significant difference of both CCI-B7.5 (Fisher's PLSD analysis; $p = 0.0222$) and CCI-A15 ($p < 0.0001$) vs. CCI-saline mice, and of CCI-B7.5 vs. CCI-A15 mice ($p < 0.0001$).

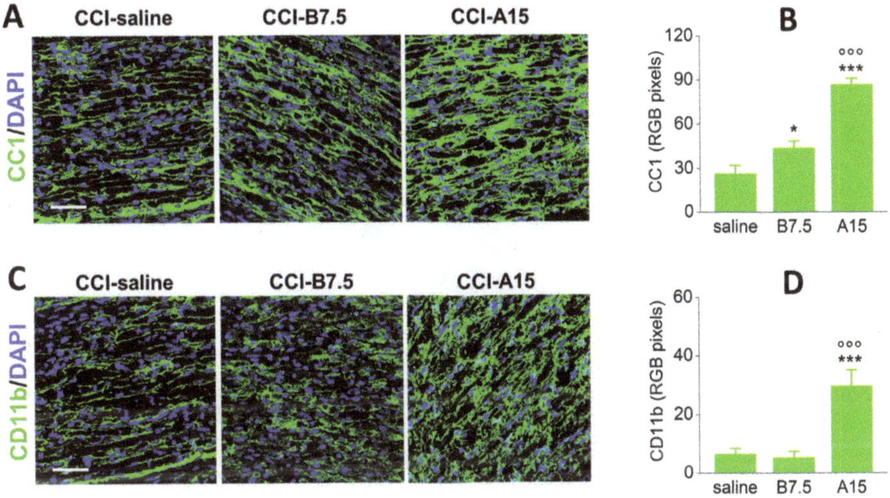

Figure 4. IF analysis of CC1 and CD11b in injured sciatic nerve. (**A**) Representative examples of confocal images at high magnification (63×) showing IF expression of CC1 (green) and its quantification by RGB analysis (**B**) in sciatic nerve sections from CCI-saline, CCI-B7.5, and CCI-A15 mice. Scale bar: 50 μm. RGB evaluation reveals an increased expression of CC1 in CCI-B7.5 and CCI-A15 mice compared to CCI-saline mice. This increase is particularly evident in CCI-A15 mice. (**C**) Representative examples of confocal images at high magnification (63×) showing IF expression of CD11b (green) and its quantification by RGB analysis (**D**) in sciatic nerve sections from CCI-saline, CCI-B7.5 and CCI-A15 mice. Scale bar: 50 μm. RGB evaluation reveals an increased expression of CD11b only in CCI-A15 mice compared to CCI-saline mice. Statistical symbols: (***) $p < 0.001$ vs. CCI-saline; (ooo) $p < 0.0001$ vs. CCI-B7.5.

Figure 4C shows the IF of CD11b (green), marker of peripheral macrophages, in the sciatic nerves from CCI mice. Compared to CCI-saline mice, the expression of macrophages was highly enhanced in CCI-A15 mice, but not in CCI-B7.5 mice group. RGB analysis and one-way ANOVA (Figure 4D) for CD11b expression indicated a significant main effect for treatment ($F_{2,24} = 14.072$; $p < 0.0001$); post hoc comparisons confirmed a significant difference of CCI-A15 vs. CCI-saline ($p = 0.0002$) and CCI-B7.5 ($p < 0.0001$).

2.6. Effect of BoNT/B on Spinal Cord after CCI

After nerve injury, activation of glial cells, both microglia and astrocytes, is observed in spinal cord. Microglia activation, characterized by phosphorylation of p38 MAP kinase (p-p38), induces the production and secretion of proinflammatory cytokines that contribute to the onset and maintenance of pain hypersensitivity.

To detect spinal microglia, we incubated transverse sections of L4/L5 spinal cord segment of CCI-saline and CCI-B7.5 mice with rat monoclonal antibody anti-CD11b, as a marker of microglia, and with rabbit polyclonal antibody anti-p-p38. Figure 5A shows the expression of microglia (CD11b; green), and their colocalization with p-p38 (red) in ipsilateral dorsal (ID) and ipsilateral ventral (IV) horns of CCI-saline and CCI-B7.5 mice. Figure 5B,C show the counting of total number of CD11b immunoresponsive (IR) cells and the number of CD11b IR cells colocalized with p-p38 (p-p38/CD11b) in ID and IV horns, respectively. One-way ANOVA for the expression of total CD11b and p-p38/CD11b IR cells indicated no significant difference between CCI-saline and CCI-B7.5 mice, both at ID horn (total CD11b: $F_{1,10} = 0.804$, $p = 0.3911$; p-p38/CD11b: $F_{1,10} = 3.586$, $p = 0.0875$) and IV horn (total CD11b: $F_{1,10} = 0.028$, $p = 0.8716$; p-p38/CD11b: $F_{1,10} = 0.000$).

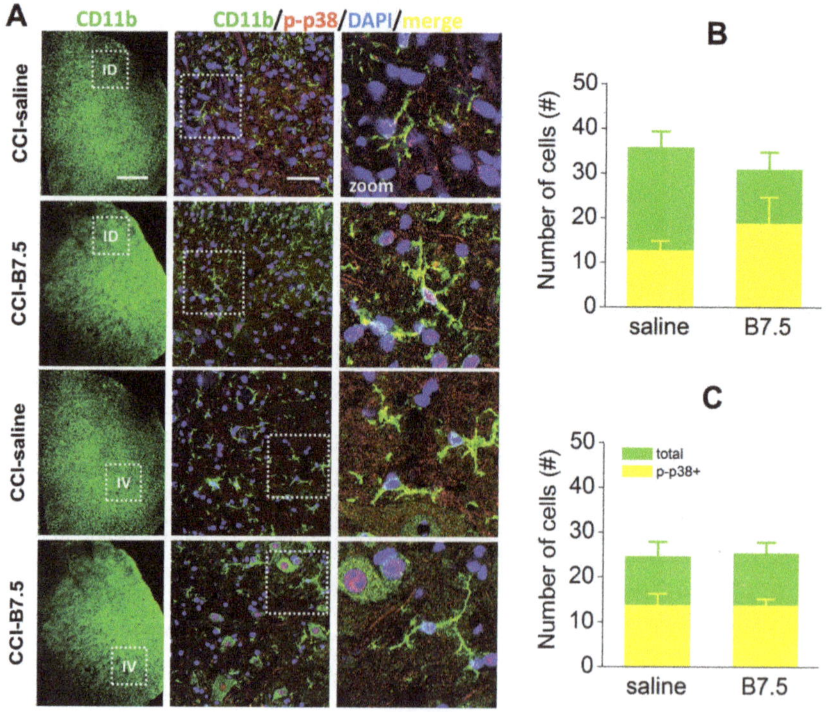

Figure 5. IF analysis of CD11b and p-p38 colocalization in ipsilateral spinal horns. (**A**) Examples of confocal images at 10× or 63× magnification showing double IF expression of CD11b (green), p-p38 (red), and CD11b/p-p38 (yellow) cells in ipsilateral dorsal (ID) and ventral (IV) horns of spinal cord sections in CCI-saline and CCI-B7.5 mice. White boxes in 10× images indicate the zone of the spinal cord sections considered for the 63× images. White boxes in 63× images indicate the zone of dorsal or ventral horns considered for further zoomed (2×) images. Scale bars: 300 μm for 10×; 50 μm for 63×. Analysis of number of cells in ipsilateral dorsal (**B**) and ventral (**C**) horns indicates no difference between CCI-saline and CCI-B7.5 mice in the counting of total CD11b and CD11b/p-p38 IR cells.

Together with microglia, astrocyte activation also plays a role in chronic pain sensitization. After damage to peripheral nerves hypertrophy and proliferation of spinal astrocytes, which are accompanied by enhanced expression of GFAP, are observed. Figure 6A shows the IF of astrocytes (GFAP; green), and their colocalization with p-p38 (red) in ID and IV horns of CCI-saline and CCI-B7.5 mice. One-way ANOVA for the expression of total GFAP and p-p38/GFAP IR cells in ID horns (Figure 6B) indicated a strong significant decrease for both total GFAP ($F_{1,10} = 59.387$, $p < 0.001$) and p-p38/GFAP ($F_{1,10} = 22.510$, $p = 0.0008$) IR cells in CCI-B7.5 compared to CCI-saline group. Unlike ID horns, in IV horns (Figure 6C) one-way ANOVA for the expression of total GFAP and p-p38/GFAP IR cells showed a significant decrease only for total GFAP ($F_{1,10} = 5.604$, $p = 0.0395$), but not for the activated p-p38/GFAP ($F_{1,10} = 2.169$, $p = 0.1715$) IR cells.

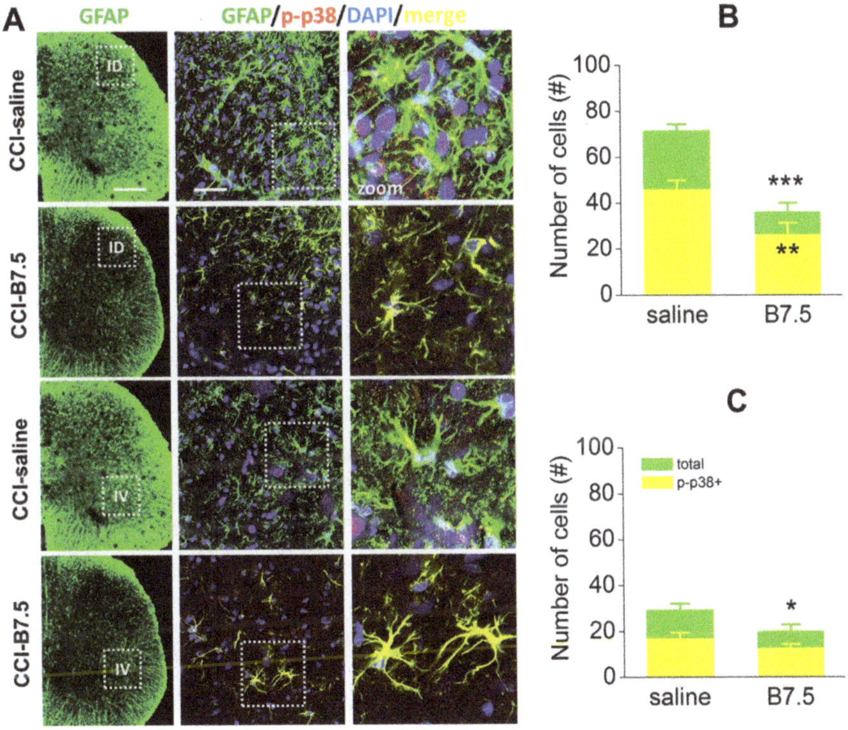

Figure 6. IF analysis of GFAP and p-p38 colocalization in ipsilateral spinal horns. (**A**) Examples of confocal images at 10× or high 63× magnification, showing double IF expression of GFAP (green), p-p38 (red) and GFAP/p-p38 (yellow) cells in ipsilateral dorsal (ID) and ventral (IV) horns of spinal cord sections in CCI-saline and CCI-B7.5 mice. White boxes in 10× images indicate the zone of the spinal cord sections considered for the 63× images. White boxes in 63× images indicate the zone of dorsal or ventral horns considered for further zoom (2×) images. Scale bars: 300 μm for 10×; 50 μm for 63×. Counting of total GFAP and GFAP/p-p38 IR cells in 63X dorsal (**B**) and ventral (**C**) horn images indicates a strong significant difference between CCI-saline and CCI-B7.5 for both total GFAP and GFAP/p-p38 IR cells in dorsal horns, and only for total GFAP IR cells in ventral horns. Statistical symbols: (***) $p < 0.001$, (**) $p < 0.01$, (*) $p < 0.05$ vs. CCI-saline.

3. Discussion

The most considerable finding of this report is the remarkable difference between the two botulinum serotypes A and B in counteracting symptoms induced by CCI neuropathy: BoNT/B, differing from BoNT/A, reduced pain sensitivity in neuropathic mice without inducing any positive effect on functional recovery. This result is particularly relevant for its clinical implications, considering that both serotypes can be alternatively used when one of them resulted in the development of immunoresistance.

A single ipl injection of BoNT/B (5 or 7.5 pg/paw) exerted an almost immediate antiallodynic effect, which started from the day after injection and lasted for at least 30 days. The long-lasting analgesic effect resulted independently from the dose considered, the maximal effect being already observed at the lower dose of 5 pg/paw. This finding is compatible with the action of BoNTs as proteolytic enzymes, which is not directly proportional to the dose administered.

In the past years, analgesic effects mainly of BoNT/A, but also of BoNT/B, have been reported in several pain models [3,4,17,26]. Interestingly, it was also demonstrated that BoNT/A, in addition to its analgesic effects, is able to accelerate functional rehabilitation in CCI-mice [11]. On the contrary, the present results show that BoNT/B not only did not improve but also slowed down functional recovery of mice, as shown by significant differences between CCI-BoNT/B and CCI-saline mice in walking track analysis.

Differences in functional recovery between the two BoNTs serotypes may depend on different modulation by BoNTs of the processes favorable, or unfavorable, to the nerve regeneration. Table 1 shows a summary of changes in the expression of protein markers, associated to peripheral nerve injury, in the different experimental groups.

Table 1. Summary of differences in the expression of biological markers associated to peripheral nerve injury in CCI-A15 and CCI-B7.5 vs. CCI-saline mice.

Target	Marker	CCI-A15	CCI-B7.5
Non-myelinating SCs	GFAP	↑	↓
Myelinating SCs	S100b	=	=
Peripheral myelin	P0	↓	↓↓
Peripheral myelin	PMP22	↓↓↓	↓↓
Mast cells	CC1	↑↑↑	↑
Macrophages	CD11b	↑↑↑ [1]	=

[1] Upward arrows, downward arrows, or equal sign indicate, respectively, enhanced, reduced, or equal expression of corresponding markers in CCI-BoNTs vs. CCI-saline mice. One, two, or three arrows indicate significant difference: $p < 0.05$ (↑), $p < 0.01$ (↑↑), or $p < 0.001$ (↑↑↑).

After peripheral nerve injury, resident mast cells are found along the axons and juxtaposed to free nerve endings; they are activated from bacteria, viruses, and neuropeptides, including substance P, NGF, TNF-α, IL-1β, and many others. Activated mast cells degranulate and release a variety of proinflammatory mediators, including histamine, leukotrienes, and chemokines, which contribute to recruitment of neutrophils. Neutrophils, in turn, release several substances that help recruitment of activated hematogenous macrophages to the site of injury into degenerating nerve [25]; supplementation of resident macrophages by infiltrating activated hematogenous macrophages leads to a rapid elimination of myelin debris, making the nerve regeneration easier. Macrophages not only remove axon and myelin debris, but also participate in the production of mitogenic factors for SCs [23,27].

With respect to saline, BoNT/A increased the expression of markers related to proliferation of mast cells, of macrophages, and of SCs, which may support an early clearance of fragmented myelin and of its debris [8,24], an important precondition for the axonal regeneration after peripheral nerve injury [28]. In parallel, BoNT/A reduced the expression of P0 and PMP22 myelin peripheral proteins and the presence of the myelin ovoids, which characterize peripheral nerves in CCI-saline mice, indicating an anticipation of myelin phagocytosis processes in CCI mice [24].

A different pattern was obtained in CCI-BoNT/B mice (Table 1). With respect to saline, BoNT/B reduced proliferation of SCs (GFAP; but not S100β), did not increase the expression of macrophages, and increased only the expression of mast cells, even if to a lesser extent than BoNT/A. Instead, similarly to BoNT/A, BoNT/B reduced the expression of P0 and PMP22. However, the finding that the functional recovery appears slowed down in CCI-BoNT/B mice with respect to CCI-BoNT/A mice, could indicate that myelin phagocytosis, which *per se* should facilitate the nerve regeneration, is not sufficient if not accompanied by other relevant processes, e.g., the increased proliferation of macrophages and SCs observed in CCI-BoNT/A. In this regard, we should consider that activated mast cells at the periphery release different proinflammatory cytokines that directly stimulate receptors on axons or cell bodies, and may result in neuronal activation. Some released factors, such as chemokines, serve as chemoattractants and activators for other immune cells, such as neutrophils and leukocytes [29], which help the recruitment of hematogenous macrophages at the site of injured nerve [25]. The modest increase of mast cells, not accompanied by an enhancement of macrophages observed in CCI-BoNT/B mice, could indicate a reduced pro-regenerative effect of this serotype. On the other hand, it has to be considered that neurofilaments in BoNT/B appear particularly disorganized and deranged, similarly to saline nerves, while the cytoskeleton of BoNT/A-treated nerves are much more structurally organized.

Regarding the SC marker S100β, we found a similar expression in all CCI mice groups. This result seems to be in contrast with Cobianchi et al. [30] where BoNT/A-injected regenerating nerves showed a higher expression of S100β with respect to saline-injected regenerating nerves. The discrepancy is only apparent because the higher expression of S100β was detected in distal portion of crushed nerve. In the proximal portion of crushed nerve, as in the present experimental conditions, the expression of S100β in BoNT/A-injected nerves does not differ from saline-injected nerves, also in Cobianchi et al. [30].

After damage to the PNS, spinal microglia cell density increases through the migration of these cells from other sites and through local proliferation. In response to traumatic nerve injury, microglia exhibit variable alterations in function and morphology, from a resting state, where the cell body is small with long and thin processes, into an activated state, in which cells present an amoeboid form [31]. Microglial recruitment and activation in spinal cord is accompanied by proliferation and activation of astrocytes. Compared with the microglial response, astrocyte proliferation begins relatively late, progresses slowly, and is sustained for a longer period [32].

By IF analysis, we revealed that, compared to CCI-saline mice, CCI-B7.5 mice displayed no difference in the expression of resting and phosphorylated microglia, both in dorsal and ventral horns. On the other hand, in CCI-B7.5 mice, the toxin exerted a strong effect on the astrocytes of dorsal horn, resulting in lower abundance and activation. Unlike dorsal horn, in ipsilateral ventral horn of CCI-B7.5 mice, astrocytes, even if decreased in number, showed still a strong activation, as indicated by the intense expression of phosphorylated astrocytes and by their morphology.

Previous studies have already shown that, after ligature of sciatic nerve, glial activation in spinal cord can be reduced by peripheral administration of BoNT/A [13]. In fact, Vacca et al. [33] have shown that treatment with BoNT/A induces significant reduction of activated and not activated glial cells (both microglia and astrocytes) in dorsal and ventral horns of mice. This effect can be explained by indirect but also by direct action of BoNT/A on spinal cord. Marinelli and colleagues [12] showed that BoNT/A, injected into plantar surface of injured paws of CCI-mice, is transported from the peripheral nerve endings to the spinal cord, where it can be transcytosed by nociceptive fibers to astroglial cells.

Our results showed that, as BoNT/A, also BoNT/B might act at both peripheral and central levels. Previous studies have already suggested possible transsynaptic/transcytotic effects of ipl BoNT/B, which would be transported centrally to inhibit spinal activation and affect nociceptive processes [17,18].

The target of enzymatic activity for BoNT/B, i.e., the protein VAMP2, was found expressed in sensory neurons located in laminae I-VI and X of the spinal cord [34,35]. Analgesic effect of BoNT/B observed in the behavioral tests may be explained by considering its proteolytic activity on VAMP2 protein, which blocks the release of excitatory substances from primary afferents of dorsal horn neurons. Moreover, a contribution to the analgesic effect of BoNT/B may be due to the reduction of astrogliosis at the dorsal horn of spinal cord in CCI-B7.5 mice, as already reported for BoNT/A [33]. In particular, a possible direct action of BoNT/B on dorsal horn astrocytes, probably by transcytosis, could inhibit the glutamate release from astroglial cells and, consequently, contribute to the reduction of pain. Effectively, the possibility that BoNTs can be transcytosed to astrocytes has been already suggested, at least for BoNT/A [23], as it has also been demonstrated, the ability of BoNT/B to inhibit the release of glutamate by astrocyte cultures [36].

In conclusion, results of IF experiments associated with behavioral and functional data indicate that BoNT/B exerts analgesic effects on allodynia, similarly to BoNT/A, but does not exert beneficial action on functional recovery of the injured hindlimb, reproducing only some of the effects induced by BoNT/A on structural alterations in CCI-injured nerves. Finally, at spinal cord level, reactive astrogliosis is still present in ventral horns of CCI-B7.5 mice, where terminals of motoneurons are prevalently localized, an effect that could contribute to the impairment of functional recovery.

Although further research will be needed to clarify and better understand the molecular mechanism underlying the different effects of BoNT/A and BoNT/B in neuropathic pain, data presented in this study show clearly that the two botulinum serotypes are not fully interchangeable. This result is particularly relevant in view of a therapeutic approach aimed at neutralizing the neuropathy induced by peripheral nerve injury; in fact, while both toxins are able to act as analgesics, BoNT/B, differently from BoNT/A, does not induce a parallel acceleration of functional recovery of the injured limb.

4. Materials and Methods

4.1. Animals

CD1 male mice (Charles River, Como, Italy) were used in the present study. Upon arrival, the animals were housed in groups of four in standard breeding cages (21 × 21 × 12 cm), at constant temperature (22 ± 1 °C), under 12 h light/dark cycle (07:00 a.m.–07:00 p.m.), with food and water ad libitum. At the time of surgery, they were approximately 3 months old and weighed 40–45 g. Experiments were carried out from 10:00 a.m. to 02:00 p.m. Experimenters were blind with regard to which treatment group each subject belonged. All the experiments were conducted in accordance with the Italian National Law (DL 26/2014), with the European Union Council Directive of 22 September 2010 (2010/63/EU), with the NIH guidelines on animal care, and with the ethical guidelines of the Committee for Research and Ethical Issues of IASP [37].

4.2. Surgical Procedure

Following the procedure originally proposed by Bennett and Xie [38], adapted to mice, CCI of sciatic nerve was used as model of peripheral nerve injury that can evoke neuropathic pain symptoms. Surgery was performed under anesthesia induced by intraperitoneal (ip) injection of a mixture of ketamine (100 mg/kg) and xylazine (5 mg/kg) purchased from Sigma-Aldrich (St. Louis, MO, USA). The CCI was obtained by means of three unilateral ligatures of sciatic nerve. The middle third of the right sciatic nerve was exposed through a 1.5 cm longitudinal skin incision. Three ligatures (7-0 prolene, Ethicon) were tied loosely around the nerve. The wound was then closed with silk suture (4-0 vicryl, Ethicon) and the mouse was allowed to recover in a heated cage until all reflexes were normalized. The injured and uninjured hindpaws were named as ipsilateral and contralateral hindpaws, respectively.

4.3. Pharmacological Treatments and Experimental Groups

Isolated and purified 150 kDa di-chain BoNT/A and /B were a kind gift from Prof. C. Montecucco and Prof. O. Rossetto (University of Padova). The toxins were frozen in liquid nitrogen and stored at −80 °C in 10 mM NaHEPES, 150 mM NaCl, pH 7.2. Stock solutions were tested for activity in the ex vivo mouse hemidiaphragm model, and in the in vitro cleavage of SNAP-25 for BoNT/A and

VAMP/synaptobrevin for BoNT/B, respectively. Injectable solutions of BoNTs were freshly made by dilution in saline (0.9% NaCl).

After verification of the onset of neuropathy at day 3 post CCI (D3), CCI mice were randomly assigned to different groups according to their experimental use. At D5, selected solutions of BoNTs (BoNT/B = 5 or 7.5 pg/mouse, indicated as B5 or B7.5, respectively; BoNT/A = 15 pg/mouse, indicated as A15) or saline (0.9% NaCl) were ipl injected into plantar surface of the injured hindpaw. Doses of BoNT/A and /B were chosen on the basis of neurotoxicity (LD50: 0.5–1.0 $\times$ 10^{-6} mg/kg) and previous studies [11,19,39,40]. These studies showed that BoNT/B is more toxic than BoNT/A (see also [41]), therefore, doses of BoNT/B higher than 7.5 pg/paw were not tested. Behavioral investigations were carried out in CCI-saline, CCI-B5, and CCI-B7.5 mice (n = 10 mice/group). Immunofluorescence (IF) analysis was carried out on sciatic nerve of naïve, CCI-saline, CCI-B7.5 and, for comparison, on nerves of CCI-A15 mice (n = 3 mice/group), and on spinal cord of CCI-saline and CCI-B7.5 mice (n = 3 mice/group).

4.4. Behavioral Tests

4.4.1. Measurement of Mechanical Nociceptive Threshold

The onset of CCI-induced neuropathy was assessed by measuring the threshold of both hindpaws to normally non-noxious punctuate mechanical stimuli. The hindpaw nociceptive threshold, measured by an automatic von Frey apparatus (Dynamic Plantar Aesthesiometer, Ugo Basile, Italy), was expressed as the force (in grams) at which mice withdrew their paws in response to the mechanical stimulus. For habituation, mice were placed in plastic cages with a wire net floor 5 min before the experiment. The mechanical stimulus was applied to the mid-plantar surface of the hindpaw to induce a slight pressure to the skin. At each testing day, ipsi- and contralateral withdrawal thresholds were taken as mean of three consecutive measurements per paw with 10 s interval between each measurement. Mice were tested each day from D3 to D7, every two days from D10 to D21, and every ten days from D31 to D101.

4.4.2. Measurement of Weight Bearing

Weight bearing on the two hindlimbs was determined by incapacitance test (Linton Instrumentation, Norfolk, UK). The apparatus used was adapted for mice with a strain gauge/amplifier resolution of 0.03 g, and a strain gauge/amplifier accuracy of 0.1 g. Mice were carefully placed in an angled Plexiglas chamber positioned with hindpaws on the two separate force plates. Care was taken to ensure that the animal weight was directed onto the force plates, and not dissipated through the walls of the chamber. The force exerted by each hindlimb (measured in grams) was automatically averaged over a 5 s period and, for each animal, measurement was repeated three times with 5 min interval. Mice were tested the same day of the measurement of mechanical nociceptive, with weight bearing performed before and with 1 h of rest between the two tests. The weight bearing was calculated by the equation

$$[\text{ipsilateral weight}/(\text{ipsilateral weight} + \text{contralateral weight})] \times 100$$

4.4.3. Walking Footprint Analysis and Sciatic Static Index

The gradual recovery of the paw functionality was monitored by analyzing individual free-walking patterns and by measuring several footprint parameters to calculate the sciatic static index (SSI). Footprints were recorded by dipping in black ink the hindpaws of mice and leaving them to freely walk along a Perspex runaway corridor (15 $\times$ 5 $\times$ 50 cm) lined with white paper. Footprint parameters were calculated from at least five footprints recorded on three different walking track runaways. Mice were tested at D11, D19, and every ten days from D32 to D102. SSI was evaluated using the equation proposed by Baptista et al. [42]:

$$SSI = +101.3 \times (ITS\text{-}CTS)/CTS - 54.03 \times (IPL\text{-}CPL)/CPL - 9.5$$

considering ITS and CTS as the toe spreads, i.e., the distance between 1st to 5th digit, of the ipsilateral and contralateral hindpaw, and IPL and CPL as the paw length, i.e., the distance between the tip of the third toe and the most posterior aspect of the ipsilateral and contralateral hindpaw. Based on this equation, a value of SSI close to 0 corresponds to normal function, while a value close to −100 is equivalent to complete functional loss.

4.5. *Immunohistochemistry Assays*

4.5.1. Immunostaining of Sciatic Nerve

At D7, mice assigned to sciatic nerve immunostaining were anaesthetized with a mixture of ketamine (100 mg/kg, ip) and xylazine (5 mg/kg, ip) purchased from Sigma-Aldrich (St. Louis, MO, USA) and the lesioned part of the ipsilateral sciatic nerve, including ligatures, were removed immediately before perfusion and kept in immersion for 48 h in paraformaldehyde (PFA; Sigma-Aldrich, Milan, Italy) 4% in 0.1 M phosphate-buffer saline (PBS; Sigma-Aldrich, Milan, Italy), pH 7.2, room temperature. Nerves were cryoprotected with a solution of 30% (w/v) sucrose in PBS, then stored at −80 °C until sectioning.

Longitudinal sections (25 µm thick) of sciatic nerves segment, including the portion with ligature, were cut on cryostat microtome and mounted directly on slides. For IF staining, sciatic nerves sections were washed three times in PBS, and then incubated overnight in Triton (0.3% in PBS; Sigma-Aldrich) with the following primary antibodies in different combinations: mouse anti-GFAP (monoclonal; 1:100; Sigma-Aldrich); rabbit anti-PMP22 (polyclonal; 1:100; Sigma-Aldrich); chicken anti-P0 (polyclonal; 1:100; Millipore, Vimodrone, Italy); rabbit anti-NF200 (polyclonal; 1:100; Sigma-Aldrich); mouse anti-S100β (polyclonal; 1:100; Sigma-Aldrich); rat anti-CD11b (monoclonal; 1:100; Bio-Rad, Segrate, Italy); mouse anti-CC1 (monoclonal; 1:100; Santa Cruz, Segrate, Italy). Afterwards, sections were washed three times with PBS, and incubated for 2 h at room temperature, in Triton with one of the following secondary antibodies: donkey anti-mouse fluorescein-conjugated (FITC; 1:100; Jackson ImmunoResearch, West Grove, PA, USA); goat anti-rabbit fluorescein-conjugated (FITC; 1:100; Santa Cruz); goat anti-rabbit rhodamine-conjugated (TRITC; 1:100; Jackson ImmunoResearch); donkey anti-chicken rhodamine-conjugated (TRITC; 1:100; Jackson ImmunoResearch). Sections were washed three times in PBS, incubated in PBS with the nuclear marker Hoechst 33258 (1:1000; Sigma-Aldrich) for 5 min, washed again three times in PBS, mounted with glycerol/PBS 3:1 mounting medium, and cover slipped.

4.5.2. Immunostaining of Spinal Cord

At D7, mice assigned for spinal cord immunostaining were anaesthetized with chloral hydrate (500 mg/kg ip; Sigma-Aldrich, Italy) and transcardiacally perfused with saline (100 mL) followed by PFA (100 mL). After perfusion, the entire spinal cord of each animal was removed and kept in PFA for 24 h. Spinal cords were cryoprotected with a solution of 30% (w/v) sucrose in PBS, then stored at −80 °C until sectioning.

Transverse sections (40 µm thick) of L4/L5 spinal cord segment were cut on a cryostat microtome and collected in PBS for free-floating double IF procedures. Ipsi- and contralateral side of sections were recognized by marking the spinal cord with a notch on the contralateral side before mounting spinal cord trunk on the chuck of the cryostat. Sections were first incubated overnight in Triton with different combinations of the following primary antibodies: mouse anti-GFAP (monoclonal; 1:100; Sigma-Aldrich); rat anti-CD11b (monoclonal; 1:100; Bio-Rad); rabbit anti-p-p38 (polyclonal; 1:100; Santa Cruz). Afterward, sections were washed three times in PBS, and incubated for 2 h at room temperature in Triton, with one of the following secondary antibodies: donkey anti-mouse or anti-rat fluorescein-conjugated (FITC; 1:100; Jackson ImmunoResearch); goat anti-rabbit rhodamine-conjugated (TRITC; 1:100; Jackson ImmunoResearch). Sections were washed three times in PBS, incubated in PBS with the nuclear marker Hoechst 33258 (DAPI; 1:1000; Sigma-Aldrich) for 5 min, washed again three times in PBS, mounted on slides with glycerol/PBS 3:1, and cover slipped.

4.5.3. Confocal IF Analysis

Low (10×) magnification images of spinal cord sections, and high (63×) magnification images of spinal cord and sciatic nerve sections, were captured by laser scanning confocal microscopy (TCS SP5 microscope, Leica Microsystem, Buccinasco, Italy) connected to digital camera diagnostic instruments operated by I.A.S. software (Delta Systems, Bergamo, Italy).

In sciatic nerve sections, only the part of nerve including the ligature was used. The analysis of IF staining (in term of emitted fluorescence) was performed by using the ImageJ software (version 1.41, National Institutes of Health, Bethesda, MA, USA). The fluorescence was quantified with RGB (red, green, blue) method, which uses brightness values for calculation [43]. The IF images were analyzed in three mice, considering three nerve sections per mouse.

In spinal cord sections, to quantify glial cells immunoreactivity (IR), IF images of the ipsilateral side of the dorsal horn (medial portion of laminae I–IV) and ventral horn (dorsolateral column, lamina IX) from three spinal cord sections per mouse were examined. Quantification was performed using the ImageJ software. Image contrast was adjusted such that the background level just disappeared, and the cell bodies and processes appeared without boundaries; the same cutoff level was used for all images. To quantify GFAP and CD11b IR-cells, and their colocalization with p-p38, the number of positive cells was counted in three mice, considering three spinal cord sections per mouse.

4.6. Data Analysis

Data are expressed as mean ± SEM. Statistical analysis of results from behavioral analysis was performed by two-way ANOVA for repeated measure, followed by Tukey–Kramer post hoc comparison. Statistical analysis of results from RGB pixels analysis of IF were performed by one-way ANOVA followed by Fisher PLSD post hoc comparison.

Acknowledgments: This publication was made possible thanks to the cooperation with the Regione Lazio, as part of the "Distretto Tecnologico delle Bioscienze" and supported by FILAS Regione Lazio Funds for "Sviluppo della Ricerca sul Cervello". V.V. was supported by a fellowship from "Fondazione Umberto Veronesi". We thank the Animal Facility of the CNR/IRCCS Santa Lucia Foundation.

Author Contributions: F.P. conceived the experiments; A.F., S.M., F.D.A. and V.V. designed the experiments; A.F., F.D.A. performed the experiments; A.F. and S.L. analyzed the data; S.L., F.P. and S.M. contributed reagents/materials/analysis tools; S.L. and F.P. wrote the paper.

Conflicts of Interest: The authors declare no conflict of interest.

References

1. Cairns, B.E.; Gazerani, P. Botulinum neurotoxin A for chronic migraine headaches: Does it work and how? *Pain Manag.* **2014**, *4*, 377–380. [CrossRef] [PubMed]
2. Luvisetto, S.; Gazerani, P.; Cianchetti, C.; Pavone, F. Botulinum toxin type A as a therapeutic agent against headache and related disorders. *Toxins* **2015**, *7*, 3818–3844. [CrossRef] [PubMed]
3. Matak, I.; Lackovic, Z. Botulinum toxin A, brain and pain. *Prog. Neurobiol.* **2014**, *119–120*, 39–59. [CrossRef] [PubMed]
4. Pellett, S.; Yaksh, T.L.; Ramachandran, R. Current status and future directions of botulinum neurotoxins for targeting pain processing. *Toxins* **2015**, *7*, 4519–4563. [CrossRef] [PubMed]
5. Rossetto, O.; Pirazzini, M.; Montecucco, C. Botulinum neurotoxins: Genetic, structural and mechanistic insights. *Nat. Rev. Microbiol.* **2014**, *12*, 535–549. [CrossRef] [PubMed]

6. Rossetto, O.; Pirazzini, M.; Montecucco, C. Current gaps in basic science knowledge of botulinum neurotoxin biological actions. *Toxicon* **2015**, *107*, 59–63. [CrossRef] [PubMed]
7. Montecucco, C.; Rasotto, M.B. On botulinum neurotoxin variability. *MBio* **2015**, *6*, e02131-14. [CrossRef] [PubMed]
8. Han, J.; Pluhackova, K.; Böckmann, R.A. The Multifaceted Role of SNARE Proteins in Membrane Fusion. *Front. Physiol.* **2017**, *8*, 5. [CrossRef] [PubMed]
9. Schiavo, G.; Matteoli, M.; Montecucco, C. Neurotoxins affecting neuroexocytosis. *Physiol. Rev.* **2000**, *80*, 717–766. [CrossRef] [PubMed]
10. Luvisetto, S.; Marinelli, S.; Cobianchi, S.; Pavone, F. Anti-allodynic efficacy of botulinum neurotoxin A in a model of neuropathic pain. *Neuroscience* **2007**, *145*, 1–4. [CrossRef] [PubMed]
11. Marinelli, S.; Luvisetto, S.; Cobianchi, S.; Makuch, W.; Obara, I.; Mezzaroma, E.; Caruso, M.; Straface, E.; Przewlocka, B.; Pavone, F. Botulinum neurotoxin type A counteracts neuropathic pain and facilitates functional recovery after peripheral nerve injury in animal models. *Neuroscience* **2010**, *171*, 316–328. [CrossRef] [PubMed]
12. Marinelli, S.; Vacca, V.; Ricordy, R.; Uggenti, C.; Tata, A.M.; Luvisetto, S.; Pavone, F. The analgesic effect on neuropathic pain of retrogradely transported botulinum neurotoxin A involves Schwann cells and astrocytes. *PLoS ONE* **2012**, *7*, e47977. [CrossRef] [PubMed]
13. Mika, J.; Rojewska, E.; Makuch, W.; Korostynski, M.; Luvisetto, S.; Marinelli, S.; Pavone, F.; Przewlocka, B. The effect of botulinum neurotoxin A on sciatic nerve injury-induced neuroimmunological changes in rat dorsal root ganglia and spinal cord. *Neuroscience* **2011**, *175*, 358–366. [CrossRef] [PubMed]
14. Zychowska, M.; Rojewska, E.; Makuch, W.; Luvisetto, S.; Pavone, F.; Marinelli, S.; Przewlocka, B.; Mika, J. Participation of pro- and anti-nociceptive interleukins in botulinum toxin A-induced analgesia in a rat model of neuropathic pain. *Eur. J. Pharmacol.* **2016**, *791*, 377–388. [CrossRef] [PubMed]
15. Chen, S. Clinical uses of botulinum neurotoxins: Current indications, limitations and future developments. *Toxins* **2012**, *4*, 913–939. [CrossRef] [PubMed]
16. Bentivoglio, A.R.; Del Grande, A.; Petracca, M.; Ialongo, T.; Ricciardi, L. Clinical differences between botulinum neurotoxin type A and B. *Toxicon* **2015**, *107*, 77–84. [CrossRef] [PubMed]
17. Sikandar, S.; Gustavsson, Y.; Marino, M.J.; Dickenson, A.H.; Yaksh, T.L.; Sorkin, L.S.; Ramachandran, R. Effects of intraplantar botulinum toxin-B on carrageenan-induced changes in nociception and spinal phosphorylation of GluA1 and Akt. *Eur. J. Neurosci.* **2016**, *44*, 1714–1722. [CrossRef] [PubMed]
18. Marino, M.J.; Terashima, T.; Steinauer, J.J.; Eddinger, K.A.; Yaksh, T.L.; Xu, Q. Botulinum toxin B in the sensory afferent: Transmitter release, spinal activation, and pain behavior. *Pain* **2014**, *155*, 674–684. [CrossRef] [PubMed]
19. Luvisetto, S.; Marinelli, S.; Lucchetti, F.; Marchi, F.; Cobianchi, S.; Rossetto, O.; Montecucco, C.; Pavone, F. Botulinum neurotoxins and formalin-induced pain: Central vs. peripheral effects in mice. *Brain Res.* **2006**, *1082*, 124–131. [CrossRef] [PubMed]
20. Huang, P.P.; Khan, I.; Suhail, M.S.; Malkmus, S.; Yaksh, T.L. Spinal botulinum neurotoxin B: Effects on afferent transmitter release and nociceptive processing. *PLoS ONE* **2011**, *6*, e19126.
21. Park, H.J.; Marino, M.J.; Rondon, E.S.; Xu, Q.; Yaksh, T.L. The effects of intraplantar and intrathecal botulinum toxin type B on tactile allodynia in mono and polyneuropathy in the mouse. *Anesth. Analg.* **2015**, *121*, 229–238. [CrossRef] [PubMed]
22. Pavone, F.; Ueda, I. Is BoNT/B useful for pain treatment? *Pain* **2014**, *155*, 649–650. [CrossRef] [PubMed]
23. Dubový, P. Wallerian Degeneration and Peripheral Nerve Conditions for Both Axonal Regeneration and Neuropathic Pain Induction. *Ann. Anat.* **2011**, *193*, 267–275. [CrossRef] [PubMed]
24. Vargas, M.E.; Barres, B.A. Why Is Wallerian Degeneration in the CNS So Slow? *Annu. Rev. Neurosci.* **2007**, *30*, 153–179. [CrossRef] [PubMed]
25. Thacker, M.A.; Clark, A.K.; Marchand, F.; McMahon, S.B. Pathophysiology of peripheral neuropathic pain: Immune cells and molecules. *Anesth. Analg.* **2007**, *105*, 838–847. [CrossRef] [PubMed]
26. Pavone, F.; Luvisetto, S. Botulinum neurotoxin for pain management: Insights from animal models. *Toxins* **2010**, *2*, 2890–2913. [CrossRef] [PubMed]
27. Perry, V.H.; Brown, M.C. Macrophages and nerve regeneration. *Curr. Opin. Neurobiol.* **1992**, *2*, 679–682. [CrossRef]

28. Barrette, B.; Hébert, M.A.; Filali, M.; Lafortune, K.; Vallières, N.; Gowing, G.; Julien, J.P.; Lacroix, S. Requirement of Myeloid Cells for Axon Regeneration. *J. Neurosci.* **2008**, *28*, 9363–9376. [CrossRef] [PubMed]
29. Moalem, G.; Tracey, D.J. Immune and inflammatory mechanisms in neuropathic pain. *Brain Res. Rev.* **2006**, *51*, 240–264. [CrossRef] [PubMed]
30. Cobianchi, S.; Jaramillo, J.; Luvisetto, S.; Pavone, F.; Navarro, X. Botulinum neurotoxin A promotes functional recovery after peripheral nerve injury by increasing regeneration of myelinated fibers. *Neuroscience* **2017**, *359*, 82–91. [CrossRef] [PubMed]
31. Calvo, M.; Bennett, D.L. The mechanisms of microgliosis and pain following peripheral nerve injury. *Exp. Neurol.* **2012**, *234*, 271–282. [CrossRef] [PubMed]
32. Scholz, J.; Woolf, C.J. The Neuropathic Pain Triad: Neurons, Immune Cells and Glia. *Nat. Neurosci.* **2007**, *10*, 1361–1368. [CrossRef] [PubMed]
33. Vacca, V.; Marinelli, S.; Luvisetto, S.; Pavone, F. Botulinum toxin A increases analgesic effects of morphine, counters development of morphine tolerance and modulates glia activation and μ opioid receptor expression in neuropathic mice. *Brain Behav. Immun.* **2013**, *32*, 40–50. [CrossRef] [PubMed]
34. Jacobsson, G.; Piehl, F.; Meister, B. VAMP-1 and VAMP-2 Gene Expression in Rat Spinal Motoneurones: Differential Regulation after Neuronal Injury. *Eur. J. Neurosci.* **1998**, *10*, 301–316. [CrossRef] [PubMed]
35. Li, J.Y.; Edelmann, L.; Jahn, R.; Dahlström, A. Axonal transport and distribution of synaptobrevin I and II in the rat peripheral nervous system. *J. Neurosci.* **1996**, *16*, 137–147. [PubMed]
36. Jeftinija, S.D.; Jeftinija, K.V.; Stefanovic, G. Cultured astrocytes express proteins involved in vesicular glutamate release. *Brain Res.* **1997**, *750*, 41–47. [CrossRef]
37. Zimmermann, M. Ethical guidelines for investigations of experimental pain in conscious animals. *Pain* **1983**, *16*, 109–110. [CrossRef]
38. Bennett, G.J.; Xie, Y.K. A peripheral mononeuropathy in rat that produces disorders of pain sensation like those seen in man. *Pain* **1988**, *33*, 87–107. [CrossRef]
39. Luvisetto, S.; Rossetto, O.; Montecucco, C.; Pavone, F. Toxicity of botulinum neurotoxins in central nervous system of mice. *Toxicon* **2003**, *41*, 475–481. [CrossRef]
40. Luvisetto, S.; Marinelli, S.; Rossetto, O.; Montecucco, C.; Pavone, F. Central injection of botulinum neurotoxins: Behavioural effects in mice. *Behav. Pharmacol.* **2004**, *15*, 233–240. [CrossRef] [PubMed]
41. Aoki, K.R. A comparison of the safety margins of botulinum neurotoxin serotypes A, B, and F in mice. *Toxicon* **2001**, *39*, 1815–1820. [CrossRef]
42. Baptista, A.F.; Gomes, J.R.; Oliveira, J.T.; Santos, S.M.; Vannier-Santos, M.A.; Martinez, A.M. A New Approach to Assess Function after Sciatic Nerve Lesion in the Mouse—Adaptation of the Sciatic Static Index. *J. Neurosci. Meth.* **2007**, *161*, 259–264. [CrossRef] [PubMed]
43. Fu, Y.; Lam, A.; Sato, I.; Okabe, T.; Sato, Y. Reflectance and Fluorescence Spectral Recovery via Actively Lit RGB Images. *IEEE Trans. Pattern Anal. Mach. Intell.* **2016**, *38*, 1313–1326. [CrossRef] [PubMed]

toxins

MDPI

Review

Botulinum Toxin Type A—A Modulator of Spinal Neuron–Glia Interactions under Neuropathic Pain Conditions

Ewelina Rojewska, Anna Piotrowska, Katarzyna Popiolek-Barczyk and Joanna Mika *

Department of Pain Pharmacology Institute of Pharmacology, Polish Academy of Sciences, 31-343 Krakow, Poland; rojewska@if-pan.krakow.pl (E.R.); anna.piotrowskamurzyn@gmail.com (A.P.); popiolek@if-pan.krakow.pl (K.P.-B.)

* Correspondence: joasia272@onet.eu

Received: 9 March 2018; Accepted: 30 March 2018; Published: 2 April 2018

Abstract: Neuropathic pain represents a significant clinical problem because it is a chronic condition often refractory to available therapy. Therefore, there is still a strong need for new analgesics. Botulinum neurotoxin A (BoNT/A) is used to treat a variety of clinical diseases associated with pain. Glia are in continuous bi-directional communication with neurons to direct the formation and refinement of synaptic connectivity. This review addresses the effects of BoNT/A on the relationship between glia and neurons under neuropathic pain. The inhibitory action of BoNT/A on synaptic vesicle fusion that blocks the release of miscellaneous pain-related neurotransmitters is known. However, increasing evidence suggests that the analgesic effect of BoNT/A is mediated through neurons and glial cells, especially microglia. In vitro studies provide evidence that BoNT/A exerts its anti-inflammatory effect by diminishing NF-κB, p38 and ERK1/2 phosphorylation in microglia and directly interacts with Toll-like receptor 2 (TLR2). Furthermore, BoNT/A appears to have no more than a slight effect on astroglia. The full activation of TLR2 in astroglia appears to require the presence of functional TLR4 in microglia, emphasizing the significant interaction between those cell types. In this review, we discuss whether and how BoNT/A affects the spinal neuron–glia interaction and reduces the development of neuropathy.

Keywords: BoNT/A; astroglia; interleukins; microglia; TLR2; TLR4; Snap-23

---

1. The Therapeutic Effect of Bont/A—Powerful Analgesic Agent against Neuropathic Pain

Neuropathic pain is caused by damage or injury to the nerves, and it is commonly experienced in the human and animal populations, involving a huge number of pathological conditions. Recent clinical and experimental research has shown that neuroimmune factors significantly influence the modulation of the pain development process [1–4]. The mechanism of the development and persistence of chronic pain remains an important clinical problem. Current knowledge does not allow us to fully assess the process and identify its most crucial elements. As suggested by data available from the International Association for the Study of Pain, one out of every five Europeans suffers from chronic pain of various origins and must make lifestyle changes for that reason. An additional problem is posed by the lack of appropriate therapy for these disorders. The treatment of neuropathic pain is a therapeutic challenge, and many pharmacological and non-pharmacological interventions have been suggested, with unsatisfying results [5–9]. Pharmacological medicaments include non-steroidal anti-inflammatory drugs, antidepressants, anticonvulsants, and opioids [6]. However, their use increases the risk of adverse events, as well as reductions in analgesic efficacy. The mechanism of this loss in efficacy is also not sufficiently understood to fully counteract this phenomenon and effectively treat pain. More effective treatments based on new targets and mechanisms of action are still being sought. This is the case for botulinum toxin A (BoNT/A), the use and application of which is increasing and becoming more widespread with time. BoNT/A is one of seven different BoNT types originating from *Clostridium botulinum* and is the most poisonous substance known to man [10], but, paradoxically, it has been widely used in the clinic, and its importance as a therapeutic agent is rising [11–18]. The well-defined mechanism of BoNT/A action is based on preventing release of the neurotransmitter acetylcholine from presynaptic nerve terminals through fragmentation of the protein SNAP-25 [19]. BoNT/A inhibits the release not only of acetylcholine but also of other neurotransmitters and neuropeptides, such as substance P and the calcitonin gene-related peptide (CGRP) [20–22]. The toxin also blocks conductivity in the autonomic system through sensory fibers and reduces the majority of substances acting on nociceptors [23]. Therefore, scientists are using it for clinical applications, including therapy for neuropathic pain.

BoNT/A has been used in medical practice since 1989, when it was first included in the medication list by The Food and Drug Administration in the United States. A year later, the report of the American Academy of Neurology stated that BoNT/A injections are efficient in treating blepharospasms, facial spasticity, tremor, hyperhidrosis, hypersalivation, and wrinkle correction [24]. The evidence for the efficacy of BoNT/A in neuropathic pain relief in humans was first presented by Klein in 2004 [25] in relation to neuropathic pain linked to multiple sclerosis, neuralgia and peripheral neuropathy. BoNT/A has been successfully used in clinical practice for the treatment of many types of headaches [16,26], migraine [14,27,28], arthritic pain [29], cerebral palsy with serious acute sialadenitis [29], and recently also in small-fiber neuropathy [30], trigeminal neuralgia [11,17,31] and refractory joint pain [18]. Presently, BoNT/A usage has been extended to many medical conditions, including in urological, gastroenterological, and surgical contexts [32]. BoNT/A is often used to reduce spasticity in a neurorehabilitation setting and to treat other disorders, including complex regional pain syndrome with focal dystonia and phantom limb [12,13]. Many papers suggest that the use of BoNT/A represents a novel therapeutic strategy, especially for neuropathic pain, whenever widely use pharmacological agents have been ineffective [29,30,33]. Animal studies, including ours, support the clinical observations [31,34–39]. Interestingly, BoNT/A also increases morphine-induced analgesia and prevents the development of morphine tolerance upon long-term treatment [40,41]. Despite its wide application in medicine, its mechanisms of action are still not fully understood. Several lines of evidence indicate the crucial role of neuron–glia interactions in the development and progression of neuropathic pain. Since an analgesic action of BoNT/A has been demonstrated, the question concerning the role of this toxin in the modulation of neuron–glia interactions arises. This review addresses the effects of BoNT/A on the relationship between glial and neuronal cells in treating neuropathic pain.

2. Mechanism-Based Evidence for the Analgesic Actions of Bont/A

The peripheral sensory neurons conduct nociceptive information, which enters the spinal cord dorsal horn and then from the spinal projection is conveyed to supraspinal structures (such as the brainstem, thalamus, somatosensory cortex, insular cortex and anterior cingulate cortex) via ascending pathways. Nerve injury form pre- and postsynaptic long-term plasticity within the brain structures, which contributes to emotional and motivational aspects of neuropathic pain condition. Studies using human brain imaging and genetically modified mice have shown that neuropathy is largely due to long-term plastic changes within the sensory pathways [42,43]. In the nervous system, neuronal activity is mediated by synaptic release of neurotransmitters. Under resting conditions, synaptic vesicles are delivered to plasma membrane and may undergo constitutive exocytosis after fusion with newly synthesized proteins in the membrane without uniquely identifiable regulators [44–46]. In contrast to constitutive the regulated exocytosis is under the strict control of calcium signals present only in activated neurons experiencing a rise in calcium concentration. During this process, the probability of vesicle fusion rises dramatically by increasement of cytosolic calcium level, which is caused by the opening of voltage-gated calcium channels in response to the presence of an action potential at a nerve terminal [19,47,48]. In vivo studies showed that fast-regulated exocytosis requires the interaction of a members of protein superfamily, called SNAREs (soluble *N*-ethylmaleimide-sensitive factor attachment protein receptors), which are small cytoplasmically exposed membrane proteins. In regulated exocytosis, relevant SNAREs include synaptobrevin/VAMP (located on the membrane of the vesicle) and syntaxin-1 and SNAP-25 and/or its analogue SNAP-23 (localized on the plasma membrane), which create a complex representing the minimal mechanism required for fusion [49]. Increased calcium concentration (caused by calcium influx through voltage-gated calcium channels), is detected by synaptotagmin, and triggers fusion of docked synaptic vesicles, resulting in neurotransmitter release. Fusion is driven by a progressive zippering of vesicle and SNAREs proteins to form a strong four-helix bundle. Thus, the assembly of a SNARE complex represents crucial steps for nociceptive transmission between neuronal cells in the presence of neuropathic pain. Blockage of synaptic neurotransmission is strictly due to an inhibition of neurotransmitter release via vesicle-regulated exocytosis, and BoNT/A represents a powerful tool for the investigation of the involvement of SNAREs in exocytosis [35,50].

The involvement of BoNT/A in pain modulation mechanisms was first described by Cui et al., 2004 [51], who studied the effects of this toxin in inflammatory pain caused by formalin administration. Acting via SNAP-25, BoNT/A strongly inhibits the neuronal release of neurotransmitters and neuropeptides involved in nociceptive transmission, such as glutamate [51], substance P [20] and CGRP [21,52]. The authors demonstrated that single subcutaneous administration of BoNT/A into the paw after formalin injection reduced paw swelling and hypersensitivity to pain, and this effect was associated with inhibition of pronociceptive factors. In 2006, Luvisetto et al. [53], using a murine model of inflammatory pain, demonstrated that BoNT/A may act not only on the peripheral but also on the central nervous system (CNS). The analgesic effect of BoNT/A was also demonstrated in other inflammatory pain models, such as administration of carrageenan and capsaicin into the paw [34]. The authors suggested that intraarticular administration of BoNT/A is a promising method for the treatment of arthritis. The effects of BoNT/A were also studied in visceral pain models; it was also shown that intravenous administration of BoNT/A caused analgesia in an acetic acid-induced bladder pain model in rats [54]. In 2008, Antonucci et al. [55] suggested that the effects of BoNT/A might be due to retrograde transport or to the effect of transcytosis. Beneficial effects of BoNT/A were also observed in numerous clinical studies under neuropathic pain [11–18,30,31,38,39,56,57]. Several studies, including those conducted by our group, have shown that intraplantar injections of BoNT/A are also effective for treating neuropathic pain [31,35,36,38,40,58]. The results showed that BoNT/A diminished neuropathic pain by suppressing the secretion of neurotransmitters from neurons. Interesting results were obtained by the group of Vacca [40,41], who showed that administration of BoNT/A increased morphine antinociceptive action and countered morphine-induced tolerance after chronic treatment. These data suggest that BoNT/A is not only a potent analgesic but might also be useful as a component of multimodal pain therapy.

Attention has been paid to older works showing that radiolabeled BoNT/A injected into the cat gastrocnemius muscle is detected in the spine 24–38 h after administration [59,60]. Antonucci et al. [55] suggested retrograde transport and transcytosis as a mechanism by which BoNT/A acts not only at the administration site but also at the distant areas that project to the infusion region. In 2012, Marinelli et al. [61] used a murine model of neuropathy to demonstrate that BoNT/A injected intraplantarly may migrate from the site of administration into the sciatic nerve, DRG and spinal cord. Evidenced provided by Cui et al. [51] showed that analgesic BoNT/A action is correlated with modulation of central sensitization process, while BoNT/A has no impact on acute pain. Proposed mechanism of BoNT/A action is that toxin inhibits the release of neurotransmitters from peripheral nerve endings and reduces peripheral sensitization. Following this process, the afferent input to the spinal cord is damped and central sensitization is reduced, which suggest indirectly role of BoNT/A in this process. However, direct mechanism is also possible, as it was already shown that BoNT/A might be transported via retrograde transport along the nociceptive neurons [55]. Based on those hypotheses, peripherally applied BoNT/A gains access to CNS and directly inhibits neurotransmitters release onto dorsal horn neurons.

In a 2016 paper by Zychowska et al. [39], intraplantar injections of BoNT/A not only relieved neuropathic pain-related behaviours but also restored the neuroimmune balance disturbed after nerve injury. BoNT/A diminished CCI-induced level of IL-1β and IL-18 within the spinal cord and/or the DRG, and in parallel, it enhanced the levels of the anti-nociceptive interleukins IL-1RA and IL-10. Obtained data suggest that BoNT/A, in addition to altering neuronal function, can also influence spinal microglial cells [38,39]; however, it is still unclear whether those BoNT/A actions are mediated in a direct or indirect manner. The latest in vitro research by Piotrowska et al. 2017 [62] shed new light on the analgesic effect of BoNT/A and suggested a possible direct impact of this toxin on microglia in the CNS (Figure 1).

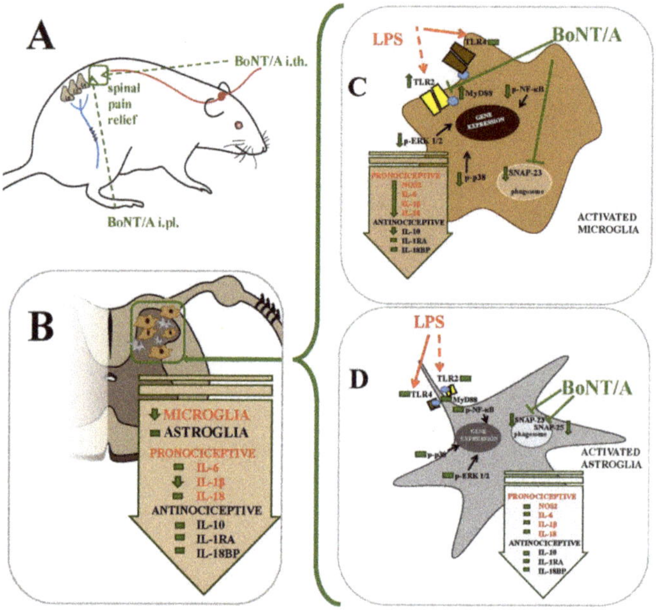

Figure 1. Suggested mechanism of botulinum toxin type A action under neuropathic pain conditions. (**A**) Intrathecal (*i.th.*) as well as intraplantar (*i.pl.*) injections of BoNT/A relief pain in animal models of neuropathy. Recent evidence suggests the possible retrograde transport and transcytosis of BoNT/A, which might be at least partially responsible for its analgesic effect. (**B**) Peripheral administration of BoNT/A reduced spinal microglial, but not astroglial, activation after sciatic nerve injury. (**C**,**D**) The data obtained from in vitro studies revealed that BoNT/A can directly influence microglial cells and it is achieved through the modulation of TLR2 receptor, SNARE proteins and intracellular pathways in microglial cells. BoNT/A diminishes LPS-induced phosphorylation of p38, ERK1/2, and NF-κB and reduces the release of pro-inflammatory factors, such as IL-1β, IL-18, IL-6, and anti-inflammatory IL-10 in microglia. No effects of BoNT/A on astroglia were observed. Mechanism of BoNT/A in glial cells is related to activation of TLRs, type 2 and 4. Complete activation of TLR2 in astroglia requires the presence of the microglial TLR4 receptor. Glial cross-talk may explain the lack of effect of BoNT/A on astroglia and it was suggested that the molecular target of BoNT/A is TLR2. See detailed description in the text **Abbreviations:** SNAP, synaptosomal-associated protein; TLR, Toll-like receptor; MyD, myeloid differentiation primary response gene; ERK1/2, extracellular-signal-regulated kinase 1/2; NF-κB, nuclear factor-κB; NOS2, inducible nitric oxide synthase; IL, interleukin; LPS, lipopolysaccharide, BoNT/A, botulinum toxin serotype A.

3. Far Beyond the Neurons—The Role of Glial Cells in Bont/A-Induced Analgesia

BoNT/A affects both SNAP-25 and -23 in neuronal cells; however, it was recently suggested that BoNT/A is also able to cleave SNAPs in astroglia and microglia [63,64]. Within the CNS, glial cells seem to play a crucial role in neuronal homeostasis [2,4,65,66]. Two main types of glial cells are present: macroglia (which include astroglia, oligodendrocytes and radial cells, including Bergmann and Müller cells) and microglia. Under physiological conditions, glial cells account for 70% of cells, and resting microglia account for only 5–20% of cells [3]. It is now obvious that glial cells are an important component of neural tissue and play a crucial role in the synthesis, release and uptake of many factors. The contribution of astroglia and microglia in the progression of neuropathy is well known [67,68]; however, the role of other macroglial cells (oligodendrocytes and radial cells) is still not well established. Under neuropathic pain, activated astroglia and microglia play a role in synaptic transmission based on the presence of similar receptors, ion channels, transporters and intracellular signaling cascades to neurons [66,68]. Glial cells are also capable of conducting active communication with neighboring neurons by gap junctions [69–71] and synapses [72–74].

Astroglia represent the most abundant cell population in the nervous system and are critical in maintaining the homeostasis of their surrounding environment by regulating the concentrations of the neurotransmitters, ions, and proteins in the synaptic cleft. Activation of astroglia as a result of peripheral neuropathy occurs approximately four days after microglial activation and persists until 12 weeks or longer after the injury, thus suggesting that astroglia are involved in the persistence of pain [68,75,76]. The direct influence of BoNT/A on astroglia was unclear, since the study by Parpura et al. (1995) [64] showed the expression of some of the SNARE protein complexes but not that of SNAP-25. The authors analyzed post-nuclear astroglial cell membrane extract, not the whole lysates as in Piotrowska et al. 2017 [62]. The authors, using in vitro primary cell culture studies, have demonstrated that astroglial cells possess both mRNA and protein for the SNAREs SNAP-25 and SNAP-23 [62]. These data correlate well with the study of Marinelli et al. (2012) [61] showing that BoNT/A exerts analgesic effects on neuropathic pain through the cleavage of SNAP-25 in spinal astroglia. Interestingly, in vitro studies gave evidence that BoNT/A did not influence pro-nociceptive factors (IL-1β, IL-6, IL-18, and NOS2) or anti-nociceptive factors (IL-1RA, IL-10, and IL-18BP) in LPS-stimulated astroglial cell cultures [62] (Figure 1). The authors revealed that BoNT/A does not affect the activation of MAPKs, p38 and ERK1/2, or NF-κB pathways in LPS-treated primary astroglial cell cultures. Moreover, they showed no changes in TLR2 and TLR4 expression, the adaptors for which initiate the activation of NF-κB and MAPK cascades in astroglia, which is required for the production of nociceptive factors [77]. Surprisingly, BoNT/A appears to have no more than a slight direct effect on astroglia.

Recently, some authors have suggested that the molecular mechanism of BoNT/A action involves microglia [38,41]. Microglial cells are highly dynamic immune cells, which are responsible for the maintenance of homeostasis in the CNS [66,78]. They are known to dynamically modulate neuronal functions under neuropathic pain. They are the first cell type to become spinally activated following peripheral nerve injury [76] and remain active for several weeks [66,79–81]. Several reports have provided evidence that inhibitors of microglial activation, such as minocycline, propentofylline, and pentoxifylline, might largely limit the development of neuropathic pain [38,51,78,82–84] and those effects are due to reduced activation of microglial cells, which entails the inhibition of numerous cytokine secretion [85–87]. In 2011, Mika et al. [38] showed that a single intraplantar administration of BoNT/A, after nerve injury, attenuated neuropathic pain-related behaviors in neuropathic rats and, in parallel, reduced spinal microglial activation. The results provide evidence that BoNT/A, in addition to having an impact on neuronal functions, can also influence the activation of microglia; therefore, the involvement of these non-neuronal cells in BoNT/A action should also be regarded. Although in vivo studies have shown that BoNT/A influences the activation of microglial cells in rat and mouse neuropathic pain models [38,41], it was not clear if that occurred in a direct or indirect manner. The well-characterized molecular targets of BoNT/A action are superfamily of SNARE proteins.

The studies of Hepp et al. 1999 [63] suggested that in microglia, SNAP-25 is replaced by SNAP-23. SNAP-23 is structurally and functionally similar to SNAP-25 and binds tightly to multiple syntaxins and synaptobrevins/VAMPs. It is a crucial component of the high-affinity receptor for the general membrane fusion machinery and is an important regulator of transport vesicle docking and fusion. In 2017, Piotrowska et al. [62] using in vitro primary cell culture, demonstrated the presence of both mRNA and protein for SNAP-23, but not for SNAP-25, in microglia. The in vitro studies correspond well with in vivo data obtained by Marinelli et al. (2012) [61], where the authors did not observe staining for cleaved SNAP-25 protein co-localized with microglia. Therefore, it seems that SNAP-23, not SNAP-25, plays an important role in the effects of BoNT/A on microglia.

Zychowska et al. (2016) [39] showed that BoNT/A injection reverts the neuro-immune changes after sciatic nerve injury. In vitro studies with glial cell cultures [62] revealed the inhibitory action of BoNT/A on the intracellular cascades, which is possibly involved in changes in the expression of many nociceptive factors. BoNT/A prevents the LPS-induced upregulation of pro-nociceptive factors (IL-1β, IL-18, NOS2) through the modulation of intracellular pathways activation (NF-κB, p38 and ERK1/2) and increases the expression of TLR2 and its adaptor protein MyD88 in microglia (Figure 1). These results can be compared with those published in 2015 by Kim et al. [88] who showed that BoNT/A inhibited LPS-upregulated NO production in RAW264.7 macrophages by blocking the activation of ERK and p38.

Recently, many papers have shown that the inhibition of the MAPK family members (namely p38 and ERK1/2) leads to lower rates of neuropathy in animal models, down-regulated pro-nociceptive factors and enhanced opioid efficiency [84,89–96]. The in vitro results of Piotrowska et al. (2017) have shown that BoNT/A decreased the LPS-induced activation of p38 and ERK1/2 in microglia; similar results were obtained in the monocyte/macrophage cell line RAW264.7 by Kim et al. (2015) [88]. Many studies have shown an important role for the NF-κB pathway in nociception and microglial cell activation [94–99]. In vitro results of Piotrowska et al. (2017) [62] revealed that BoNT/A reduced NF-κB phosphorylation in LPS-treated microglia. It has been shown that the inhibition of NF-κB with a potent inhibitor, parthenolide, diminished the symptoms of neuropathic pain, and, moreover, it potentiated morphine-induced analgesia and reduced the levels of pro-nociceptive factors produced by microglial cells (such as IL-1β, IL-18, NOS2) [95].

Among the numerous receptors expressed by microglial cells, the family of TLR receptors, especially subtypes 2 and 4, represents a possible link between microglia activation and nerve injury and illustrate an essential role of those cells in the development of neuropathy [100–103]. The TLRs are a type of receptor, which are important for pathogen recognition. Activation of those receptors leads to the initiation of direct antimicrobial pathways, expression of co-stimulatory factors, and release of cytokines via NF-κB and/or MAPK signaling pathways. The TLRs family recognize pathogen-associated molecular patterns (PAMPs), expression of which is characteristic for infectious agents [104,105]. The TLRs can also discern danger-associated molecular patterns (DAMPs), products of nerve injury [106]. It has been confirmed that TLR2 or TLR4 knockout mice have less microglial activation after nerve injury and fewer neuropathic pain symptoms [100,101,103,107]. Piotrowska et al. (2017) [62] revealed that LPS induced a decrease in TLR4 in microglia. Recently, studies using macrophages revealed that BoNT/A is sensed by TLR2, but not by TLR4 [88]. In turn, BoNT/A increased the TLR2 level in LPS-stimulated microglia. It has been demonstrated that TLR4 activation is mediated by dimerization of adaptor proteins (MyD88 or TRIF), but TLR2 uses only MyD88 [108]. Our data have proven that BoNT/A administration rescues downregulated by LPS level of MyD88 in microglia [62]. Recently, an interaction between TLR signaling and SNARE proteins has been suggested. In 2014, Nair-Gupta et al. [109] showed that MyD88-dependent TLR signaling is involved in the phosphorylation of SNAP-23 present on the phagosome in dendritic cells. The phosphorylated SNAP-23 protein stabilizes SNARE complexes, which leads to fusion with the endosomal recycling compartment and ultimately to cross-presentation. In our opinion, we observed a similar phenomenon in microglia: these cells act as key players in the immune response in the CNS. Microglia are the resident innate immune cells and within CNS they are responsible for the early control of infections and for the recruitment of cells of the adaptive immune system, which are required for pathogen clearance [110]. Thus, it seems that the microglial TLR/MyD88/NF-κB cascade contributes to the decrease of SNAP-23. Recently, it has been suggested that microglia are characterized by heightened expression of TLRs and by a stronger response to LPS compared to astroglia [111]. Furthermore, in 2012 Holm et al. [111] discovered that the response of astroglial cells to TLR2 agonists is completely dependent on the presence of functional TLR4 in microglial cells. The activation of TLR4 by LPS induces a synthesis of closely related TLR2 [112]. In 2017, Piotrowska et al. [62] did not observe changes in expression of the analyzed factors, with the exception of SNAP-23 and SNAP-25, after BoNT/A treatment in LPS-stimulated astroglia. The authors suggested that TLR2 is another important molecular target for BoNT/A. In sum, BoNT/A exerts its anti-inflammatory action by inhibiting signaling pathways (such as NF-κB, p38 and ERK1/2) activation in microglia; very importantly, it can directly interact with TLR2. Based on the current state of knowledge, we can hypothesize that the full activation of astroglial TLR2 requires the presence of functional TLR4 in microglia, which emphasizes the significant cross-talk between those cells types within the CNS.

4. Conclusions

Further investigation concerning the action of BoNT/A in the CNS is needed and will provide priceless information to help understand the pathophysiology of neuropathic pain. The literature provides evidence that BoNT/A, in addition to having an impact on neuronal functions, can also influence the activation of microglia; therefore, the involvement of these non-neuronal cells in the BoNT/A mechanism of action should also be regarded as an important component of its analgesic effects. However, BoNT/A appears to have no more than a slight direct effect on astroglia. In our opinion, BoNT/A is a powerful modulator of neuron–glia interactions in the CNS in the context of neuropathic pain. More research into BoNT/A as a treatment for neuropathy is warranted because it could be an attractive alternative for patients who do not respond positively to other drugs.

Acknowledgments: This work was supported by the National Science Centre, Poland grant HARMONIA 5 2013/10/M/NZ4/00261, and statutory funds of the Institute of Pharmacology Polish Academy of Sciences. The English language in the manuscript was edited by American Journal Experts.

Author Contributions: E.R., A.P., K.P.-B. and J.M. made substantial contributions to the conception and design of the study, and were involved in drafting the manuscript or revising it critically. All authors made substantial contributions to the acquisition and interpretation of data and have given final approval of the version for publication.

Conflicts of Interest: The authors declare no conflict of interest.

References

1. Austin, P.J.; Moalem-Taylor, G. The neuro-immune balance in neuropathic pain: Involvement of inflammatory immune cells, immune-like glial cells and cytokines. *J. Neuroimmunol.* **2010**, *229*, 26–50. [CrossRef] [PubMed]
2. Mika, J.; Zychowska, M.; Popiolek-Barczyk, K.; Rojewska, E.; Przewlocka, B. Importance of glial activation in neuropathic pain. *Eur. J. Pharmacol.* **2013**, *716*, 106–119. [CrossRef] [PubMed]
3. Watkins, L.R.; Milligan, E.D.; Maier, S.F. Glial activation: A driving force for pathological pain. *Trends Neurosci.* **2001**, *24*, 450–455. [CrossRef]
4. Watkins, L.R.; Maier, S.F. GLIA: A novel drug discovery target for clinical pain. *Nat. Rev. Drug Discov.* **2003**, *2*, 973–985. [CrossRef] [PubMed]
5. Gibson, W.; Wand, B.M.; O'Connell, N.E. Transcutaneous electrical nerve stimulation (TENS) for neuropathic pain in adults. *Cochrane Database Syst. Rev.* **2017**, *2017*, CD011976. [CrossRef] [PubMed]
6. Hatch, M.N.; Cushing, T.R.; Carlson, G.D.; Chang, E.Y. Neuropathic pain and SCI: Identification and treatment strategies in the 21st century. *J. Neurol. Sci.* **2017**, *384*, 75–83. [CrossRef] [PubMed]
7. Çakici, N.; Fakkel, T.M.; van Neck, J.W.; Verhagen, A.P.; Coert, J.H. Systematic review of treatments for diabetic peripheral neuropathy. *Diabet. Med.* **2016**, *33*, 1466–1476. [CrossRef] [PubMed]

8. Tamburin, S.; Lacerenza, M.R.; Castelnuovo, G.; Agostini, M.; Paolucci, S.; Bartolo, M.; Bonazza, S.; Federico, A.; Formaglio, F.; Giusti, E.M.; et al. Italian Consensus Conference on Pain in Neurorehabilitation (ICCPN) Pharmacological and non-pharmacological strategies in the integrated treatment of pain in neurorehabilitation. Evidence and recommendations from the Italian Consensus Conference on Pain in Neurorehabilitation. *Eur. J. Phys. Rehabil. Med.* **2016**, *52*, 741–752. [PubMed]
9. Boldt, I.; Eriks-Hoogland, I.; Brinkhof, M.W.G.; de Bie, R.; Joggi, D.; von Elm, E. Non-pharmacological interventions for chronic pain in people with spinal cord injury. *Cochrane Database Syst. Rev.* **2014**, *11*, CD009177. [CrossRef] [PubMed]
10. Johnson, E.A. Clostridial toxins as therapeutic agents: Benefits of nature's most toxic proteins. *Annu. Rev. Microbiol.* **1999**, *53*, 551–575. [CrossRef] [PubMed]
11. Castillo-Álvarez, F.; Hernando de la Bárcena, I.; Marzo-Sola, M.E. Botulinum toxin in trigeminal neuralgia. *Med. Clin. (Barc)* **2017**, *148*, 28–32. [CrossRef] [PubMed]
12. Alviar, M.J.M.; Hale, T.; Dungca, M. Pharmacologic interventions for treating phantom limb pain. *Cochrane Database Syst. Rev.* **2016**, *10*, CD006380. [CrossRef] [PubMed]
13. Bruno, V.A.; Fox, S.H.; Mancini, D.; Miyasaki, J.M. Botulinum Toxin Use in Refractory Pain and Other Symptoms in Parkinsonism. *Can. J. Neurol. Sci.* **2016**, *43*, 697–702. [CrossRef] [PubMed]
14. Cho, S.-J.; Song, T.-J.; Chu, M.K. Treatment Update of Chronic Migraine. *Curr. Pain Headache Rep.* **2017**, *21*, 26. [CrossRef] [PubMed]
15. Cuadrado, M.L.; García-Moreno, H.; Arias, J.A.; Pareja, J.A. Botulinum neurotoxin type-A for the treatment of atypical odontalgia. *Pain Med.* **2016**, *17*, 1717–1721. [CrossRef] [PubMed]
16. Kleen, J.K.; Levin, M. Injection Therapy for Headache and Facial Pain. *Oral Maxillofac. Surg. Clin. N. Am.* **2016**, *28*, 423–434. [CrossRef] [PubMed]
17. Lunde, H.M.B.; Torkildsen, Ø.; Bø, L.; Bertelsen, A.K. Botulinum Toxin as Monotherapy in Symptomatic Trigeminal Neuralgia. *Headache* **2016**, *56*, 1035–1039. [CrossRef] [PubMed]
18. Wu, T.; Song, H.; Dong, Y.; Ye, Y.; Li, J. Intra-articular injections of botulinum toxin a for refractory joint pain: A systematic review and meta-analysis. *Clin. Rehabil.* **2017**, *31*, 435–443. [CrossRef] [PubMed]
19. Montecucco, C.; Molgó, J. Botulinal neurotoxins: Revival of an old killer. *Curr. Opin. Pharmacol.* **2005**, *5*, 274–279. [CrossRef] [PubMed]
20. Welch, M.J.; Purkiss, J.R.; Foster, K. A Sensitivity of embryonic rat dorsal root ganglia neurons to Clostridium botulinum neurotoxins. *Toxicon* **2000**, *38*, 245–258. [CrossRef]
21. Durham, P.L.; Cady, R.; Cady, R.; Blumenfeld, A.J. Regulation of Calcitonin Gene-Related Peptide Secretion from Trigeminal Nerve Cells by Botulinum Toxin Type A: Implications for Migraine Therapy. *Headache* **2004**, *44*, 35–43. [CrossRef] [PubMed]
22. Krämer, H.H.; Angerer, C.; Erbguth, F.; Schmelz, M.; Birklein, F. Botulinum toxin A reduces neurogenic flare but has almost no effect on pain and hyperalgesia in human skin. *J. Neurol.* **2003**, *250*, 188–193. [CrossRef] [PubMed]
23. Burstein, R.; Zhang, X.C.; Levy, D.; Aoki, K.R.; Brin, M.F. Selective inhibition of meningeal nociceptors by botulinum neurotoxin type A: Therapeutic implications for migraine and other pains. *Cephalalgia* **2014**, *34*, 853–869. [CrossRef] [PubMed]
24. Brodsky, M.A.; Swope, D.M.; Grimes, D. Diffusion of botulinum toxins. *Tremor Other Hyperkinet. Mov.* **2012**, *2*, 319–322. [CrossRef]
25. Klein, A.W. The therapeutic potential of botulinum toxin. *Dermatol. Surg.* **2004**, *30*, 452–455. [PubMed]
26. Wheeler, A.H. Botulinum toxin A, adjunctive therapy for refractory headaches associated with pericranial muscle tension. *Headache* **1998**, *38*, 468–471. [CrossRef] [PubMed]
27. Binder, W.J.; Brin, M.F.; Blitzer, A.; Schoenrock, L.D.; Pogoda, J.M. Botulinum toxin type A (BOTOX) for treatment of migraine headaches: An open-label study. *Otolaryngol. Head Neck Surg.* **2000**, *123*, 669–676. [CrossRef] [PubMed]
28. Ashkenazi, A. Botulinum toxin type a for chronic migraine. *Curr. Neurol. Neurosci. Rep.* **2010**, *10*, 140–146. [CrossRef] [PubMed]
29. Yuan, R.Y.; Sheu, J.J.; Yu, J.M.; Chen, W.T.; Tseng, I.J.; Chang, H.H.; Hu, C.J. Botulinum toxin for diabetic neuropathic pain: A randomized double-blind crossover trial. *Neurology* **2009**, *72*, 1473–1478. [CrossRef] [PubMed]

30. Ranoux, D.; Attal, N.; Morain, F.; Bouhassira, D. Botulinum toxin type A induces direct analgesic effects in chronic neuropathic pain. *Ann. Neurol.* **2008**, *64*, 274–283. [CrossRef] [PubMed]
31. Kitamura, Y.; Matsuka, Y.; Spigelman, I.; Ishihara, Y.; Yamamoto, Y.; Sonoyama, W.; Kuboki, T.; Oguma, K. Botulinum toxin type a (150 kDa) decreases exaggerated neurotransmitter release from trigeminal ganglion neurons and relieves neuropathy behaviors induced by infraorbital nerve constriction. *Neuroscience* **2009**, *159*, 1422–1429. [CrossRef] [PubMed]
32. Arbizu, R.A.; Rodriguez, L. Use of Clostridium botulinum toxin in gastrointestinal motility disorders in children. *World J. Gastrointest. Endosc.* **2015**, *7*, 433–437. [CrossRef] [PubMed]
33. Intiso, D.; Basciani, M.; Santamato, A.; Intiso, M.; Di Rienzo, F. Botulinum toxin type a for the treatment of neuropathic pain in neuro-rehabilitation. *Toxins* **2015**, *7*, 2454–2480. [CrossRef] [PubMed]
34. Bach-Rojecky, L.; Lacković, Z. Antinociceptive effect of botulinum toxin type a in rat model of carrageenan and capsaicin induced pain. *Croat. Med. J.* **2005**, *46*, 201–208. [PubMed]
35. Luvisetto, S.; Rossetto, O.; Montecucco, C.; Pavone, F. Toxicity of botulinum neurotoxins in central nervous system of mice. *Toxicon* **2003**, *41*, 475–481. [CrossRef]
36. Luvisetto, S.; Marinelli, S.; Cobianchi, S.; Pavone, F. Anti-allodynic efficacy of botulinum neurotoxin A in a model of neuropathic pain. *Neuroscience* **2007**, *145*, 1–4. [CrossRef] [PubMed]
37. Marinelli, S.; Luvisetto, S.; Cobianchi, S.; Makuch, W.; Obara, I.; Mezzaroma, E.; Caruso, M.; Straface, E.; Przewlocka, B.; Pavone, F. Botulinum neurotoxin type A counteracts neuropathic pain and facilitates functional recovery after peripheral nerve injury in animal models. *Neuroscience* **2010**, *171*, 316–328. [CrossRef] [PubMed]
38. Mika, J.; Rojewska, E.; Makuch, W.; Korostynski, M.; Luvisetto, S.; Marinelli, S.; Pavone, F.; Przewlocka, B. The effect of botulinum neurotoxin A on sciatic nerve injury-induced neuroimmunological changes in rat dorsal root ganglia and spinal cord. *Neuroscience* **2011**, *175*, 358–366. [CrossRef] [PubMed]
39. Zychowska, M.; Rojewska, E.; Makuch, W.; Luvisetto, S.; Pavone, F.; Marinelli, S.; Przewlocka, B.; Mika, J. Participation of pro- and anti-nociceptive interleukins in botulinum toxin A-induced analgesia in a rat model of neuropathic pain. *Eur. J. Pharmacol.* **2016**, *791*, 377–388. [CrossRef] [PubMed]
40. Vacca, V.; Marinelli, S.; Eleuteri, C.; Luvisetto, S.; Pavone, F. Botulinum neurotoxin A enhances the analgesic effects on inflammatory pain and antagonizes tolerance induced by morphine in mice. *Brain Behav. Immun.* **2012**, *26*, 489–499. [CrossRef] [PubMed]
41. Vacca, V.; Marinelli, S.; Luvisetto, S.; Pavone, F. Botulinum toxin A increases analgesic effects of morphine, counters development of morphine tolerance and modulates glia activation and μ opioid receptor expression in neuropathic mice. *Brain Behav. Immun.* **2013**, *32*, 40–50. [CrossRef] [PubMed]
42. Tsuda, M.; Koga, K.; Chen, T.; Zhuo, M. Neuronal and microglial mechanisms for neuropathic pain in the spinal dorsal horn and anterior cingulate cortex. *J. Neurochem.* **2017**, *141*, 486–498. [CrossRef] [PubMed]
43. Zhuo, M.; Wu, G.; Wu, L.J. Neuronal and microglial mechanisms of neuropathic pain. *Mol. Brain* **2011**, *4*, 31. [CrossRef] [PubMed]
44. Wasser, C.R.; Kavalali, E.T. Leaky synapses: Regulation of spontaneous neurotransmission in central synapses. *Neuroscience* **2009**, *158*, 177–188. [CrossRef] [PubMed]
45. Choi, B.J.; Imlach, W.L.; Jiao, W.; Wolfram, V.; Wu, Y.; Grbic, M.; Cela, C.; Baines, R.A.; Nitabach, M.N.; McCabe, B.D. Miniature Neurotransmission Regulates Drosophila Synaptic Structural Maturation. *Neuron* **2014**, *82*, 618–634. [CrossRef] [PubMed]
46. Molgó, J.; Siegel, L.S.; Tabti, N.; Thesleff, S. A study of synchronization of quantal transmitter release from mammalian motor endings by the use of botulinal toxins type A and D. *J. Physiol.* **1989**, *411*, 195–205. [CrossRef] [PubMed]
47. Rossetto, O.; Seveso, M.; Caccin, P.; Schiavo, G.; Montecucco, C. Tetanus and botulinum neurotoxins: Turning bad guys into good by research. *Toxicon* **2001**, *39*, 27–41. [CrossRef]
48. Katz, E.; Ferro, P.A.; Cherksey, B.D.; Sugimori, M.; Llinas, R.; Uchitel, O.D. Effects of Ca2+ channel blockers on transmitter release and presynaptic currents at the frog neuromuscular junction. *J. Physiol.* **1995**, *486*, 695–706. [CrossRef] [PubMed]
49. Südhof, T.C.; Rothman, J.E. Membrane fusion: Grappling with SNARE and SM proteins. *Science* **2009**, *323*, 474–477. [CrossRef] [PubMed]
50. Pantano, S.; Montecucco, C. The blockade of the neurotransmitter release apparatus by botulinum neurotoxins. *Cell. Mol. Life Sci.* **2014**, *71*, 793–811. [CrossRef] [PubMed]

51. Cui, M.; Khanijou, S.; Rubino, J.; Aoki, K.R. Subcutaneous administration of botulinum toxin a reduces formalin-induced pain. *Pain* **2004**, *107*, 125–133. [CrossRef] [PubMed]
52. Meng, J.; Wang, J.; Lawrence, G.; Dolly, J.O. Synaptobrevin I mediates exocytosis of CGRP from sensory neurons and inhibition by botulinum toxins reflects their anti-nociceptive potential. *J. Cell Sci.* **2007**, *120*, 2864–2874. [CrossRef] [PubMed]
53. Luvisetto, S.; Marinelli, S.; Lucchetti, F.; Marchi, F.; Cobianchi, S.; Rossetto, O.; Montecucco, C.; Pavone, F. Botulinum neurotoxins and formalin-induced pain: Central vs. peripheral effects in mice. *Brain Res.* **2006**, *1082*, 124–131. [CrossRef] [PubMed]
54. Chuang, Y.C.; Yoshimura, N.; Huang, C.C.; Chiang, P.H.; Chancellor, M.B. Intravesical botulinum toxin a administration produces analgesia against acetic acid induced bladder pain responses in rats. *J. Urol.* **2004**, *172 (4 Pt 1)*, 1529–1532. [CrossRef] [PubMed]
55. Antonucci, F.; Rossi, C.; Gianfranceschi, L.; Rossetto, O.; Caleo, M. Long-Distance Retrograde Effects of Botulinum Neurotoxin A. *J. Neurosci.* **2008**, *28*, 3689–3696. [CrossRef] [PubMed]
56. Foster, K.A.; Bigalke, H.; Aoki, K.R. Botulinum neurotoxin—From laboratory to bedside. *Neurotox. Res.* **2006**, *9*, 133–140. [CrossRef] [PubMed]
57. Jabbari, B. Botulinum neurotoxins in the treatment of refractory pain. *Nat. Clin. Pract. Neurol.* **2008**, *4*, 676–685. [CrossRef] [PubMed]
58. Bach-Rojecky, L.; Relja, M.; Lacković, Z. Botulinum toxin type A in experimental neuropathic pain. *J. Neural Transm. Vienna Austria 1996* **2005**, *112*, 215–219. [CrossRef] [PubMed]
59. Habermann, E. 125I-labeled neurotoxin from clostridium botulinum A: Preparation, binding to synaptosomes and ascent to the spinal cord. *Naunyn Schmiedebergs Arch. Pharmacol.* **1974**, *281*, 47–56. [CrossRef] [PubMed]
60. Wiegand, H.; Erdmann, G.; Wellhöner, H.H. 125I-Labelled botulinum a neurotoxin: Pharmacokinetics in cats after intramuscular injection. *Naunyn. Schmiedebergs. Arch. Pharmacol.* **1976**, *292*, 161–165. [CrossRef] [PubMed]
61. Marinelli, S.; Vacca, V.; Ricordy, R.; Uggenti, C.; Tata, A.M.; Luvisetto, S.; Pavone, F. The Analgesic Effect on Neuropathic Pain of Retrogradely Transported botulinum Neurotoxin A Involves Schwann Cells and Astrocytes. *PLoS ONE* **2012**, *7*, e47977. [CrossRef] [PubMed]
62. Piotrowska, A.; Popiolek-Barczyk, K.; Pavone, F.; Mika, J. Comparison of the Expression Changes after Botulinum Toxin Type A and Minocycline Administration in Lipopolysaccharide-Stimulated Rat Microglial and Astroglial Cultures. *Front. Cell. Infect. Microbiol.* **2017**, *7*, 147. [CrossRef] [PubMed]
63. Hepp, R.; Perraut, M.; Chasserot-Golaz, S.; Galli, T.; Aunis, D.; Langley, K.; Grant, N.J. Cultured glial cells express the SNAP-25 analogue SNAP-23. *Glia* **1999**, *27*, 181–187. [CrossRef]
64. Parpura, V.; Fang, Y.; Basarsky, T.; Jahn, R.; Haydon, P.G. Expression of synaptobrevin II, cellubrevin and syntaxin but not SNAP-25 in cultured astrocytes. *FEBS Lett.* **1995**, *377*, 489–492. [CrossRef] [PubMed]
65. DeLeo, J.A.; Yezierski, R.P. The role of neuroinflammation and neuroimmune activation in persistent pain. *Pain* **2001**, *90*, 1–6. [CrossRef]
66. Popiolek-Barczyk, K.; Mika, J. Targeting the microglial signaling pathways: New insights in the modulation of neuropathic pain. *Curr. Med. Chem.* **2016**, *23*, 2908–2928. [CrossRef] [PubMed]
67. Colburn, R.W.; DeLeo, J.A.; Rickman, A.J.; Yeager, M.P.; Kwon, P.; Hickey, W.F. Dissociation of microglial activation and neuropathic pain behaviors following peripheral nerve injury in the rat. *J. Neuroimmunol.* **1997**, *79*, 163–175. [CrossRef]
68. Colburn, R.W.; Rickman, A.J.; Deleo, J.A. The effect of site and type of nerve injury on spinal glial activation and neuropathic pain behavior. *Exp. Neurol.* **1999**, *157*, 289–304. [CrossRef] [PubMed]
69. Nedergaard, M. Direct signaling from astrocytes to neurons in cultures of mammalian brain cells. *Science* **1994**, *263*, 1768–1771. [CrossRef] [PubMed]
70. Roh, D.H.; Yoon, S.Y.; Seo, H.S.; Kang, S.Y.; Han, H.J.; Beitz, A.J.; Lee, J.H. Intrathecal injection of carbenoxolone, a gap junction decoupler, attenuates the induction of below-level neuropathic pain after spinal cord injury in rats. *Exp. Neurol.* **2010**, *224*, 123–132. [CrossRef] [PubMed]
71. Zündorf, G.; Kahlert, S.; Reiser, G. Gap-junction blocker carbenoxolone differentially enhances NMDA-induced cell death in hippocampal neurons and astrocytes in co-culture. *J. Neurochem.* **2007**, *102*, 508–521. [CrossRef] [PubMed]
72. Haber, M.; Murai, K.K. Reshaping neuron-glial communication at hippocampal synapses. *Neuron Glia Biol.* **2006**, *2*, 59–66. [CrossRef] [PubMed]

73. Panatier, A.; Vallée, J.; Haber, M.; Murai, K.K.; Lacaille, J.C.; Robitaille, R. Astrocytes are endogenous regulators of basal transmission at central synapses. *Cell* **2011**, *146*, 785–798. [CrossRef] [PubMed]
74. Oliet, S.H.R.; Panatier, A.; Piet, R.; Mothet, J.P.; Poulain, D.A.; Theodosis, D.T. Neuron-glia interactions in the rat supraoptic nucleus. *Prog. Brain Res.* **2008**, *170*, 109–117. [PubMed]
75. Romero-Sandoval, A.; Chai, N.; Nutile-McMenemy, N.; DeLeo, J.A. A comparison of spinal Iba1 and GFAP expression in rodent models of acute and chronic pain. *Brain Res.* **2008**, *1219*, 116–126. [CrossRef] [PubMed]
76. Tanga, F.Y.; Raghavendra, V.; DeLeo, J.A. Quantitative real-time RT-PCR assessment of spinal microglial and astrocytic activation markers in a rat model of neuropathic pain. *Neurochem. Int.* **2004**, *45*, 397–407. [CrossRef] [PubMed]
77. Kawai, T.; Akira, S. The role of pattern-recognition receptors in innate immunity: Update on toll-like receptors. *Nat. Immunol.* **2010**, *11*, 373–384. [CrossRef] [PubMed]
78. Mika, J. Modulation of microglia can attenuate neuropathic pain symptoms and enhance morphine effectiveness. *Pharmacol. Rep.* **2008**, *60*, 297–307. [PubMed]
79. Clark, A.K.; Gentry, C.; Bradbury, E.J.; McMahon, S.B.; Malcangio, M. Role of spinal microglia in rat models of peripheral nerve injury and inflammation. *Eur. J. Pain* **2007**, *11*, 223–230. [CrossRef] [PubMed]
80. Coyle, D.E. Partial peripheral nerve injury leads to activation of astroglia and microglia which parallels the development of allodynic behavior. *Glia* **1998**, *23*, 75–83. [CrossRef]
81. Zychowska, M.; Rojewska, E.; Przewlocka, B.; Mika, J. Mechanisms and pharmacology of diabetic neuropathy—Experimental and clinical studies. *Pharmacol. Rep.* **2013**, *65*, 1601–1610. [CrossRef]
82. Amin, A.R.; Attur, M.G.; Thakker, G.D.; Patel, P.D.; Vyas, P.R.; Patel, R.N.; Patel, I.R.; Abramson, S.B. A novel mechanism of action of tetracyclines: Effects on nitric oxide synthases. *Proc. Natl. Acad. Sci. USA* **1996**, *93*, 14014–14019. [CrossRef] [PubMed]
83. Colovic, M.; Caccia, S. Liquid chromatographic determination of minocycline in brain-to-plasma distribution studies in the rat. *J. Chromatogr. A* **2003**, *791*, 337–343. [CrossRef]
84. Mika, J.; Osikowicz, M.; Rojewska, E.; Korostynski, M.; Wawrzczak-Bargiela, A.; Przewlocki, R.; Przewlocka, B. Differential activation of spinal microglial and astroglial cells in a mouse model of peripheral neuropathic pain. *Eur. J. Pharmacol.* **2009**, *623*, 65–72. [CrossRef] [PubMed]
85. Lundblad, R.; Ekstrøm, P.; Giercksky, K.E. Pentoxifylline improves survival and reduces tumor necrosis factor, interleukin-6, and endothelin-1 in fulminant intra-abdominal sepsis in rats. *Shock* **1995**, *3*, 210–215. [CrossRef] [PubMed]
86. Mika, J.; Osikowicz, M.; Makuch, W.; Przewlocka, B. Minocycline and pentoxifylline attenuate allodynia and hyperalgesia and potentiate the effects of morphine in rat and mouse models of neuropathic pain. *Eur. J. Pharmacol.* **2007**, *560*, 142–149. [CrossRef] [PubMed]
87. Sweitzer, S.M.; Schubert, P.; DeLeo, J.A. Propentofylline, a glial modulating agent, exhibits antiallodynic properties in a rat model of neuropathic pain. *J. Pharmacol. Exp. Ther.* **2001**, *297*, 1210–1217. [PubMed]
88. Kim, Y.J.; Kim, J.-H.; Lee, K.-J.; Choi, M.-M.; Kim, Y.H.; Rhie, G.; Yoo, C.-K.; Cha, K.; Shin, N.-R. Botulinum Neurotoxin Type A Induces TLR2-Mediated Inflammatory Responses in Macrophages. *PLoS ONE* **2015**, *10*, e0120840. [CrossRef] [PubMed]
89. Jin, S.X.; Zhuang, Z.Y.; Woolf, C.J.; Ji, R.R. p38 mitogen-activated protein kinase is activated after a spinal nerve ligation in spinal cord microglia and dorsal root ganglion neurons and contributes to the generation of neuropathic pain. *J. Neurosci.* **2003**, *23*, 4017–4022. [PubMed]
90. Tsuda, M.; Mizokoshi, A.; Shigemoto-Mogami, Y.; Koizumi, S.; Inoue, K. Activation of p38 Mitogen-Activated Protein Kinase in Spinal Hyperactive Microglia Contributes to Pain Hypersensitivity Following Peripheral Nerve Injury. *Glia* **2004**, *45*, 89–95. [CrossRef] [PubMed]
91. Ma, W.; Quirion, R. The ERK/MAPK pathway, as a target for the treatment of neuropathic pain. *Expert Opin. Ther. Targets* **2005**, *9*, 699–713. [CrossRef] [PubMed]
92. Rojewska, E.; Popiolek-Barczyk, K.; Jurga, A.M.; Makuch, W.; Przewlocka, B.; Mika, J. Involvement of pro- and antinociceptive factors in minocycline analgesia in rat neuropathic pain model. *J. Neuroimmunol.* **2014**, *277*, 57–66. [CrossRef] [PubMed]
93. Rojewska, E.; Piotrowska, A.; Makuch, W.; Przewlocka, B.; Mika, J. Pharmacological kynurenine 3-monooxygenase enzyme inhibition significantly reduces neuropathic pain in a rat model. *Neuropharmacology* **2016**, *102*, 80–91. [CrossRef] [PubMed]

94. Mika, J.; Popiolek-Barczyk, K.; Rojewska, E.; Makuch, W.; Starowicz, K.; Przewlocka, B. Delta-opioid receptor analgesia is independent of microglial activation in a rat model of neuropathic pain. *PLoS ONE* **2014**, *9*, e104420. [CrossRef] [PubMed]
95. Popiolek-Barczyk, K.; Kolosowska, N.; Piotrowska, A.; Makuch, W.; Rojewska, E.; Jurga, A.M.; Pilat, D.; Mika, J. Parthenolide relieves pain and promotes M2 microglia/macrophage polarization in rat model of neuropathy. *Neural Plast.* **2015**, *2015*. [CrossRef] [PubMed]
96. Piotrowska, A.; Kwiatkowski, K.; Rojewska, E.; Makuch, W.; Mika, J. Maraviroc reduces neuropathic pain through polarization of microglia and astroglia—Evidence from in vivo and in vitro studies. *Neuropharmacology* **2016**, *108*, 207–219. [CrossRef] [PubMed]
97. Ma, W.; Bisby, M. a Increased activation of nuclear factor kappa B in rat lumbar dorsal root ganglion neurons following partial sciatic nerve injuries. *Brain Res.* **1998**, *797*, 243–254. [CrossRef]
98. Meunier, A.; Latrémolière, A.; Dominguez, E.; Mauborgne, A.; Philippe, S.; Hamon, M.; Mallet, J.; Benoliel, J.J.; Pohl, M. Lentiviral-mediated targeted NF-κB blockade in dorsal spinal cord glia attenuates sciatic nerve injury-induced neuropathic pain in the rat. *Mol. Ther.* **2007**, *15*, 687–697. [CrossRef] [PubMed]
99. Miyoshi, K.; Obata, K.; Kondo, T.; Okamura, H.; Noguchi, K. Interleukin-18-Mediated Microglia/Astrocyte Interaction in the Spinal Cord Enhances Neuropathic Pain Processing after Nerve Injury. *J. Neurosci.* **2008**, *28*, 12775–12787. [CrossRef] [PubMed]
100. Jurga, A.M.; Rojewska, E.; Piotrowska, A.; Makuch, W.; Pilat, D.; Przewlocka, B.; Mika, J. Blockade of toll-like receptors (TLR2, TLR4) attenuates pain and potentiates buprenorphine analgesia in a rat neuropathic pain model. *Neural Plast.* **2016**, *2016*. [CrossRef] [PubMed]
101. Kim, D.; Kim, M.A.; Cho, I.-H.; Kim, M.S.; Lee, S.; Jo, E.-K.; Choi, S.-Y.; Park, K.; Kim, J.S.; Akira, S.; et al. A critical role of toll-like receptor 2 in nerve injury-induced spinal cord glial cell activation and pain hypersensitivity. *J. Biol. Chem.* **2007**, *282*, 14975–14983. [CrossRef] [PubMed]
102. Lehnardt, S.; Massillon, L.; Follett, P.; Jensen, F.E.; Ratan, R.; Rosenberg, P.A.; Volpe, J.J.; Vartanian, T. Activation of innate immunity in the CNS triggers neurodegeneration through a Toll-like receptor 4-dependent pathway. *Proc. Natl. Acad. Sci. USA* **2003**, *100*, 8514–8519. [CrossRef] [PubMed]
103. Tanga, F.Y.; Nutile-McMenemy, N.; DeLeo, J.A. The CNS role of Toll-like receptor 4 in innate neuroimmunity and painful neuropathy. *Proc. Natl. Acad. Sci. USA* **2005**, *102*, 5856–5861. [CrossRef] [PubMed]
104. Borrello, S.; Nicolò, C.; Delogu, G.; Pandolfi, F.; Ria, F. TLR2: A crossroads between infections and autoimmunity? *Int. J. Immunopathol. Pharmacol.* **2011**, *24*, 549–556. [CrossRef] [PubMed]
105. Medzhitov, R.; Preston-Hurlburt, P.; Janeway, C.A. A human homologue of the Drosophila toll protein signals activation of adaptive immunity. *Nature* **1997**, *388*, 394–397. [CrossRef] [PubMed]
106. Liu, T.; Gao, Y.-J.; Ji, R.-R. Emerging role of Toll-like receptors in the control of pain and itch. *Neurosci. Bull.* **2012**, *28*, 131–144. [CrossRef] [PubMed]
107. Miyake, K. Innate immune sensing of pathogens and danger signals by cell surface Toll-like receptors. *Semin. Immunol.* **2007**, *19*, 3–10. [CrossRef] [PubMed]
108. Kigerl, K.A.; de Rivero Vaccari, J.P.; Dietrich, W.D.; Popovich, P.G.; Keane, R.W. Pattern recognition receptors and central nervous system repair. *Exp. Neurol.* **2014**, *258*, 5–16. [CrossRef] [PubMed]
109. Nair-Gupta, P.; Baccarini, A.; Tung, N.; Seyffer, F.; Florey, O.; Huang, Y.; Banerjee, M.; Overholtzer, M.; Roche, P.A.; Tampé, R.; et al. TLR signals induce phagosomal MHC-I delivery from the endosomal recycling compartment to allow cross-presentation. *Cell* **2014**, *158*, 506–521. [CrossRef] [PubMed]
110. Beauvillain, C.; Donnou, S.; Jarry, U.; Scotet, M.; Gascan, H.; Delneste, Y.; Guermonprez, P.; Jeannin, P.; Couez, D. Neonatal and adult microglia cross-present exogenous antigens. *Glia* **2008**, *56*, 69–77. [CrossRef] [PubMed]
111. Holm, T.H.; Draeby, D.; Owens, T. Microglia are required for astroglial toll-like receptor 4 response and for optimal TLR2 and TLR3 response. *Glia* **2012**, *60*, 630–638. [CrossRef] [PubMed]
112. Lin, Y.; Lee, H.; Berg, A.H.; Lisanti, M.P.; Shapiro, L.; Scherer, P.E. The lipopolysaccharide-activated Toll-like receptor (TLR)-4 induces synthesis of the closely related receptor TLR-2 in adipocytes. *J. Biol. Chem.* **2000**, *275*, 24255–24263. [CrossRef] [PubMed]

toxins

MDPI

Article

The Effect of Botulinum Neurotoxin Serotype a Heavy Chain on the Growth Related Proteins and Neurite Outgrowth after Spinal Cord Injury in Rats

Ya-Fang Wang, Fu Liu, Jing Lan, Juan Bai and Xia-Qing Li *

Department of Pathophysiology, Shanxi Medical University, Taiyuan 030001, China; 041510570@b.sxmu.edu.cn (Y.-F.W.); 031513156@b.edu.cn (F.L.); 041410136@b.sxmu.edu.cn (J.L.); 041510569@sxmu.edu.cn (J.B.)

* Correspondence: xqli2013@sxmu.edu.cn; Tel.: +86-135-4632-8095

Received: 23 November 2017; Accepted: 31 January 2018; Published: 2 February 2018

Abstract: (1) Background: The botulinum toxin A (BoNT-A) heavy chain (HC) can stimulate the growth of primary motor neurites. (2) Methods: A recombinant BoNT/A HC was injected locally plus interval intrathecal catheter of BoNT/A HC to rats with ipsilateral semi-dissociated lumbar spinal cord injuries (SCIs). First, 2D gel with a silver nitrate stain was applied to detect the general pattern of protein expression. Growth associated protein 43 (GAP-43) and superior cervical ganglion 10 (SCG10) were chosen to represent the altered proteins, based on their molecular weight and pI, and were used to further detect their expression. Meanwhile, the neuronal processes were measured. The measurements of thermal hyperalgesia and grasp power at the ipsilateral hindlimb were used to evaluate spinal sensory and motor function, respectively. (3) Results: The local injection of BoNT/A HC followed by its intrathecal catheter intervally altered the spinal protein expression pattern after an SCI; protein expression was similar to normal levels or displayed a remarkable increase. The changes in the expression and distribution of phosphorylated growth associated protein 43(p-GAP 43) and superior cervical ganglion 10 (SCG 10) indicated that the administration of BoNT/A HC to the SCI significantly amplified the expression of p-GAP43 and SCG10 ($p < 0.05$). Meanwhile, the positive immunofluorescent staining for both p-GAP43 and SCG10 was mainly present near the rostral aspect of the injury, both in the cytoplasm and the neuronal processes. Moreover, the outgrowth of neurites was stimulated by the BoNT/A HC treatment; this was evident from the increase in neurite length, number of branches and the percentage of cells with neuronal processes. The results from the spinal function tests suggested that the BoNT/A HC did not affect sensation, but had a large role in improving the ipsilateral hindlimb grasp power ($p < 0.05$). (4) Conclusions: The local injection with the intermittent intrathecal administration of BoNT/A heavy chain to rats with SCI increased the local expression of GAP-43 and SCG 10, which might be affiliated with the regeneration of neuronal processes surrounding the injury, and might also be favorable to the relief of spinal motor dysfunction.

Keywords: botulinum neurotoxins; botulinum neurotoxin serotype A; heavy chain; botulinum neurotoxin serotype a heavy chain (BoNT/A HC); spinal cord injury (SCI); nerve regeneration; growth associated protein 43 (GAP-43); superior cervical ganglion 10 (SCG10); neuronal processes; neural regeneration

Key Contribution: This is a preliminary and breakthrough explore for the effect of botulinum neurotoxin serotype A heavy chain on neuritogenesiis in vivo. The local application of BoNT-A heavy chain to the site of spinal cord injury might be helpful for relief of structural damage and dysfunction.

1. Introduction

A spinal cord injury (SCI) is a devastating condition characterized by a sudden loss of spinal functions distal to the level of trauma, including sensory, motor, and autonomic function. These effects are due to various traumatic or non-traumatic factors. The regenerative capacity of the injured spinal cord is extremely limited in adult mammals [1,2]. Patients suffer various disabilities which greatly impact quality of life [3]. The deficiency of spinal regenerative ability after an SCI has been attributed to various alterations in the local microenvironment, including: (1) the accumulation of many inhibitory factors by the degeneration of neurons, axon, and myelin; and (2) the lack of a sufficient number of upregulated or activated neuritogenic-associated genes and proteins [4–8]. At present, although there are many attempts for the treatment of the SCI, such as IL-6, stem cell transplantation [9,10], etc. few are actually available for clinical practice. Therefore, endeavors towards new strategies to revitalize neuritogenic ability following spinal injuries are being continuously made.

Botulinum toxin A (BoNT/A) is one of seven botulinum toxins (categorized based on serologic features) and is one of the most potent toxins known [11–14]. The toxicity of BoNT/A is due to its selective binding to the membranous receptor located on the presynaptic membrane of the motor endplate. This leads to the cleavage of the synaptosomal-associated protein 25 kDa (or SNAP-25) which blocks the release of the neurotransmitter acetylcholine contained in the vesicles [15,16]. This results in the paralysis of skeletal muscle. Patients die of severe respiratory failure due to a lack of respiratory muscle contractions [17]. Besides the aforementioned mechanisms of BoNT/A, it has been verified that it can also inhibit or block the release of other components in synaptic vesicles of different neurons, such as the calcitonin gene related peptide (CGRP) and substance P in sensory neurons [18–22]. Because of the actions of BoNT/A on neurotransmitters, it has been used as therapy to relieve hyper-reactive muscle dysfunctions (e.g., torticollis and hemifacial spasm), various types of chronic pain, hyperhidrosis, etc. [23,24].

Structurally, BoNT/A consists of two polypeptide chains linked by a disulfide bond. The longer chain (MW = 100 kDa) is called a heavy chain (HC) of BoNT-A; it is mainly responsible for binding to target cells and mediating the endocytosis of the toxin. The other chain with a smaller molecular weight is a light chain (LC, MW = 50 kDa). The LC is a zinc-dependent proteolytic enzyme which contributes to the cleavage of SNAP-25 at the neuromuscular junction [15,25,26]. It had been observed by some investigators that new axonal branches formed around skeletal muscles that had been paralyzed by BoNT/A for three to four months [27–29]. Meanwhile, the observations in vitro showed that BoNT/A was able to promote neuritogenesis in mouse motor neuron cultures [30]. The observation of neurite sprouting associated with BoNT/A in vivo or in vitro could not simply be attributed to the toxic role of BoNT-A. Moreover, the observations form Coffield's lab also showed that the isolated binding domain heavy chain (BoNT/A HC) has the same role as BoNT/A [30]. The signal pathways relating to the binding of the heavy chain and the receptor might also be a reasonable alternative explanation.

In our previous studies, the increased phosphorylation of Akt and ERK1/2 (growth- and survival-related intracellular signal proteins) was paralleled with neuritogenesis when adding BoNT/A heavy chain into neuro-2a cell cultures (data published in Chinese). In that study, an obvious increase in phosphorylated-ERK 1/2 was seen between one to five hours after adding 1 nmol/L of BoNT/A HC ($p < 0.05$), and an increased protein level of phosphorylated-Akt was observed mainly at 15 and 60 min ($p < 0.05$). Based on the results, it was concluded that the BoNT-A heavy chain stimulates neuritogenesis. The neuritogenic mechanism of it on Neuro-2a cells might be due to the activation of ERK1/2 and Akt phosphorylation. Meanwhile, it is reasonably presumed that BoNT/A heavy chain exerted its biological roles by modulating many intracellular signals and proteins expression, some of which may be involved in neural growth and regeneration; others are possibly related to growth inhibition. Among of these proteins, growth-associated protein-43 (GAP-43) and superior cervical ganglion 10 (SCG 10) have already been evidenced to be closely related to trhe axonal growth and neural regeneration [31–33]. Therefore, commercial recombinant BoNT/A HC was applied in this study to explore the effect of BoNT/A HC on the expression of some selective growth-associated proteins, as well as its role in neurite outgrowth in rat lumbar SCI model in vivo. Meanwhile, the motor and sensory functions of the ipsilateral hindlimb were evaluated after BoNT/A HC treatment as a therapeutic regent.

2. Results

2.1. Unilateral Lumbar SCI Model and Spinal Function Evaluation

Observations of the SCI two days after surgery showed that it was located within the left lumbar area (Figure 1A,B). The control values for the grasp power and thermal hyperalgesia were obtained one day prior to the SCI. Two days after the SCI, both motor and sensory function appeared remarkably impaired (Figure 1C,D), i.e., the value of grasp power on grip test appeared dropped, which indicated the dysfunction of nervous control on skeletal muscle in hindlimbs, which might be related to the lesion of the corticospinal tract at lumbar spinal level, and also contributed in the appearance of the draging of the ipsilateral hindlimb.

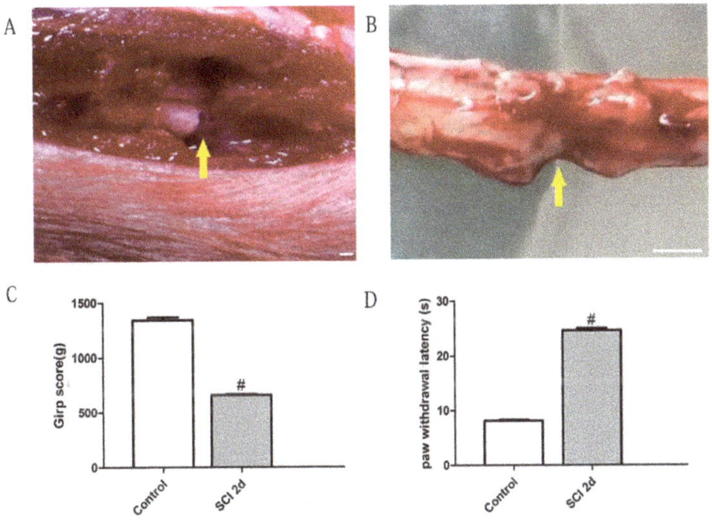

Figure 1. An observation of lumbar spinal cord injury (SCI) and spinal function testing. (**A**) The SCI was made by the tip of a pair of fine forceps. A clear unilateral defection was seen in the field (arrow explanation). (**B**) The lesion was located in the lumbar area when the whole spinal cord was exposed (both two arrows point to the same damaged area). (**C**,**D**) There was an obvious ipsilateral drop in the grip score and a prolonged hind-paw withdrawal latency greater than 25 s ($^{\#}$ $p < 0.05$ versus the control group; bar = 5 mm).

2.2. The Alteration of Local Protein Expression after SCI and the Effect of BoNT/A HC on It

Two-dimensional electrophoresis with silver nitrate staining showed that the general expression of protein in SCIs was altered compared to that of the control group. The major changes noted after injury were that some protein dots were lighter in color or smaller in size, while others appeared simultaneously denser or increased. Furthermore, the proteins with either increased or decreased expression appeared as a single dot or a dot group. After administration of the BoNT/A HC, the alterative expression of proteins demonstrated some interesting phenomena: some of the protein dots with increased expression tended to decrease towards the levels seen in the control group, whereas some dots with increased expression either further increased remarkably or went down in expression. It was noted that the protein dots that were 35–45 kDa (isoelectric point of 4 to 5) and 18–25 kDa in molecular weight (isoelectric point 7) had an interesting appearance: their expression was increased after the SCI, and then this increase became much more significant after treatment with BoNT/A HC (Figure 2).

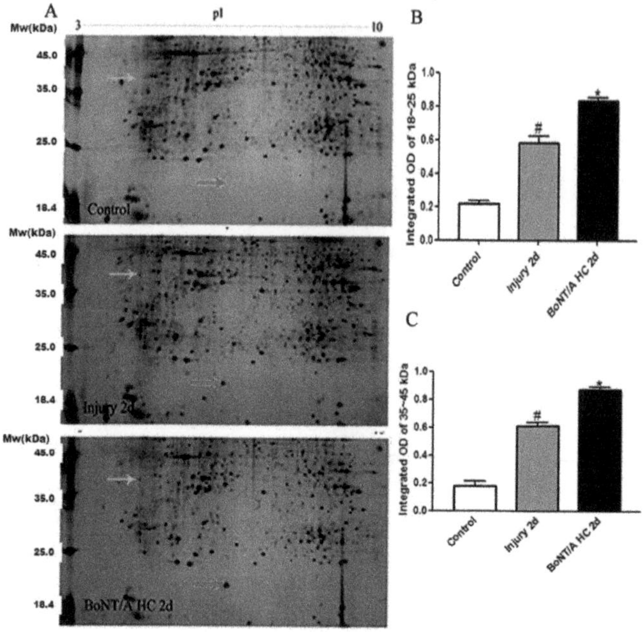

Figure 2. The two-dimensional gel with silver nitrate staining. (**A**) The images show that the protein dots change to molecular weights of approximately 18–45 kDa. Red and green arrows point to the dots with obvious alterative expression in the different groups. (**B**) The integrated OD value for protein expression ($n = 4$/each group) appeared at approximately 18–25 kDa. (**C**) The integrated OD value for protein expression appeared at approximately 35–45 kDa. Results were statistically significant ($^{\#}$ $p < 0.05$, vs. control group; * $p < 0.05$, vs. both control & injury groups).

2.3. *Effects of BoNT/A Heavy Chain on the Expression of Selective Growth-Associated Proteins*

According to the profile of the 2D gel from different group, two dots from the molecular weight (MW) between 35 and 45 kDa, Isoelectric point (pI) around 4–5 and the MW between 18 and 25 kDa, pI around 7 were selected as the aimed proteins. Based mainly on the molecular weight of some growth-associated proteins, GAP43 (MW = 43 kDa) and SCG10 (MW = 20.8 kDa) were selected as target proteins for the BoNT/A HC treatment intervention. Both SDS-PAGE and a Western blot showed that the expression of p-GAP43 and SCG10 were increased two days after the SCI while using GAPDH as a loading control. However, the increase declined as time post-injury increased, even dropping below the level of the control group two weeks after the injury. With the BoNT/A HC injection, there was a much greater increase of the expressions of the two proteins. The increase was significant compared with SCI-only samples during the corresponding period ($p < 0.05$). In comparison, SCG10 had a more increased expression than p-GAP43 after administration of BoNT-A HC; this was based on the semi-quantification of both protein bands on the Western blot. The expression level of SCG10 was almost two times greater than that of control groups and 75% greater than SCI-only groups at four weeks post-injury. Meanwhile, the expression of p-GAP43 was also increased after BoNT/A heavy chain treatment, but the change was not as dramatic as in SCG10 (Figure 3).

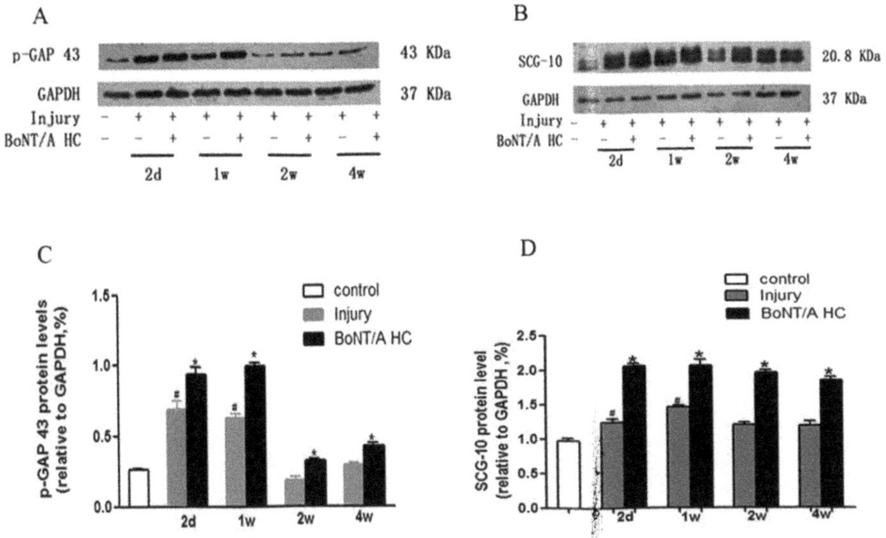

Figure 3. The effect of BoNT-A heavy chain (HC) on the expression of p-GAP43 and SCG10. The Western blot bands for both: p-GAP43 (**A**); and SCG10 (**B**) at different periods (two days, one week, two weeks, and four weeks). The semi-quantification analysis (4 sample/each group) of: p-GAP43 (**C**); and SCG10 (**D**). Results were statistically significant ($^{\#}$ $p < 0.05$, vs. the control group; * $p < 0.05$, vs. both the control and the injury groups).

2.4. The Distribution of Positive GAP43 and SCG10 Immunofluorescence at the Injured Area after Administration of the BoNT/A HC

Results showed that in a normal spinal cord both GAP43 and SCG10 are evident in only a few cells with weak positive expression. Under the microscope, the positive immunofluorescence of GAP43 and SCG10 at the injury area was consistent with the results of the Western blot. The distributive features of the two proteins appeared very similar. The positive GAP43 and SCG10 expression was mainly within the cell body. These cells were very evident during the immunofluorescence of both proteins; they were found in the caudal and rostral parts of the injury area two to seven days after the injury, with or without BoNT/A HC administration. With BoNT/A HC treatment, however, the immunopositivity of both proteins appeared more intense than the SCI-only groups after two weeks post-injury. Furthermore, with BoNT/A heavy chain treatment, the positive staining was observed not only within the cytoplasm but also in the cellular processes; this made the processes easily identifiable. Comparably, the neuronal processes were much more obvious in the immunofluorescence of SCG10 than of GAP43 (Figure 4). Both Western blot and immunofluorescence results imply that SCG10 might be an important growth-associated protein affected by the BoNT/A HC. The positive SCG10 neuronal processes were used as the target for the measurement of neurite length and number after in vivo administration of BoNT/A HC.

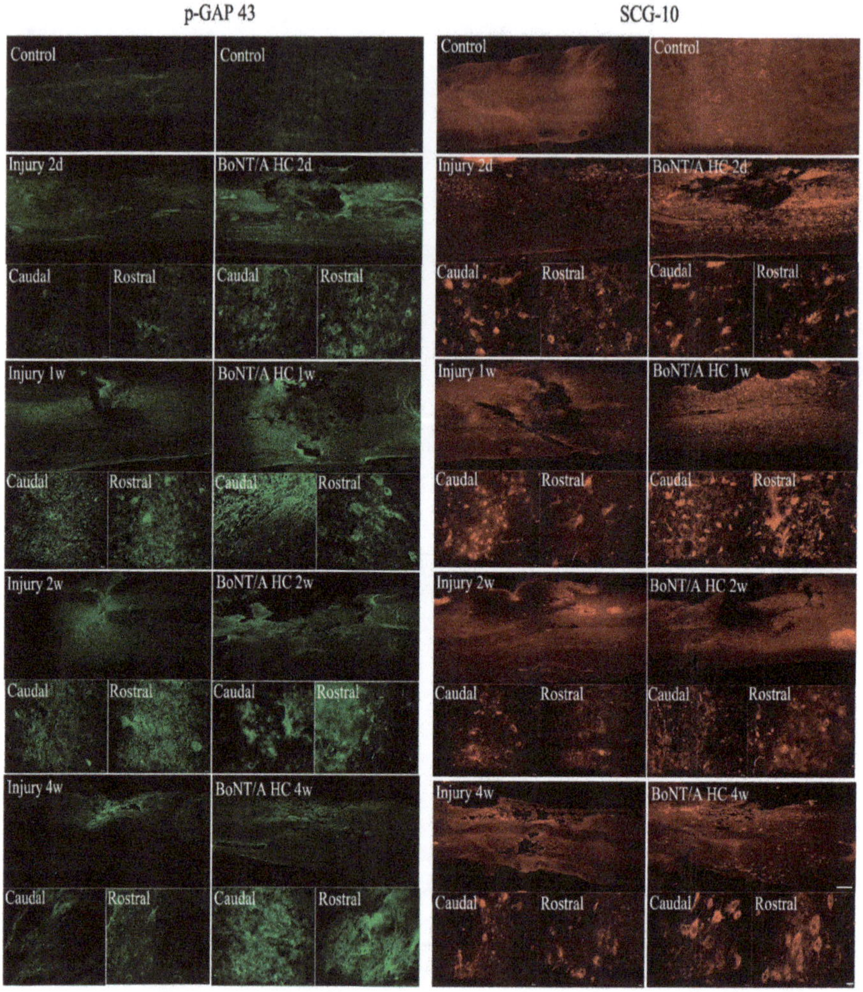

Figure 4. A comparison of the immunofluorescence of GAP43 (Green) and SCG10 (Red) at the spinal injury site. The scale bars were set at 500 μm (on the long rectangular image at right bottom; and 20 μm (short rectangular image at right bottom; lower sections are the magnified images from rostral and caudal sites of the corresponding upper one. Each group consists of one long rectangular and two short rectangular images), respectively.

2.5. The Measurement of SCG 10 Positive Neuronal Processes

Based on immunofluorescence, the length and number of neuronal processes with SCG10 positivity at the caudal and rostral areas of injury were imaged and measured using ImageJ software (a free software from https://imagej.nih.gov/ij/). (The number of SCG 10 positive neurons was various from group to group, but the variation between group and group, especially SCI and BoNT/A HC treatment group, was not significant ($p > 0.05$). The calculation appeared as 35–45 (in controls), 55–65 (in SCI 2 d), 80–90 (SCI 1 w), 90–100 (SCI 2 w), 80–90 (SCI 4 w), 70–80 (with BoNT/A HC 2 d), 100–105 (with BoNT/A HC 1 w), 100–105 (with BoNT/A HC 2 w) and 90–100 (with BoNT/A HC 4 w). SCG10 positive processes were scattered, short, and not easily identified one week after the SCI; this was true even regarding the positive cells that were clearly observed in that time. With lasting post-injury time (four weeks), these neuronal processes eventually disappeared in the SCI-only group. In contrast, the number of neuronal processes significantly increased when BoNT/A HC was given. The total length of positive SCG10 neurites reached 400 μm in four weeks, and the process branches were observed to increase even two weeks after injury. The increase in neuronal number was almost three times greater than control and SCI-only groups ($p < 0.05$) (Figure 5). Additionally, the percentage of positive SCG10 cells with identified neurites was higher than in SCI-only groups at the corresponding time ($p < 0.05$) (Figure 5). These results indicate that BoNT/A HC was able to stimulate the re-growth of neuronal processes after an SCI, as previously seen in vitro studies.

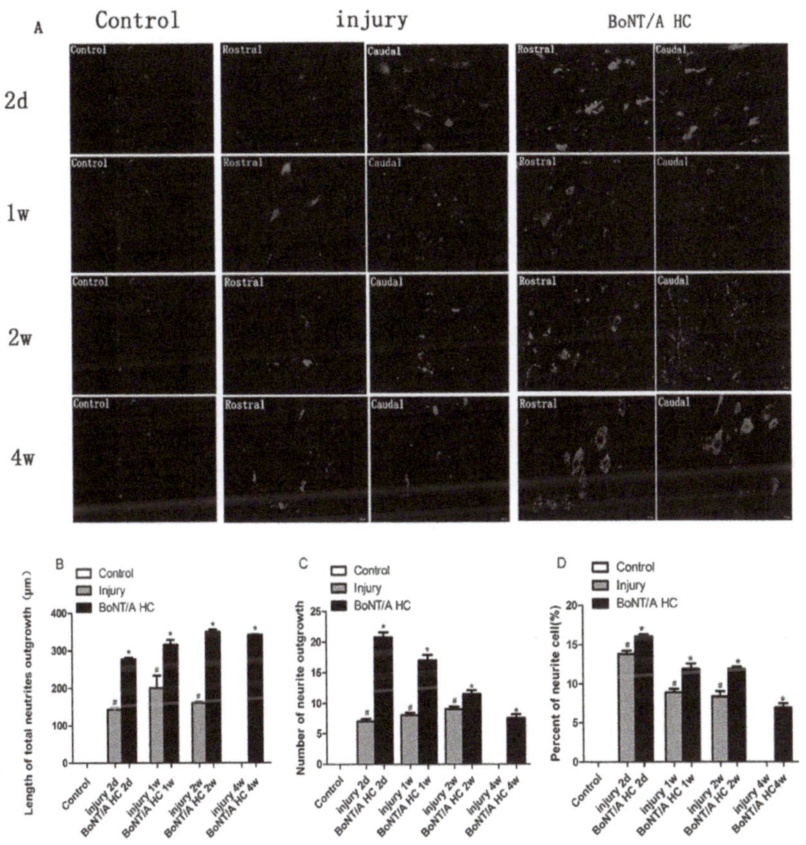

Figure 5. The effects of BoNT/A HC on the neurite outgrowth. (**A**) The visualization of neuronal processes and their variation in different groups using SCG10 immunofluorescence. A quantitative comparison of the: total length (**B**); number (**C**); and the percentage of neurons with visualized processes in all SCG10 positive cells (**D**). Results were statistically significant ($^{\#}$ $p < 0.05$, vs. control group; * $p < 0.05$, vs. both control and injury groups); Bar = 20 μm.

2.6. The Amelioration of Motor and Sensory Function by BoNT/A HC Treatment Based on SCI

The ipsilateral hindlimb motor function was evaluated using grip testing at two days, one week, two weeks, and four weeks post-SCI. Results showed that there was a significant drop in grip scores, which indicated that there was some damaged motor function of the ipsilateral hindlimb after the SCI.

However, rats administered with BoNT/A HC treatment showed relatively higher scores than those in the SCI-only group ($p < 0.05$), though their scores were not as high as those of the control group (Figure 6).

The test for thermal hyperalgesia was used to assess sensory function. The results indicated that the paw withdrawal latency (PWTL) was prolonged after an SCI, with or without the application of BoNT/A HC, and there was no significant difference between the SCI groups and the BoNT/A HC treatment groups (Table 1).

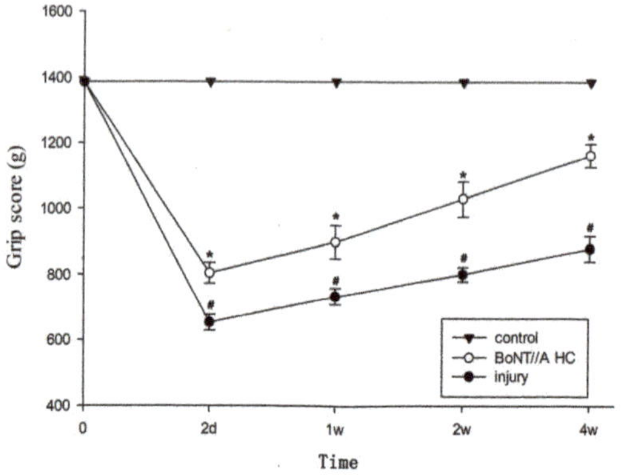

Figure 6. The motor function changes in the ipsilateral hindlimb after BoNT/A HC treatment. Results were statistically significant ($^{\#}$ $p < 0.05$, vs. control group; * $p < 0.05$, vs. injury group).

Table 1. Comparison of thermal pain thresholds at different time points in different groups.

Groups	0 d	2 d	1 w	2 w	4 w
Control	8.5 ± 0.2	8.5 ± 0.2	8.3 ± 0.1	7.8 ± 0.2	8.2 ± 0.2
Injury	8.5 ± 0.2	22.8 ± 1.0 #	22.1 ± 0.9 #	22.4 ± 1.0 #	21.5 ± 0.9 #
BoNT/A HC	8.5 ± 0.2	24.4 ± 0.3	24.5 ± 0.3	24.1 ± 0.4	22.5 ± 0.9

# $p < 0.05$, vs. control group.

3. Discussion

The stimulatory effect of BoNT/A HC on neurite outgrowth has previously been verified in vitro. In this work, the intermittent administration of BoNT/A HC through intrathecal injection on a lumbar unilateral SCI rat model was used to determine the role of BoNT/A HC in the local expression of growth-associated proteins. It was then explored whether, in vitro, BoNT/A HC was able to promote re-growth by upregulating the expression of growth-associated proteins after an SCI. Unlike the peripheral nervous system (PNS), the central nervous system (CNS) is deficient in its ability to regenerate after injury [34,35]. Based on previous research, the CNS has difficulty regenerating due to the abundance of myelin inhibitory factors and the shortage of macrophages [6]. Another possible explanation is the limited or arrested initiation of intrinsic neuron growth programs in the injured CNS [7]. Because the spine is part of the CNS, most patients suffer from severe spinal dysfunction and lifelong disability due to various pathogeneses when SCIs develop. Therefore, one of the principal foci of regenerative medicine after an SCI is to explore strategies and methods which can influence the improvement of the spinal microenvironment (e.g., the exclusion of myelin inhibitory factors) or revive the intrinsic regenerative ability of neuron itself [36].

The human recombinant BoNT/A HC used in this study is a non-toxic peptide, unlike the original potential holotoxin. The results evident after treatment with BoNT/A HC can be explained by its ability to bind to membranes and the activation of related intracellular signals upon the attachment of the heavy chain to the receptor. A previous study from the same research team has demonstrated that the BoNT/A HC had a stimulatory role in promoting neurite outgrowth in Neuro-2a cell cultures. It is known that the basis for neurogenesis and neuritogenesis is the synthesis of proteins; even the myelin inhibitory factors that accumulate after SCI can be regarded as a secondary phospholipoprotein. Therefore, it can be assumed that there is a significant modification in protein expression after an SCI, and the administration of the BoNT/A HC following an SCI should have an input in protein expression. Some definite results were obtained from this study. First, the application of BoNT/A HC reversed the alterations caused by the SCI, such as the increased expression of some proteins when the SCI developed. When the BoNT/A HC was given at the same time as the injury established, the increase dropped towards the levels of the controls, which is consistent with our previous study (published in Chinese). Briefly, the main difference in the previous study are as foolows: (1) the SCI model was established with a modified needle inserted into the lumbar spinal cord at the same anatomical location as this study; and (2) different doses of BoNT/A heavy chain (2 μg, 4 μg, 6 μg and 8 μg) was injected one-time into the spinal cord cavity while the injury made. The second result observed in this study is that BoNT/A HC treatment magnified the expression of some proteins evident from the SCI, for example, the expression of GAP43 and SCG10 were obviously increased after BoNT/A HC treatment. In this study, the selection of GAP43 and SCG10 as markers (to detect the efficiency of BoNT/A HC on stimulating protein regeneration) is based on the changes of protein molecular weight on the two-dimensional gel and the Western blot. In fact, the levels of both GAP43 and SCG10 displayed a certain elevation shortly after the SCI (two days post-injury), but these declined as the post-injury period progressed. However, when the SCI model was treated with BoNT/A HC, both proteins exhibited a continuous increased expression until the end of the experiment.

The increased expression of GAP43 after injury has been considered by most researchers to be actively involved in axonal regeneration [37–41]. GAP43 is mainly involved in the sprouting and regeneration of mature axons in their phosphorylated form. Its expression was upregulated following nerve injury. SCG10, also known as stathmin-like 2 (STMN2) protein, is another regenerative protein [42]. It is mainly involved in axonal microtubule dynamics and protein transport [43–45]. The initial increase in GAP43 and SCG10 expression after the SCI, without the application of BoNT/A HC, can be explained as a limited regenerative response after spinal cord injuries, however the response ceased when the injury continued to exist. The mechanism might be related to the intervention of myelin inhibitory factors binding to their specific receptors. The continuous enhancement of GAP43 and SCG10 expression when BoNT/A HC is applied is evidence of the recombinant peptide's involvement in promoting nerve regeneration after injury. The study also gave an outline of the role BoNT/A HC plays in stimulating the in vivo sprouting of neuronal processes. When BoNT/A HC treatment was administered during the SCI's development, the length and the number of neuronal process around injury site (in both its rostral and caudal parts) increased compared to measurements in the SCI-only group. The percentage of neurons with processes was also greater than that in the SCI-only group. Additionally, it was found that the spinal motor function at the ipsilateral hindlimb was improved due to the efficiency of BoNT/A HC in the upregulation of growth-associated proteins and in the promotion of neuronal process re-growth. The ineffectiveness of BoNT/A HC on improving spinal sensory function might be attributed to the difference in the expression of the heavy chain binding receptor in sensory neurons. Besides, direct damage of the sensory neurons in injury location might contribute to the difference of sensory and motor after SCI with or without BoNT/A HC treatment. Therefore, more detailed information about these should be explored after all in the future.

4. Conclusions

The local injection with intermittent intrathecal administration of BoNT/A heavy chain to rats with SCI increased the local expression of GAP-43 and SCG 10, which might be affiliated with the regeneration of neuronal processes surrounding the injury, and might also be favorable to the relief of spinal motor dysfunction. The exact role and mechanism in vivo of BoNT/A heavy after nervous injury need to be verified in the future.

5. Materials and Methods

5.1. Establishing the Rat Spinal Cord Hemi-Section Injury Model

All experimental procedures were done in accordance with the National Institute of Health's Guide for the Care and Use of Laboratory Animals, and were approved by the Ethics Committee of Animal Research at Shanxi Medical University (IACUC2017-001) on 20 January 2017. Every effort was made to minimize animal suffering and the number of animals sacrificed.

Sprague-Dawley rats (6–7 weeks old, and weighing between 200 and 220 g) were provided by Beijing Haidian Experimental Animal Farm (No. SCXK (Beijing) 2014-0013). As there is no difference regarding spinal cord injury study, male rats were used in this research. The rats were deeply anaesthetized with 1% pentobarbital sodium (at a dose of 4 mL/kg body weight) and given a laminectomy at vertebral level $T_9/_{10}$ to expose the spinal cord. Briefly, the T_9 and T_{10} vertebrae were first orientated using the iliac crest as an anatomical landmark. The lumbar spinal cord was exposed by removing the T9 vertebra dorsally. A unilateral (left) lumbar spinal injury was achieved by nipping against the left side of the dorsal median vein with the tip of a pair of fine forceps. Left hindlimb paralysis was regarded as the sign of success in achieving a unilateral SCI. Meanwhile, the loss of motor function (based on hindlimb grasp power measurement) and the abnormality of sensory function (based on an assay of thermal hyperalgesia) after surgery were used to evaluate the severity of spinal cord function impact. The animals were placed in a temperature-controlled (24 °C ± 1 °C) chamber under a 12 h light/dark cycle. Standard amounts of food and tap water were given daily.

5.2. BoNT/A Heavy Chain Administration and Groups

Recombinant BoNT-A HC was purchased from List Biological Laboratories Inc. (Campbell, CA, USA).

Intermittent administration of BoNT/A HC applied in the study was done via two routes: (1) local application of the BoNT/A HC directly onto injury site (4 μg/μL in 16 μL saline); and (2) administration of BoNT/A HC via a lumbar intrathecal catheter [46]. After establishing the rat model, 2 μg/μL of BoNT/A HC were administered every week to the SCI in the BoNT/A HC treatment groups. Animals were divided into the following groups, with six rats in each group: (1) the control (or pseudo surgery) group for which the skin incisions were made, the laminae were cut, and the spinal cords were exposed but not injured; (2) the SCI-only group for which unilateral (left side) lumbar spinal cord injuries were made (to prevent the vehicle intervention on BoNT/A heavy chain, the same volume of sterile saline was applied in SCI-only animal with same method and period); and (3) the SCI with BoNT/A HC treatment, in which BoNT/A HC was administered every week, and the injury was made. This group was further divided into four groups (with six rats each) based on different periods post-injury, i.e., two days, one week, two weeks and four weeks. The groups of animals are summarized in Table 2.

Table 2. Number and Groups of Animals.

Name of Group	Pseudo Surgery	SCI without BoNT/A HC				SCI with BoNT/A HC			
Time	0	2 d	1 wk	2 wks	4 wks	2 d	1 wk	2 wks	4 wks
No. of animals	6	6	6	6	6	6	6	6	6

5.3. Two-Dimensional Gel Electrophoresis

The spinal cords were fully exposed when the experiment's period was completed. Then, the segment of the cord containing the spinal lesion center and the rostral and caudal area (6 mm in total) was collected. Spinal protein was extracted using a pre-cooled lysis buffer (urea: 21 g, thiourea: 7.9 g, DTE: 0.5 g, Tris: 0.5 g, in 50 mL of DD H_2O). The protein concentration was determined using the Bradford protein assay.

For the two-dimensional gel, two 150 mg protein samples from each group were loaded onto IPG strips (NL) for first-dimension isoelectric focusing (IEF). The IPG strips were then washed and equilibrated in a 2D equilibration buffer, and then they underwent a 12.5% sodium dodecyl sulfate polyacrylamide gel vertical electrophoresis. After that, the gel was stained with 0.1% silver nitrate. The gel was imaged and analyzed with the Bio-Rad gel imaging system. Some interesting protein dots from different group were chosen and compared upon their changes on size and density at the same level of molecular weight and the isoelectric point (pI). For statistical analysis, two gels were prepared. The selective dots were circled and assessed by the integrated optional density (IOD) using ImageJ software in a double-blinded way and two people who were not related to the study were asked to do the assessment. In this way, four values four each dot were obtained and analyzed.

5.4. SDS-PAGE and Western Blot

Twenty micrograms of protein homogenates were subjected to 15% sodium dodecyl sulfate polyacrylamide gel electrophoresis. Subsequently, the proteins were transferred onto polyvinylidene difluoride (PVDF) membranes for Western blotting. The PVDF membranes were blocked with 5% non-fat milk powder in a TBST wash buffer (Tris buffered saline containing 1% Tween-20) for 1 h at room temperature. The selective primary antibodies were applied onto the membrane and incubated at 4 °C overnight. These antibodies were the following: rabbit anti-phosphorylated GAP43 antibody (1:3000, Thermo Fisher, Waltham, MA, USA); rabbit anti-SCG10 polyclonal antibody (1:1000, Thermo Fisher, Waltham, MA, USA); and rabbit anti-GAPDH polyclonal antibody (1:5000, Bioword, Nanjing, China). The following day, the membranes were incubated with HRP-conjugated secondary antibodies (goat anti-rabbit IgG, 1:1000, Bioword, Nanjing, China) for 1 h at room temperature. The membranes were then immersed into the EasySee Western blot kit (DW101, TRAN, Beijing, China; A solution: B solution = 1; 1 plus 2 μL C solution) and made to undergo the reaction for 3 min in dark. X-ray film which corresponded to the membrane was developed in a darkroom. The protein bands were imaged and analyzed for the variation in integrated optional density (IOD), while GAPDH bands as a loading control, with Bio-Rad gel imaging system.

5.5. Immunofluorescence Staining

At the set time point, rats from each group were anesthetized lethally with 1% pentobarbital sodium. They then underwent a 30 min transcardial perfusion with ice-cold 4% paraformaldehyde for fixation purposes. A 1 cm segment of spinal cord containing the lesion center was dissected out. The samples were post-fixed in the same fixatives for another hour and subsequently immersed in a 30% sucrose solution at 4 °C overnight. After being embedded onto an OCT compound, a section of spinal cord 16 μm in thickness across the lesion site was cut dorsal-coronary-longitudinally by cryostat (1950-Cryostat, Leca, Nussloch, Germany).

The sections were penetrated with 0.1% Triton-X100 for 10 min, washed three times with 0.1 mol/L PBS buffer, and blocked with a blocking buffer (10% goat or donkey serum and 0.1% Triton X-100 in PBS) for 1 h. Primary antibodies (as previously listed) were incubated with the section at 4 °C overnight. The following day, the sections were incubated with Alexa Fluoro-594-labeled goat anti-rabbit IgG (1:500; Life Technologies, Shanghai, China) and Alexa Fluoro-488-labeled donkey anti-rabbit IgG (1:500; Life Technologies, Shanghai, China) in the dark for 1 h, at room temperature. The sections were then mounted with an antifade mountant with DAPI (2-(4-amidinophenyl)-1H-indole-6-carboxamidine, Life Technologies, Grand Island, NY, USA). These were then checked and photographed under a fluorescence microscope (Olympus IX71, Tokyo, Japan).

5.6. Measurement of Neuronal Processes

The immunofluorescence staining of SCG 10 was applied to 6–8 sections each samples. Approximately 5–7 of images were captured of each section. The imaging area was mainly at the periphery of the spinal cord lesion. The measurements included the total length of neurites, the number of neurites, and percentage of cells with neurites in all the immunofluorescence positive cells in the image. These were taken using ImageJ software. The identification of neurites was determined and confirmed according to literature [47]. Neurites were traced from the cell body to the end of the process, and the total length was calculated for each process. Neurites were distinguished according to their soma diameter; this meant that only neurites with a length greater than the maximum diameter of the cell would be considered a real neurite.

5.7. Behavioral Evaluation

Six rats in each group were used for assessment of motor and sensory function of ipsilateral hindlimb. Alteration in sensory and motor function at the ipsilateral hindlimb of rats with an SCI or an SCI with BoNT/A HC treatment were evaluated using the thermal hyperalgesia test and the grip power test, respectively. The thermal hyperalgesia test was completed using thermal stimulation of the PWTL by the paw thermal radiation stimulation tester (SERIES 8; RWD Life Science). The response time (in seconds) for the ipsilateral paw to withdraw because of the thermal stimulus was recorded. In fact, the response time represented the latency of the stimulation of the rat's foot (accurate to 0.1 s). To avoid tissue damage caused by long time thermal stimulation, 25 s was regarded as the maximum time of PWTL. At every time point, the average value was obtained using at least three measurements. A 10 min interval was suggested between taking these measurements. The values from three or more assessments was applied to calculate the average $\pm$ SD at a certain time point.

The grip test was performed using the rats grip tester based on the manufacturer's instructions (YLS-13A, Zhishuduobao, Baoding, China). First, wrap two fore-limbs and one counter-lateral hindlimb with tape, leaving the ipsilateral hind-limb free. Then, the rat was placed gently on the grasping force tester, the rat's tail was grabbed and dragged backwards. The power (in grams) of the ipsilateral hind paw in holding the grip was automatically recorded by the instrument as the maximum rat grip power; this stands for its motor function. The value was the average of three measurements, with 15 min intervals between each measurement.

5.8. Statistical Analysis

The data were expressed as mean and standard error (SEM). The protein bands or protein spots were quantified by ImageJ software. Data were analyzed using GraphPad Prism 5.0 software and one-way ANOVA was used to analyze the significance. $p < 0.05$ was considered statistically significant.

Acknowledgments: We are grateful for the financial support by National Natural Science Foundation of China (81171178) and the grant for returned overseas of Shanxi Province of China (2012047). We would like to express our thanks to all of the graduates who were involved in the projects. In addition, we sincerely appreciate Julie A. Coffield at the University of Georgia for the knowledge introduction of BoNTs.

Author Contributions: Y.-F.W. wrote the main manuscript. Y.W. and J.L. performed experiments and collected samples. Y.W., J.B. and F.L. analyzed data and prepared figures. X.-Q.L. and Y.W. designed experiment. X.-Q.L. offered the financial support to the project. All authors approved the final version of the paper.

Conflicts of Interest: All of the authors declare no conflict of interest.

References

1. Silver, J.; Miller, J.H. Regeneration beyond the glial scar. *Nat. Rev. Neurosci.* **2004**, *5*, 146–156. [CrossRef] [PubMed]
2. Giger, R.J.; Hollis, E.R.; Tuszynski, M.H. Guidance molecules in axon regeneration. *Cold Spring Harb. Perspect. Biol.* **2010**, *2*, 1–21. [CrossRef] [PubMed]
3. Simpson, L.A.; Eng, J.J.; Hsieh, J.T.C.; Wolfe, D.L.; Team, T.S. The health and life priorities of individuals with spinal cord injury: A systematic review. *J. Neurotrauma* **2012**, *29*, 1548–1555. [CrossRef] [PubMed]
4. Ferguson, T.A.; Son, Y.J. Extrinsic and intrinsic determinants of nerve regeneration. *J. Tissue Eng.* **2011**, *2*, 1–12. [CrossRef] [PubMed]

5. Baldwin, K.T.; Giger, R.J. Insights into the physiological role of CNS regeneration inhibitors. *Front. Mol. Neurosci.* **2015**, *8*, 1–8. [CrossRef] [PubMed]
6. Geoffroy, C.G.; Zheng, B. Myelin-associated inhibitors in axonal growth after CNS injury. *Curr. Opin. Neurobiol.* **2014**, *27*, 31–38. [CrossRef] [PubMed]
7. He, Z. Intrinsic control of axon regeneration. *J. Biomed. Res.* **2010**, *24*, 2–5. [CrossRef]
8. Mckerracher, L.; Rosen, K.M. MAG, myelin and overcoming growth inhibition in the CNS. *Front. Mol. Neurosci.* **2015**, *8*, 1–6. [CrossRef] [PubMed]
9. Amemori, T.; Ruzicka, J.; Romanyuk, N.; Jhanwaruniyal, M.; Sykova, E.; Jendelova, P. Comparison of intraspinal and intrathecal implantation of induced pluripotent stem cell-derived neural precursors for the treatment of spinal cord injury in rats. *Stem Cell Res. Ther.* **2015**, *6*, 257–268. [CrossRef] [PubMed]
10. Yang, P.; Qin, Y.; Bian, C.; Zhao, Y.; Zhang, W. Intrathecal delivery of il-6 reactivates the intrinsic growth capacity of pyramidal cells in the sensorimotor cortex after spinal cord injury. *PLoS ONE* **2015**, *10*, 1–12. [CrossRef] [PubMed]
11. Zhang, P.; Ray, R.; Singh, B.R.; Ray, P. Mastoparan-7 rescues botulinum toxin-A poisoned neurons in a mouse spinal cord cell culture model. *Toxicon* **2013**, *76*, 37–43. [CrossRef] [PubMed]
12. Zichel, R.; Mimran, A.; Keren, A.; Barnea, A.; Steinberger-Levy, I.; Marcus, D.; Turgeman, A.; Reuvenyet, S. Efficacy of a potential trivalent vaccine based on Hc fragments of botulinum toxins A, B, and E produced in a cell-free expression system. *Clin. Vaccine Immunol.* **2010**, *17*, 784–792. [CrossRef] [PubMed]
13. Rossetto, O.; Pirazzini, M.; Montecucco, C. Botulinum neurotoxins: Genetic, structural and mechanistic insights. *Nat. Rev. Microbiol.* **2014**, *12*, 535–549. [CrossRef] [PubMed]
14. Meunier, F.A.; Lisk, G.; Sesardic, D.; Dolly, J.O. Dynamics of motor nerve terminal remodeling unveiled using SNARE-cleaving botulinum toxins: The extent and duration are dictated by the sites of SNAP-25 truncation. *Mol. Cell. Neurosci.* **2003**, *22*, 454–466. [CrossRef]
15. Dolly, O. Synaptic transmission: Inhibition of neurotransmitter release by Botulinum toxins. *Headache* **2003**, *43*, 16–24. [CrossRef]
16. Jankovic, J. Botulinum toxin in clinical practice. *J. Neurol. Neurosurg. Psychiatry* **2004**, *75*, 951–957. [CrossRef] [PubMed]
17. Beske, P.H.; Hoffman, K.M.; Machamer, J.B.; Eisen, M.R.; McNutt, P.M. Use-dependent potentiation of voltage-gated calcium channels rescues neurotransmission in nerve terminals intoxicated by botulinum neurotoxin serotype A. *Sci. Rep.* **2017**, *7*, 15862. [CrossRef] [PubMed]
18. Durham, P.L.; Cady, R.; Cady, R. Regulation of Calcitonin Gene-Related Peptide Secretion From Trigeminal Nerve Cells by Botulinum Toxin Type A: Implications for Migraine Therapy. *Headache* **2004**, *44*, 35–43. [CrossRef] [PubMed]
19. Guo, B.L.; Zheng, C.X.; Sui, B.D.; Li, Y.Q.; Wang, Y.Y.; Yang, Y.L. A closer look to botulinum neurotoxin type A-induced analgesia. *Toxicon* **2013**, *71*, 134–139. [CrossRef] [PubMed]
20. Aoki, K.R. Review of a Proposed Mechanism for the Antinociceptive Action of Botulinum Toxin Type A. *Neurotoxicology* **2005**, *26*, 785–793. [CrossRef] [PubMed]
21. Jeynes, L.C.; Gauci, C.A. Evidence for the use of botulinum toxin in the chronic pain setting: A review of the literature. *Pain Pract.* **2008**, *8*, 269–276. [CrossRef] [PubMed]
22. Aoki, K.R. Future aspects of botulinum neurotoxins. *J. Neural Trans.* **2008**, *115*, 567–573. [CrossRef] [PubMed]
23. Thenganatt, M.A.; Fahn, S. Botulinum toxin for the treatment of movement disorders. *Curr. Neurol. Neurosci. Rep.* **2012**, *12*, 399–409. [CrossRef] [PubMed]
24. Foster, L.; Clapp, L.; Erickson, M.; Jabbari, B. Botulinum toxin A and chronic low back pain: A randomized, double-blind study. *Neurology* **2001**, *56*, 1290–1293. [CrossRef] [PubMed]
25. Ayyar, B.V.; Tajhya, R.B.; Beeton, C.; Atassi, M.Z. Antigenic sites on the H N domain of botulinum neurotoxin A stimulate protective antibody responses against active toxin. *Sci. Rep.* **2015**, *5*, 15776. [CrossRef] [PubMed]
26. Humeau, Y.; Doussau, F.; Grant, N.J.; Poulain, B. How botulinum and tetanus neurotoxins block neurotransmitter release. *Biochimie* **2002**, *82*, 427–446. [CrossRef]
27. Juzans, P.; Comella, J.X.; Molgo, J.; Faille, L.; Angaut-Petit, D. Nerve terminal sprouting in botulinum type-A treated mouse levator auris longus muscle. *Neuromuscul. Disord.* **1996**, *6*, 177–185. [CrossRef]
28. Foran, P.G.; Davletov, B.; Meunier, F.A. Getting musclesmoving again after botulinum toxin: Novel therapeuti challenges. *Trends Mol. Med.* **2003**, *9*, 291–299. [CrossRef]

29. Ko, C.P. Do nerve terminal sprouts contribute to functional recovery from botulinum neurotoxin A? *J. Physiol.* **2008**, *586*, 3021. [CrossRef] [PubMed]
30. Coffield, J.A.; Yan, X. Neuritogenic actions of botulinum neurotoxin A on cultured motor neurons. *J. Pharmacol. Exp. Ther.* **2009**, *330*, 352–358. [CrossRef] [PubMed]
31. Mori, N.; Morii, H. SCG10-related neuronal growth-associated proteins in neural development, plasticity, degeneration, and aging. *J. Neurosci. Res.* **2002**, *70*, 264–273. [CrossRef] [PubMed]
32. Pellier-Monnin, V.; Astic, L.; Bichet, S.; Riederer, B.M.; Grenningloh, G. Expression of SCG10 and stathmin proteins in the rat olfactory system during development and axonal regeneration. *J. Comp. Neurol.* **2001**, *433*, 239–254. [CrossRef] [PubMed]
33. Holahan, M.R. A Shift from a Pivotal to Supporting Role for the Growth-Associated Protein (GAP-43) in the Coordination of Axonal Structural and Functional Plasticity. *Front. Cell. Neurosci.* **2017**, *11*, 1–19. [CrossRef] [PubMed]
34. Goldberg, J.L.; Klassen, M.P.; Hua, Y.; Barres, B.A. Amacrine-signaled loss of intrinsic axon growth ability by retinal ganglion cells. *Science* **2002**, *296*, 1860–1864. [CrossRef] [PubMed]
35. Fernandes, K.J.; Fan, D.P.; Tsui, B.J.; Cassar, S.L.; Tetzlaff, W. Influence of the axotomy to cell body distance in rat rubrospinal and spinal motoneurons: Differential regulation of gap-43, tubulins, and neurofilamentm. *J. Comp. Neurol.* **1999**, *414*, 495–510. [CrossRef]
36. Fagoe, N.D.; Heest, J.V.; Verhaagen, J. Spinal cord injury and the neuron-intrinsic regeneration-associated gene program. *Neuromol. Med.* **2014**, *16*, 799–813. [CrossRef] [PubMed]
37. Lieberman, A.R. The axon reaction: A review of the principal features of perikaryal responses to axon injury. *Int. Rev. Neurobiol.* **1971**, *14*, 49–124. [PubMed]
38. Grafstein, B. The nerve cell body response to axotomy. *Exp. Neurol.* **1975**, *48*, 32–51. [CrossRef]
39. Skene, J.H.; Willard, M. Axonally Transported Proteins Associated with Axon Growth in Rabbit Central and Peripheral Nervous Systems. *J. Cell Biol.* **1981**, *89*, 96–103. [CrossRef] [PubMed]
40. Skene, J.H. Axonal growth-associated proteins. *Annu. Rev. Neurosci.* **1989**, *12*, 127–156. [CrossRef] [PubMed]
41. Tetzlaff, W.; Alexander, S.W.; Miller, F.D.; Bisby, M.A. Response of facial and rubrospinal neurons to axotomy: Changes in mrna expression for cytoskeletal proteins and gap-43. *J. Neurosci.* **1991**, *11*, 2528–2544. [PubMed]
42. Shin, J.E.; Geisler, S.; Diantonio, A. Dynamic regulation of SCG10 in regenerating axons after injury. *Exp. Neurol.* **2014**, *252*, 1–11. [CrossRef] [PubMed]
43. Ozon, S.; Maucuer, A.; Sobel, A. The stathmin family—Molecular and biological characterization of novel mammalian proteins expressed in the nervous system. *Eur. J. Biochem.* **2010**, *248*, 794–806. [CrossRef]
44. Riederer, B.M.; Pellier, V.; Antonsson, B.; Paolo, G.D.; Stimpson, S.A.; Lütjens, R.; Catsicas, S.; Grenningloh, G. Regulation of microtubule dynamics by the neuronal growth-associated protein SCG 10. *Proc. Natl. Acad. Sci. USA* **1997**, *94*, 741–745. [CrossRef] [PubMed]
45. Wang, J.; Shan, C.; Cao, W.; Zhang, C.; Teng, J.; Chen, J. SCG10 promotes non-amyloidogenic processing of amyloid precursor protein by facilitating its trafficking to the cell surface. *Hum. Mol. Genet.* **2013**, *22*, 4888–4900. [CrossRef] [PubMed]
46. Prado, W.A. Antinociceptive potency of intrathecal morphine in the rat tail flick test: A comparative study using acute lumbar catheter in rats with or without a chronic atlanto-occipital catheter. *J. Neurosci. Methods* **2003**, *129*, 33–39. [CrossRef]
47. Ulmann, L.; Rodeau, J.L.; Danoux, L.; Contet-Audonneau, J.L.; Pauly, G.; Schlichter, R. Dehydroepiandrosterone and neurotrophins favor axonal growth in a sensory neuron-keratinocyte coculture model. *Neuroscience* **2009**, *159*, 514–525. [CrossRef] [PubMed]

toxins

MDPI

Review

Correction of Malocclusion by Botulinum Neurotoxin Injection into Masticatory Muscles

Hyun Seok [1] and Seong-Gon Kim [2,*]

1 Department of Oral and Maxillofacial Surgery, Chungbuk National University Hospital, Cheongju 28644, Korea; sok8585@hanmail.net
2 Department of Oral and Maxillofacial Surgery, College of Dentistry, Gangneung-Wonju National University, Gangneung 25457, Korea
* Correspondence: kimsg@gwnu.ac.kr; Tel.: +82-33-640-2468

Received: 1 December 2017; Accepted: 31 December 2017; Published: 2 January 2018

Abstract: Botulinum toxin (BTX) is a neurotoxin, and its injection in masticatory muscles induces muscle weakness and paralysis. This paralytic effect of BTX induces growth retardation of the maxillofacial bones, changes in dental eruption and occlusion state, and facial asymmetry. Using masticatory muscle paralysis and its effect via BTX, BTX can be used for the correction of malocclusion after orthognathic surgery and mandible fracture. The paralysis of specific masticatory muscles by BTX injection reduces the tensional force to the mandible and prevents relapse and changes in dental occlusion. BTX injection in the anterior belly of digastric and mylohyoid muscle prevents the open-bite and deep bite of dental occlusion and contributes to mandible stability after orthognathic surgery. The effect of BTX injection in masticatory muscles for maxillofacial bone growth and dental occlusion is reviewed in this article. The clinical application of BTX is also discussed for the correction of dental malocclusion and suppression of post-operative relapse after mandibular surgery.

Keywords: botulinum neurotoxin; masticatory system; maxillofacial bone; dental occlusion; orthognathic surgery

Key contribution: BTX injection into masticatory muscles affects the maxillofacial bony growth and dental occlusion. In clinical practices, BTX injection has been used for reducing post-operative relapse after mandibular surgery.

---

1. Introduction

For the correction of malocclusion, the understanding of growth and development is a key component. Broken harmony between the maxilla and the mandible during growth influences dental occlusion [1]. Most discrepancies in growth are under genetic control [2]. However, the interaction between muscles and the skeleton is the front line in the battlefield of growth. For these reasons, many orthodontists have used orthopedic appliances to correct abnormal jaw bone growth.

Dental occlusion is located in the border between the buccal shelf and the tongue. A patient with a narrow dental arch is treated using the appliance, which shields the action of the buccinator muscles. To prevent tongue thrust habit, an appliance can be used for treating anterior open-bite. In the case of pediatric mandibular prognathism, a chin cap, high-pull headgear, and other types of functional appliances have been used to restrain forward growth of the mandible. However, these efforts have often not achieved their treatment goals because most patients have shown relapse [3]. Compared to young patients, the results of orthodontic treatment are poor in aged patients because of slow bony remodeling and periodontal problems [4]. In the case of maxillary molar area, 20–30% of relapse has been reported between one and three years after treatment [5,6]. As the reasons of malocclusion are many, such as genetics, environmental and habitual factors, clinicians should consider all contributing factors [7]. Generally, relapse after treatment is associated with the severity of disease. Accordingly, intensive maintenance is required for patients needing large corrections [8].

If certain treatments can strengthen or weaken the power of specific muscles, they may replace unpleasant long-term usage of orthopedic appliances. Botulinum toxin is produced by bacterium and can weaken the power of specific muscles. If the rationale of the orthopedic appliance treatment is applied, BTX can be a highly effective treatment option for the correction of malocclusion-associated problems. Accordingly, recent knowledge regarding BTX on facial bone growth is reviewed in this article. Additionally, several frontier clinical applications of BTX are discussed.

Botulinum toxin-A (BTX) is a family of BTX and is most commonly used in clinical practice [9]. BTX reversibly reduces muscle activity and induces muscle paralysis by inhibiting the release of acetylcholine in presynaptic membrane of nerve terminal [10]. This treatment degrades synaptosomal-associated protein of 25 kDa (SNAP-25), which is required for acetylcholine secretion and release [11]. This paralytic effect of BTX has been used in various fields of oral and maxillofacial regions for the treatment of facial muscle spasms, muscle myalgia, temporomandibular disorder, masticatory muscle hypertrophy, and cosmetic purposes [12,13]. A therapeutic dose of BTX can be safely used in masticatory muscles with few complications [14].

The BTX injection in masticatory muscles influences balanced masticatory activity, including food mastication, swallowing, and breathing [15]. The BTX injection can disturb the balanced masticatory muscle activity and lead to masticatory muscle weakness and decreased mastication activity [16]. The paralytic effect of BTX in masticatory muscles influences maxillofacial bone growth when administered in the growth phase [17]. In animal studies, BTX injection in masticatory muscles has an effect on various portions of maxillofacial bone growth that are muscle-related areas and significantly decreased size and morphology [18]. The unilateral masticatory muscle weakness by BTX injection induces the maxillofacial bone hypoplasia and facial asymmetry [19]. The decrease of masticatory muscle function and bite force contributes to the changes of molar tooth eruption state and potentially affects dental occlusion [19,20].

In this review, we introduced the balanced masticatory muscle function in normal masticatory activity and the role of masticatory muscles in the masticatory system. We investigated the effect of the BTX injection in masticatory muscles on the changes of maxillofacial bone growth, dental eruption, and occlusion. We also suggested the therapeutic application of BTX for the recovery and correction of dental occlusion.

2. Balanced Muscle Power in the Masticatory System

The masticatory system is a complex functional unit composed of the maxillofacial bones, masticatory muscles, teeth, tongue, and temporomandibular joint (TMJ) [21]. This system is supplied by vascular and neuromuscular supports for function and activity [22], is controlled by the neurological system and cooperatively interacts with head and neck musculatures, ligaments, salivary gland, lips, palate, and cheek [23]. Mastication activity is highly organized and controlled neuromuscular activity that is integrated with the various masticatory system components [21]. The neurologically coordinated mastication system effectively regulates mandible movement and contracture of surrounding tissue [24]. The balanced muscle function and jaw movement contributes to normal masticatory activities, such as food intake, digestion, mastication, speech, and swallowing [15].

Mastication is a highly complex and organized neuromuscular activity involved with bone, muscles, teeth, and surrounding structure [22]. This activity requires the movement of jaw and TMJ, and masticatory muscle activity [21]. Balanced masticatory muscle activity is effectively regulated by the central nervous system [24]. The sensory input from the receptors in teeth, periodontal ligament, and TMJ is received to the brain stem and cortex through the afferent nerve [25]. The brain stem and cortex organizes this sensory input and provides motor activity output through efferent nerve fiber in masticatory muscles [24]. The integrated muscle functions are possible by the control of the central pattern generator (CPG) in the brain stem [24]. The masticatory CPG is located between rostral poles of trigeminal and facial motor nucleus and composed of several nuclei, such as nucleus ambigus, nucleus tracti solitary [26]. A neural signal from the hypothalamus activates neurons in the medulla oblongata through the nucleus tracti solitari and elicits masticatory activity [27]. The motor activity of CPG regulates the contracture of certain muscles and the relaxation of others [28]. The CPG regulates the rhythm and timing of muscle activity such that the activities of chewing, swallowing, and breathing can be effectively performed [23].

Mastication is rhythmic and repetitive chewing action and the beginning of digestion [24]. The muscles activated during mastication are temporalis, masseter, medial and lateral pterygoid, and suprahyoid musculatures [15]. These masticatory muscles are innervated with the trigeminal nerve and receive motor activity through the trigeminal motor nucleus [15]. Each of the masticatory muscles is attached on both sides of mandible and correspondingly activated according to the jaw movement and chewing phase [29]. In the opening phase of mandible, the inferior head of lateral pterygoid and digastric muscle are activated, and the digastric muscle acts in the rotation of mandible [30]. The temporalis, masseter, and medial pterygoid muscles involve the closing phase of mandible and act on clenching and chewing the food bolus [15]. Food mastication activity is also supported by the function of the lip, tongue, and buccinators [22]. The lip and perioral muscles involve the intake of food to the oral cavity, and maintain the sealing of mouth during mastication [31]. The tongue and buccinators contribute to effective chewing by repositioning food on the occlusal surface of teeth [31].

Normal mastication activity and masticatory muscle function can influence the maxillofacial bone morphology [32]. Mandible has symmetrical bone morphology, being a mirror image [27]. This bone connects with the cranial bone by the articulation of TMJ [29]. In addition, mandible can be moved by the symmetric movement of TMJ and activation of both sides of masticatory muscles [33]. Disruption of this harmonious masticatory muscle function and movement of mandible affects the symmetric growth of maxillofacial bones [34]. In functional matrix theory, maxillofacial mandibular bone growth can be affected by attached muscle activity and surrounding soft tissue [35]. The balancing of masticatory muscle function and activity can affect harmonious maxillofacial bone morphology, jaw movement, proper dental occlusion, and TMJ function [33,36].

3. Broken Balance Muscle Function by BTX Injection and Its Effects on Maxillofacial Growth

Balanced masticatory muscle function is closely related with maxillofacial bone growth and development [32,35]. Impaired masticatory muscle activity affects the reduced growth of the craniofacial bone structure [37,38]. Animal studies that have masticatory muscle hypofunction by soft food diet, muscle myotomy, and motor nerve denervation show reduced growth of maxillofacial bone [37,39–41]. Masticatory muscle hypofunction affects the bone mass, size, and length [42,43], and also affects the composition of the trabecular bone and thickness of the cortical bone [44]. The maxillofacial bone growth can be affected by the paralytic effect of BTX when it is administered in masticatory muscles [45]. BTX is a neurotoxin that reversibly reduces muscle activity without tissue damage [12]. BTX injection in masticatory muscle can disturb the balance and symmetric growth of maxillofacial bone in growing rats [36], and affects the change of craniofacial bone dimension and composition [18,46].

3.1. The Changes of Maxillofacial Bone Growth by BTX Injection in Masticatory Muscles

BTX injection in masseter muscles decreases muscle activity and affects the maxillofacial bone growth in animal studies [16,45]. Masseter muscle is attached to the zygomatic arch and inserted to the ramus and angle of mandible [47]. With the use of unilateral BTX injection in rabbit masseter muscle, the bone volumes of zygomatic and mandibular bone are significantly reduced [43]. In addition, with BTX injection in the masseter of growing rat, the mandibular length and ramus height are also significantly reduced (Figures 1 and 2) [17]. The unilateral injection of BTX in masseter muscle induces the growth retardation of mandible (Figure 2) [17,18,48] and causes mandible deviation and facial asymmetry in adult rats (Figure 2c,d) [36]. The BTX injection in temporalis muscle also affects craniofacial bone growth. The temporalis muscle extends from the temporal bone and to the coronoid process of mandible [18]. Rats that received BTX in unilateral temporalis muscles had a significantly reduced skull base dimension [18], and the premaxilla, maxilla, and zygomatic arch dimensions were also decreased [18]. These previous animal studies show that the hypofunction of masticatory muscle by BTX injection affects the growth potential of the involved craniofacial bone and induces morphological changes in facial bone growth [17,43].

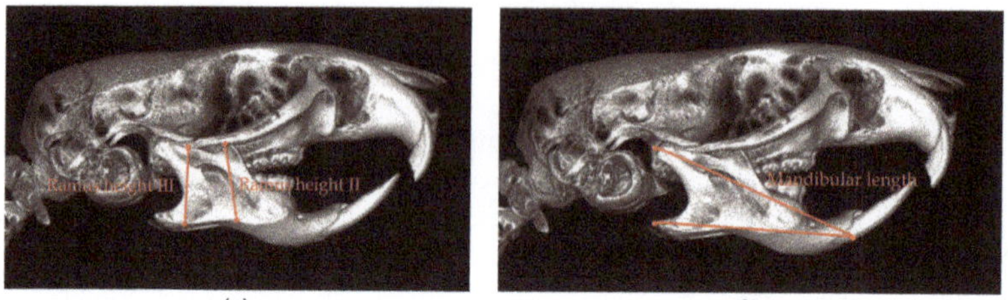

(**a**) (**b**)

Figure 1. Anthropometric measurement of ramus height and mandible length. (**a**) Ramus height II is the distance between the zygomatic arch and inferior point of antegonial notch; ramus height III is the distance between the temporozygomatic suture of zygomatic arch and inferior point of mandible; (**b**) Mandible length is the distance between posterior point of mandible condyle and anterior point of mandible crest in mandible incisor.

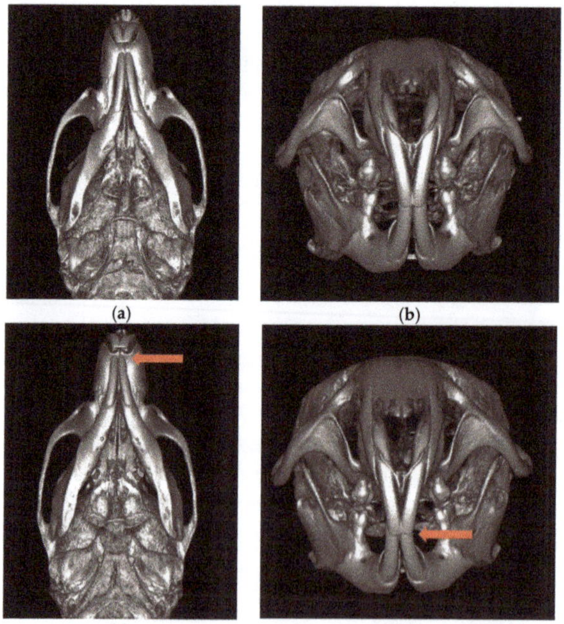

(**c**) (**d**)

Figure 2. Unilateral Botulinum toxin (BTX) injection to the right masseter muscle induces the retardation of mandible and facial asymmetry. (**a**,**b**) The control group with saline injection to the right masseter muscle; (**c**,**d**) the experimental group with BTX injection to the right masseter muscle (red arrow; the deviation of the mandible midline to the BTX injection side).

Masticatory muscle function has an important role in maintaining the bone density and quality of skeleton [49]. Decreased muscle function affects the bone metabolism and remodeling [50], and increases osteoclastic activity and accelerates bone resorption [51]. Muscle paralysis contributes to the disruption of bone homeostasis and leads to bone degradation and morphological changes [50]. Masticatory hypofunction with a soft food diet affects the internal bone structure of mandible in growing rats [44] and shows the thinner cortical bone and reduced bone density in the mandible ramus region [44]. These changes are also observed in the BTX application in masticatory muscle. The paralytic effect of BTX in masseter muscle influences the structural changes of mandible in rat [19]. The BTX-injected side of the mandible shows the significantly reduced bone mineral content and cortical bone thickness [19,52], and the proportion of the trabecular bone area is also reduced [19]. The rats that were BTX-injected in both masseter and temporalis show significantly reduced the trabecular bone in the alveolar and condylar bone region [53]. BTX injection in temporalis muscle of rat reduces the bone mineral density in the bones associated with temporalis muscle [46].

3.2. The Effect of BTX on the Growth of the Mandibular Condyle and Condylar Cartilage

BTX injection into the masticatory muscle may influence the growth of the mandibular condyle [54]. BTX injection into the masseter muscle in mice shows the significantly reduced condylar head width [55], and the distance between the medial and lateral margins of the condylar head is also significantly reduced in growing rats [43]. In BTX injection into the masseter and temporalis muscles, the bone volume is reduced in the BTX-injected side of the condyle [53]. The BTX injection into the masticatory muscle is also related to the bone density and quality of the condyle [53,54].

In animal research, trabecular bone density and condyle thickness are significantly reduced by the BTX injection into the masseter muscle [18], and the marrow cavity and trabecular spacing area are significantly increased [53,55]. The osteoclast activity and bone turnover are decreased in the subchondral area of the condyle [55], which suggests that BTX has sufficient paralytic effects to affect condyle development and induce bony hypoplasia or mandible deviation [17,18,43]. Masticatory muscle hypofunction induced by BTX injection not only negatively affects condylar growth, size, and volume, but also bone density and quality [55].

The detailed mechanism for the change of the condylar cartilage has been unclear. BTX injection of the masticatory muscle influences the temporomandibular joint via altering masticatory loading and causes structural and cellular changes in the condylar cartilage [48]. The growing rat, after receiving a BTX injection into the masseter muscle, shows significantly thinner condylar cartilage compared to the non-injected side [46]. This structural change of the condylar cartilage is associated with a decrease in cellular proliferation and division in the proliferative zone of the cartilage [55]. Unilateral BTX injection in the masseter muscle leads to an increase in the apoptotic process and a decrease in cellular proliferation in the proliferative zone of the cartilage [48]. Decreases in chondrocyte proliferation and proteoglycan secretion are observed in the BTX injection side of the cartilage [55]. Additionally, this change is a cellular response to the decrease in loading on the condylar surface [55]. This result indicates that the muscle paralysis caused by BTX injection may have an inhibitory effect on condylar cartilage proliferation [56].

3.3. The Effect of Masticatory Hypofunction by BTX on Dental Occlusion

Masticatory muscle hypofunction caused by BTX injection decreases the bite force and affects the dental occlusion and tooth eruption [19,20]. The masseter muscle volume and weight are significantly reduced by BTX injection [19], and the maximum bite force is also decreased [57]. The weakness of the bite force is directly related to the loading on the occlusal surface and the eruption state of the tooth [45]. In animal research, rats receiving BTX injection in the masseter muscle show decreased masseter muscle size and weight and overeruptions of the lower molars and incisors [19]. Furthermore, the maxilla and mandibular molar height are also increased after BTX injection into the masseter muscle [17]. Masticatory muscle weakness caused by BTX injection affects the tooth eruption state [19,20], and this tooth overeruption can affect the facial morphological changes, such as anterior open-bite, increased anterior facial height, and dolichofacial morphology [58,59].

4. Clinical Application of BTX

The application of BTX on the perioral area has been performed for cosmetic purposes or for the treatment of temporomandibular disorder [12]. Recently, BTX application has been tried to prevent post-operative relapse after orthognathic surgery. Post-operative relapse has been reported after orthognathic surgery [60]. The main reason for post-operative relapse is the memory of masticatory muscles in their preoperative position [61]. When muscles and connective tissues are extended by jaw bone movement, the stretch receptor will be activated and attempt to restore its original length [62]. Accordingly, the prevention of postoperative relapse has been designed to resist muscular tension.

Considering that post-operative relapse after orthognathic surgery is induced by the muscular tension, the strategy for reducing muscular tension can be an effective treatment option. In this aspect, BTX injection can be a solution for the postoperative relapse. Though the literature on this issue is scarce, there are several articles on the correction of open-bite after the treatment of trauma. The open-bite can be frequently found in bilateral mandibular angle fractures and the chin is depressed by the contracture of the digastric muscles [63]. Most patients can be corrected by open reduction and intermaxillary fixation. When patients do not receive the open reduction in time, reduced segments might be unstable due to the tensional force of the digastric muscles. Similar to BTX injection, radiofrequency therapy is also effective for reducing muscular power and volume. Targeting the anterior belly of the digastric muscle, the application of radiofrequency therapy is effective for correcting post-traumatic open-bite [64]. Based on this finding, similar cases have been treated by 20-unit BTX injections into the anterior belly of the digastric muscle [65]. When the patient is in the state of open-bite, the anterior belly of the digastric muscle receives the tensional force according to the counterclockwise rotation of the mandible in the course of treatment (Figure 3). Accordingly, the mandible has a tendency of clockwise rotation after reduction, and this mechanism will contribute to relapse after treatment. In fact, BTX injection into the anterior belly of the digastric muscle has been shown to be successful, and there has been no relapse after injection (Figure 4) [65]. As improper injection of BTX in the neck may induce such complications as dysphagia, the precise localization of injection site may be important to avoid these complications [66].

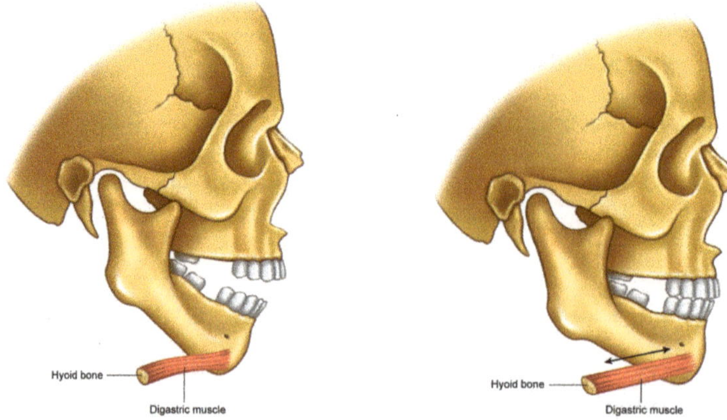

Figure 3. Schematic illustration of relapse mechanism after open-bite correction. During the correction of anterior open-bite, the mandible was rotated in a counterclockwise direction and the anterior belly of the digastric muscle was lengthened. Accordingly, the tensional force was generated and the relapse of the open-bite could have occurred during relieving the tensional force.

In the case of malocclusion patients, the anterior open bite has been frequently observed, and this protocol can be applied for these patients. The treatment of the open bite has been challenging because it has multiple etiological factors [67]. The open bite can be caused by the imbalance of the growth between the mandible and the maxilla, airway obstruction, para-functional habits, and trauma [68]. In the case of mandibular prognathism, approximately 30% of patients show an open bite [69]. These skeletal open-bite patients show clockwise rotation of the mandible and higher anterior facial height [70]. The patients with mandibular prognathism and open bite can be corrected by surgical treatment, and the mandible is moved backward and counterclockwise after the operation [71]. Postoperative anterior open bite is caused by unstable condylar position and muscular pull [72]. Postoperative anterior open bite after orthognathic surgery is a kind of relapse, and its rate has been reported at 10 to 15% [73,74]. Many kinds of modifications have been introduced for minimizing postoperative relapse. Overcorrection is overtreatment, rather than therapeutic movement, considering repositioning of jaw bones. Distal cutting of the mandibular proximal segment has been done to reduce the tension applied on the pterygomasseteric sling after the posterior movement of the mandible. If the surgeon modifies the design of osteotomy, the amount and the type of muscles attached to each sectioned bony segment can be changed. By adapting vertical ramus osteotomy design, postoperative relapse may be reduced [75]. Myotomy, as a preventive measure of the postoperative relapse, is an aggressive approach that targets the muscle directly. Most literature claims that these modifications have been successful in reducing postoperative relapse. However, cutting additional bone and myotomy have higher rates of complications, such as bleeding and nerve damage. A number of clinicians are concerned that the duration of the therapeutic effects of BTX is temporary. However, BTX application for the prevention of postoperative relapse can be promising, considering that the greatest amount of relapse (47.8%) has been observed during the early postoperative period [76].

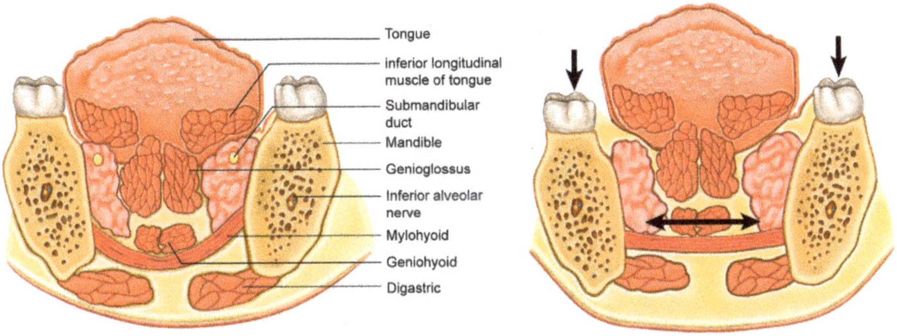

Figure 4. Schematic illustration of relapse mechanism after deep bite correction. During the correction of deep bite, the mandible was moved in a downward direction and the mylohyoid muscle was lengthened. Accordingly, the tensional force was generated and the relapse of the deep bite could have occurred while relieving the tensional force.

"Deep bite" is the opposite of open-bite. The status of malocclusion has been frequently found in mandibular retrognathism [77]. For the surgical correction of this malocclusion, the position of the mandible usually moves downward and the myohyoid muscle receives tension [78] (Figure 4). Accordingly, relapse after treatment occurs at a high frequency, regardless of treatment protocol [79,80]. There has been comparative study on this issue. BTX has been given to the myohyoid muscle to reduce tension after surgery [60]. When compared to untreated control, the BTX application group has shown significantly higher positional stability. Myotomy for the suprahyoid muscles also showed an increase in stability after the mandibular advancement, and these findings can be interpreted in that the tensional force of the suprahyoid muscles is a contributing factor for skeletal relapse [61]. Considering the complications of suprahyoid muscle myotomy [81], BTX injection is a relatively simple and effective treatment.

In the course of orthognathic surgery, patients usually prefer the intra-oral approach to the trans-buccal approach. However, compared to bi-cortical screws fixation, single plate fixation is less rigid fixation [82]. Patients who received bi-cortical screw fixation may open their mouth immediately after operation. In the case of single plate fixation, patients may be asked about intermaxillary fixation for three to four weeks. In our preliminary study [83], the patients (n = 7) received BTX-A injection into their masseter muscles along with two weeks of intermaxillary fixation. This group was compared to the patients (n = 11) who did not receive BTX treatment and the same period of intermaxillary fixation. The incidence of plate fractures was 14.3% in the BTX-injected group and 31.8% in the untreated control group (Figure 5). As the plate fracture is largely a fatigue type of fracture induced by the action of the masticatory muscles, reduced muscle power by BTX application may prevent the plate fracture. Though postoperative relapse has not been assessed, it may be reduced by BTX injection. To draw definite conclusions, further follow-up studies will be required.

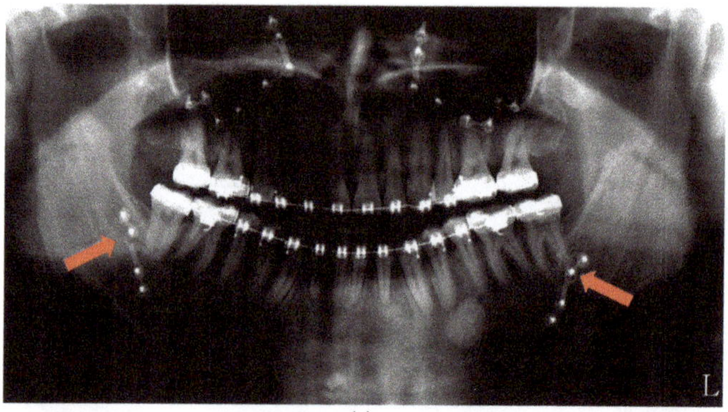

(**a**)

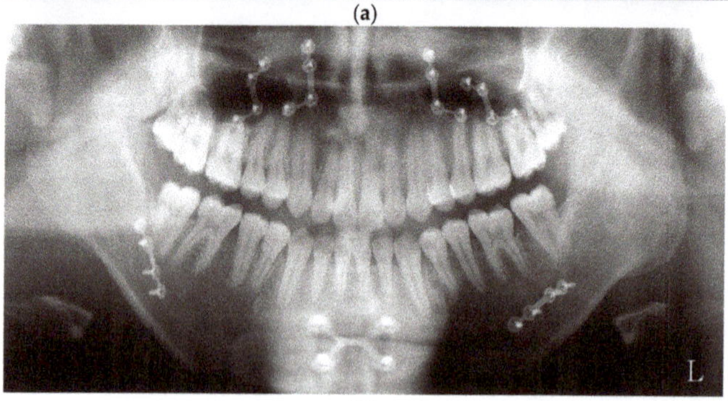

(**b**)

Figure 5. BTX treatment after orthognathic surgery. (**a**) Single plate fixation group after orthognathic surgery without BTX treatment (plate fracture in red arrow); (**b**) BTX injection group in both masseter muscles after orthognathic surgery.

The application of BTX in pediatric patients has been rare. In the progress of growth, the size of muscle fibers increases [84]. In experimental research, BTX prevents the exercise-induced increase in muscle fiber size of young rats via reduction in contractile activity [85]. When the upward movement of the maxillary posterior teeth is affected by posterior impaction, overbite in the anterior teeth can be increased, and anterior open bite can be corrected [86]. Accordingly, posterior bite block can be considered nonsurgical treatment of open bite [87]. If the open bite is caused by tongue thrust habit, tongue spurs can be used to control the force generated by tongue muscles [88].

When the parafunctional habit is intervened in the early stage of growth, irreversible open bite can be prevented [89]. The correction of open bite in the children is mainly composed of functional appliance that can shield the action of perioral musculatures [89]. Though many types of functional appliances have been introduced, their therapeutic effects have not been promising due to study design limitations [90].

BTX injection into perioral muscle has been considered a relatively safe treatment. Except for periocular injection, complications related to BTX injection have been rarely reported. Recently, a case of temporary blindness has been reported after BTX injection into the masseter muscle [91]. The blindness after BTX injection may be induced by intravascular introduction of BTX [92]. When BTX is introduced into the vessel, it may induce myocardial infarction and pulmonary embolism via pro-thrombotic effect [93]. When an ocular event is observed after BTX injection, early injection of steroid may be helpful for relieving retinal pressure [94]. To avoid intravascular introduction of BTX, BTX should not be diluted too much and a small-sized needle should be used. Deep injection may increase the probability of intravascular introduction of BTX. There is no difference in the therapeutic effect between intradermal and intramuscular injection of BTX [95]. To prevent systemic effects of BTX injection, the clinician should make every effort to minimize diffusion and vascular introduction of BTX after injection.

5. Conclusions

Balanced masticatory muscle function is a key component of maxillofacial bone growth and development. The dysfunction of masticatory muscle influences the retardation of facial bone growth and disruption of dental occlusion. The BTX injection to the masticatory muscle induces reversible paralysis and weakness of muscle power. The injection of BTX in masticatory muscle disrupts the balanced function of mastication and can influence maxillofacial bone growth and dental occlusion when administered during the growth phase. The weakness of masticatory muscle activity by BTX induces the hypoplasia of maxillofacial bone in the zygoma, temporal bone, mandible, and condyle area, and the alteration of the tooth occlusion state.

Clinically, the paralysis of masticatory muscle by BTX has an effect on maintaining mandible stability and preventing changes in dental occlusion after orthognathic and mandible fracture surgery. BTX injection in digastric muscle reduces the tensional force of mandible and prevents the counterclockwise rotation of mandible and open-bite of teeth. The BTX injection in mylohyoid muscle also prevents the deep bite of teeth and postoperative relapse after orthognathic surgery. Compared with a surgery-only patient, the patient in our clinic who received BTX in both masseter muscles after orthognathic surgery showed more stable dental occlusion. The BTX injection is an effective method for the correction of dental occlusion by inducing specific masticatory muscle paralysis without major complications. In an animal growth study, the injection of BTX in masticatory muscle has an effect on the growth potential of the maxillofacial bones. Additionally, this treatment could be an effective tool for the correction of facial bone and dental occlusion in the pediatric patient. Further study will be necessary for the therapeutic use of BTX in orthopedic treatment to correct abnormal jaw bone growth and malocclusion.

Acknowledgments: This work was carried out with the support of the "Cooperative Research Program for Agriculture Science and Technology Development (Project No. PJ01121404)" Rural Development Administration, Republic of Korea.

Author Contributions: Seong-Gon Kim conceived and designed the review; Seong-Gon Kim and Hyun Seok write the first draft and reviewed and wrote the paper. All of the authors read and approved the final version of the manuscript.

Conflicts of Interest: The authors declare no conflict of interest.

References

1. Janson, G.; Laranjeira, V.; Rizzo, M.; Garib, D. Posterior tooth angulations in patients with anterior open bite and normal occlusion. *Am. J. Orthod. Dentofac. Orthop.* **2016**, *150*, 71–77. [CrossRef] [PubMed]
2. Mossey, P. The heritability of malocclusion: Part 1—Genetics, principles and terminology. *Br. J. Orthod.* **1999**, *26*, 103–113. [CrossRef] [PubMed]
3. Freeman, C.S.; McNamara, J.A.; Baccetti, T.; Franchi, L.; Graff, T.W. Treatment effects of the bionator and high-pull facebow combination followed by fixed appliances in patients with increased vertical dimensions. *Am. J. Orthod. Dentofac. Orthop.* **2007**, *131*, 184–195. [CrossRef] [PubMed]
4. Tanne, K.; Yoshida, S.; Kawata, T.; Sasaki, A.; Knox, J.; Jones, M. An evaluation of the biomechanical response of the tooth and periodontium to orthodontic forces in adolescent and adult subjects. *Br. J. Orthod.* **1998**, *25*, 109–115. [CrossRef] [PubMed]
5. Sugawara, J.; Baik, U.B.; Umemori, M.; Takahashi, I.; Nagasaka, H.; Kawamura, H.; Mitani, H. Treatment and posttreatment dentoalveolar changes following intrusion of mandibular molars with application of a skeletal anchorage system (SAS) for open bite correction. *Int. J. Adult Orthod. Orthognath. Surg.* **2002**, *17*, 243–253.
6. Baek, M.S.; Choi, Y.J.; Yu, H.S.; Lee, K.J.; Kwak, J.; Park, Y.C. Long-term stability of anterior open-bite treatment by intrusion of maxillary posterior teeth. *Am. J. Orthod. Dentofac. Orthop.* **2010**, *138*, 396.e1–396.e9. [CrossRef]
7. Burford, D.; Noar, J.H. The causes, diagnosis and treatment of anterior open bite. *Dent. Update* **2003**, *30*, 235–241. [CrossRef] [PubMed]
8. Marzouk, E.S.; Kassem, H.E. Evaluation of long-term stability of skeletal anterior open bite correction in adults treated with maxillary posterior segment intrusion using zygomatic miniplates. *Am. J. Orthod. Dentofac. Orthop.* **2016**, *150*, 78–88. [CrossRef] [PubMed]
9. Pearce, L.B.; Borodic, G.E.; First, E.R.; MacCallum, R.D. Measurement of botulinum toxin activity: Evaluation of the lethality assay. *Toxicol. Appl. Pharmacol.* **1994**, *128*, 69–77. [CrossRef] [PubMed]
10. Rossetto, O.; Pirazzini, M.; Montecucco, C. Botulinum neurotoxins: Genetic, structural and mechanistic insights. *Nat. Rev. Microbiol.* **2014**, *12*, 535–549. [CrossRef] [PubMed]
11. Moon, Y.M.; Kim, M.K.; Kim, S.G.; Kim, T.W. Apoptotic action of botulinum toxin on masseter muscle in rats: Early and late changes in the expression of molecular markers. *Springerplus* **2016**, *5*, 1–11. [CrossRef] [PubMed]
12. Kim, H.S.; Yun, P.Y.; Kim, Y.K. A clinical evaluation of botulinum toxin-A injections in the temporomandibular disorder treatment. *Maxillofac. Plast. Reconstr. Surg.* **2016**, *38*, 5. [CrossRef] [PubMed]
13. Baş, B.; Ozan, B.; Muğlali, M.; Çelebi, N. Treatment of masseteric hypertrophy with botulinum toxin: A report of two cases. *Med. Oral Patol. Oral Cir. Bucal* **2010**, *15*, 649–652. [CrossRef]
14. Mahant, N.; Clouston, P.; Lorentz, I. The current use of botulinum toxin. *J. Clin. Neurosci.* **2000**, *7*, 389–394. [CrossRef] [PubMed]
15. Thexton, A.J. Mastication and swallowing: An overview. *Br. Dent. J.* **1992**, *173*, 197–206. [CrossRef] [PubMed]
16. Park, S.Y.; Park, Y.W.; Ji, Y.J.; Park, S.W.; Kim, S.G. Effects of a botulinum toxin type A injection on the masseter muscle: An animal model study. *Maxillofac. Plast. Reconstr. Surg.* **2015**, *37*, 10. [CrossRef] [PubMed]
17. Tsai, C.Y.; Chiu, W.C.; Liao, Y.H.; Tsai, C.M. Effects on craniofacial growth and development of unilateral botulinum neurotoxin injection into the masseter muscle. *Am. J. Orthod. Dentofac. Orthop.* **2009**, *135*, 142.e1–142.e6. [CrossRef]
18. Babuccu, B.; Babuccu, O.; Yurdakan, G.; Ankaral, H. The effect of the botulinum toxin-A on craniofacial development: An experimental study. *Ann. Plast. Surg.* **2009**, *63*, 449–456. [CrossRef] [PubMed]
19. Tsai, C.Y.; Huang, R.Y.; Lee, C.M.; Hsiao, W.T.; Yang, L.Y. Morphologic and bony structural changes in the mandible after a unilateral injection of botulinum neurotoxin in adult rats. *J. Oral Maxillofac. Surg.* **2010**, *68*, 1081–1087. [CrossRef] [PubMed]
20. Navarrete, A.L.; Rafferty, K.L.; Liu, Z.J.; Ye, W.; Greenlee, G.M.; Herring, S.W. Botulinum neurotoxin type a in the masseter muscle: Effects on incisor eruption in rabbits. *Am. J. Orthod. Dentofac. Orthop.* **2013**, *143*, 499–506. [CrossRef] [PubMed]
21. Ahlgren, J. Mechanism of mastication. *Acta Odontol. Scand.* **1966**, *24*, 44–45.
22. Soboļeva, U.; Lauriņa, L.; Slaidiņa, A. The masticatory system—An overview. *Stomatologija* **2005**, *7*, 77–80. [PubMed]

23. Dellow, P.; Lund, J. Evidence for central timing of rhythmical mastication. *J. Physiol.* **1971**, *215*, 1–13. [CrossRef] [PubMed]
24. Lund, J.P. Mastication and its control by the brain stem. *Crit. Rev. Oral Biol. Med.* **1991**, *2*, 33–64. [CrossRef] [PubMed]
25. Gibbs, C.H.; Messerman, T.; Reswick, J.B.; Derda, H.J. Functional movements of the mandible. *J. Prosthet. Dent.* **1971**, *26*, 604–620. [CrossRef]
26. Morquette, P.; Lavoie, R.; Fhima, M.D.; Lamoureux, X.; Verdier, D.; Kolta, A. Generation of the masticatory central pattern and its modulation by sensory feedback. *Prog. Neurobiol.* **2012**, *96*, 340–355. [CrossRef] [PubMed]
27. Nakamura, Y.; Yanagawa, Y.; Morrison, S.F.; Nakamura, K. Medullary reticular neurons mediate neuropeptide Y-induced metabolic inhibition and mastication. *Cell Metab.* **2017**, *25*, 322–334. [CrossRef] [PubMed]
28. Nozaki, S.; Iriki, A.; Nakamura, Y. Localization of central rhythm generator involved in cortically induced rhythmical masticatory jaw-opening movement in the guinea pig. *J. Neurophysiol.* **1986**, *55*, 806–825. [CrossRef] [PubMed]
29. Neeman, H.; McCall, W.; Plesh, O.; Bishop, B. Analysis of jaw movements and masticatory muscle activity. *Comput. Methods Programs Biomed.* **1990**, *31*, 19–32. [CrossRef]
30. Wood, W.; Takada, K.; Hannam, A. The electromyographic activity of the inferior part of the human lateral pterygoid muscle during clenching and chewing. *Arch. Oral Biol.* **1986**, *31*, 245–253. [CrossRef]
31. Horio, T.; Kawamura, Y. Effects of texture of food on chewing patterns in the human subject. *J. Oral Rehabilit.* **1989**, *16*, 177–183. [CrossRef]
32. Kiliaridis, S. Masticatory muscle influence on craniofacial growth. *Acta Odontol. Scand.* **1995**, *53*, 196–202. [CrossRef] [PubMed]
33. Cho, J.W.; Park, J.H.; Kim, J.W.; Kim, S.J. The sequential management of recurrent temporomandibular joint ankylosis in a growing child: A case report. *Maxillofac. Plast. Reconstr. Surg.* **2016**, *38*, 39. [CrossRef] [PubMed]
34. Choi, J.W.; Kim, B.H.; Kim, H.S.; Yu, T.H.; Kim, B.C.; Lee, S.H. Three-dimensional functional unit analysis of hemifacial microsomia mandible—A preliminary report. *Maxillofac. Plast. Reconstr. Surg.* **2015**, *37*, 28. [CrossRef] [PubMed]
35. Moss, M.L.; Rankow, R.M. The role of the functional matrix in mandibular growth. *Angle Orthod.* **1968**, *38*, 95–103. [PubMed]
36. Chen, Z.; Chen, Z.; Zhao, N.; Shen, G. An animal model for inducing deviation of the mandible. *J. Oral Maxillofac. Surg.* **2015**, *73*, 2207–2218. [CrossRef] [PubMed]
37. Ulgen, M.; Baran, S.; Kaya, H.; Karadede, I. The influence of the masticatory hypofunction on the craniofacial growth and development in rats. *Am. J. Orthod. Dentofac. Orthop.* **1997**, *111*, 189–198. [CrossRef]
38. Kim, J.H.; Lee, S.C.; Kim, C.H.; Kim, B.J. Facial asymmetry: A case report of localized linear scleroderma patient with muscular strain and spasm. *Maxillofac. Plast. Reconstr. Surg.* **2015**, *37*, 29. [CrossRef] [PubMed]
39. Bouvier, M.; Hylander, W.L. The effect of dietary consistency on gross and histologic morphology in the craniofacial region of young rats. *Am. J. Anat.* **1984**, *170*, 117–126. [CrossRef] [PubMed]
40. Navarro, M.; Delgado, E.; Monje, F. Changes in mandibular rotation after muscular resection. Experimental study in rats. *Am. J. Orthod. Dentofac. Orthop.* **1995**, *108*, 367–379. [CrossRef]
41. Phillips, C.; Shapiro, P.A.; Luschei, E.S. Morphologic alterations in macaca mulatta following destruction of the motor nucleus of the trigeminal nerve. *Am. J. Orthod.* **1982**, *81*, 292–298. [CrossRef]
42. Tsai, C.; Yang, L.; Chen, K.; Chiu, W. The influence of masticatory hypofunction on developing rat craniofacial structure. *Int. J. Oral Maxillofac. Surg.* **2010**, *39*, 593–598. [CrossRef] [PubMed]
43. Matic, D.B.; Yazdani, A.; Wells, R.G.; Lee, T.Y.; Gan, B.S. The effects of masseter muscle paralysis on facial bone growth. *J. Surg. Res.* **2007**, *139*, 243–252. [CrossRef] [PubMed]
44. Bresin, A.; Kiliaridis, S.; Strid, K.G. Effect of masticatory function on the internal bone structure in the mandible of the growing rat. *Eur. J. Oral Sci.* **1999**, *107*, 35–44. [CrossRef] [PubMed]
45. Rafferty, K.L.; Liu, Z.J.; Ye, W.; Navarrete, A.L.; Nguyen, T.T.; Salamati, A.; Herring, S.W. Botulinum toxin in masticatory muscles: Short-and long-term effects on muscle, bone, and craniofacial function in adult rabbits. *Bone* **2012**, *50*, 651–662. [CrossRef] [PubMed]

46. Tsai, C.Y.; Shyr, Y.M.; Chiu, W.C.; Lee, C.M. Bone changes in the mandible following botulinum neurotoxin injections. *Eur. J. Orthod.* **2010**, *33*, 132–138. [CrossRef] [PubMed]
47. Raadsheer, M.; Kiliaridis, S.; Van Eijden, T.; Van Ginkel, F.; Prahl-Andersen, B. Masseter muscle thickness in growing individuals and its relation to facial morphology. *Arch. Oral Biol.* **1996**, *41*, 323–332. [CrossRef]
48. Kim, J.Y.; Kim, S.T.; Cho, S.W.; Jung, H.S.; Park, K.T.; Son, H.K. Growth effects of botulinum toxin type a injected into masseter muscle on a developing rat mandible. *Oral Dis.* **2008**, *14*, 626–632. [CrossRef] [PubMed]
49. Forwood, M.; Turner, C. Skeletal adaptations to mechanical usage: Results from tibial loading studies in rats. *Bone* **1995**, *17*, S197–S205. [CrossRef]
50. Poliachik, S.L.; Bain, S.D.; Threet, D.; Huber, P.; Gross, T.S. Transient muscle paralysis disrupts bone homeostasis by rapid degradation of bone morphology. *Bone* **2010**, *46*, 18–23. [CrossRef] [PubMed]
51. Ausk, B.J.; Huber, P.; Srinivasan, S.; Bain, S.D.; Kwon, R.Y.; McNamara, E.A.; Poliachik, S.L.; Sybrowsky, C.L.; Gross, T.S. Metaphyseal and diaphyseal bone loss in the tibia following transient muscle paralysis are spatiotemporally distinct resorption events. *Bone* **2013**, *57*, 413–422. [CrossRef] [PubMed]
52. Park, Y.W.; Kim, S.G.; Jo, Y.Y. S100 and p65 expression are increased in the masseter muscle after botulinum toxin-A injection. *Maxillofac. Plast. Reconstr. Surg.* **2016**, *38*, 33. [CrossRef] [PubMed]
53. Kün-Darbois, J.D.; Libouban, H.; Chappard, D. Botulinum toxin in masticatory muscles of the adult rat induces bone loss at the condyle and alveolar regions of the mandible associated with a bone proliferation at a muscle enthesis. *Bone* **2015**, *77*, 75–82. [CrossRef] [PubMed]
54. Kün-Darbois, J.D.; Manero, F.; Rony, L.; Chappard, D. Contrast enhancement with uranyl acetate allows quantitative analysis of the articular cartilage by microct: Application to mandibular condyles in the BTX rat model of disuse. *Micron* **2017**, *97*, 35–40. [CrossRef] [PubMed]
55. Dutra, E.H.; O'Brien, M.H.; Lima, A.; Kalajzic, Z.; Tadinada, A.; Nanda, R.; Yadav, S. Cellular and matrix response of the mandibular condylar cartilage to botulinum toxin. *PLoS ONE* **2016**, *11*, e0164599. [CrossRef] [PubMed]
56. Matthys, T.; Dang, H.A.H.; Rafferty, K.L.; Herring, S.W. Bone and cartilage changes in rabbit mandibular condyles after 1 injection of botulinum toxin. *Am. J. Orthod. Dentofac. Orthop.* **2015**, *148*, 999–1009. [CrossRef] [PubMed]
57. Ahn, K.Y.; Kim, S.T. The change of maximum bite force after botulinum toxin type A injection for treating masseteric hypertrophy. *Plast. Reconstr. Surg.* **2007**, *120*, 1662–1666. [CrossRef] [PubMed]
58. Kwon, T.G.; Park, H.S.; Ryoo, H.M.; Lee, S.H. A comparison of craniofacial morphology in patients with and without facial asymmetry—A three-dimensional analysis with computed tomography. *Int. J. Oral Maxillofac. Surg.* **2006**, *35*, 43–48. [CrossRef] [PubMed]
59. Kiliaridis, S.; Mejersjö, C.; Thilander, B. Muscle function and craniofacial morphology: A clinical study in patients with myotonic dystrophy. *Eur. J. Orthod.* **1989**, *11*, 131–138. [CrossRef] [PubMed]
60. Mücke, T.; Löffel, A.; Kanatas, A.; Karnezi, S.; Rana, M.; Fichter, A.; Haarmann, S.; Wolff, K.D.; Loeffelbein, D.J. Botulinum toxin as a therapeutic agent to prevent relapse in deep bite patients. *J. Craniomaxillofac. Surg.* **2016**, *44*, 584–589. [CrossRef] [PubMed]
61. Carlson, D.S.; Ellis, E.; Dechow, P.C.; Nemeth, P.A. Short-term stability and muscle adaptation after mandibular advancement surgery with and without suprahyoid myotomy in juvenile macaca mulatta. *Oral Surg. Oral Med. Oral Pathol.* **1989**, *68*, 135–149. [CrossRef]
62. Carlson, D.S.; Ellis, E.; Dechow, P.C. Adaptation of the suprahyoid muscle complex to mandibular advancement surgery. *Am. J. Orthod. Dentofac. Orthop.* **1987**, *92*, 134–143. [CrossRef]
63. Haskell, R. Applied surgical anatomy. In *Rowe and Williams' Maxillofacial Injuries*, 2nd ed.; Wiliams, J.L., Rowe, N.L., Eds.; Churchill Livingstone: Edinburgh, UK, 1994; pp. 12–14.
64. Choi, S.-S.; Rotaru, H.; Kim, S.G. Treatment of post-traumatic open bite by radiofrequency. *Br. J. Oral Maxillofac. Surg.* **2007**, *45*, 311–313. [CrossRef] [PubMed]
65. Seok, H.; Park, Y.T.; Kim, S.G.; Park, Y.W. Correction of post-traumatic anterior open bite by injection of botulinum toxin type A into the anterior belly of the digastric muscle: Case report. *J. Korean Assoc. Oral Maxillofac. Surg.* **2013**, *39*, 188–192. [CrossRef] [PubMed]
66. Zdilla, M.J. Screening for variations in anterior digastric musculature prior to correction of post-traumatic anterior open bite by injection of botulinum toxin type A: A technical note. *J. Korean Assoc. Oral Maxillofac. Surg.* **2015**, *41*, 165–167. [CrossRef] [PubMed]

67. Park, J.H.; Yu, J.; Chae, J.M. Lateral open bite and crossbite correction in a class III patient with missing maxillary first premolars. *Am. J. Orthod. Dentofac. Orthop.* **2017**, *152*, 116–125. [CrossRef] [PubMed]
68. Greenlee, G.M.; Huang, G.J.; Chen, S.S.H.; Chen, J.; Koepsell, T.; Hujoel, P. Stability of treatment for anterior open-bite malocclusion: A meta-analysis. *Am. J. Orthod. Dentofac. Orthop.* **2011**, *139*, 154–169. [CrossRef] [PubMed]
69. Ellis, E.; McNamara, J.A. Components of adult class III open-bite malocclusion. *Am. J. Orthod.* **1984**, *86*, 277–290. [CrossRef]
70. Turkkahraman, H.; Cetin, E. Comparison of two treatment strategies for the early treatment of an anterior skeletal open bite. *J. Orofac. Orthop.* **2017**, *78*, 338–347. [CrossRef] [PubMed]
71. Ismail, I.; Leung, Y. Anterior open bite correction by Le Fort I osteotomy with or without anterior segmentation: Which is more stable? *Int. J. Oral Maxillofac. Surg.* **2017**, *46*, 766–773. [CrossRef] [PubMed]
72. Yoshioka, I.; Khanal, A.; Tominaga, K.; Horie, A.; Furuta, N.; Fukuda, J. Vertical ramus versus sagittal split osteotomies: Comparison of stability after mandibular setback. *J. Oral Maxillofac. Surg.* **2008**, *66*, 1138–1144. [CrossRef] [PubMed]
73. Chen, C.M.; Lai, S.S.T.; Wang, C.H.; Wu, J.H.; Lee, K.T.; Lee, H.E. The stability of intraoral vertical ramus osteotomy and factors related to skeletal relapse. *Aesthet. Plast. Surg.* **2011**, *35*, 192–197. [CrossRef] [PubMed]
74. Nihara, J.; Takeyama, M.; Takayama, Y.; Mutoh, Y.; Saito, I. Postoperative changes in mandibular prognathism surgically treated by intraoral vertical ramus osteotomy. *Int. J. Oral Maxillofac. Surg.* **2013**, *42*, 62–70. [CrossRef] [PubMed]
75. Choi, S.H.; Cha, J.Y.; Park, H.S.; Hwang, C.J. Intraoral vertical ramus osteotomy results in good long-term mandibular stability in patients with mandibular prognathism and anterior open bite. *J. Oral Maxillofac. Surg.* **2016**, *74*, 804–810. [CrossRef] [PubMed]
76. Silva, I.; Suska, F.; Cardemil, C.; Rasmusson, L. Stability after maxillary segmentation for correction of anterior open bite: A cohort study of 33 cases. *J. Craniomaxillofac. Surg.* **2013**, *41*, e154–e158. [CrossRef] [PubMed]
77. Lux, C.J.; Dücker, B.; Pritsch, M.; Komposch, G.; Niekusch, U. Occlusal status and prevalence of occlusal malocclusion traits among 9-year-old schoolchildren. *Eur. J. Orthod.* **2009**, *31*, 294–299. [CrossRef] [PubMed]
78. Danz, J.; Greuter, C.; Sifakakis, I.; Fayed, M.; Pandis, N.; Katsaros, C. Stability and relapse after orthodontic treatment of deep bite cases—A long-term follow-up study. *Eur. J. Orthod.* **2012**, *36*, 522–530. [CrossRef] [PubMed]
79. Xi, T.; Schreurs, R.; van Loon, B.; de Koning, M.; Bergé, S.; Hoppenreijs, T.; Maal, T. 3D analysis of condylar remodelling and skeletal relapse following bilateral sagittal split advancement osteotomies. *J. Craniomaxillofac. Surg.* **2015**, *43*, 462–468. [CrossRef] [PubMed]
80. Al Yami, E.A.; Kuijpers-Jagtman, A.M.; van't Hof, M.A. Stability of orthodontic treatment outcome: Follow-up until 10 years postretention. *Am. J. Orthod. Dentofac. Orthop.* **1999**, *115*, 300–304. [CrossRef]
81. Papageorge, M.B.; Doku, H.C. Postoperative infection following suprahyoid myotomy performed in conjunction with sagittal osteotomy of the mandible: Report of a case. *J. Oral Maxillofac. Surg.* **1987**, *45*, 460–462. [CrossRef]
82. Erkmen, E.; Şimşek, B.; Yücel, E.; Kurt, A. Three-dimensional finite element analysis used to compare methods of fixation after sagittal split ramus osteotomy: Setback surgery-posterior loading. *Br. J. Oral Maxillofac. Surg.* **2005**, *43*, 97–104. [CrossRef] [PubMed]
83. Shin, S.H.; Kim, S.G.; Park, Y.W.; Kim, M.K.; Kweon, K.J. The effect of Botulinum toxin-A injection on patients with orthognathic surgery. In Proceedings of the 56th Congress of the Korean Association of Maxillofacial Plastic and Reconstructive Surgeons, Seoul, Korea, 3–4 November 2017; p. 31.
84. Allen, D.L.; Roy, R.R.; Edgerton, V.R. Myonuclear domains in muscle adaptation and disease. *Muscle Nerve* **1999**, *22*, 1350–1360. [CrossRef]
85. Smith, H.; Merry, T. Voluntary resistance wheel exercise during post-natal growth in rats enhances skeletal muscle satellite cell and myonuclear content at adulthood. *Acta Physiol.* **2012**, *204*, 393–402. [CrossRef] [PubMed]
86. Janson, G.; Crepaldi, M.V.; de Freitas, K.M.S.; de Freitas, M.R.; Janson, W. Evaluation of anterior open-bite treatment with occlusal adjustment. *Am. J. Orthod. Dentofac. Orthop.* **2008**, *134*, 10.e1–10.e9. [CrossRef] [PubMed]

87. Vela-Hernández, A.; López-García, R.; García-Sanz, V.; Paredes-Gallardo, V.; Lasagabaster-Latorre, F. Nonsurgical treatment of skeletal anterior open bite in adult patients: Posterior build-ups. *Angle Orthod.* **2016**, *87*, 33–40. [CrossRef] [PubMed]
88. Giuntini, V.; Franchi, L.; Baccetti, T.; Mucedero, M.; Cozza, P. Dentoskeletal changes associated with fixed and removable appliances with a crib in open-bite patients in the mixed dentition. *Am. J. Orthod. Dentofac. Orthop.* **2008**, *133*, 77–80. [CrossRef] [PubMed]
89. Moimaz, S.A.S.; Garbin, A.J.Í.; Lima, A.M.C.; Lolli, L.F.; Saliba, O.; Garbin, C.A.A.S. Longitudinal study of habits leading to malocclusion development in childhood. *BMC Oral Health* **2014**, *14*, 96. [CrossRef] [PubMed]
90. Feres, M.F.N.; Abreu, L.G.; Insabralde, N.M.; de Almeida, M.R.; Flores-Mir, C. Effectiveness of open bite correction when managing deleterious oral habits in growing children and adolescents: A systematic review and meta-analysis. *Eur. J. Orthod.* **2017**, *39*, 31–42. [CrossRef] [PubMed]
91. Chun, B.Y.; Kim, S.Y. Acute visual loss after botulinum toxin A injection in the masseter muscle. *Int. Ophthalmol.* **2017**, 1–4. [CrossRef] [PubMed]
92. Korn, B.S.; Seo, S.W.; Levi, L.; Granet, D.B.; Kikkawa, D.O. Optic neuropathy associated with botulinum a toxin in thyroid-related orbitopathy. *Ophthalmic Plast. Reconstr. Surg.* **2007**, *23*, 109–114. [CrossRef] [PubMed]
93. Coté, T.R.; Mohan, A.K.; Polder, J.A.; Walton, M.K.; Braun, M.M. Botulinum toxin type A injections: Adverse events reported to the us food and drug administration in therapeutic and cosmetic cases. *J. Am. Acad. Dermatol.* **2005**, *53*, 407–415. [CrossRef] [PubMed]
94. Tranos, P.G.; Wickremasinghe, S.S.; Stangos, N.T.; Topouzis, F.; Tsinopoulos, I.; Pavesio, C.E. Macular edema. *Surv. Ophthalmol.* **2004**, *49*, 470–490. [CrossRef]
95. Sapra, P.; Demay, S.; Sapra, S.; Khanna, J.; Mraud, K.; Bonadonna, J. A single-blind, split-face, randomized, pilot study comparing the effects of intradermal and intramuscular injection of two commercially available botulinum toxin a formulas to reduce signs of facial aging. *J. Clin. Aesthet. Dermatol.* **2017**, *10*, 34. [PubMed]

toxins

MDPI

Article

Botulinum Neurotoxin Injection for the Treatment of Recurrent Temporomandibular Joint Dislocation with and without Neurogenic Muscular Hyperactivity

Kazuya Yoshida

Department of Oral and Maxillofacial Surgery, National Hospital Organization, Kyoto Medical Center, 1-1 Mukaihata-cho, Fukakusa, Fushimi-ku, Kyoto 612-8555, Japan; kayoshid@kyotolan.hosp.go.jp; Tel.: +81-75-641-9161; Fax: +81-75-643-4325

Received: 19 February 2018; Accepted: 20 April 2018; Published: 25 April 2018

Abstract: The aim of this study was to compare treatment outcomes following intramuscular injection of botulinum neurotoxin (BoNT) in patients with recurrent temporomandibular joint dislocation, with and without muscle hyperactivity due to neurological diseases. Thirty-two patients (19 women and 13 men, mean age: 62.3 years) with recurrent temporomandibular joint dislocation were divided into two groups: neurogenic (8 women and 12 men) and habitual (11 women and 1 man). The neurogenic group included patients having neurological disorders, such as Parkinson's disease or oromandibular dystonia, that are accompanied by muscle hyperactivity. BoNT was administered via intraoral injection to the inferior head of the lateral pterygoid muscle. In total, BoNT injection was administered 102 times (mean 3.2 times/patient). The mean follow-up duration was 29.5 months. The neurogenic group was significantly ($p < 0.001$) younger (47.3 years) than the habitual group (84.8 years) and required significantly ($p < 0.01$) more injections (4.1 versus 1.7 times) to achieve a positive outcome. No significant immediate or delayed complications occurred. Thus, intramuscular injection of BoNT into the lateral pterygoid muscle is an effective and safe treatment for habitual temporomandibular joint dislocation. More injections are required in cases of neurogenic temporomandibular joint dislocation than in those of habitual dislocation without muscle hyperactivity.

Keywords: botulinum neurotoxin; temporomandibular joint dislocation; lateral pterygoid muscle; botulinum toxin therapy

Key Contribution: Botulinum neurotoxin therapy can be the first choice treatment for patients presenting with recurrent temporomandibular joint dislocation.

1. Introduction

Botulinum neurotoxin (BoNT) is produced by the gram-positive, anaerobic, spore-forming bacterium *Clostridium botulinum*, and is one of the most lethal biological toxins known to man. BoNT has seven antigenically different serotypes and exerts a paralytic action by rapidly and strongly binding to presynaptic cholinergic nerve terminals [1]. It is then internalized and ultimately inhibits the exocytosis of acetylcholine by decreasing the frequency of acetylcholine release. Without its nerve supply, the muscle fiber will deteriorate; however, the muscle will regain its strength as the nerves regenerate. The clinical applications of BoNT continue to expand in a variety of diseases such as strabismus, blepharospasm, cervical dystonia, Meige syndrome, spasmodic dysphonia, tics, tremor, and other movement disorders [2–6]. In the oral and maxillofacial region, BoNT has been used to treat oromandibular dystonia, hemifacial spasm, oral dyskinesia, synkinesis following defective healing of the facial nerve, temporomandibular disorders, bruxism, painful masseter hypertrophy, Frey's syndrome, hypersalivation, trigeminal neuralgia, myofascial pain, and for aesthetic applications, such as perioral and other wrinkles [5–8].

The dislocation of the temporomandibular joint is defined as a non-reducing displacement of the condyle in front of, and superior to, the articular eminence. Dislocation of the temporomandibular joint is not rare and is observed relatively often in the field of oral and maxillofacial surgery. The dislocation is classified according to its course (acute, recurrent, or habitual), its direction (anterior, posterior, lateral, and superior), and the affected side (bilateral and unilateral) of the jaw. If acute dislocation becomes increasingly frequent and progressively aggravating, it is classified as recurrent or habitual dislocation. Recurrent temporomandibular joint dislocation can be seen in morphological changes such as atrophic eminence, temporomandibular joint laxity, occlusal disharmony, and functional changes such as neurogenic or drug-induced muscular hypertonus [9]. Dislocation can be anterior, posterior, lateral or superior. The most commonly occurring dislocation were anterior dislocations. Fracturing often accompanies dislocation in the posterior, lateral, or superior direction. The symptoms of bilateral dislocations, which are found commonly, include a fixed-open mouth, protruding mandible, pain in the masticatory muscles and temporomandibular joint, salivation, and difficulties with speech and eating. In cases of unilateral dislocation, the mandible exhibits deviation toward the contralateral side to the dislocated condyle. These symptoms are distressing and result in severe dysarthria, dysphasia, and masticatory disturbance, and require immediate treatment.

The lateral pterygoid, or the external pterygoid, is a muscle involved in mastication and usually has two heads: the inferior (lower) head and the superior (upper) head. The lateral pterygoid has a specialized role in the mouth opening that is mediated by horizontally oriented fibers of the inferior head. When the muscles of the bilateral inferior head contract together, the condyle is pulled forward and slightly downward. The mandible can be opened or protruded. If only one of the inferior head muscles contracts, the mandible rotates about a vertical axis, passing roughly through the opposite condyle and is pulled medially towards the contralateral side. Numerous methods have been reported for inserting electromyographic electrodes into the inferior and superior heads of the lateral pterygoid muscle [10–26]. Most of these methods involve "freehand" manual needle insertion, which occasionally results in complications such as hematoma or arterial bleeding [12,13] due to maxillary artery injury. Investigators have elucidated the course of the maxillary artery and found variation in this course between populations [27–44]. Although this variation is important during injection into the lateral pterygoid muscle, almost no attention has been paid to this anatomical difference.

In 1995, Daelen et al. [45] first described botulinum toxin injection into the lateral pterygoid muscle for the treatment of habitual temporomandibular joint dislocation. Several investigators subsequently reported using BoNT therapy for recurrent temporomandibular joint dislocation. They reported that it was effective and minimal unfavorable reactions were observed [46–53]. However, almost all previous studies have been single case reports or case series. As such, there is insufficient data regarding associated complications and the detailed application of the treatment.

In this report, differences in outcomes of BoNT therapy between patients with neurogenic temporomandibular joint dislocation and other habitual dislocations are examined. Additionally, the safety of injection into the inferior head of the lateral pterygoid muscle, with respect to the course of the maxillary artery, is discussed.

2. Results

The neurogenic group was significantly ($p < 0.001$, unpaired t-test) younger (47.3 ± 20.7 years) than the habitual group (84.8 ± 5.4 years). The percentage of female patients in the habitual group (91.7%) was significantly higher ($p < 0.01$, Fisher's exact test) than the percentage in the neurogenic group (40%). The ratio of edentulous to dentate patients was significantly higher ($p < 0.01$, Fisher's exact test) in the habitual group (66.7%) than in the neurogenic group (15%).

The results of the BoNT therapy for each patient are shown in Table 1. BoNT injections were administered 102 times in total (mean: 3.2 ± 2.8 times, range: 1–12 times). The dosage of BoNT per treatment session was 50.0 ± 6.4 units and 27.7 ± 7.6 units per side (Table 1). One injection was enough to prevent another episode in 9 of 32 (28.1%) patients from the habitual group. The percent of single injections was significantly higher ($p < 0.01$, Fisher's exact test) in the habitual group (75%) than in the neurogenic group (0%). The neurogenic group required significantly ($p < 0.01$) more (4.1 ± 2.8 times) injections than the habitual group (1.7 ± 1.7 times). No significant immediate or delayed complications were observed. The mean follow-up period was 29.5 ± 19.9 months (range: 6–75 months) (Table 1).

Table 1. The results of the treatment of the BoNT injection.

Patient No.	Group	Dosage per Time (Units)	Dosage per Side (Units)	Botox Injection (Times)	Follow-Up (Months)
1	N	25	25	2	12
2	N	50	25	2	6
3	N	50	25	5	36
4	N	50	25	8	38
5	N	50	25	12	48
6	N	50	25	2	12
7	N	50	25	6	28
8	N	50	25	2	29
9	N	50	25	8	52
10	N	50	25	2	45
11	N	50	50	3	51
12	N	50	25	4	59
13	N	50	25	8	75
14	N	50	25	2	26
15	N	50	25	2	15
16	N	50	25	2	13
17	N	50	25	5	31
18	N	50	25	2	19
19	N	50	25	3	10
20	N	75	37.5	2	15
21	H	50	50	1	27
22	H	50	25	7	56
23	H	50	25	1	6
24	H	50	25	1	9
25	H	50	50	1	10
26	H	50	25	1	9
27	H	50	25	2	12
28	H	50	25	1	47
29	H	50	25	1	53
30	H	50	25	2	15
31	H	50	25	1	14
32	H	50	25	1	65
Mean (SD)		50.0 (6.4)	27.7 (7.6)	3.2 (2.8)	29.5 (19.9)

N: neurogenic group, H: habitual group.

3. Discussion

The present study is the first to report on differences in outcomes following BoNT injection into the inferior head of the lateral pterygoid muscle between patient groups presenting with neurogenic or habitual temporomandibular joint dislocation. Intramuscular injection of BoNT by the intraoral approach is very effective and causes no adverse reactions. A greater number of injections are required in cases of temporomandibular joint dislocation caused by neurological dysfunction than in those of dislocation presenting without muscle hypertonus.

3.1. Limitations

There are limitations in the interpretation of the data presented here. Significant differences in age, gender distribution, and edentulousness between two groups may bias the data and prevent adequate statistical analysis. However, these differences might represent the real characteristics of each type of dislocation.

Referral bias is another possible limitation. The author produced a website for patients with involuntary movements of the stomatognathic region [54], and within the author's department, a comprehensive range of multimodal therapies for involuntary movements of the orofacial region, including medication, muscle afferent block therapy [55–57], botulinum toxin therapy [25,26], splint therapy [58], and surgery [59,60] are offered. As the number of patients with involuntary movements presenting to the author's department is high [61], temporomandibular joint dislocation derived from oromandibular dystonia constituted the majority of cases in this study. Therefore, the number of neurogenic temporomandibular joint dislocation and related diseases may be greatly influenced by the specialty of the investigator. Briefly, neurogenic patients may be more prevalent in the Department of Neurology, while habitual dislocation may be more common in a Department of Oral and Maxillofacial Surgery or Dentistry.

Furthermore, in the current study, a control group was not included due to ethical reasons. Randomization and blinding were not included in this study. Despite ethical difficulties, in the future, evidence-based randomized control trials with a larger number of patients are required to further characterize the differences between neurogenic and simple habitual dislocation.

Radiographic examination was impossible due to the lack of compliance in patients with dementia, and also due to the involuntary movements associated with neurological diseases. Therefore, precise evaluations of temporomandibular joint dislocation, such as morphological characteristics or changes in the articular eminence, the condyle, and the temporomandibular joint disc, were lacking in this study. Additionally, dementia and involuntary movements impaired the investigation of symptoms associated with joint and muscle conditions, such as joint sounds, condylar movements, maximal mouth opening, and muscle tenderness. Although there were insufficient clinical findings in these areas, diagnosis based on the palpable dislocation of the condyle was simple and there were no issues with regard to the treatment of the dislocation. In future studies, a more precise description of symptoms, as well as radiographic examinations, are desirable.

3.2. Local Anatomy for Safe Injection

The maxillary artery, the larger terminal branch of the external carotid artery, arises behind the neck of the mandible and is initially embedded in the parotid gland. The maxillary artery passes lateral to the inferior head of the lateral pterygoid muscle or medial to the muscle (Figure 1).

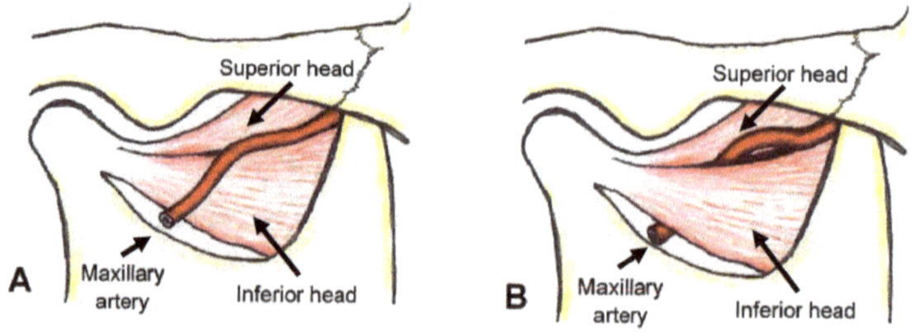

Figure 1. The lateral and medial courses of the maxillary artery to the lateral pterygoid muscle. The two main courses of the maxillary artery are lateral (**A**) and medial (**B**). In the lateral course, the maxillary artery passes lateral to the inferior head of the lateral pterygoid muscle (**A**). In the medial course, the artery passes medial to the muscle (**B**).

In 1928, Adachi [30] first reported a discrepancy in the frequency of the medial course of the maxillary artery to the inferior head of the lateral pterygoid muscle between Japanese and Caucasian populations. In 92.7% of Japanese subjects (and possibly other Asian groups), the maxillary artery passes lateral to the inferior head of the lateral pterygoid muscle (Figure 2). However, in Caucasian subjects, the artery passes medial to the muscle in a greater proportion of individuals (38%) (Figure 2).

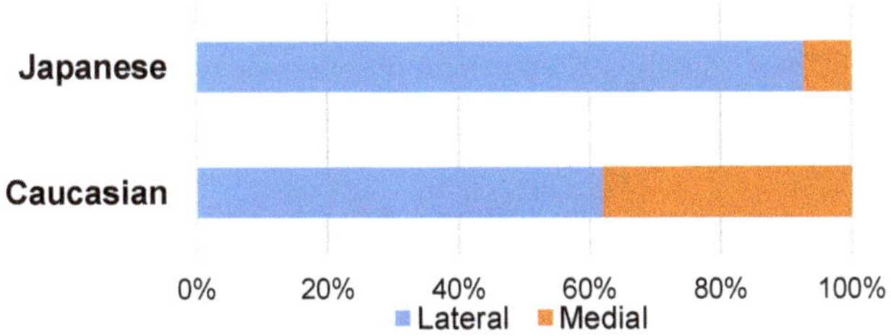

Figure 2. The frequency of the lateral and medial course of the maxillary artery in Japanese and Caucasian populations. The frequency was calculated based on the total data from previous studies in Japanese and Caucasian populations, which evaluated more than 100 cases [28,30–32,34–43]. The maxillary artery runs medially to the inferior head of the lateral pterygoid in 7.3% and 38% of Japanese and Caucasian individuals, respectively.

Operators should be aware of these differences prior to performing the procedure as there is a decreased risk of injury to the maxillary artery is if the needle is inserted only once. However, with increased needle insertion, the risk of complications such as bleeding, hematoma, and swelling increases [26]. These are related to the injury of the maxillary artery. Although most reports on BoNT injection into the lateral pterygoid muscles used the extraoral preauricular transcutaneous approach for Caucasian patients, clinicians should consider the course of the maxillary artery to minimize complication related to injuries to the artery.

3.3. Injection Methods into the Lateral Pterygoid Muscle

The inferior head of the lateral pterygoid muscle can be accessed via intraoral and extraoral transcutaneous routes (Figure 3). Various methods used for inserting electromyographic electrodes into the inferior and superior heads of the lateral pterygoid muscle have been reported [10–26]. However, the intraoral approach is preferable for several reasons [15,25,26]. First, this approach leads to less patient anxiety as it is similar to the approach employed during routine intraoral injections in dental treatment. Second, it reduces the risk of damage to the maxillary artery, and third, during the extraoral preauricular transcutaneous approach, the needle electrode could be bent or broken if the patient bites down forcefully.

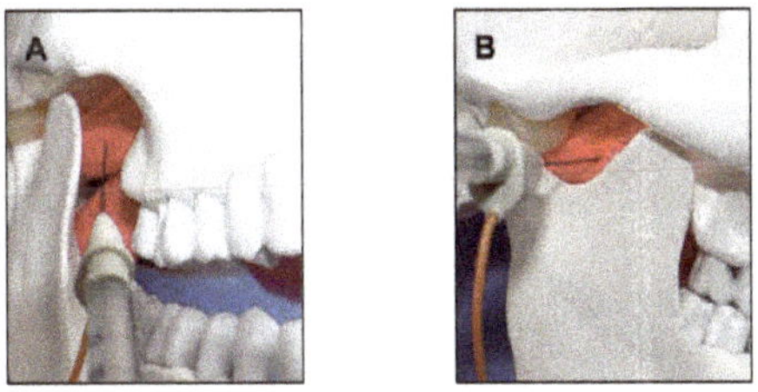

Figure 3. The intraoral (**A**) and extraoral (**B**) approaches for lateral pterygoid muscle injection.

As previously stated, the greater the number of times the needle is inserted, the greater the risk of complications and pain [15,25]. Thus, the more accurately the needle is inserted, the more likely the improvement in the patient's condition is, and the less likely complications are. BoNT therapy for oromandibular dystonia is more effective when it is administered to the jaw closing muscles than when it is administered to the lateral pterygoid muscle [62], which may reflect the anatomical complexity of the lateral pterygoid muscle and the resulting difficulty of accurate needle insertion [25,26].

Dystonia is a movement disorder that is characterized by sustained or intermittent muscle contractions that cause abnormal, often repetitive, movements, postures, or both [63]. Oromandibular dystonia is a focal type of dystonia involving the masticatory and/or lingual muscles [58,59,64,65]. Patients with oromandibular dystonia often exhibit dystonic contracture of the lateral pterygoid muscle [19–23,25,26,53,55]. Injection of BoNT into the lateral pterygoid muscle requires skill, sufficient anatomical knowledge, and experience, and such injections are rarely administered; therefore, it is difficult, practically speaking, to become skilled in this procedure [25,26]. Since 1988, the author has performed this procedure several thousand times for electromyographic studies [14–17], muscle afferent block [19,54,56,57], and BoNT therapy [25,26,53,54,64]. Recently, a method using a computer-aided design/computer-assisted manufacture-derived needle guide (Figure 4) was published [26]. The use of the needle guide allows clinicians to perform the injection procedures without any complications at skill levels that would normally require several years to achieve. The needle insertion guide has enabled development of what the author considers to be the most accurate and safe method for injecting BoNT into the inferior head of the lateral pterygoid muscle reported so far [26].

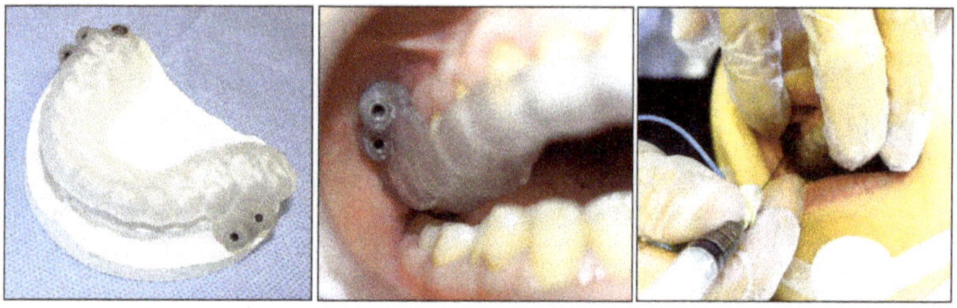

Figure 4. The needle guide using computer-aided design/computer-assisted manufacture-based data. Two points at the center of the inferior head of the lateral pterygoid muscle are selected, after checking the orientation and volume of the lateral pterygoid muscles on computed tomography [26]. A needle guide is fabricated using the stereolithographic method (**A**). The guide is inserted into the oral cavity and stabilized with the help of the teeth (**B**). A disposable hypodermic needle electrode is inserted through the metal sleeves (**C**).

It is very difficult to accurately and safely inject BoNT using the intraoral approach in patients with an extremely narrow space between the coronoid process and maxilla [25,26]. Indeed, despite repeated BoNT injections using the intraoral approach, there can be decreased beneficial effects. This might be related to the fact that BoNT is injected into a limited part of the muscle. For such patients, the extraoral preauricular percutaneous approach is an alternative option. After careful palpation of the infratemporal fossa, clinicians can insert the needle vertically into the skin [25]. The needle should be inserted 20–25 mm through the mandibular notch. After aspiration, BoNT is injected into the muscle. The correct placement of the needle is verified by evaluating the electromyographic burst during mouth opening or protrusion. If patients can open their mouth according to the clinician's instruction, confirmation of correct needle placement is easy. However, patients with severe mental impairment have to be injected under general anesthesia. In such cases, the correct placement can be verified by eliciting jaw reflex [48] or by the use of a nerve stimulator [51].

Excluding adverse effects related to injuries to the maxillary artery or the pterygoid nervous plexus, previously reported complications, which postulated diffusion of the BoNT into adjacent muscles, include transient dysphagia, painful chewing, dysarthria, nasal regurgitation, or nasal speech [66]. However, all complications were reported to subside within 2–4 weeks [66]. In this study, BoNT injections were administered more than 100 times via the intraoral route, and no immediate or delayed adverse reactions were detected.

3.4. BoNT Therapy for Recurrent Temporomandibular Joint Dislocation

Acute temporomandibular joint dislocation can be reduced using Hippocratic maneuvers: specifically, applying downward pressure on the posterior teeth and upward pressure on the chin while pushing the mandible posteriorly. However, in some cases, this requires sedation or general anesthesia. Conservative treatments of temporomandibular joint dislocation include physical therapy, chin cap, muscle relaxants, splint therapy, and instruction to avoid wide mouth opening [9]. Various surgical interventions are also used to treat this condition. These procedures include augmentation of the height of the articular eminence, reduction of the height of the eminence, intermaxillary fixation, and the injection of sclerosant or autologous blood around the temporomandibular joint [9,67].

To the best of our knowledge, the first BoNT injection for the purpose of treating habitual temporomandibular joint dislocation was described in 1995 by Daelen et al. [45]. They were also the first to propose the term "neurogenic temporomandibular joint dislocation", which was derived from neurological diseases such as multiple sclerosis or Parkinson's disease [46]. Following this study, several investigators reported using BoNT therapy for recurrent temporomandibular joint dislocation [45–53]. All these investigators reported that this treatment was effective and had minimal adverse effects.

The proper dosage of BoNT for the successful treatment of temporomandibular joint dislocation remains unclear. Although the dosage is empirical, the lowest sufficiently effective dose is the best. The frequent administration of BoNT in high doses could result in the development of antibodies. The author normally uses a 50-unit vial (Botox®). If the dislocation occurred unilaterally, 50 units were injected into the inferior head of the lateral pterygoid on the dislocated side (Table 1). If dislocation occurred bilaterally, 25 units were administered into the muscles on each side (Table 1). For patients with oromandibular dystonia, the dose of BoNT is determined according to the volume of the target muscles and the strength of the muscle contraction [25,26]. Further studies with larger samples are necessary to determine the optimal treatment dosage.

3.5. Differences in the Pathophysiology between Neurogenic and Habitual Dislocation

There are many causes of dislocation, including trauma, excessive mouth opening during yawning, dental or otorhinolaryngological examinations or treatments, vomiting, hypermobile or deranged temporomandibular joints, and involuntary movements [9]. Furthermore, dislocation can be influenced by other conditions such as neurogenic muscle hyperactivity, pathological osseous conditions affecting the articular eminence, and connective tissue disorders [9]. Therefore, it is likely that the pathophysiology of neurogenic and habitual temporomandibular joint dislocations is different. In this study, the diseases present in the neurogenic group included dystonia, Parkinson's disease, and progressive supra atrophy. One patient with oromandibular dystonia exhibited temporomandibular joint dislocation due to excessively strong muscle contraction in the lateral pterygoid muscle that subsequently resulted in the complete obstruction of the patient's upper airway [53]. For such patients, a higher dosage of BoNT and repeated injections are necessary to reduce the extraordinary muscle contraction. In these patients, the lateral pterygoid muscle showed excessively forceful involuntary contracture. Therefore, the BoNT injection must be repeated significantly more times than for the habitual group.

In elderly patients, temporomandibular joints are easily dislocated due to the atrophy of the articular eminence, joint laxity, and edentulousness. The percentage of edentulous patients was significantly higher in the habitual group than in the neurogenic group, in this study. A previous study [50] assumed that the cause of dislocation was a muscular imbalance between the jaw opening and jaw closing muscles caused by neuromuscular dysfunction. These patients rarely have hyperactive lateral pterygoids and BoNT therapy can be applied. In the habitual group, it is not forceful involuntary movements, but a disharmony between the jaw opening and jaw closing muscles, and also an atrophic articular eminence, that may result in dislocation. Although this can be treated by an eminectomy, this intervention may be ineffective due to poor health. The effects of BoNT diminishes over time; however, BoNT therapy can prevent another dislocation of the temporomandibular joint for a few months, and fibrosis around the temporomandibular joint may make another occurrence less likely.

In the past, if conservative treatment was not successful, surgical intervention was the only option [9,67]. The method described in this study should be the first choice treatment for temporomandibular joint dislocation, particularly for elderly patients who cannot tolerate conservative methods and are vulnerable to complications associated with operative procedures. If the cause of the temporomandibular joint dislocation is morphological, surgical procedures can be helpful. However, neurogenic hyperactivity of the inferior lateral pterygoid muscle cannot be relieved by surgical intervention, and BoNT injection into the inferior head of the lateral pterygoid muscle is helpful for such patients. Many clinicians have begun to recognize this therapy as an attractive option. Recently, the number of patients being referred for this treatment has been increasing rapidly.

4. Conclusions

The intramuscular injection of BoNT into the inferior head of the lateral pterygoid muscle via the intraoral route is highly effective and safe for treating patients with recurrent temporomandibular joint dislocation. This method should be the first choice in patients for whom surgical procedures are contraindicated.

5. Materials and Methods

5.1. Patients

Thirty-two patients with recurrent temporomandibular joint dislocation (19 women and 13 men; mean age with standard deviation [SD]: 62.3 ± 24.0 years), all of whom were intolerant to conservative methods, visited the author's department from July 2007 to June 2017. All the patients, or their legal guardians, provided written informed consent after listening to a detailed and complete explanation of the planned treatment. This study was performed in accordance with the Declaration of Helsinki after obtaining the approval of the institutional review board and ethics committee of the Kyoto Medical Center. The demographic characteristics of the patients are summarized in Table 2.

The diagnosis of recurrent temporomandibular joint dislocation was based on the past history and current symptoms, such as the inability to close the mouth in the intercuspal position due to an open-locked position and the palpable dislocation of the condyle from the fossa. Twenty-eight patients had bilateral, and four had unilateral, temporomandibular joint dislocation (Table 2). Although radiographic examination was impossible in most cases with dementia due to the lack of patient compliance, the diagnosis was made easily based on symptoms. Patients were divided into two groups; neurogenic (8 women and 12 men; mean age: 47.3 ± 20.7 years) and habitual (10 women and 1 man; mean age: 84.8 ± 5.4 years) (Table 2). The neurogenic group included patients with neurological disorders that are accompanied by muscular hypertonus. Muscle hyperactivity was confirmed by electromyographic examination, or from the tenderness or hardness during palpation of the lateral pterygoid muscle. The diseases present in the neurogenic group included oromandibular dystonia (20 patients), Parkinson's disease (3 patients), corticobasal degeneration (1 patient), multiple system atrophy (1 patient), and progressive supranuclear palsy (1 patient) (Table 2). The author diagnosed oromandibular dystonia based on the patients' electromyographic findings and the characteristic clinical features such as stereotypy, task-specificity, co-contraction, and morning benefit [55,58,59,64]. Other neurological diseases were diagnosed previously by qualified neurologists. Patients who had no neurological diseases accompanying muscle hyperactivity were classified as the habitual group. Ten of the twelve (83.3%) patients in the habitual group had dementia. Ten of the thirty-two (31.3%) patients were currently being prescribed psychiatric medication and had tardive dystonia. Twelve patients

(37.5%) had other dystonia in a different part of their body, including cervical dystonia (7 patients), writer's cramp (3 patients), generalized dystonia (3 patients) and blepharospasm (1 patient) (Table 2). Eleven patients (34.4%) used full dentures or were edentulous.

Table 2. The patients' demographic characteristics.

No.	Group	Age (Years)	Sex	Side	Duration (Months)	Frequency (Times/Week)	Diseases Causing Muscle Hyperactivity	Other Diseases	Denture
1	N	33	F	Uni	30	1	OMD, CD	schizophrenia	-
2	N	86	F	Bi	8	21	corticobasal degeneration, OMD	dementia, HT	+
3	N	43	M	Bi	36	3	OMD, CD, blepharospasm	depression	-
4	N	38	M	Bi	180	0.5	PD, generalized dystonia	-	-
5	N	30	M	Bi	8	1	OMD, CD	schizophrenia	-
6	N	53	M	Bi	24	2	OMD, WC	-	-
7	N	51	F	Bi	1	3	OMD, WC, CD	-	-
8	N	48	M	Bi	120	1	PD, OMD, CD	sleep apnea syndrome	-
9	N	66	M	Bi	120	2	PD, OMD	depression	-
10	N	35	F	Bi	36	7	OMD	schizophrenia	-
11	N	50	M	Uni	6	3	OMD	scoliosis	-
12	N	67	F	Bi	36	7	generalized dystonia	-	-
13	N	29	F	Bi	12	5	OMD	depression	-
14	N	35	M	Bi	10	10	OMD	panic disorder	-
15	N	19	F	Bi	6	3	OMD, CD, WC	depression	-
16	N	42	M	Bi	1	14	OMD, CD	dementia	-
17	N	21	M	Bi	60	7	generalized dystonia	hypoxia, DM	-
18	N	84	F	Bi	8	14	OMD	dementia, HT	+
19	N	64	M	Bi	6	21	multiple system atrophy, OMD	-	-
20	N	80	M	Bi	5	2	progressive supranuclear palsy, OMD	-	+
21	H	79	F	Bi	3	2	-	dementia, CI, HT	-
22	H	87	F	Uni	120	0.5	-	CI, HT, heart failure	+
23	H	87	F	Bi	1	1	-	dementia, osteoporosis, pneumonia	+
24	H	84	F	Bi	6	0.5	-	dementia	+
25	H	98	F	Uni	3	14	-	HT	-
26	H	86	F	Bi	8	21	-	dementia, HT, gastric ulcer	+
27	H	84	M	Bi	2	23	-	dementia	+
28	H	80	F	Bi	6	14	-	dementia	+
29	H	88	F	Bi	84	7	-	dementia, heart failure, breast cancer, depression	-
30	H	83	F	Bi	3	7	-	dementia, HT, pneumonia	+
31	H	85	F	Bi	6	2	-	dementia, HT	+
32	H	77	F	Bi	4	14	-	dementia, HT, CI, cervical spondylosis	-
Mean (SD)		62.3 (24.0)	-		30.0 (45.3)	6.7 (6.5)	-	-	

N: neurogenic group, H: habitual group, Bi: bilateral, Uni: unilateral, OMD: oromandibular dystonia, CD: cervical dystonia, WC: writer's cramp, PD: Parkinson's disease, HT: hypertension, DM: diabetes mellitus, CI: cerebral infarct.

5.2. Botulinum Neurotoxin (BoNT) Therapy

BoNT type A (Botox®, Allergan, Irvine, CA, USA) was reconstituted with normal saline to reach a final concentration of 2.5–5 units/0.1 mL. This procedure was normally performed using a final concentration of 2.5 units/0.1 mL. If the injection was unilateral or required a 100-units vial (Botox®), BoNT was reconstituted to 5 units/0.1 mL. The insertion point was the mucobuccal fold of the distal root of the upper second molar. After a gargle with a 50-fold diluted solution of Neostelin Green 0.2% mouthwash solution (Nippon Shika Yakuhin, Yamaguchi, Japan), a disposable hypodermic needle electrode (TECA™ MyoJect™ Luer Lock, 37 mm × 25 G, Natus Neurology Incorporated, Pleasanton, CA, USA) was angled posteriorly and superiorly by 30 degrees in relation to the occlusal plane, and medially by 20 degrees [25,26]. The needle was inserted to a depth of 20–30 mm without local anesthesia. After aspiration that the needle had not pierced a blood vessel, 25–50 units of BoNT were injected into the muscle. The correct placement of the electrode was verified by evaluating the full recruitment of electromyographic signal during mouth opening, or contralateral mandibular movement using an electromyographic apparatus (Neuropack n1, MEM-8301, Nihon Kohden, Tokyo, Japan), after amplification and filtering (low-cut filter, 10 Hz; high-cut filter, 3 kHz), and digitized with a sampling frequency of 10 kHz and 16-bit resolution [24]. The effects of BoNT manifested anywhere from 2–3 days to 1–2 weeks following treatment. Therefore, patients were vulnerable to another episode of dislocation during this time. Patients were carefully observed during this period. The injections were repeated over time if the patients showed involuntary mouth opening or experienced another dislocation. If the first injection was not sufficiently beneficial, a second injection was administered after 2 months. Successive injections must be administered, at minimum, every 3 months. Patient follow-up continued until no dislocation occurred for at least 6 months. All procedures were conducted under outpatient conditions without sedation or general anesthesia. For ethical reasons, a control group was not used in this study.

5.3. Statistical Analysis

The demographic characteristics and the results of BoNT therapy were compared between the neurogenic and habitual groups. An unpaired t-test was used to compare the data obtained from the two groups. Fisher's exact test was used to assess the statistical significance of differences in the distributions between the two groups. All analyses were performed using SPSS version 14.0 (SPSS Japan Inc., Tokyo, Japan). A value of $p < 0.05$ was considered statistically significant.

Acknowledgments: This study was supported by grants from the Japanese Ministry of Health, Labor, and Welfare (24592946 and 22111201).

Conflicts of Interest: The author declares no conflict of interest.

References

1. Simpson, L.L. The origin, structure, and pharmacologic activity of botulinum toxin. *Pharmacol. Rev.* **1981**, *33*, 155–188. [PubMed]
2. Jankovic, J.; Brin, M.F. Therapeutic uses of botulinum toxin. *N. Engl. J. Med.* **1991**, *324*, 1186–1194. [PubMed]
3. Truong, D.D.; Stenner, A.; Reichel, G. Current clinical applications of botulinum toxin. *Curr. Pharm. Des.* **2009**, *15*, 3671–3680. [CrossRef] [PubMed]
4. Hallett, M.; Albanese, A.; Dressler, D.; Segal, K.R.; Simpson, D.M.; Truong, D.; Jankovic, J. Evidence-based review and assessment of botulinum neurotoxin for the treatment of movement disorders. *Toxicon* **2013**, *67*, 94–114. [CrossRef] [PubMed]
5. Jankovic, J. An update on new and unique uses of botulinum toxin in movement disorders. *Toxicon* **2017**. [CrossRef] [PubMed]
6. Comella, C.L. Systematic review of botulinum toxin treatment for oromandibular dystonia. *Toxicon* **2018**. [CrossRef] [PubMed]

7. Laskawi, R. The use of botulinum toxin in head and face medicine: An interdisciplinary field. *Head Face Med.* **2008**, *4*, 5. [CrossRef] [PubMed]
8. Persaud, R.; Garas, G.; Silva, S.; Stamatoglou, C.; Chatrath, P.; Patel, K. An evidence-based review of botulinum toxin (Botox) applications in non-cosmetic head and neck conditions. *J. R. Soc. Med. Short Rep.* **2013**, *4*, 10. [CrossRef] [PubMed]
9. Undt, G. Temporomandibular joint eminectomy for recurrent dislocation. *Atlas Oral Maxillofac. Surg. Clin. N. Am.* **2011**, *19*, 189–206. [CrossRef] [PubMed]
10. Kamiyama, M. An electromyographic study on the function of the external pterygoid muscle. *Kokubyo Gakkai Zasshi* **1958**, *25*, 576–595. [CrossRef]
11. Mahan, P.E.; Wilkinson, T.M.; Gibbs, C.H.; Mauderli, A.; Brannon, L.S. Superior and inferior bellies of the lateral pterygoid muscle EMG activity at basic jaw position. *J. Prosthet. Dent.* **1983**, *50*, 710–718. [CrossRef]
12. Widmalm, S.E.; Lillie, J.H.; Ash, M.M., Jr. Anatomical and electromyographic studies of the lateral pterygoid muscle. *J. Oral Rehabil.* **1987**, *14*, 429–446. [CrossRef] [PubMed]
13. Koole, P.; Beenhakker, F.; Brongersma, A.J.; Boering, G. A standardized technique for the placement of electrodes in the two heads of the lateral pterygoid muscle. *J. Craniomand. Pract.* **1990**, *8*, 154–162. [CrossRef]
14. Yoshida, K.; Fukuda, Y.; Takahashi, R.; Nishiura, K.; Inoue, H. A method for inserting the EMG electrode into the superior head of the human lateral pterygoid muscle. *J. Jpn. Prosthodont. Soc.* **1992**, *36*, 88–93. [CrossRef]
15. Yoshida, K. An electromyographic study on the superior head of the lateral pterygoid muscle during mastication from the standpoint of condylar movement. *J. Jpn. Prosthodont. Soc.* **1992**, *36*, 110–120. [CrossRef]
16. Yoshida, K. Masticatory muscle responses associated with unloading of biting force during food crushing. *J. Oral Rehabil.* **1998**, *25*, 830–837. [CrossRef] [PubMed]
17. Yoshida, K. Eigenschaften der Kaumuskelaktivität während verschiedenen Unterkieferbewegungen bei Patienten mit Diskusverlagerung ohne Reposition. *Stomatologie* **1999**, *96*, 107–121.
18. Murray, G.M.; Bhutada, M.; Peck, C.C.; Phanachet, I.; Sae-Lee, D.; Whittle, T. The human lateral pterygoid muscle. *Arch. Oral Biol.* **2007**, *52*, 377–380. [CrossRef] [PubMed]
19. Yoshida, K.; Kaji, R.; Takagi, A.; Iizuka, T. Customized EMG needle insertion guide for the muscle afferent block of jaw-deviation and jaw-opening dystonias. *Oral Surg. Oral Med. Oral Pathol. Oral Radiol. Endod.* **1999**, *88*, 664–669. [CrossRef]
20. Møller, E.; Bakke, M.; Dalager, T.; Werdelin, L.M. Oromandibular dystonia involving the lateral pterygoid muscles: Four cases with different complexity. *Mov. Disord.* **2007**, *22*, 785–790. [CrossRef] [PubMed]
21. Mendes, R.A.; Upton, L.G. Management of dystonia of the lateral pterygoid muscle with botulinum toxin A. *Br. J. Oral Maxillofac. Surg.* **2008**, *47*, 481–483. [CrossRef] [PubMed]
22. Martos-Díaz, P.; Rodríguez-Campo, F.J.; Bances-Del Castillo, R.; Altura-Guillén, O.; Cho-Lee, G.Y.; de la-Plata, M.M.; Escorial-Hernandez, V. Lateral pterygoid muscle dystonia. A new technique for treatment with botulinum toxin guided by electromyography and arthroscopy. *Med. Oral Pathol. Oral Cir. Bucal* **2011**, *16*, e96–e99. [CrossRef]
23. Moscovich, M.; Chen, Z.P.; Rodriguez, R. Successful treatment of open jaw and jaw deviation dystonia with botulinum toxin using a simple intraoral approach. *J. Clin. Neurosci.* **2015**, *22*, 594–596. [CrossRef] [PubMed]
24. Fukuda, Y.; Yoshida, K.; Inoue, H.; Suwa, F.; Ohta, Y. An experimental study on inserting an EMG electrode to the superior head of the human lateral pterygoid muscle. *J. Jpn. Prosthodont. Soc.* **1990**, *34*, 902–908. [CrossRef]
25. Yoshida, K. How do I inject botulinum toxin into the lateral and medial pterygoid muscles? *Mov. Disord. Clin. Pract.* **2017**, *4*, 285. [CrossRef]
26. Yoshida, K. Computer-aided design/computer-assisted manufacture-derived needle guide for injection of botulinum toxin into the lateral pterygoid muscle in patients with oromandibular dystonia. *J. Oral Facial Pain Headache* **2018**, in press.
27. Long, J.J. The relation of the internal maxillary artery to the external pterygoid muscle. Collective investigation in the anatomical department of Trinity college, Dublin. *Trans. R. Acad. Med. Irel.* **1890**, *8*, 520–521.
28. Thomson, A. Report of the committee of collective investigation of the Anatomical Society of Great Britain and Ireland for the year 1889–1890. *J. Anat. Physiol.* **1891**, *25*, 89–101.
29. Lauber, H. Ueber einige Varietäten im Verlaufe der Arteria maxillaris interna. *Anat. Anz.* **1901**, *19*, 444–448.
30. Adachi, B. *Das Arteriensystem der Japaner*; Kyoto University: Kyoto, Japan, 1928; Volume 1, pp. 85–96.

31. Fujita, T. Über einen Fall von beiderseitig medial vom N. mandibularis verlaufender A. maxillaries interna, nebst einer Statistik der verlaufsvariatioon der Arterie. *J. Stomatol. Soc. Jpn.* **1932**, *6*, 250–252. [CrossRef]
32. Lasker, G.W.; Opdyke, D.L.; Miller, H. The position of the internal maxillary artery and its questionable relation to the cephalic index. *Anat. Rec.* **1951**, *109*, 119–126. [CrossRef] [PubMed]
33. Kijima, N. On distribution of the artery over the mandibular-joint. *Med. J. Kagoshima Univ.* **1958**, *10*, 71–83.
34. Križan, Z. Beirträge zur deskriptiven und topographischen Anatomie der A. maxillaris. *Acta Anat.* **1960**, *41*, 319–333. [CrossRef] [PubMed]
35. Ikakura, K. On the origin course and distribution of the maxillary artery in Japanese. *Kouku Kaibou Kenkyu* **1961**, *18*, 91–122.
36. Lurje, A. On the topographical anatomy of the internal maxillary artery. *Acta Anat.* **1947**, *2*, 219–231. [CrossRef]
37. Takarada, T. Anatomical studies on the maxillary artery. *J. Tokyo Dent. Coll. Soc.* **1958**, *53*, 1–20.
38. Skopakoff, C. Über die Variabilität im Verlauf der A. maxillaris. *Anat. Anz.* **1968**, *123*, 534–546. [PubMed]
39. Czerwiński, F. Variability of the course of external carotid artery and its rami in man in the light of anatomical and radiological studies. *Folia Morphol.* **1981**, *40*, 449–453.
40. Iwamoto, S.; Konishi, M.; Takahashi, Y.; Kimura, K. Some variations in the course of the maxillary artery. *J. Natl. Def. Med. Coll.* **1981**, *6*, 75–78.
41. Sashi, R. X-ray anatomy of the maxillary artery. *Akita J. Med.* **1990**, *16*, 817–831.
42. Tsuda, K. Three-dimensional analysis of arteriographs of the maxillary artery in man—Part 1: The maxillary artery and its branches. *J. Jpn. PRS* **1991**, *11*, 188–198.
43. Otake, I.; Kageyama, I.; Mataga, I. Clinical anatomy of the maxillary artery. *Okajima Folia Anat. Jpn.* **2011**, *87*, 155–164. [CrossRef]
44. Maeda, S.; Aizawa, Y.; Kumaki, K.; Kageyama, I. Variations in the course of the maxillary artery in Japanese adults. *Anat. Sci. Int.* **2012**, *87*, 187–194. [CrossRef] [PubMed]
45. Daelen, B.; Thorwirth, V.; Koch, A. Botulinumtoxin bei habituellen Luxationen Behandlung einer rezidivierenden Kiefergelenksluxation mit Botulinumtoxin A. *Mund Kiefer Gesichtschirurgie Mag.* **1995**, *22*, 11–12.
46. Daelen, B.; Thorwirth, V.; Koch, A. Treatment of recurrent dislocation of the temporomandibular joint with type A botulinum toxin. *Int. J. Oral Maxillofac. Surg.* **1997**, *26*, 458–460. [CrossRef]
47. Daelen, B.; Thorwirth, V.; Koch, A. Neurogene Kiefergelenkluxation Definition und Therapie mit Botulinumtoxin. Definition und Therapie mit Botulinumtoxin. *Nervenarzt* **1997**, *68*, 346–350. [CrossRef] [PubMed]
48. Moore, A.P.; Wood, G.D. Medical treatment of recurrent temporomandibular joint dislocation using botulinum toxin A. *Br. Dent. J.* **1997**, *183*, 415–417. [CrossRef] [PubMed]
49. Ziegler, C.M.; Haag, C.; Mühling, J. Treatment of recurrent temporomandibular joint dislocation with intramuscular botulinum toxin injection. *Clin. Oral Investig.* **2003**, *7*, 52–55. [CrossRef] [PubMed]
50. Fu, K.Y.; Chen, H.M.; Sun, Z.P.; Zhang, Z.K.; Ma, X.C. Long-term efficacy of botulinum toxin type A for the treatment of habitual dislocation of the temporomandibular joint. *Br. J. Oral Maxillofac. Surg.* **2010**, *48*, 281–284. [CrossRef] [PubMed]
51. Vázquez Bouso, O.; Forteza González, G.; Mommsen, J.; Grau, V.G.; Rodríguez Fernández, J.; Mateos Micas, M. Neurogenic temporomandibular joint dislocation treated with botulinum toxin: Report of 4 cases. *Oral Surg. Oral Med. Oral Pathol. Oral Radiol. Endod.* **2010**, *109*, e33–e37. [CrossRef] [PubMed]
52. Martínez-Pérez, D.; García Ruiz-Espiga, P. Recurrent temporomandibular joint dislocation treated with botulinum toxin: Report of 3 cases. *J. Oral Maxillofac. Surg.* **2004**, *62*, 244–246. [CrossRef] [PubMed]
53. Yoshida, K.; Iizuka, T. Botulinum toxin treatment for upper airway collapse resulting from temporomandibular joint dislocation due to jaw-opening dystonia. *J. Craniomandib. Pract.* **2006**, *24*, 217–222. [CrossRef] [PubMed]
54. Yoshida, K. Involuntary Movements of the Stomatognathic Region. Available online: https://sites.google.com/site/oromandibulardystoniaenglish/ (accessed on 19 April 2018).
55. Yoshida, K.; Kaji, R.; Kubori, T.; Kohara, N.; Iizuka, T.; Kimura, J. Muscle afferent block for the treatment of oromandibular dystonia. *Mov. Disord.* **1998**, *13*, 699–705. [CrossRef] [PubMed]
56. Yoshida, K.; Kaji, R.; Shibasaki, H.; Iizuka, T. Factors influencing the therapeutic effect of muscle afferent block for oromandibular dystonia and dyskinesia: Implications for their distinct pathophysiology. *Int. J. Oral Maxillofac. Surg.* **2002**, *31*, 499–505. [CrossRef] [PubMed]

57. Yoshida, K.; Iizuka, T. Jaw-deviation dystonia evaluated by movement-related cortical potentials and treated with muscle afferent block. *J. Craniomandib. Pract.* **2003**, *21*, 295–300. [CrossRef]
58. Yoshida, K. Sensory trick splint as a multimodal therapy for oromandibular dystonia. *J. Prosthodont. Res.* **2018**, *62*, 239–244. [CrossRef] [PubMed]
59. Yoshida, K. Surgical intervention for oromandibular dystonia-related limited mouth opening: Long-term follow-up. *J. Cranioaxillofac. Surg.* **2017**, *45*, 56–62. [CrossRef] [PubMed]
60. Yoshida, K. Coronoidotomy as treatment for trismus due to jaw-closing oromandibular dystonia. *Mov. Disord.* **2006**, *21*, 1028–1031. [CrossRef] [PubMed]
61. Yoshida, K. Multilingual website and cyberconsultations for oromandibular dystonia. *Neurol. Int.* **2018**, *10*, 7536. [CrossRef]
62. Singer, C.; Papapetropoulos, S. A comparison of jaw-closing and jaw-opening idiopathic oromandibular dystonia. *Parkinsonism Relat. Discord.* **2006**, *12*, 115–118. [CrossRef] [PubMed]
63. Albanese, A.; Bhatia, K.; Bressman, S.B.; Delong, M.R.; Fahn, S.; Fung, V.S.; Hallett, M.; Jankovic, J.; Jinnah, H.A.; Klein, C.; et al. Phenomenology and classification of dystonia: A consensus up date. *Mov. Disord.* **2013**, *28*, 863–873. [CrossRef] [PubMed]
64. Yoshida, K. Clinical and phenomelogical characteristics of patients with task-specific lingual dystonia: Possible association with occupation. *Front. Neurol.* **2017**, *8*, 649. [CrossRef] [PubMed]
65. Yoshida, K.; Kaji, R.; Kohara, N.; Murase, N.; Ikeda, A.; Shibasaki, H.; Iizuka, T. Movement-related cortical potentials before jaw excursions in patients with oromandibular dystonia. *Mov. Disord.* **2003**, *18*, 94–100. [CrossRef] [PubMed]
66. Brin, M.F.; Blitzer, A.; Herman, S.; Stewart, C. Oromnadibular dystonia: Treatment of 96 patients with botulinum toxin type A. In *Therapy with Botulinum-Toxin*; Jankovic, J., Hallett, M., Eds.; Marcel Dekker: New York, NY, USA, 1994; pp. 429–435.
67. Undt, G.; Kerner, C.; Piehslinger, E.; Rasse, M. Treatment of recurrent mandibular dislocation. Part I. Leclerc blocking procedure. *Int. J. Oral Maxillofac. Surg.* **1997**, *26*, 92–97. [CrossRef]

toxins

MDPI

Article

Botulinum Toxin A for Sialorrhoea Associated with Neurological Disorders: Evaluation of the Relationship between Effect of Treatment and the Number of Glands Treated

Domenico A. Restivo [1,*], Mariangela Panebianco [2], Antonino Casabona [3], Sara Lanza [4], Rosario Marchese-Ragona [5], Francesco Patti [6], Stefano Masiero [7], Antonio Biondi [8] and Angelo Quartarone [9]

1 Neurology Department, Garibaldi Hospital, 95100 Catania, Italy
2 Department of Molecular and Clinical Pharmacology, Institute of Translational Medicine, University of Liverpool, Liverpool L271XF, UK; dott_mariangela@hotmail.com
3 Department of Biomedical and Biotechnological Sciences, Section of Physiology, University of Catania, 95100 Catania, Italy; casabona@unict.it
4 UOC di Medicina Fisica e Riabilitazione, Comiso-Vittoria, ASP Ragusa, 97013 Ragusa, Italy; sara.lanza@asp.rg.it
5 ENT Department, University of Padova, 35121 Padova, Italy; rossmr@libero.it
6 DANA Department, "GF Ingrassia", Neuroscience Section—Multiple Sclerosis Center, University of Catania, 95100 Catania, Italy; patti@unict.it
7 School of Physical Medicine and Rehabilitation, University of Padua, 35121 Padua, Italy; stef.masiero@unipd.it
8 Department of Surgery, University of Catania, 95100 Catania, Italy; abiondi@unict.it
9 IRCCS Centro Neurolesi "Bonibo-Pulejo", via Provinciale Palermo, Contrada Casazza, 95124 Messina, Italy; aquartar@unime.it or aquartar65@gmail.com
* Correspondence: darestivo@libero.it; Tel.: +39-095-7593909

Received: 21 December 2017; Accepted: 22 January 2018; Published: 27 January 2018

Abstract: *Background*: Sialorrhoea and drooling are disabling manifestations of different neurological disorders. The aim of this study was to evaluate the effects of botulinum neurotoxin type A (BoNT/A) injection on hypersalivation in 90 patients with neurological diseases of different aetiologies, and to define the minimum number of injected salivary glands to reduce sialorrhoea. Determining the minimum number of glands that need to be engaged in order to have a significant reduction in drooling may be very useful for establishing the minimum total dosage of BoNT/A that may be considered effective in the treatment of hypersalivation. *Methods*: Twenty-five mouse units (MU) of BoNT/A (*onabotulinumtoxin A*, Botox; Allergan, Irvine, CA, USA; 100 MU/2 mL, 0.9% saline; or *incobotulinumtoxin A*, Xeomin; Merz Pharma, Germany; 100 MU/2 mL, 0.9% saline) were percutaneously injected into the parotid (p) glands and/or submandibular (s) glands under ultrasound control. On this basis, patients were divided into three groups. In group A (30 patients), BoNT/A injections were performed into four glands; in group B (30 patients), into three glands, and in group C (30 patients), into two glands. Patients treated in three glands (group B) were divided into two subgroups based on the treated glands (2 p + 1 s = 15 patients; 2 s + 1 p = 15 patients). Similarly, patients being injected in two glands (group C) were subdivided into three groups (2 p = 10 patients; 1 p + 1 s = 10 patients; 2 s = 10 patients). In patients who were injected in three and two salivary glands, saline solution was injected into the remaining one and two glands, respectively. Assessments were performed at baseline and at 2 weeks after the injections. *Results*: BoNT/A significantly reduced sialorrhoea in 82 out of 90 patients. The effect was more evident in patients who had four glands injected than when three or two glands were injected. The injections into three glands were more effective than injections into two glands. *Conclusions*: Our results have shown that BoNT/A injections induced a significant reduction in sialorrhoea in most patients (91%). In addition, we demonstrated that sialorrhoea associated with different neurological diseases was better controlled when the number of treated glands was higher.

Keywords: sialorrhoea; drooling; salivary glands; swallowing; botulinum toxin; eccrine glands; *onabotulinumtoxin A*; *incobotulinumtoxin A*

Key contribution: This study evaluated the effects of BoNT/A injection on hypersalivation in a wide number of neurologic patients and, also, it evaluate whether the number of treated glands might influence the efficacy of the treatment.

1. Introduction

Sialorrhoea or hypersalivation and drooling are known to be associated with several neurological disorders [1]. Other than a disabling social problem, hypersalivation is often associated with impairment of swallowing coordination. This condition affects about 10% of patients with cerebral palsy and post-traumatic encephalopathy [2] and 20% of patients with amyotrophic lateral sclerosis [3]. In Parkinson's disease, its frequency varies from 10% to 84% [4].

Salivation is controlled by the autonomic nervous system via cholinergic nerve fibres. In healthy adults, the parotid (p) and submandibular (s) glands—the major salivary glands—account for about 95% of the total salivary secretion. The remaining 5% is produced by the lingual and minor glands [5].

Traditional treatment of excessive drooling includes anticholinergic oral drugs, surgical intervention and local irradiation of salivary glands [6,7]. However, these treatments are poorly tolerated, are invasive and are often ineffective in a number of patients. In fact, systemic anticholinergic drugs are often ineffective and produce unacceptable side effects such as blurred vision, urinary retention, and cardiac arrhythmia. Surgical intervention and local irradiation of salivary glands have been performed, but these are invasive procedures that are often unacceptable to patients and their caregivers.

Recently, the percutaneous injection of botulinum neurotoxin type A (BoNT/A) into salivary glands has been shown to be effective in abolishing excessive sialorrhoea associated with several neurological disorders [8–13]. In addition, studies on botulinum neurotoxin type B (BoNT/B) in patients affected with cervical dystonia have shown a relatively high incidence of dry mouth [14]. This suggests that BoNT/B may be more effective in the treatment of hypersalivation than BoNT/A [14]. However, in our country, BoNT/B treatment can be performed only in patients unresponsive to BoNT/A.

The rationale for the use of BoNT/A in this condition is the selective block of presynaptic release of acetylcholine from the cholinergic endings supplying eccrine salivary glands [15,16]. Usually, the effect of this treatment lasts several months. Although encouraging, the results of these studies were obtained from a restricted number of subjects. Moreover, in previous studies, a correlation between the number of glands treated and the amount of salivation reduction was not investigated.

The aim of the present study was thus to evaluate the effects of BoNT/A injection on hypersalivation in a wide number of patients with different neurological disorders and, in addition, to evaluate whether the number of treated glands might influence the efficacy of the treatment. The determination of the minimum number of glands that should be engaged in order to have a significant drooling reduction may be very useful for establishing the minimum total dosage of BoNT/A that may be considered effective in the treatment of hypersalivation.

2. Results

In evaluating the effects of BoNT/A, we detected four different levels of responsiveness to the treatment. We scored from 3 (good responders with a reduction of 75% in the roll weight) to 0 (no response; when weights of the wet rolls did not change); intermediate and poor responders were scored with 2 or 1, respectively, when the reduction of their roll weights was equal to 50% or 25% (see Table 1).

Table 1. The demographic characteristics of the 90 neurological patients with hypersalivation treated with BoNT/A injections into different salivary glands. Abbreviations: PD, Parkinson disease; ALS, amyotrophic lateral sclerosis; BI, brain injury; CP, cerebral palsy; s, submandibular; p, parotids; Inco = incobotulinum toxin A; Ona = onabotulinumtoxin A.

Patient	Age	Sex	Disease	Injected Glands	Effects (2 Weeks)	Type of Toxin	Group
1	40	F	CP	2p-2s	2	Ona	A
2	56	F	PD	2p-2s	3	Inco	A
3	73	M	PD	2p-2s	3	Inco	A
4	71	M	PD	2p-2s	3	Inco	A
5	67	F	Stroke	2p-2s	2	Ona	A
6	72	M	Stroke	2p-2s	3	Ona	A
7	63	M	PD	2p-2s	3	Ona	A
8	65	F	PD	2p-2s	3	Ona	A
9	50	M	BI	2p-2s	2	Ona	A
10	28	M	Stroke	2p-2s	3	Ona	A
11	55	M	PD	2p-2s	3	Ona	A
12	55	F	Stroke	2p-2s	3	Ona	A
13	67	F	PD	2p-2s	3	Ona	A
14	72	M	PD	2p-2s	2	Ona	A
15	63	M	PD	2p-2s	3	Ona	A
16	65	F	Stroke	2p-2s	2	Ona	A
17	73	M	PD	2p-2s	3	Ona	A
18	71	M	PD	2p-2s	3	Inco	A
19	67	M	BI	2p-2s	1	Inco	A
20	55	M	PD	2p-2s	3	Inco	A
21	63	M	PD	2p-2s	3	Ona	A
22	65	M	PD	2p-2s	3	Ona	A
23	50	F	Stroke	2p-2s	3	Ona	A
24	45	F	CP	2p-2s	3	Ona	A
25	19	F	CP	2p-2s	3	Ona	A
26	71	M	PD	2p-2s	0	Ona	A
27	72	M	PD	2p-2s	2	Inco	A
28	66	M	Stroke	2p-2s	3	Inco	A
29	18	M	BI	2p-2s	3	Ona	A
30	18	M	CP	2p-2s	3	Ona	A
31	61	M	PD	2p-1s	1	Ona	B
32	59	M	ALS	2p-1s	0	Ona	B
33	71	M	PD	2p-1s	2	Ona	B
34	48	M	PD	2p-1s	1	Ona	B
35	55	M	BI	2p-1s	2	Inco	B
36	67	M	PD	2p-1s	2	Inco	B
37	72	F	Stroke	2p-1s	2	Inco	B
38	55	F	ALS	2p-1s	2	Inco	B
39	63	M	Stroke	2p-1s	2	Ona	B
40	65	M	Stroke	2p-1s	2	Ona	B
41	50	M	PD	2p-1s	1	Ona	B
42	67	F	PD	2p-1s	2	Inco	B
43	70	M	PD	2p-1s	2	Inco	B
44	53	M	PD	2p-1s	3	Inco	B
45	22	M	CP	2p-1s	1	Ona	B
46	53	M	ALS	1p-2s	1	Inco	B
47	47	M	Stroke	1p-2s	2	Inco	B
48	59	F	PD	1p-2s	2	Inco	B
49	72	M	Stroke	1p-2s	2	Inco	B

Table 1. *Cont.*

Patient	Age	Sex	Disease	Injected Glands	Effects (2 Weeks)	Type of Toxin	Group
50	61	F	PD	1p-2s	1	Ona	B
51	18	F	CP	1p-2s	2	Inco	B
52	21	M	CP	1p-2s	2	Inco	B
53	18	F	CP	1p-2s	2	Ona	B
54	69	M	PD	1p-2s	2	Inco	B
55	49	F	CP	1p-2s	3	Inco	B
56	29	F	CP	1p-2s	2	Ona	B
57	46	F	CP	1p-2s	2	Ona	B
58	68	F	ALS	1p-2s	0	Ona	B
59	29	F	CP	1p-2s	2	Ona	B
60	57	M	Stroke	1p-2s	2	Ona	B
61	66	F	ALS	2p	0	Inco	C
62	38	M	BI	2p	1	Ona	C
63	66	F	ALS	2p	1	Ona	C
64	38	M	BI	2p	1	Ona	C
65	36	M	CP	2p	2	Ona	C
66	28	M	CP	2p	1	Inco	C
67	63	M	ALS	2p	1	Ona	C
68	71	F	Stroke	2p	2	Inco	C
69	70	M	ALS	2p	1	Ona	C
70	69	M	Stroke	2p	1	Ona	C
71	58	M	Stroke	2s	1	Inco	C
72	61	M	PD	2s	1	Inco	C
73	70	F	ALS	2s	1	Inco	C
74	65	F	ALS	2s	0	Ona	C
75	25	F	Stroke	2s	1	Ona	C
76	22	M	CP	2s	1	Ona	C
77	37	M	BI	2s	1	Inco	C
78	54	M	BI	2s	1	Ona	C
79	70	M	Stroke	2s	1	Ona	C
80	59	M	Stroke	2s	1	Ona	C
81	22	M	CP	1p-1s	1	Ona	C
82	24	M	CP	1p-1s	1	Inco	C
83	49	F	ALS	1p-1s	0	Inco	C
84	21	M	CP	1p-1s	1	Ona	C
85	73	M	PD	1p-1s	1	Inco	C
86	69	F	PD	1p-1s	0	Ona	C
87	26	F	CP	1p-1s	1	Ona	C
88	68	M	Stroke	1p-1s	1	Ona	C
89	65	F	Stroke	1p-1s	0	Ona	C
90	34	M	BI	1p-1s	1	Ona	C

Eighty-two out of 90 patients (91%) were responders to the treatment. In almost all patients, sialorrhoea was dramatically reduced at 2 weeks (mean dental roll weight before BoNT/A: 0.8 ± 0.08 g; mean dental roll weight 2 weeks after BoNT/A: 0.25 ± 0.1 g). Only 8 (8.8%) out of 90 patients did not benefit from the treatment. Patients with injections into four, three and two glands showed large differences over the three groups (Figure 1 $F_{2,87} = 48.78$; $p < 0.000001$), with the highest average score being observed for the four-gland group (2.63 ± 0.13) and lower scores recorded for the three-gland group (1.73 ± 0.13) and for the two-gland group (0.9 ± 0.09). Significant differences were also observed for each paired comparison (four glands vs. three glands: $p = 0.000003$; four glands vs. two glands: $p < 0.000001$; three glands vs. two glands: $p < 0.000007$).

The narrow bars inserted in Figure 1 represent the scores recorded when injections were unevenly distributed between parotid and submandibular glands. No significant differences were detected and all the scores were similar regardless of which glands were most engaged.

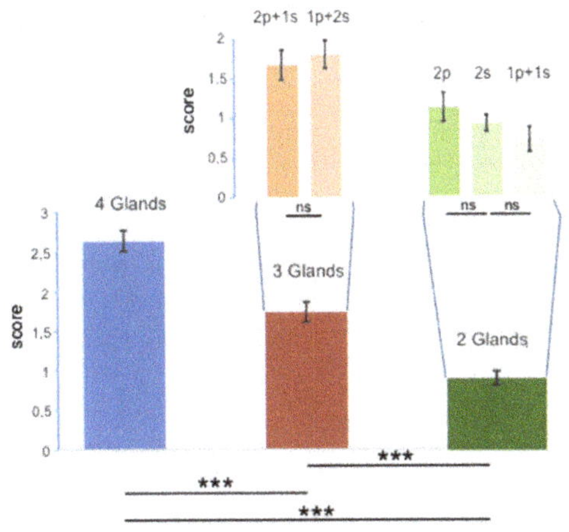

Figure 1. Values of scores obtained over the groups with injections into four, three and two glands (large bars) and in the groups where injections were unevenly distributed between parotid (p) and submandibular (s) glands (narrow bars). The error bars represent the standard error, *** indicates differences with $p < 0.00001$, and ns indicates no statistical differences.

Although the score for *incobotulinum toxin* was higher than the score for *onabotulinumtoxin*, the type of toxin did not produce significant differences when the score was measured over the entire sample of patients ($N = 90$; $F_{1,84} = 2.47$; $p = 0.12$), and no interaction was observed between the number of glands engaged and the type of toxin ($F_{2,84} = 2.76$; $p = 0.069$). This is reported in Figure 2.

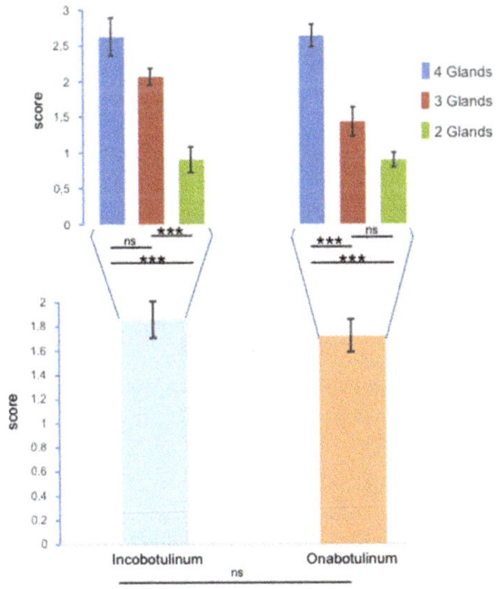

Figure 2. Values of scores observed with respect to the two types of toxins injected (incobotulinum and onabotulinum). Large bars represent the results obtained from the entire sample of patients; the narrow bars show the subdivision over the groups with injections into four, three and two glands. The error bars represent the standard error, *** indicates differences with $p < 0.00001$, and ns indicates no statistical differences.

When the dataset was separated into two subsamples associated with each toxin, significant differences were observed over the three groups for both the effect of *incobotulinumtoxin* ($F_{2,30} = 22.45$; $p < 0.000001$) and *onabotulinumtoxin* ($F_{2,54} = 40.14$; $p < 0.000001$). The largest influence was detected in group A and, except for the comparison between group A and group B for *incobotulinumtoxin* and between group B and C for *onabotulinumtoxin*, the other paired comparisons were statistically different.

The overall effect of disease was statistically significant ($F_{4,85} = 6.68$; $p < 0.0001$). The Bonferroni multiple comparison showed that the main contribution to this result was provided by the paired differences between ALS and CP ($p = 0.0033$), PD ($p < 0.0001$) and stroke ($p = 0.0022$).

Only one patient complained of dysphagia 7 days after BoNT/A injection, which disappeared within 15 days; another two patients had a hematoma at the site of injection, which needed compressive bondage for 2 h.

3. Discussion

This is the first randomized, blinded study exploring the relationship between the effect of BoNT/A injections and the number of salivary glands injected.

Our results showed that BoNT/A injections induced a dramatic reduction of sialorrhoea in almost all patients (91%). The reduction of sialorrhoea was evident 2 weeks after the injection. However, the production of saliva was still enough that swallowing of both foods and drink in all patients was not impaired. In fact, parotid and submandibular glands together account for about 95% of the total salivary secretion. The remaining 5% is produced by the lingual and minor glands [5].

The effect of salivation reduction was more significant in patients with four glands treated than patients with three or two glands treated. Patients treated in three glands showed a more significant reduction in hypersalivation than patients treated in two glands. In patients treated in three glands, no significant differences were observed between injections into one parotid and two submandibular glands and injections into one submandibular gland and two parotid glands. In patients treated in two glands, no significant differences were observed among patients who were injected into two parotids, two submandibular glands or one parotid and one submandibular gland, respectively.

Otherwise, we cannot exclude that the beneficial effect was due to the different total doses that were used. Both dose and number of injected glands may have a synergic effect in reducing hypersalivation.

It is noteworthy that the score recorded for the *incobotulinumtoxin A* tended to be higher than the *onabotulinumtoxinA*, and the two toxins showed slightly different effects over the groups. In fact, as both of the toxins influenced the score of patients treated in four and two glands, *incobotulinumtoxin A* differentiated the scores associated with patients treated in three and two glands, while *onabotulinumtoxin A* exhibited an effect between patients treated in four and three glands. Thus, the overall influence of BoNT/A derived from a differentiated effect of the single toxins.

The major number of injected glands did not produce any side effects and the dose of BoNT/A used for each gland was safe in all patients. This treatment has the advantage that it avoids the use of oral anticholinergic medications, which has previously been administered in most patients for the symptomatic therapy of the sialorrhoea.

However, this study did not establish whether BoNT/A parotid injections are superior to BoNT/A submandibular injections in reducing hypersalivation. In fact, when only two parotids or two submandibular glands were injected (Group C, 2p and 2s patients, respectively), no significant differences were observed.

In addition, our findings have shown that injections in patients with sialorrhoea associated with ALS were less effective than in patients with PD, stroke, BI or CP. A possible explanation for these differences may reside in a different saliva composition (more prevalence of mucinoses component in the saliva of patients with ALS) or with a more impaired oral/preparatory phase of swallowing in ALS, with consequent major saliva pooling in the mouth. However, further studies specifically focused on this topic and involving a larger number of ALS patients are needed before drawing definitive conclusions.

Our study demonstrated that sialorrhoea due to different neurological diseases may be successfully managed with injections into four or at least three salivary glands. This treatment is safe, simple and highly effective.

4. Materials and Methods

4.1. Patients

A consecutive series of 117 patients with neurological disorders arising from different aetiologies was screened in our hospital from January 2005 to December 2016 for hypersalivation. Out of these 117 patients with sialorrhoea, ninety subjects (59 men and 31 women; mean age: 53.4 ± 17.6 years) who had experienced a high frequency and severity of hypersalivation and drooling in the preceding 6 months satisfied all of the inclusion/exclusion criteria and were enrolled in the study (Figure 3). We included those patients who had wet rolls with a roll-weight at least ten times heavier than the dry rolls. Thirty out of 90 patients were affected by Parkinson disease (PD), 11 were suffering from amyotrophic lateral sclerosis (ALS), 21 were affected by stroke, 8 by brain injury (BI) and 20 by cerebral palsy (CP). Table 1 shows the demographic characteristics of these 90 patients.

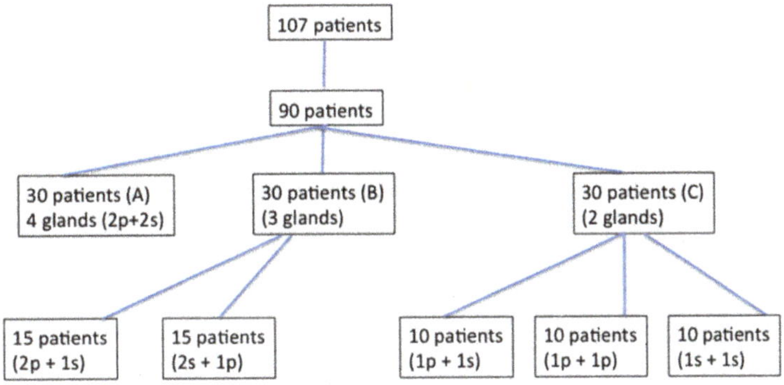

Figure 3. Study profile.

4.2. Inclusion criteria

(1) Accepting to participate in the study; (2) age ≥ 18 and ≤ 75 years; (3) the diagnosis of one of the following neurological disorders often associated with hypersalivation and/or drooling: diagnosis of PD, stroke, ALS, CP, or BI; (4) severely disabling sialorrhoea lasting for at least 6 months.

4.3. Exclusion criteria

The presence of other neurological diseases or the inability to give informed consent because of cognitive impairment.

All patients gave their written informed consent to the BoNT/A treatment after the approval of the local ethics committee.

4.4. Treatment

Twenty-five mouse units (MU) of botulinum neurotoxin type A (BoNT/A; Botox, [*onabotulinumtoxin A*], Allergan, Irvine, CA, USA; 100 MU/2 mL, 0.9% saline; or twenty-five mouse units (MU) of BoNT/A, Xeomin [*incobotulinumtoxin A*], Merz Pharma, Frankfurt, Germany; 100 MU/2 mL, 0.9% saline) were injected into each parotid gland using a 27G 3/4 needle.

The submandibular glands were also injected with 25 MU each. Out of 90 patients, 57 patients were treated with *onabotulinumtoxin A* and 33 patients with *incobotulinumtoxin A*. The total number of patients treated with *onabotulinumtoxin A* injections was more than the number of patients treated with *incobotulinumtoxin A* because the latter was introduced later on. BoNT/A was percutaneously injected in all patients into the salivary glands under ultrasound control using a linear electronic probe 7.5 MHz (Aloka 650-SSD), which allowed the operator to accurately inject into the targeted salivary gland. Injections were performed once in all patients. Before injection, patients underwent an objective assessment of sialorrhoea and then they were randomised into three groups according to the number of treated glands. The number of glands that were injected was randomly assigned using a computer-generated list. Patients were divided into three groups (group A, B, and C). In group A (N = 30 patients; 10 females and 20 males; age range: 18–73 years), BoNT/A injections were performed into four glands (2p + 2s); in group B (N = 30 patients; 12 females and 18 males; age range: 18–72 years), BoNT/A injections were performed into three glands (2p + 1s, N = 15 patients; 2s + 1p, N = 15 patients) and in group C (30 patients; 10 females and 20 males; age range: 21–73 years), BoNT/A was injected into two glands (1p + 1s, N = 10 patients; 2p, N = 10 patients; 2s, N = 10 patients). In patients with four salivary glands treated, the total dose of botulinum toxin injected was 100 MU (25 UI for each gland). In patients with three and two salivary glands injected, the total dose was 75 MU and 50 MU (25 MU per gland), respectively. In patients injected into three and two salivary glands, an equal amount of saline solution was injected into the remaining one and two glands, respectively.

4.5. Assessment

Assessments were made at the same time of the day for each visit and patients were seated upright. Patients were inhibited from eating or drinking one hour before each assessment. Assessments were performed by a physician examiner who was blinded to the treatment allocation at baseline, and then at 2 weeks after the injection. All patients were blinded to their treatment allocation. Both treating and physician examiners reported their evaluations in separate case report forms. Hypersalivation was measured with six dental rolls placed in six different areas of the mouth and then retained there for 5 min. The difference in weight between the dry and wet rolls was calculated. The procedure was repeated after 15 min. The mean value of these consecutive assessments was taken as the final value.

4.6. Statistical analysis

Likert's transformation was obtained to change the qualitative results of BoNT/A injection into salivary glands into a score ranging from 0 (no effect) to 3 (maximum effect = 75% reduction of sialorrhoea). Two-way analysis of variance (ANOVA) was performed to evaluate the effect of the number of glands receiving toxin injection and the type of toxin. One-way ANOVA was applied to the two subgroups with injections into three glands (2p + 1s, 1p + 2s; N = 15 for each group) and the three subgroups with injections into two glands (2p, 2s, 1p + 1s; N = 10 for each group). An additional one-way ANOVA was used to estimate the effect of disease on the score value. For the ANOVA with three levels, the multiple comparisons were adjusted by Bonferroni correction. The data are expressed as means and standard errors, and the results were considered significant when $p < 0.05$. Statistical analyses were performed using SYSTAT version 11 (Systat Inc., Evaston, IL, USA).

Author Contributions: D.A.R., R.M.-R., and S.M. conceived and designed the experiments; D.A.R., F.P., S.L., A.Q. performed the experiments; A.C., A.B., and M.P. analyzed the data; A.C. wrote the paper.

Conflicts of Interest: The authors declare no conflict of interest. We had no founding sponsor.

References

1. Banerjee, K.J.; Glasson, C.; O'Flaherty, S.J. Parotid and submandibular botulinum toxin a injections for sialorrhoea in children with cerebral palsy. *Dev. Med. Child. Neurol.* **2006**, *48*, 883–887. [CrossRef] [PubMed]

2. Banfi, P.; Ticozzi, N.; Lax, A.; Guidugli, G.A.; Nicolini, A.; Silani, V. A review of options for treating sialorrhea in amyotrophic lateral sclerosis. *Respir. Care* **2015**, *60*, 446–454. [CrossRef] [PubMed]
3. Borg, M.; Hirst, F. The role of radiation therapy in the management of sialorrhoea. *Int. J. Radiat. Oncol. Biol. Phys.* **1998**, *41*, 1113–1119. [CrossRef]
4. Dias, B.L.; Fernandes, A.R.; Maia Filho, H.S. Sialorrhea in children with cerebral palsy. *J. Pediatr.* **2016**, *92*, 549–558. [CrossRef] [PubMed]
5. Fuster Torres, M.A.; Berini Aytes, L.; Gay Escoda, C. Salivary gland application of botulinum toxin for the treatment of sialorrhea. *Med. Oral Patol. Oral Cir. Bucal.* **2007**, *12*, E511–E517. [PubMed]
6. García Ron, A.; Miranda, M.C.; Garriga Braun, C.; Jensen Verón, J.; Torrens Martinez, J.; Diez Hanbino, M.P. Efficacy and safety of botulinum toxin in the treatment of sialorrhea in children with neurological disorders. *An. Pediatr.* **2012**, *77*, 289–291. [CrossRef] [PubMed]
7. Jeung, I.S.; Lee, S.; Kim, H.S.; Yeo, C.K. Effect of botulinum toxin a injection into the salivary glands for sialorrhea in children with neurologic disorders. *Ann. Rehabil. Med.* **2012**, *36*, 340–346. [CrossRef] [PubMed]
8. Lagalla, G.; Millevolte, M.; Capecci, M.; Provinciali, L.; Ceravolo, M.G. Botulinum toxin type a for drooling in Parkinson's disease: A double-blind, randomized, placebo-controlled study. *Mov. Disord.* **2006**, *5*, 704–707. [CrossRef] [PubMed]
9. Lovato, A.; Restivo, D.A.; Ottaviano, G.; Marioni, G.; Marchese-Ragona, R. Botulinum toxin therapy: Functional silencing of salivary disorders. *Acta Otorhinolaryngol. Ital.* **2017**, *37*, 168–171. [PubMed]
10. McGeachan, A.J.; Mcdermott, C.J. Management of oral secretions in neurological disease. *Pract. Neurol.* **2017**, *17*, 96–103. [CrossRef] [PubMed]
11. Naumann, M.; Jost, W.H.; Toyka, K.V. Botulinum toxin in the treatment of neurological disorders of the autonomic nervous system. *Arch. Neurol.* **1999**, *56*, 914–916. [CrossRef] [PubMed]
12. Porta, M.; Gamba, M.; Bertacchi, G.; Vaj, P. Treatment of shialorrhoea with ultrasound guided botulinum toxin type a injection in patients with neurological disorders. *J. Neurol. Neurosurg. Psychiatry* **2001**, *70*, 538–540. [CrossRef] [PubMed]
13. Potulska, A.; Friedman, A. Controlling sialorrhoea: A treatment options. *Expert Opin. Pharmacother.* **2005**, *6*, 1551–1554. [CrossRef] [PubMed]
14. Dashtpour, K.; Bhidayasiri, R.; Chen, J.J.; Jabbari, B.; Lew, M.; Torres-Russotto, D. RimabotulinumtoxinB in sialorrhoea: Systematic review of clinical trials. *J. Clin. Mov. Disord.* **2017**, *6*. [CrossRef]
15. Reid, S.M.; Johnstone, B.R.; Westbury, C.; Rawicki, B.; Reddihough, D.S. Randomized trial of botulinum toxin injections into the salivary glands to reduce drooling in children with neurological disorders. *Dev. Med. Child. Neurol.* **2008**, *50*, 123–128. [CrossRef] [PubMed]
16. Srivanitchapoom, P.; Pandey, S.; Hallett, M. Drooling in parkinson's disease: A review. *Parkinsonism Relat. Disord.* **2014**, *20*, 1109–1118. [CrossRef] [PubMed]

toxins

MDPI

Review

Therapeutic Approaches of Botulinum Toxin in Gynecology

Marius Alexandru Moga [1], Oana Gabriela Dimienescu [1,*], Andreea Bălan [1], Ioan Scârneciu [1], Barna Barabaş [2] and Liana Pleş [3]

[1] Department of Medical and Surgical Specialties, Faculty of Medicine, Transilvania University of Brasov, Brasov 500019, Romania; moga.og@gmail.com (M.A.M.); dr.andreeabalan@gmail.com (A.B.); urologie_scarneciu@yahoo.com (I.S.)

[2] Department of Fundamental Disciplines and Clinical Prevention, Faculty of Medicine, Transilvania University of Brasov, Brasov 500019, Romania; barabas.mihail@gmail.com

[3] Clinical Department of Obstetrics and Gynecology, The Carol Davila University of Medicine and Pharmacy, Bucharest 020021, Romania; plesliana@gmail.com

* Correspondence: dimienescu.oana@gmail.com; Tel.: +40-0268-412-185

Received: 31 March 2018; Accepted: 19 April 2018; Published: 21 April 2018

Abstract: Botulinum toxins (BoNTs) are produced by several anaerobic species of the genus *Clostridium* and, although they were originally considered lethal toxins, today they find their usefulness in the treatment of a wide range of pathologies in various medical specialties. Botulinum neurotoxin has been identified in seven different isoforms (BoNT-A, BoNT-B, BoNT-C, BoNT-D, BoNT-E, BoNT-F, and BoNT-G). Neurotoxigenic Clostridia can produce more than 40 different BoNT subtypes and, recently, a new BoNT serotype (BoNT-X) has been reported in some studies. BoNT-X has not been shown to actually be an active neurotoxin despite its catalytically active LC, so it should be described as a putative eighth serotype. The mechanism of action of the serotypes is similar: they inhibit the release of acetylcholine from the nerve endings but their therapeutically potency varies. Botulinum toxin type A (BoNT-A) is the most studied serotype for therapeutic purposes. Regarding the gynecological pathology, a series of studies based on the efficiency of its use in the treatment of refractory myofascial pelvic pain, vaginism, dyspareunia, vulvodynia and overactive bladder or urinary incontinence have been reported. The current study is a review of the literature regarding the efficiency of BoNT-A in the gynecological pathology and on the long and short-term effects of its administration.

Keywords: botulinum toxin; chronic pelvic pain; overactive detrusor; vaginism

Key Contribution: This review highlights the efficiency of BoNT-A in the gynecological pathology (vaginism, vulvodynia, chronic pelvic pain or urinary tract disorders) pointing out the effects of BoNT-A after the first injection and during the follow up period.

1. Introduction

The incidence of chronic pelvic pain in women is constantly increasing, and is approximately 15% worldwide [1]. Jarell et al. [2] defined chronic pelvic pain as pain not related to gastrointestinal problems, menstruation or sexual activity, with a complex etiology. Chronic pelvic pain affects both women and men through common mechanisms, involving the central nervous system. The result is a regional pain syndrome that affects the entire pelvis. The triggers may be relatively benign, but individuals predisposed to chronic pelvic pain syndrome develop a series of sensory abnormalities and may perceive normal sensations as increased, until the point of unbearable pain and dysphoria. It is also associated with psychological, sexual, social and behavioral problems [2,3]. Other sequelae of this pathology include: decreased physical activity, impairment of social and family relationships, depression and accompanying vegetative signs such as sleep and appetite dysfunctions [4]. Potentially beneficial drugs include medroxyprogesterone depot or hormone therapy, but only in association with behavioral therapy [5,6]. Several treatments including conventional or homeopath drugs have been proposed for the management of this pathology. Medicinal plant supplements are therapeutic alternatives, when traditional interventions (surgery, anti-inflammatory or antalgic medication) fail to manage the disease [7]. Medicinal herbs have various effects on the women reproductive system, being used worldwide, in several pathologies including vulvodynia, vaginism, chronic pelvic pain of unknown etiology or urinary tract pathologies [3]. A study conducted in six European countries in 2016 pointed that several plants, such as *Plantago psyllium*, *Prunus Africana* or *Equisetum arvense*, could be used in the treatment of chronic pelvic pain of gynecological or urinary origin. Even if medicinal herbs are frequently used worldwide, new studies are mandatory to propose new drugs [7].

Another alternative to the treatment of several gynecological diseases, more studied nowadays, is Botulinum toxin (BoNT). Botulinum Toxin A (BoNT-A) has been used to treat various gynecological pathologies such as: chronic pelvic pain, vaginism, dyspareunia and urinary incontinence with overactive bladder or sphincter dyssynergia. This article is a review of the current published data regarding the administration of BoNT in gynecological pathology, but, to recommend the wider use of this treatment, it is essential to carry out more research. BoNT/A1 and BoNT/B1 are the only BoNT types used for clinical purposes and BoNT-A is the most studied isoform for therapeutic purposes. Clinical trials on this topic have defined the safety and tolerability profile of BoNT-A [8]. All patients from the clinical studies injected with BoNT-A understood the possible undesirable effects of the treatment, giving their approval through signing the informed consent [9]. The incidence of adverse effects was observed to be approximately 25% in the BoNT-A treated groups compared to 15% in the control group. Among the side effects of the treatment with BoNT-A, the most frequently mentioned was the focal weakness, erythema, edema or hyperesthesia [10]. BoNT-A is used in various fields of medicine: dermatology, motion disorders, ophthalmic disorders, and gastrointestinal disorders, as well as in urogynecology pathologies, having high efficiency with minimal adverse effects. Table 1 summarizes the clinical applications of BoNT in medicine [11].

Regarding the use of other serotypes, such as BoNT-B, it has been used to induce human muscle paralysis but, according to Sloop and coworkers' research, the paralysis resulting from BoNT-B is not as efficient as the one resulting from BoNT-A [12].

Table 1. Clinical uses of BoNT-A.

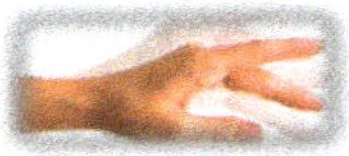	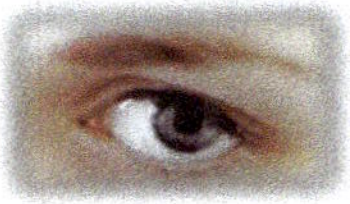	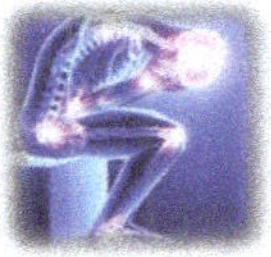	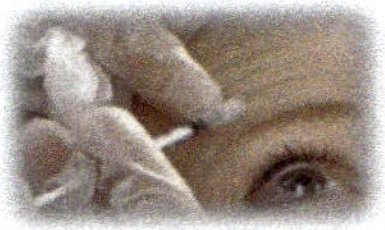	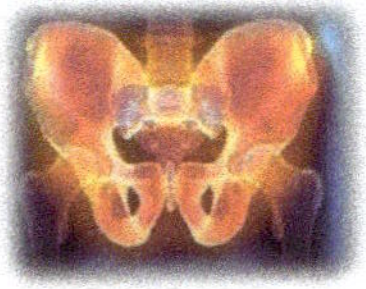	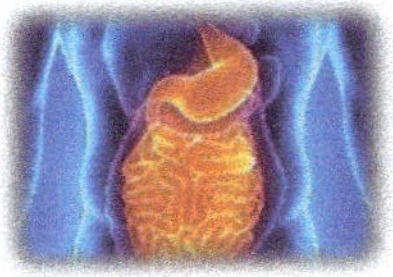	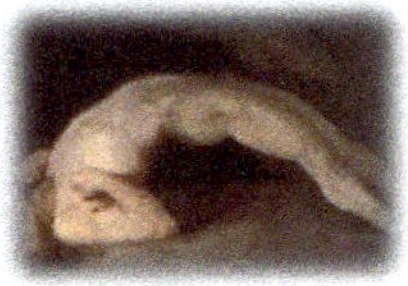
Neuromuscular Disorders	Ophthalmic Disorders	Chronic Pain	Cosmetic and Dermatological Applications	Pelvic floor Disorders	Gastrointestinal Disorders	Spasticity
Idiopathic/secondary focal dystonia	Misalignment	Tension headache	Wrinkles	Anismus	Achalasia	Stoke induced spasticity
Hemifacial Spasm/post-facial nerve palsy synkinesis	Paralytic strabismus	Cervicogenic headache	Face rejuvenation	Vaginismus	Bruxism	Cephalic tetanus
Tremor (essential, writing, palatal or cerebellar)	Therapeutic ptosis for corneal protection	Migraine	Hypersecretory disorders (hyperhidrosis, sialorrhea)	Detrusor sphincter dyssynergia	Temporomandibular joint dysfunction	Multiple sclerosis
Tic disorders	Restrictive or myogenic strabismus	Lower back ache	Glabellar frown	Chronic anal fissures	Palatal myoclonus	Traumatic brain injury
Myokymia	Upper eyelid retraction	Tennis elbow	Vertical platysma bands	Perineal muscles spasm	Esophageal diverticulosis	Cerebral palsy
Neuromyotonia	Duane's syndrome	Myofascial pain	Browlift	Vulvodynia	Laryngeal disorders	Spinal cord injury

2. Botulinum Toxin

BoNT are proteic neurotoxins produced by anaerobic sporulated bacteria of the *Clostridium* genus. Pirazzini et al. [13,14] described in a comprehensive review four different clostridial groups (Clostridium *Botulinum* groups I–IV, *Clostridium baratii* and *Clostridium butyricum*) that are known to produce the seven serotypes of BoNTs (BoNT-A to BoNT-G) [15]. Based on the amino-acid sequences, the serotypes are divided into subtypes, being more than 40 BoNT subtypes identified [16].

The first neurotoxin serotypes were identified in 1919 (BoNT-A and BoNT-B) and the last one in the year 1969 (BoNT-G) [16–18]. In 2017, Zhang et al. described a new BoNT-serotype (BoNT-X) [19]. The particularity of this serotype is that can cleave VAMP4 (which mediates vesicle fusion between endosome and TGN) [20,21] and Ykt6—an atypical SNARE without transmembrane domain (an essential protein in yeast, involved in membrane fusion events such as ER-Golgi, intra-Golgi, autophagosome formation) [22]. Zornetta et al. [23] also described in 2016 the first non-Clostridial botulinum like toxin (BoNT-Wo) identified from *Weissella oryzae* (an anaerobe isolated from fermenting rice) [24]. The particularity of this toxin is that it cleaves the VAMP at a single site (a unique Trp-Trp peptide bond, localized within the juxtamembrane segment of VAMP). Recently, Zhang et al. reported another Botulinum Neurotoxin-like toxin in the *Enterococcus faecium* strain isolated from cow feces (BoNT-En) [25]. BoNT-En cleaves two proteins that mediate synaptic vesicle exocytosis in neurons: SNAP-25 and VAMP-2.

BoNT consists of two chains: a heavy chain of 100 kDa and a light chain of 50 kDa linked by a disulfide bond which is extending from the heavy chain and surrounds the light chain like "a belt" [26]. The heavy chain contains a N-terminal HC that mediates the translocation of the LC (which acts as a protease, cleaving various proteins of BoNT-A, -C and -E cleave SNAP-25; BoNT-B, -D, -F and -G cleave VAMP1, -2 and -3; and BoNT C cleaves syntaxin 1) into the endosomal membranes. The cleavage of one of the three SNARE proteins prevents neurotransmitter release from neurons by blocking the fusion of synaptic vesicles to plasma membranes [13,27,28]. Table 2 summarizes the BoNT serotypes, subtypes, the target SNARE proteins, and their intracellular compartments.

After exceeding the intestinal barrier, BONTs spread into the extracellular fluids, entering the lymphatic system, followed by spreading into the blood circulation [29], without crossing the blood barrier. BoNTs can bind to any neurons, but they are distributed primarily to the peripheral nerve terminals [14]. The molecular mechanism of BoNTs inside nerve terminals is described in Figure 1.

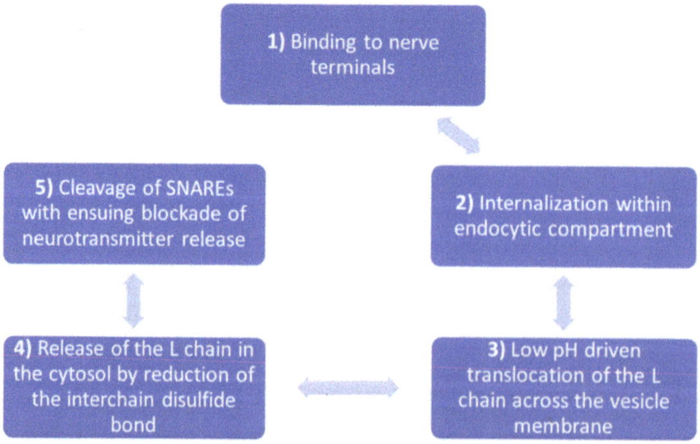

Figure 1. The five steps of BoNTs' mechanism of action inside nerve terminal.

Table 2. Classification of BoNTs.

Origin		BoNT Serotype	Target Substrate	Bont Subtype	Substrate Localization
C. *Botulinum* group I		A	SNAP-25	A1; A2; A3; A4; A5; A6; A7; A8; A9; A10; A(B); Ab; Af; Af84	Presynaptic plasma membrane
		B	VAMP	B1; B2; B3; B5(Be); B6; B7; Bf	Synaptic vesicle
		F	$VAMP_1$, $VAMP_2$	F1; F2; F3; F4; F5	Synaptic vesicle
		X	$VAMP_4$, $VAMP_5$, Ykt6	-	Synaptic vesicle
C. *Botulinum* group II		B	VAMP	B4	Synaptic vesicle
		E	SNAP 25	E1; E2; E3; E6; E7; E8; E9; E10	Presynaptic plasma membrane
		F	$VAMP_1$, $VAMP_2$	F6	Synaptic vesicle
C. *Botulinum* group III		C	SNAP 25, Syntaxin 1A, Syntaxin 1b	C; CD;	Presynaptic plasma membrane
		D	$VAMP_1$, $VAMP_2$	D; DC	Synaptic vesicle
C. *Botulinum* group IV (C. *argentinese*)		G	$VAMP_1$, $VAMP_2$	G	Synaptic vesicle
Other organisms producing BoNTs	C. *Butyricum*	E	SNAP 25	E4; E5	Presynaptic plasma membrane
	C. *Baratii*	F	$VAMP_1$, $VAMP_2$	F4	Synaptic vesicle
	Enterococcus faecium strain	En	$VAMP_2$, SNAP25	-	Synaptic vesicle
	Weissella oryzae SG25T	Wo	$VAMP_2$	-	Synaptic vesicle

The first step is binding to the presynaptic vesicle membrane of the nerve terminals, through HC domain, to two independent receptors: a PSG receptor and a protein receptor of the synaptic vesicle (glycosylated SV2 in case of BoNT-A1 and BoNT E1, synaptotagmin I/II for BoNT-B1, BoNT-DC and BoNT-G) [30–34]. The next step involves internalization of BoNT, through dual binding with synaptic vesicle receptors and PSG. Following this process, the strength of BoNT interactions with the membrane increases [13,14,33].

The third step of the process, namely translocation has been extensively studied. The vesicular ATPase proton pump generates a transmembrane pH gradient, to translocate the L-chain from the synaptic vesicle into the cytosol. ATPase inhibitors are an important component, because they block completely the nerve termination intoxications by BONTs [35–40]. After translocation, the L chain is released on the cytosolic side of the membrane. However, this process requires the inter-change disulfide bond to be reduced, because the BONTs that possess reduced inter-chain disulfide bonds do not form channels. Fisher et al. described in their paper the importance of reduction in the inter-chain disulfide bon that needs to take place at any stage before the exposure to the cytosol. It is necessary because it prevents the L-chain translocation. Several enzymatic systems (thioredoxins and glutaredoxins) are involved in the reduction of protein disulfide bond, having a major role in the release of L chain into the neuronal cytosol [41]. After the enzymatic system reduction of the disulfide bond, the toxin can interact with the target proteins [40,42–45].

The final step of the BoNTs mechanism is the cleavage of SNARE proteins with ensuing blockade of neurotransmitter release. The L chains of all BoNTs are specific metalloproteases for one of the SNARE proteins: VAMP, SNAP25 or syntaxin. BONT-A and -E cleave SNAP25; BONT-B, -D, -F, and -G cleave VAMP; and BONT-C targets syntaxin and SNAP25. The result of the proteolytic actions is the prolonged inhibition of the neurotransmitter release, followed by neuroparalysis [13,46,47].

BoNT-A is used in medicine in a wide range of muscular dysfunctions because it acts on nerve endings and inhibits the release of acetylcholine in synaptic spaces, preventing muscle spasm [48]. BoNTs acts on chronic pain, spasm and dystonia and could be successfully used to relieve these symptoms [49,50]. Of all BoNT serotypes, BoNT-A specifically cleaves SNAP-25 and thus prevents the release of acetylcholine in the synaptic space. As the synapses are blocked by the action of the toxin, the neuron will form new ones, a process known as sprouting [26,51]. A systematized description of the mechanism of BoNT-A in pain inhibition can be observed in Figure 2.

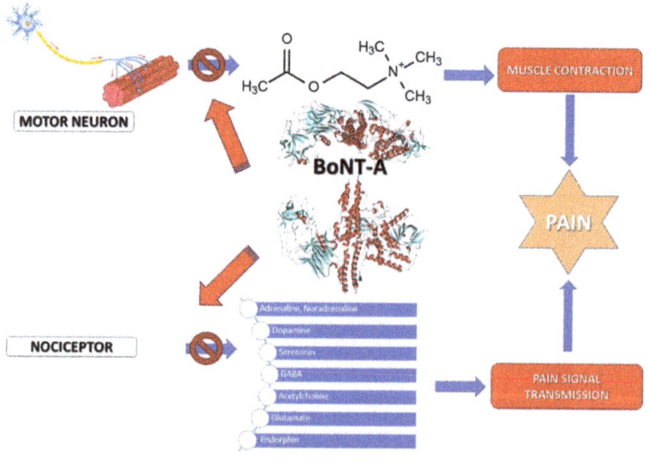

Figure 2. Mechanism of action of BoNT-A in pain. Inhibition of acetylcholine and neurotransmitter released from motor neuron and nociceptor by BoNT-A reduces pain by inhibiting the pain signal transmission.

3. Review of the Literature Regarding the Gynecologic Indications for the Use of BoNT-A

3.1. Use of BoNT-A in the Treatment of Vaginism

The term "vaginism" describes the involuntary, recurrent or persistent contraction of the perineal muscles that surround the outer third of the vagina. It occurs during sexual intercourse and/or penetration with a swab or vaginal speculum during a gynecological examination. This involuntary contraction of the perineal muscles can aggravate or even make sexual life impossible [52].

The severity of vaginism could be classified according to the Lamont Scale, depending on the presenting symptoms and pain during the gynecology exams. Vaginismus was first described in 1978 by Lamont, who divided the pathology into four degrees [53]:

- 1st degree:
    - Levator and perineal spasm relieved with reassurance
    - Able to tolerate vaginal exam
- 2nd degree:
    - the perineal spasm is maintained through the gynecology exam
    - Unable to relax for the pelvic exam
- 3rd degree:
    - Spasm of the levator muscle
    - Elevation of buttocks to avoid the gynecology exam
- 4th degree:
    - Perineal and levator spasm
    - Adduction of thighs, elevation of buttocks, unable to tolerate the pelvic exam.

Depending on the severity degree, there are cases when penetration with vaginal swabs or vaginal speculum is allowed, but, in severe cases, penetration with any gynecological instrument or sexual intercourse is impossible [54]. Kegel exercises, relaxation and physical examination are considered the first line treatment in this pathology. In addition, voluntary control of perineal muscle contraction is a key factor in the successful treatment of vaginism [53]. Anxiolytic therapeutic agents and local treatments (lubricants and anesthetic creams) have been used as pharmacological treatments of this pathology, but approximately 10% of patients do not find amelioration in the symptoms [54].

Because of the numerous unresponsive cases to the conventional treatment, several authors investigated the effect of BoNT in this pathology [54–57]. The first case of vaginismus treated with BoNT-A was described in 1977 [58] and since then it had been carried out multiple studies.

A retrospective study from 2004 included 24 women aged 19–34 years with 3rd- or 4th-degree vaginism, without previous treatment [54]. Prior to injection, 500 U BoNT-A was diluted with 1.5 mL of saline solution and a total dose of 150–400 U was injected equally into levator ani muscles, in three points on each side, under sedation with Midazolam and with Oxygen administration. For the first cases, 150–200 U BoNT-A was used, with the dose gradually increased for the following patients, up to 400 U. Patients were monitored on average for 12 months and the conclusions showed that: 95.8% of the patients did not show any resistance or showed reduced resistance to post-injection vaginal examinations, 75% achieved satisfactory sexual intercourse after the first injection and 16.7% had mild pain at penetration after the first injection. In addition, recurrent vaginism in patients treated with BoNT-A was not detected.

In a case-control study, the efficiency of BoNT use in the treatment of vaginism was investigated [55]. The cohort consisted of thirteen cases of women diagnosed with vaginism, with an average age of 26.6 years. The cohort was divided into two groups: eight patients suffering from vaginism and five patients diagnosed with vaginism prior to the treatment, considered the control group. The first group was injected with 25 U of BoNT diluted in 1 mL of saline in each bulbospongiosus muscle. The controllers were injected with saline solution. After the injection, the patients were followed for an average of 3.3 months. The results obtained were encouraging: improvements were observed, and, in all cases, sexual life became possible or satisfactory. However, recurrences of vaginism have also been reported. There were no improvements in the control group.

To point out the utility of BoNT-A in the treatment of vaginismus secondary to vulvar vestibulitis syndrome, Bertolasi et al. recruited 39 women whose electromyography (EMG) recordings in the levator ani muscle had showed reduced resting and reduced inhibition during exercise [56]. The patients were injected with BoNT-A into repeated cycles under the guidance of EMG and were followed for an average of 105 ($\pm$50) weeks. Four weeks after each cycle, the women underwent EMG evaluations, vaginal examinations, evaluation of bowel and bladder symptoms completed VAS and the female sexual function index scale (FSFI). The results of the questionnaires were satisfactory at the first follow up (at four weeks after the first injection of BoNT-A) and the results maintained, with the increase in the number of subsequent injections. At the end of the follow-up period, 63.2% of the patients were completely cured, 15.4% requested re-injections and 15.4% dropped out the study before finishing it.

Another retrospective study that pointed out the use of BoNT-A in the treatment of vaginism was conducted on a cohort of 20 patients that have been treated with BoNT-A injections during 2005–2009 [57]. The patients were divided according to the severity of vaginism: 12 women with primary vaginism, 5 women with secondary vaginism and 3 women with severe dyspareunia. Initially, low doses of BoNT-A were used, and then the doses increased from 100 U to 150 U, diluted in 2 mL saline solution, injected under sedation (15–20 mL of bupivacaine 0.25% with epinephrine 1: 200.000) in several points along each side of the vagina (into the bulbocavernosus, pubococcygeus and puborectalis muscles). At the time of the study, 16 patients managed to have sexual intercourse in two weeks to three months after the injection and a patient was considered a failure because not even the smallest penetration dilator could ever be used. Patients continued to have a low degree of discomfort and vaginal burns during early sexual intercourse attempts, but this problem disappeared within a few weeks of completing the treatment with BoNT-A.

Table 3 summarizes the clinical studies regarding the use of BoNT-A in the treatment of vaginism.

Table 3. Studies of BoNT-A in the treatment of vaginism.

Author	Study Design	Number of Cases	Treatment Regimen	Outcome Measures	Follow-Up	Results
Ghazizadeh [54]	Retrospective study	24	Dilution: 500 U of BoNT-A diluted with 1.5 mL of normal saline solution. Dose: 150–200 U injected first; the dose gradually increased the total dose of 400 U * Dysport, Ipsen Ltd., Maidenhead, UK	• Vaginal muscles resistance	12.37 months	• 23 patients had vaginal examinations 1-week post injection that showed little or no vaginismus • 18 patients achieved satisfactory intercourse after the first injection • 4 patients had mild pain • 1 patient needed a second injection; 1 patient refused vaginal examination and did not attempt to have coitus
Shafik [55]	Case-control study	13	BoNT group: A single injection; dose and dilution: 25 U diluted in 1 mL saline solution Control group: saline solution	• Satisfaction of intromission	3.3 months	• All the symptoms at patients injected with BT improved. • There was no recurrence during the follow-up period • Control subjects did not improve
Bertolasi [56]	Prospective study	39	Repeated cycles at 4 weeks of botulinum neurotoxin injected into levator ani. * Dysport, Ipsen Ltd., Maidenhead, UK	• Possibility of sexual intercourse; • levator ani EMG hyperactivity; • Lamont scores, VAS, FSFI	105 (±50 SD) weeks	• At 4 weeks after the first cycle the primary outcome improved, as did the secondary outcomes • When follow-up ended, 63.2%—were completely recovered; 15.4% still needed reinjections and 15.4% had dropped out the study
Pacik [57]	Retrospective study	20	Dose: 100 to 150 U of BoNT-A; Dilution: 100 U of BoNT-A diluted in 2 mL of saline; * Allergan, Inc., Irvine, CA, USA.	• Possibility of having intercourse	Time of follow up not reported	• 80% of patients achieved intercourse in maximum 3 months • 15% of patients continued the injections (maximum 6 dilators); • 5% of patient did not respond to treatment (unable to advance beyond the first dilator)
Pacik [59]	Clinical trial	241	Dose: 100 U of BoNT-A; Dilution: 2 mL of saline; * onabotulinumtoxinA; Allergan, Irvine, CA, USA	• Pain and anxiety scores; • time to achieve intercourse • untoward effects.	1 month, 3 months, 6 months, 1 year	• 71% reported at a median of 2.5-week pain-free intercourse; 2.5% were unable to achieve intercourse during follow up • 26.6% were lost within 1 year after treatment. • 1.24% developed mild temporary stress incontinence, 0.41% temporary excessive vaginal dryness

3.2. Use of BoNT in the Treatment of Vulvodynia

Vulvodynia is a sexual dysfunction manifested by vulvar pain and orgasmic difficulties that cause a difficult sexual life. Women affected by this pathology receive only symptomatic treatment, anti-inflammatory and analgesic drugs, while psychotherapy can treat the fear of pain [60]. In modern medicine, BoNT could be used to treat this pathology when other treatments fail. It acts through a permanent neuromuscular blockage and muscle function recovery is achieved by forming new neuromuscular junctions [61]. The etiology of vulvodynia is not fully known, although it has been extensively researched. The factors involved in this pathology could be: inflammatory, genetic, infectious, hormonal or mechanical [62,63]. These factors induce modifications through three different pathways: sexual function, nervous system pain and pelvic floor muscles [64].

Yoon et al. performed a study regarding the use of BoNT-A in the treatment of vulvodynia [60]. The cohort consisted of seven women with genital pain that were injected with 20–40 U BoNT-A. All patients reported that the pain decreased after injections and the subjective pain score improved from 8.3 to 1.4, with no recurrences (the follow-up period was 4–24 months) Patients have also reported that, after treatment, no significant pain or discomfort occurred during or after sexual intercourse. In 2009, Petersen et al. evaluated in a randomized, double blinded, placebo-controlled study, the efficacy of BoNT-A injection in 32 women with vulvodynia and compared the results with a control group of 32 women [63]. Twenty units of BoNT were diluted in 0.5 mL saline solution and injected into bulbospongious muscles, while, for control cases, 0.5 mL saline solution was used. Both groups achieved a significant reduction in pain and the conclusion was that BoNT-A did not reduce the pain, does not improve sexual function and does not influence the quality of life compared to the placebo group.

Vulvodynia is a syndrome defined by a sharp pain in the vulva that does not have a well-defined cause which makes it very difficult to treat. The most common clinical form of vulvodynia is the provoked vestibulodynia, also named vulvar vestibulitis [65]. BoNT-A administered in high doses appears to have found utility in the treatment of this pathology that does not have a known organic substrate. Pelletier et al. administered BoNT-A to a group of 20 women aged 18–60 with provoked vulvodynia [66]. Each patient was injected with 50 U of BoNT-A into the bulbospongious muscles under EMG guidance. After three months, 80% of patients confirmed a decrease in pain intensity, and quality of life and sexual life improved significantly in the first six months. A retrospective study compared the effects of different doses of BoNT-A and Gabapentin in patients with vulvodynia also concluded that the symptoms of the patients injected with BoNT-A, measured through VAS scale were significantly improved in the group treated with Gabapentin (an anti-epileptic drug, that is also used to treat neuropathic pain) [67,68]. In Table 4 are summarized the clinical studies regarding the use of BoNT-A in the treatment of vulvodynia.

One of the causes of the occurrence of vulvodynia is the aberrant increase in the number of nociceptors. Intraepithelial neural hyperplasia associated with hypersensitivity of peripheral nociceptors generates a strong pain in the vestibule. BoNT was successfully used in this pathology. The pain is released through blocking the release of acetylcholine from parasympathetic neurons and from sympathetic post-ganglionar neurons. BoNT has been also used, with a beneficial effect on dyspareunia. These effects could be explained by two theories: the first refers to the decrease of the pelvic muscular hypertonicity and implicitly of the pain, by paralyzing the musculature. The second mechanism is the blockade of neurotransmission at nociceptive receptors in the submucosal layers of the vestibule [69].

Table 4. Studies of BoNT-A in treatment of vulvodynia.

Author	Study Design	Number of Cases	Treatment Regimen	Outcome Measures	Follow-Up	Results
Yoon [60]	Retrospective study	7	Dilution: 20 U of the BoNT diluted in saline solution; Dose: 20 U of BoNT-A * Botox, Allegran, Inc., Irvine, CA, USA	• VAS (before and 2 weeks after each administration)	4–24 months	• The subjective pain score improved from 8.3 to 1.4, and no one has experienced a recurrence. No adverse effects were observed; • In 2 cases, pain decreased after one injection; 5 cases needed injections twice; • Patients reported subjective improvement in sexual; life and having no significant pain or discomfort during or after intercourse.
Petersen [63]	Randomized, double blinded, placebo-controlled study	32 cases 32 placebo	Dilution: 100 U of BoNT-A diluted in 2.5 mL saline solution; Dose: 20 U of the BoNT diluted or 0.5 mL of saline (placebo) * Botox, Allergan	• VAS, FSFI; FSDS; • Manifest Female Sexual Dysfunction; • Demographic Questionnaire; • SF-36	3, 6, 9, and 12 months	• Both groups: significantly pain reduction ($p < 0.001$); • No significantly improvements on the FSFI score until the second follow up visit ($p = 0.635$); • Compared to the group treated with BoNT-A, in the placebo group it was observed higher decrease of the sexual distress until the second follow-up ($p = 0.044$).
Pelletier [66]	Retrospective study	20	Dilution: 1 mL: 50 U BoNT-A diluted in 1 mL saline; Dose: 50 UIBoNT diluted * Botox; Allergan, Courbevoie, France	• VAS; • FSFI; • DLQI	3, 6 months	• 16 patients reported improved VAS scores; • At the 3 months follow up visit, 13 patients reported possibility of sexual intercourse; • After the 6 months follow up visit, QoL and sexual function reported to be satisfactory.
Jeon [67]	Retrospective study	73	Dose: 40 to 100 U BoNT-A (11 patients) 300 to 600 mg Gabapentin (62 patients) * Botox, Allegran Inc., Irvine, CA, USA	• VAS	6 to 24 months	• Gabapentin group: the VAS score decreased from 8.6 to 3.2 after treatment ($p < 0.001$); • BoNT-A group: the VAS score decreased from 8.1 to 2.5 ($p < 0.001$).

3.3. Use of BoNT-A in the Treatment of Chronic Pelvic Pain

A persistent pelvic pain, lasting more than six months, which can be conceptualized as a syndrome of somatic functional pain or as a regional pain syndrome defines chronic pelvic pain [5].

One of the causes of chronic pelvic pain syndrome is the spasm of the pelvic muscles, especially the spasm of the levator ani. Myofascial pain and spasm are defined as regional muscular pain characterized by the presence of trigger points. These are hypersensitive points distributed on the levator ani surface, which once touched, cause pain. The pain resulting from reaching these trigger points appears to result from the excessive release of acetylcholine and other neurogenic inflammatory substances from the neuromuscular junction. The management of pelvic floor muscle spasm requires a multidisciplinary approach and treatment strategies including the use of steroids, non-steroidal anti-inflammatory drugs, muscle relaxants, antidepressants, neuromodulators, selective norepinephrine reuptake inhibitors and injection of various substances into the triggering points such as local anesthetics, steroids and BoNT [70–72].

Adelowo et al. designed in 2013 a retrospective study on a cohort of 31 patients to evaluate the role of injections with BoNT-A in the levator ani muscle in women with refractory pelvic myofascial pain [73]. The pain was assessed during palpation of the pelvic floor muscles using a scale of 0 to 10, 10 being the most severe pain possible. Patient reassessment occurred before six weeks after injection and again after $\geq$6 weeks post injection. Thirty-one patients met the eligibility criteria but two were lost during follow-up. Overall, 79.3% of the patients reported on the re-evaluation a pain relief, while 20.7% reported an improvement in symptoms. The conclusion of this study was that BoNT-A injection into the levator ani proved to be effective for women with refractory myofascial pelvic pain, with only a few limited side effects. In 2006 a double-blind randomized study was conducted to estimate the utility of BoNT versus placebo in women that have reported pelvic spasms and chronic pelvic pain lasting more than two years [74]. Thirty women were injected with 80 U of BoNT while 30 with saline solution in the pelvic floor muscles. Their subjective symptoms (dysmenorrhea, dyspareunia and pelvic pain of non-menstrual origin) were quantified with VAS scores (Visual analog scales). VAS is a measurement instrument used to document the symptoms severity in different patients and to assess the effectiveness of therapy in those patients [75]. The pain of the pelvic floor was measured by vaginal manometry. After six months, the patients were re-evaluated and the conclusion was that the reduction of pelvic spasm could reduce some types of pelvic pain. BoNT-A reduces pelvic floor hypertonia more than placebo, so it could be used in women with refractory pain.

Gajraj et al. presented a case of a 60-year-old woman presenting a four-year-long pelvic pain with leg irradiation and irradiation in the vagina and rectum, aggravated by clinostats [76]. The pain was assessed at a level of 4–8 out of 10 on the VAS pain scale. Physical examinations did not reveal any focal neurological signs. The vaginal examination showed sensitivity and tenderness in the right anterior and right posterior lateral regions. The patient was injected in the internal obturator muscle with 0.25% bupivacaine, resulting in a 90% reduction in pain for 12 h. Progressive and postprocedural mean scores on the VAS scale were 7 out of 10 and 1 out of 10, respectively. After a subsequent BoNT-A injection, the patient again reported a 90% decrease in pain for more than three months. In addition, after BoNT injection, there were no adverse effects such as motor weakness, and intestinal or bladder disorders. Therefore, BoNT-A has also shown its efficiency in this case.

Twelve women aged 18–55 years old, with objective hypertonia of the pelvic floor muscles for at least two years and chronic pelvic pain were recruited for testing the utility of BoNT [77]. Forty units of BoNT-A in three different dilutions were administered bilaterally in the puborectal and pubococcygeal muscles under conscious sedation. The results were favorable and uninfluenced by dilution. VAS pain scores improved for the cases with dyspareunia, but non-menstrual pelvic pain experienced insignificant reductions. At four weeks after treatment, it was observed a decrease with 37% in resting pressure measured through pelvic muscle manometer, reduction that decreased until 25% at 12 weeks. In addition, the quality of life scores improved.

A prospective study on women with refractory chronic pelvic pain and pelvic muscle spasm was conducted in 2015 to demonstrate the role of BoNT-A in the treatment of these dysfunctions [78]. BoNT-A injections in spastic pelvic muscles (up to 300 U) were performed through needle electromyographic guidance. Of the 28 women enrolled in the study, 21 qualified for analysis. The average age of the cases was 22–50 years and the comorbidities included interstitial cystitis/bladder pain syndrome in 42.9% of cases and vulvodynia in 66.7% of cases. Overall, 61.9% of subjects have reported improvement in the overall response assessment at four weeks and 80.9% at 8, 12 and 24 weeks post injection compared to baseline. Post-injection adverse reactions were also reported, including worsening of the following pre-existing conditions: constipation (28.6%), stress urinary incontinence (4.8%), fecal incontinence (4.8%) and urinary incontinence (4.8%). The conclusion of this study is consistent with the findings of other studies on this topic and suggests that BoNT could be useful in the treatment of pelvic floor muscle spasm and chronic pelvic pain, refractory to other therapies.

Levator ani syndrome is defined by chronic or recurrent episodes of rectal pain and affects approximately 6.6% of adults. There is no consensus on the pathophysiology of this painful syndrome, although the chronic hypertonia of pelvic floor muscles is the most common explanation [79]. Therefore, through the muscle spasm, the use of BoNT-A was attempted in the treatment of levator ani syndrome, however, without favorable results. Rao et al. conducted a randomized, placebo-controlled study on 12 cases with levator ani syndrome [80]. After BoNT-Administration into the anal sphincter, the duration and intensity of pain and the mean frequency remained unchanged compared to the baseline. The conclusion of the authors was that BoNT-A injections into the sphincter ani is secure but is not effective in relieving anorectal pain associated with this syndrome. Table 5 summarizes the clinical studies regarding the use of BoNT-A in the treatment of chronic pelvic pain and pelvic floor muscle spasm treatment.

Jhang J-F et al. [81] described in their research from 2015 a possible mechanism of BoNT-A on chronic pelvic pain. In several experimental studies involving both rats and humans, membrane receptors TRVP-1 and P2X3 have been observed to be up-regulated in the neuropathic pain. Xiao L. et al. concluded that a possible mechanism of BoNT-A is the reduction of TRPV-1 expression in spinal neurons of rats with hyperalgesia [82]. Muscular spasm seems to be usually associated with chronic pelvic pain [83,84] and the reduction of pain may also reduce the spasm. Myelinated and unmyelinated fibers (group III and IV, respectively) are nociceptors found in muscles, which can be sensitized by bradykinins, prostaglandin E, substance P, calcitonin gene-related peptide (CGRP) [85] and ATP [86]. BoNT-A is supposed to inhibit their release [85] and the activation of spinal cord neurons that are responsible for the pain transmission [87–89]. BoNT-A could also inhibit the spinal motor neurons alpha and gamma, mechanism through which pelvic muscle spasm could be stopped [85]. It is important to continue the research in this area and to investigate the mechanism of action and the effects of BoNT-A in the treatment of chronic pelvic pain.

Table 5. Studies of BoNT-A in chronic pelvic pain and pelvic floor muscle spasm treatment.

Author	Study Design	Number of Cases	Treatment Regimen	Outcome Measures	Follow-Up	Results
Adelowo [73]	Retrospective cohort study	31	Dose: 100–300 U BoNT-A * Botox, Allergan Inc. Irvine, CA, USA	• Patient-reported tenderness on levator palpation; • patient-reported symptom improvement; • time to and number of repeat injections; • complications	<6 weeks post-injection (visit 1) and ≥6 weeks post injection (visit 2).	• 93.5% completed the first follow-up visit; 79.3% reported improvement in pain and 20.7% reported no improvement. • Median pain with levator palpation was significantly lower than before injection ($p < 0.0001$). • 58.0% had a second follow-up visit with a median pain score lower than before injection ($p < 0.0001$); the median time to repeat injection was 4.0 (3.0–7.0) months; 10.3% women—de-novo urinary retention, 6.9%-fecal incontinence, 10.3%-constipation and/or rectal pain; all side effects resolved spontaneously.
Abott [74]	Double-blinded, randomized, placebo-controlled trial.	60	Cases: 80 U BoNT-A (20 units/mL) Placebo: 4 mL of saline solution * Botox, Allergan Westport, Ireland	• Dysmenorrhea; dyspareunia; dyschezia; • Non-menstrual; pelvic pain assessed VAS scale	0, 1, 2, 3, 4, 5 and 6 months	• In case of dyspareunia and non-menstrual pain, it was observed that VAS score improved in the group treated with BoNT (66 vs. 12 and 51 vs. 22 respectively; also, the pelvic floor pressure decreased (49 vs. 32) • Dyspareunia was reduced in the placebo group (64 vs. 27);
Jarvis [77]	Prospective study	12	Dose: 40 U BoNT; Dilutions: 10 U/mL; 20 U/mL; and 100 U/mL. * Allergan (Gordon, New South Wales, Australia).	• VAS; SF-12; EQ-5D; • Pelvic floor muscles manometry; • Sexual activity scores	2, 4, 8 and 12 weeks post-treatment	• In case of dyspareunia and dysmenorrhea, VAS scores improved (80 vs, 28; $p = 0.01$, respectively 67 vs. 28; $p = 0.03$). • SF-12, EQ-5D and sexual activity scores were improved until week 12.
Morrissey [78]	Prospective pilot open-label study	21	Dose: up to 300 U BoNT-A Administration: using needle electromyography guidance, from a transperineal approach, to localize spastic pelvic floor muscles * Botox; Allergan, Irvine, CA, USA	• VAS scores for pain and dyspareunia; • QoL and sexual function; • GRA scale for pelvic pain; pelvic floor tone and tenderness; • vaginal manometry.	6 months (4, 8, 12, and 24 weeks after injections)	• 61.9% of subjects reported improvement on GRA at 4 weeks and 80.9% at 8, 12, and 24 weeks post injection, compared with baseline; 58.8%, 68.8%, 80% and 83.3% reported less dyspareunia at 4, 8, 12, and 24 weeks, respectively. VAS score improved at weeks 12 (5.6, $p = 0.011$) and 24 (5.4, $p = 0.004$) compared with baseline (7.8); Sexual dysfunction as measured by the FSDS significantly improved; SF-12 showed improved QoL in the physical composite score at all post injections visits (42.9, 44, 43.1, and 45.5 vs 40 at baseline; $p < 0.05$), • Vaginal manometry—decrease in resting pressures and in maximum contraction pressures at all follow-up visits ($p < 0.05$); Digital assessment of PFM showed decreased tenderness on all visits • Reported post-injection adverse effects: worsening of the following preexisting conditions: constipation (28.6%), stress urinary incontinence (4.8%), fecal incontinence (4.8%), and new onset stress urinary incontinence (4.8%).
Rao [80]	Randomized, placebo-controlled study	12	Cases: 100 U of BoNT-A intra sphincterian (anal) at 3 months intervals; Placebo: saline solution * Botox; Allergan Pharmaceuticals, Los Angeles, CA, USA)	• Daily frequency; • VAS; • balloon expulsion; anorectal manometry, pudendal nerve latency tests	NR	• The VAS score did not improve ($p = 0.31$) compared with baseline; • At 3 months follow up, the mean VAS pain score was decreased: 6.79 vs. 7.08 ($p = 0.25$); • Rectal sensory thresholds, anal sphincter pressures, balloon expulsion times, pudendal nerve latency did not decrease after BoNT-A or placebo

3.4. Inferior Urinary System Dysfunctions

3.4.1. Use of BoNT in the Treatment of Interstitial Cystitis (the Painful Bladder Syndrome)

BoNT-A injections into the urethral sphincter have been used in the treatment of lower urinary tract dysfunctions in the last 20 years to reduce bladder emptying, urethral and residual urine pressures [90,91]. The pathogenesis of interstitial cystitis is still uncertain, but there is a hypothesis that asserts that this pathology arises from neurogenic inflammation that activates bladder afferent nerves and causes bladder hypersensitivity [92]. Painful bladder syndrome is a clinical syndrome characterized by pain with supra-pubian localization caused by bladder filling associated with increased urinary frequency both day and night in the absence of proven urinary infection. There is currently no standard treatment [93], but there are studies in the literature that confirm the efficiency of BoNT-A in the management of interstitial cystitis, which has an antinociceptive effect on the visceral afferent nervous fibers [94].

Giannantoni A. et al. selected a group of seven women and instilled them with 200 U BoNT-A diluted in 100 mL of saline, without any anesthesia, to analyze the utility of this treatment in bladder painful syndrome [94]. The exclusion criterion for the cohort was detrusor overactivity. The solution was injected intravesical and maintained for 40 min and the results were evaluated after one week, one month and three months. However, the results were discouraging because short-term benefits were found for four of seven patients. The explanation consists in the molecular weight of BoNT-A that does not allow it to pass the epithelial barrier to the bladder to reach sub-urothelium and to act on nerve endings. Therefore, the intravesical instillation of diluted BoNTs is not an effective treatment in this pathology.

As the intravesical instillation of BoNT-A has not been found to be convenient, studies on this subject have further been conducted and it has been found that increased amounts of sensory fibers are located into the bladder trigonum. To evaluate the tolerability and efficiency of BoNT-A injections in patients with painful bladder syndrome that are refractory to standard treatment, Pinto et al. conducted a study on 17 patients (16 women and one man), which were investigated before treatment and one, three six, and nine months later [93]. All patients received 10 intra-trigonal injections with 10 U BoNT-A, diluted in 1 mL saline (a total of 100 U). The results were favorable: the pain level decreased, the urinary frequency decreased and O'Leary-Sant score increased. Therefore, the authors concluded that intra-trigonal injections with BoNT-A are useful in treating interstitial cystitis, also called painful bladder syndrome.

Satisfactory results were also obtained in the treatment of vesical dysfunctions, by injecting BoNT-A into the bladder wall [95]. Fifteen patients received 200 U BoNT-A diluted in 20 mL saline under general anesthesia and cystoscopic guidance. To evaluate the results, VAS pain scale and drainage charts were recorded, while urodynamic studies were realized before injections and at 1, 3, 5 and 12 months after the treatment. Overall, 86.6% of patients have reported an improvement after one and three months. In 26.6% of cases, at the five months follow up visit, it was observed that the effects persisted; nevertheless, the urinary frequency during day and night was increased. Twelve months after the treatment, the pain reappeared in all patients. Nine patients claimed dysuria one month after treatment.

Kuo et al. conducted a study on 10 patients to demonstrate the efficiency of suburothelial injection of BoNT-A in the management of chronic interstitial cystitis [96]. They injected 100 U of BoNT-A suburothelial in 20 places on five patients.Five other patients were injected with another 100 U of BoNT-A at the trigonal area of the bladder. However, the therapeutic results were disappointing because no favorable evolution was observed after three months of treatment. Carl et al. conducted a pilot study involving 29 patients with painful bladder syndrome and injected them with BoNT-A, to demonstrate that it is useful in the treatment of this pathology [97]. The toxin was injected submucosally, into the trigonal area, and the results contrary to those obtained by Kuo et al. [96], suggested that BoNT-A has an antinociceptive effect on the bladder afferent nerves in patients with chronic interstitial cystitis. The authors did not experience systemic side effects during and after treatment.

A single center, prospective, non-randomized study was conducted in 2007 by Ramsay et al. to evaluate the efficiency, tolerability and safety of BoNT-A when injected intravesical at patients with interstitial cystitis [98]. Eleven women with average age of 56 years were injected with BoNT-A. The conclusion of the study was that a significant symptoms reduction had been observed at about 10–14 weeks after injection. Another prospective study based on the safety and effects of BoNT-A repeatedly administered to patients with bladder painful syndrome, was conducted on a cohort of 16 patients [99]. They were exposed to four cycles of intratrigonal injections with BoNT-A. A second injection was administered at the three-month follow up visit. Complications such as urinary tract infections or bladder hypersensitivity were evaluated at different intervals. Improvement occurred after approximately 9.9 months (±2.4 months). No total remission of symptoms was seen in any of the patients and 5 of the 16 patients had uncomplicated urinary tract infections. The studies that are pointing out the usefulness of BoNT-A in interstitial cystitis treatment are summarized is Table 6.

Apostolidis et al. proposed a possible mechanism of action of BoNT in the treatment of detrusor activity, but further research is needed to determine the significant effects of BoNT-A in this pathology [100,101]. Karsenty et al. [102] conducted a study in 2008 that pointed out that BoNT-A could also action through inhibition of other neurotransmitters, receptors or neuropeptides. A review from 2016 [103] identified a possible mechanism for the effects of BoNT-A in the treatment of inferior urinary system dysfunctions. Several studies in vivo and vitro included in this research, highlighted that BoNT-A injections into detrusor could decrease the levels of capsaicin receptor TRPV1 and purinergic receptor P2X3 (whose expression is increased) in the suburothelial nerve fibers [104–107]. Patients with detrusor overactivity have shown increased densities of substance P and CGRP, according to Smet et al. [108]. Following those observations, several studies on animals identified a possible mechanism of action of BoNT-A, which consists of the reduced release of CGRP in rat model [109] and an inhibition of SP with reduced activation of P2X3 and TRPV1 receptors in suburothelium and detrusor muscle in guinea pig model [110], leading to peripheral denervation. However, future research must be conducted to clarify the proposed mechanism and the role of BoNT-A therapy in case of inferior urinary system dysfunctions.

Table 6. Studies of BoNT in interstitial cystitis.

Author	Study Design	Number of Cases	Treatment Regimen	Outcome Measures	Follow-Up	Results
Pinto [93]	Prospective study	17	Dose: 100 U of Botulin toxin Administration: bladder trigone only, under cystoscopy guidance * Botox (Allergan, Inc., Irvine, CA, USA)	• 3-day voiding chart; • VAS • O'Leary-Sant score • pressure flow study and flowmetry	9 months	• Pain score decreased at 1 month follow up visit and 3 months follow up visit (from 5.7 to 2.2 and 1.9) ($p < 0{,}01$); • At the end of the study, 41.17% of patients reported increased urinary frequency with lower threshold of pain and O'Leary-Sant score; • All patients reported subjective improvement.
Giannantoni [94]	Prospective Study	7	Dose: 200 U BoNT-A, diluted in 100 mL saline, without any form of anesthesia. Administration: intravesical instillation, retained in the bladder for 40 mi * Botox (Allergan, Inc., Irvine, CA, USA)	• voiding diary; urodynamic; • Visual Analog Scale for pain assessment	3 months	• At baseline mean day- and night-time urinary frequencies were 9.1 and 4.6, respectively. Mean VAS score was 6.5. On urodynamics, mean bladder capacity was 270.4 mL. • No patients showed any impairment of bladder emptying • 1 week after treatment, mean day and night-time urinary frequency fell to 7.4 and to 3.3; • VAS score significantly dropped to 3.5 ($p < 0.05$). VAS score improvement was particularly marked in 4 patients • Maximum cystometric capacity was 321.4 mL. • Symptoms and urodynamic parameters did not change in 3/7 patients; • No local or systemic side effects were reported during or after instillation
Giannantoni [95]	Prospective study	15	Dose: 200 U BoNT-A diluted in 20 mL saline; * Botox (Allergan, Inc., Irvine, CA, USA)	• 3-day voiding chart; • pain visual analog scale; • urodynamics	12 months	• at follow up visit from 1 and 3 months, 86.6% of patients reported improvement in the symptoms; decreased urinary frequency and VAS score; • At the last follow up visit all patients reported re-apparition of pain; • Complication: in 9 cases after 1 month, 4 cases at the 3-month visit and in 2 cases at 5-month visit, the patients reported dysuria.

Table 6. *Cont.*

Author	Study Design	Number of Cases	Treatment Regimen	Outcome Measures	Follow-Up	Results
Kuo [96]	Prospective study	10	Dose: In 5 patients, 100 U of BoNT-A; additional 100 U BoNT-A into the trigone in the other 5 patients. Administration: suburothelial into 20 sites * Botox, Allergan Inc. Irvine, CA, USA	• number of daily urinations; • urodynamic changes functional bladder capacity; • bladder pain;	3 months	• functional bladder capacity significantly increased (155 after injection vs. 77 mL at baseline, $p < 0.001$) • VAS scores and frequency of daily urinations were decreased • urinary frequency and bladder pain were improved after the 3 months follow up visit in 2 patients • The urodynamic results (cystometric capacity) were improved (287 vs. 210 mL, $p = 0.05$).
Carl [97]	Two center pilot study	29	Dose:500 U BoNT-A diluted in 3 mL saline Administration: injected through a rigid cystoscope into 20–25 sites submucosally in the trigone and bladder floor. * Dysport® (Ipsen Pharma, Ettlingen, Germany	• Daytime frequency; nycturia; urgency; • Pain (VAS score) • Urodynamic evaluation	6 months	• Daytime frequency, nycturia, urgency and pain by VAS scale decreased by 50%, 75%, 43% and 81%, respectively, 6 weeks after treatment ($p < 0.05$); • maximal cystometric capacity increased from 282 to 360 mL; bladder compliance increased from 13 mL/cm$H_2$0 to 23 mL/cmH_2O; Two patients suffered from temporary hematuria, 3 patients had residual urine of more than 100 cc and 1 patient showed urinary retention
Ramsay [98]	Prospective study	11	Dose: 200–300 U-BoNT-A; Administration: BoNT was injected in 20–30 different sites (10 U per site) into the suburothelium of the bladder * source of toxin not reported	• BFLUTS; KHQ; • 24-h voiding frequency chart; • Filling and voiding urodynamics; • Urodynamic variables PIP1	14 weeks	• Baseline BFLUTS score 132.Improved to 118 at 6 weeks (19%, $p = 0.07$); improvement was maintained at 10 weeks (score=109, 22%, $p = 0.03$) and 14 weeks (score=105, 27%, $p = 0.01$); • Frequency improved post injection to 12 at 6 weeks ($p = 0.57$), 10 at 10 weeks ($p = 0.01$) and 10.5 at 14 weeks ($p = 0.03$); • FDV improved from 96 to 174 mls ($p = 0.04$); MCC improved from 200 to 258 mls ($p = 0.16$); BFLUTS improved at 6 weeks ($p = 0.009$) and 10 weeks ($p = 0.009$); PIP1 increased from 39 to 46 ($p = 0.9$).
Pinto [99]	Prospective study	16	Dose: 100 U BoNT-A Administration: 4 consecutive injections of BoNT-A injected intratrigonal under cystoscopic guidance * Botox (Allergan, Inc., Irvine, CA, USA)	• VAS • Voiding dysfunction; O'Leary-Sant score; • Urinary tract infections	12 months	• VAS score and O'Leary-Sant score decreased; • urinary frequency increased; • quality of life scores was similar after each injection; • The effects of BoNT-A lasted an average of 9.9 ± 2.4 months.

3.4.2. Use of BoNT-A in Urinary Incontinence through Neurogenic Overactive Bladder and Idiopathic Overactive Bladder

Urinary incontinence through both neurogenic (NOB) and idiopathic bladder hyperactivity (IOB) is a lower urinary tract dysfunction that affects many women with a prevalence of approximately 25% of the cases worldwide [111]. Bladder overactivity is defined by increased urinary frequency, feeling of urge and nycturia and could be associated with urinary incontinence. Anticholinergic therapy is essential in the treatment of overactive bladder but it also requires lifestyle and behavioral changes. If symptoms do not improve with anticholinergic therapy and lifestyle changes, urodynamic studies and cystourethroscopy are required [112]. Studies confirm the usefulness of intravesical injections with BoNT-A in women with overactive bladder (OB). After the injection of BoNT-A to the patients with neurogenic or idiopathic detrusor overactivity, there was observed a reduction in bladder detrusor pressure during both involuntary and voluntary contractions, which confirmed the BoNT-A influences the motor detrusor innervation. BoNT-A prevents the release of neurotransmitters such as Ach and in addition it acts on adenosine triphosphate (ATP), substance P and glutamate, decreasing the number of sensory receptors and nerves growth factor (NGF) in the bladder wall. These mechanisms of action may explain the utility of BoNT-A in the treatment of urinary incontinence through bladder overactivity [86].

During the period 2005–2009, 99 patients with OB were enrolled in a prospective, randomized, double-blind, placebo-controlled comparative trial [113]. Patients received a single injection with BoNT-A (50 U, 100 U or 150 U) into the vesical muscle. Three months after administration, a 50% improvement from baseline in urge and urinary incontinence was noticed. The 100 U and 150 U doses of BoNT were well tolerated and, in both cases, improvement was recorded. However, injections of 100 U showed reasonable efficiency with a lower post-voiding residual volume risk.

A comparative study between the response of patients with neurogenic detrusor overactivity and idiopathic detrusor overactivity to the first of administration of BoNT-A into the vesical detrusor was performed in 2005 by Popat et al. [114]. The study included 44 patients with neurogenic bladder overactivity and 31 with idiopathic bladder overactivity. The first group received 300 U BoNT-A and the second group received 200 U BoNT-A. The results were compared 4 and 16 weeks after injection: patients with idiopathic bladder overactivity responded to BoNT-A as well as those with neurogenic bladder overactivity and, despite the lower dose of toxin used, the results were similar.

Schmid et al. conducted a prospective study on 180 cases (135 women) to report the efficiency of a reduced dose (100 U) of BoNT-A injected into the bladder detrusor in case of patients with IOB [115]. Eighty-seven percent of patients experienced an improvement in urodynamic parameters: the urge completely disappeared in 75% of cases and the urinary incontinence disappeared in 84% of patients within two weeks. The frequency of urination decreased from 15 to 7 mictions and no more than 5 to 2 mictions per night were reported.

Brubaker et al. compared a group of 28 women with refractory urge through idiopathic bladder overactivity (200 U BoNT-A administered in the detrusor) with a placebo group of 15 women with the same pathology [116]. Sixty percent of the patients treated with BoNT-A have reported improved symptoms, effects that lasted approximately 373 days, respectively 62 days or less in the placebo cases. In the BoNT-A group, many patients with increased post-voiding residual volume (43%) and urinary tract infection were found in those with an increased post-voiding residual volume (75%).

Khanlow et al. conducted a study based on the effects of intravesical administration of BoNT-A in the management of refractory idiopathic bladder overactivity. Patients were properly informed about the improvement of life quality, the duration of re-injection and the risks for intermittent auto-catheterization. A cohort of 81 patients were injected with 200 U BoNT-A intravesically [117]. After BoNT-A injections, it was observed a significant improvement in the quality of life sustained by repeated injections. In 43% of cases treated with BoNT-A, auto-catheterization was required.

To describe the mid-term outcomes and adaptation of patients to BoNT-A therapy as a management strategy for women with refractory idiopathic bladder overactivity, Dowson et al. developed a cohort of 100 women who received BoNT-A injections as follows: all patients received an injection, 53 received 2, 20 received 3, 13 received 4, 10 received 5, 5 received 6, 3 received 7, 1 received 8, 1 received 9 and 1 received 10 injections [118]. Thirty-seven percent of patients completed the study after the first two injections and 11% of patients required intermittent auto-catheterization. As a possible complication, in 35% of patients, catheterization was required after the first administration of BoNT-A and in 21% of cases bacteriuria was detected. A review paper from 2016 investigated the use of BoNT in adults with urgency urinary incontinence and idiopathic overactive bladder. The conclusions of the study were that 22.9% to 55% cases regained complete continence and showed a significant improvement in the quality of life after treatment [119]. Detailed and comparative studies are found in Table 7.

Table 7. Studies of BoNT in overactive bladder.

Author	STUDY DESIGN	Number of Cases	Treatment Regimen	Outcome Measures	Follow-Up	Results
Le Normand [113]	Prospective, randomized, double-blind, placebo-controlled comparative study	99	Dose: 50 U, 100 U or 150 U BoNT-A Administration: intradetrusor injection * Botox (Allergan, Inc., Irvine, CA, USA)	• Clinical and urodynamic variables; • Quality of life (QoL)	day 8; 1, 3, 5, and 6 months	• after three months >50% improvement in urgency and urge urinary incontinence in 65% and 56% of patients who respectively received 100 U ($p = 0.086$) and 150 U ($p = 0.261$) BoNTA—>75% improvement in 40% of patients of both groups (100 U [$p = 0.058$] and 150 U [$p = 0.022$]); • Complete continence: in 55% and 50% patients after 100 UI and 150 U BoNTA treatment at month 3; • QoL improved up to the 6-month visit; 3 patients with postvoid residuals >200 mL in the 150 U group and a few urinary tract infections.
Popat [114]	Prospective, open label study	75	Dose: 300 U (NOB) or 200 U (IOB) of BoNT Administration: injected into the bladder * Botox (Allergan, Inc., Irvine, CA, USA)	• urodynamic maximum cystometric capacity; • maximum detrusor pressure during filling; • number of incontinence episodes; • frequency of voids;	1 month and 4 months	• At 4 months, cystometric capacity increased in NOB and IOB cases treated with BoNT (229.1 to 427.0 mL, $p < 0.0001$, respectively 193.6 to 327.1 1 mL, $p = 0.0008$; • Decreased maximum detrusor pressure during filling in NOB and IOB (60.7 to 26.1 cm H_2O, $p < 0.0001$, respectively 62.1 to 45.1 cm H_2O, $p = 0.027$); • Frequency decreased in NOB and IOB patients (12.3 to 6.6 voids/24 h, $p < 0.0001$, respectively 13.6 to 8.3, $p = 0.0002$); • Urgency decreased in NOB and IOB (7.5 to 1.44 episodes/24 h, $p < 0.0001$, respectively 10.9 to 4.9, $p < 0.0001$)
Schmid [115]	Prospective study	180 (45 men, 135 women)	Dose: 100 U of BTX-A into the detrusor at 30 different sites. Reinjection: 52/180 of patients were reinjected after the effect had diminished (time interval between two treatments was mean 11 months) * Botox (Allergan, Inc., Irvine, CA, USA)	• Urgency, frequency, maximal cystometric capacity (MCBC) • volume at first and strong desire to void (FDV, UV) • detrusor compliance (DC), postvoiding residual volume (PVR), • QoL assessment	After 4, 12 and 36 weeks	• 87% of patients showed a significant ($p > 0.001$) improvement of their bladder function urgency completely disappeared in 75% and incontinence in 84% within 2 weeks; • frequency decreased from 15 to 7 micturition and nycturia from 5 to 2; MCBC increased from mean 245 to 395 mL; FDV increased from mean 127 to 218 mL; strong desire to void from mean 215 to 312 mL; • QoL assessment revealed a significant subjective improvement in all urge-related items; side effects: 6 temporary urine retentions and 16 urinary infections.

Table 7. *Cont.*

Author	STUDY DESIGN	Number of Cases	Treatment Regimen	Outcome Measures	Follow-Up	Results
Brubaker [116]	Randomized, double-blind, placebo controlled, review	43	Dose: 200 U BoNT dissolved in 6 mL saline Placebo: 3 mL saline. * Botox (Allergan, Inc., Irvine, CA, USA)	• frequency of incontinence episodes; • symptom and quality of life measures (PGISC); • the duration and occurrence of voiding dysfunction	12 months	• 60% of the cases injected with BoNT-A reported improved PGISC scores • post-void residual urine increased in 43% of cases • urinary tract infection rate increased in the cases with increased post-void residual urine
Khanlow [117]	Prospective, open label study	81	Dose: 200 U BoNT-A Administration: intradetrusor injections at 20 sites per injection * Botox (Allergan, Inc., Irvine, CA, USA)	• UDI • IIQ	NR	• Mean UDI and IIQ scores improved after injection 1 in all patients (56 to 26 and 59 to 21), after injection 2 in 29.6% of cases (52 to 30 and 51 to 24), after injection 3 in 16.04% of cases (40 to 19 and 43 to 17), after injection 4 in 7.40% (44 to 17 and 61 to 15) and after injection 5 in 4.93% (51 to 17 and 63 to 14). • In 43% of cases, self-catheterization was requested
Dowson [118]	Prospective study	100	Dose: 200 U BoNT-A Administration: into suburothelium or detrusor muscle under cystoscopic guidance * Onabotulinumtoxin A; Allergan Ltd., Marlow, Buckinghamshire, UK	• QoL measures; • voiding diary; • residual volume; • complications	To five BoNT-A injections.	• 37% of patients completed the study after the second administration of BoNT-A (13% of cases reported poor efficacy and 11% due to the need of intermittent self-catheterization) • In 35% of cases, the need of self-catheterization was seen after the first administration of BoNT-A. • The period between administration of BoNT doses was ~322 days

4. Conclusions and Future Perspectives

In this paper, we reveal several pathologies from the gynecological field for which BoNT treatment can be used. Most of these dysfunctions have been shown to be refractory to conventional treatments, but the results after single or repeated cycles of BoNT-A were favorable and the symptoms improved.

The dosage used ranged from 40 U to 400 U in single administration. In some cases, repeated injection cycles were necessary, depending on the symptomatology and the scores obtained after the patients completed standardized questionnaires. The improvement of the symptomatology was objectively certified Susing standardized questionnaires before and after a certain period post-injection.

When compared to BoNT-B, we observed that BoNT-A is used more often with good results, especially because the paralysis resulting from BoNT-B is not as efficient as the one of BoNT-A. It is also desirable to carry out further studies to reach consensus on the optimal BoNT-A dose and administration protocol to create a standardized treatment.

In conclusion, this review highlights that BoNT could be successfully used in treating symptoms of gynecological dysfunctions refractory to conventional treatments, having few side effects and high efficacy.

Author Contributions: M.A.M., O.G.D., A.B. and P.L. together initiated, designed, and drafted the manuscript. O.G.D., A.B., I.S. and B.B contributed to the literature collection. I.S, B.B. and P.L.drew the figures. All authors revised the manuscript. All authors read and approved the final manuscript.

Conflicts of Interest: The authors declare no conflict of interest.

Abbreviations

The following abbreviations are used in the manuscript:

Ach	acetylcholine
BFLUTS	Bristol female low urinary tract symptoms
BoNT	botulinum toxin
BoNT A	botulinum toxin type A
BoNT B	botulinum toxin type B
CISC	intermittent self-catheterization
DC	detrusor compliance
EMG	electromyography
EQ 5D	a standardized instrument for use as a measure of health outcome
FSDS	female sexual distress scale
IIQ	Incontinence inventory questionnaire
IOB	idiopathic overactive bladder
KHQ	King's Health Questionnaire
LC	Light chain
MCBC	maximal cystometric capacity
NGF	nerves growth factor
NOB	neurogenic overactive bladder
OB	overactive bladder
PFM	pelvic floor muscle
PGISC	patient global impression of symptom control
PVR	postvoiding residual volume
QoL	quality of life
SNARE	Soluble NSF(N-ethylmaleimide-sensitive factor) Attachment Protein) REceptor
SF12	physical and mental health summary scales
SNAP	Synaptosomal-associated protein 25
TRPV	transient receptor potential cation channels ("V" is for vanilloid type)
UDI	urinary distress inventory
VAS	visual analog scale
VAMP	vesicle associated membrane protein

References

1. Ahangari, A. Prevalence of chronic pelvic pain among women: An updated review. *Pain Physician* **2014**, *17*, E141–E147. [PubMed]
2. Jarrell, J.F.; Vilos, G.A.; Allaire, C.; Burgess, S.; Fortin, C.; Gerwin, R.; Lapensée, L.; Lea, R.H.; Leyland, N.A.; Martyn, P.; et al. Consensus guidelines for the management of chronic pelvic pain. *J. Obstet. Gynaecol. Can.* **2005**, *27*, 781–826. [CrossRef] [PubMed]
3. Akour, A.; Kasabri, V.; Afifi, F.U.; Bulatova, N. The use of medicinal herbs in gynecological and pregnancy-related disorders by Jordanian women: A review of folkloric practice vs. evidence-based pharmacology. *Pharm. Biol.* **2016**, *54*, 1901–1918. [CrossRef] [PubMed]
4. Rapin, A.J.; Morgan, M.L. Chronic Pelvic Pain. In *Handbook of Women's Sexual and Reproductive Health*; Issues in Women's Health; Springer: Boston, MA, USA, 2002; pp. 217–229. Available online: https://link.springer.com/chapter/10.1007/978-1-4615-0689-8_12#citeas (accessed on 20 September 2017). [CrossRef]
5. Speer, L.M.; Mushkabar, S.; Erbele, T. Chronic Pelvic Pain in Women. *Am. Fam. Physician* **2016**, *93*, 380–387. [PubMed]
6. Baranowski, A.P. Chronic pelvic pain. *Best Pract. Res. Clin. Gastroenterol.* **2009**, *23*, 593–610. [CrossRef] [PubMed]
7. Restani, P.; Di Lorenzo, C.; Garcia-Alvarez, A.; Badea, M.; Ceschi, A.; Egan, B.; Dima, L.; Lude, S.; Maggi, F.M.; Marculescu, A.; et al. Adverse Effects of Plant Food Supplements Self-Reported by Consumers in the PlantLIBRA Survey Involving Six European Countries. *PLoS ONE* **2016**, *11*, e0150089. [CrossRef] [PubMed]
8. Said, S.Z.; Meshkinpour, A.; Carruthers, A.; Carruthers, J. Botulinum Toxin A. *Am. J. Clin. Dermatol.* **2003**, *4*, 609–616. [CrossRef] [PubMed]
9. Dima, L.; Repanovici, A.; Purcaru, D.; Rogozea, L. Informed consent and e-communication in medicine. *Rev. Romana Bioet.* **2014**, *12*, 37–46.
10. Naumanna, M.; Albaneseb, A.; Heinenc, F.; Molenaersd, G.; Relja, M. Safety and efficacy of botulinum toxin type A following long-term use. *Eur. J. Neurol.* **2006**, *13*, 35–40. [CrossRef] [PubMed]
11. Nigam, P.K.; Anjana, N. Botulinum toxin. *Indian J. Dermatol.* **2010**, *55*, 8–14. [CrossRef] [PubMed]
12. Sloop, R.R.; Cole, R.A.; Escutin, R.O. Human response to botulinum toxin injection: Type B compared with type A. *Neurology* **1997**, *49*. [CrossRef]
13. Pirazzini, M.; Rossetto, O.; Eleopra, R.; Montecucco, C. Botulinum Neurotoxins: Biology, Pharmacology and Toxicology. *Pharmacol. Rev.* **2017**, *69*, 200–235. [CrossRef] [PubMed]
14. Rossetto, O.; Pirazzini, M.; Montecucco, C. Botulinum neurotoxins: Genetic, structural and mechanistic insights. *Nat. Rev. Microbiol.* **2014**, *12*, 535–549. [CrossRef] [PubMed]
15. Hill, K.K.; Smith, T.J. Genetic diversity within Clostridium botulinum serotypes, botulinum neurotoxin gene clusters and toxin subtypes. *Curr. Top. Microbiol. Immunol.* **2013**, *364*, 1–20. [CrossRef] [PubMed]
16. Burke, G.S. Notes on Bacillus botulinus. *J. Bacteriol.* **1919**, *4*, 555–570. [PubMed]
17. Gimenez, D.; Ciccarelli, A.S. Another type of Clostridium botulinum. *Zentralbl. Bakteriol.* **1970**, *215*, 221–224.
18. Chai, Q.; Arndt, J.W.; Dong, M.; Tepp, W.H.; Johnson, E.A.; Chapman, E.R.; Stevens, R.C. Structural basis of cell surface receptor recognition by botulinum neurotoxin B. *Nature* **2006**, *444*, 1096–1100. [CrossRef] [PubMed]
19. Zhang, S.; Masuyer, G.; Zhang, J.; Shen, Y.; Lundin, D.; Henriksson, L.; Miyashita, S.I.; Martínez-Carranza, M.; Dong, M.; Stenmark, P. Identification and characterization of a novel botulinum neurotoxin. *Nat. Commun.* **2017**, *8*, 14130. [CrossRef] [PubMed]
20. Steegmaier, M.; Klumperman, J.; Foletti, D.L.; Yoo, J.S.; Scheller, R.H. Vesicle-associated membrane protein 4 is implicated in trans-Golgi network vesicle trafficking. *Mol. Biol. Cell.* **1999**, *10*, 1957–1972. [CrossRef] [PubMed]
21. Brandhorst, D.; Zwilling, D.; Rizzoli, S.O.; Lippert, U.; Lang, T.; Jahn, R. Homotypic fusion of early endosomes: SNAREs do not determine fusion specificity. *Proc. Natl. Acad. Sci. USA* **2006**, *103*, 2701–2706. [CrossRef] [PubMed]
22. Daste, F.; Galli, T.; Tareste, D. Structure and function of longin SNAREs. *J. Cell. Sci.* **2015**, *128*, 4263–4272. [CrossRef] [PubMed]

23. Zornetta, I.; Azarnia Tehran, D.; Arrigoni, G.; Anniballi, F.; Bano, L.; Leka, O.; Zanotti, G.; Binz, T.; Montecucco, C. The first non Clostridial botulinum-like toxin cleaves VAMP within the juxtamembrane domain. *Sci. Rep.* **2016**, *6*, 30257. [CrossRef] [PubMed]
24. Tanizawa, Y.; Fujisawa, T.; Mochizuki, T.; Kaminuma, E.; Suzuki, Y.; Nakamura, Y.; Tohno, M. Draft Genome Sequence of Weissella oryzae SG25T, Isolated from Fermented Rice Grains. *Genome Announc.* **2014**, *2*. [CrossRef] [PubMed]
25. Zhang, S.; Lebreton, F.; Mansfield, M.J.; Miyashita, S.I.; Zhang, J.; Schwartzman, J.A.; Tao, L.; Masuyer, G.; Martínez-Carranza, M.; Stenmark, P. Identification of a Botulinum Neurotoxin-like Toxin in a Commensal Strain of Enterococcus faecium. *Cell Host Microbe.* **2018**, *23*, 169–176. [CrossRef] [PubMed]
26. Kukreja, R.; Singh, B.R. The botulinum toxin as a therapeutic agent: Molecular and pharmacological insights. *Res. Rep. Biochem.* **2015**, *5*, 173–183. [CrossRef]
27. Azarnia Tehran, D.; Pirazzini, M.; Leka, O.; Mattarei, A.; Lista, F.; Binz, T.; Rossetto, O.; Montecucco, C. Hsp90 is involved in the entry of clostridial neurotoxins into the cytosol of nerve terminals. *Cell. Microbiol.* **2017**, *19*. [CrossRef] [PubMed]
28. Montal, M. Botulinum neurotoxin: A marvel of protein design. *Annu. Rev. Biochem.* **2010**, *79*, 591–617. [CrossRef] [PubMed]
29. Matac, I.; Lackovic, Z. Botulinum toxin A, brain and pain. *Prog. Neurobiol.* **2014**, *119–120*, 39–59. [CrossRef] [PubMed]
30. Gallagher, J.; Ackerman, A. Botulinum toxin: From Molecule to Medicine. In *Botulinum Toxin Cosmetic and Clinical Applications*; Wiley Online Library: Chichester, UK, 2017; pp. 37–51. Available online: https://onlinelibrary.wiley.com/doi/10.1002/9781118661833.ch3 (accessed on 7 April 2018).
31. Pickett, A.; Perrow, K. Towards new uses of botulinum toxin as a novel therapeutic tool. *Toxins* **2011**, *3*, 63–81. [CrossRef] [PubMed]
32. Simpson, L.L. The life history of a botulinum toxin molecule. *Toxicon* **2013**, *68*, 40–59. [CrossRef] [PubMed]
33. Montecucco, C. How do tetanus and botulinum toxins bind to neuronal membranes? *Trends Biochem. Sci.* **1986**, *11*, 314–317. [CrossRef]
34. Rummel, A. Double receptor anchorage of botulinum neurotoxins accounts for their exquisite neurospecificity. *Curr. Top. Microbiol. Immunol.* **2013**, *364*, 61–90. [CrossRef] [PubMed]
35. Pirazzini, M.; Rossetto, O.; Bolognese, P.; Shone, C.C.; Montecucco, C. Double anchorage to the membrane and intact inter-chain disulfide bond are required for the low pH induced entry of tetanus and botulinum neurotoxins into neurons. *Cell. Microbiol.* **2011**, *13*, 1731–1743. [CrossRef] [PubMed]
36. Colasante, C.; Rossetto, O.; Morbiato, L.; Pirazzini, M.; Molgó, J.; Montecucco, C. Botulinum neurotoxin type A is internalized and translocated from small synaptic vesicles at the neuromuscular junction. *Mol. Neurobiol.* **2013**, *48*, 120–127. [CrossRef] [PubMed]
37. Simpson, L.L.; Coffield, J.A.; Bakry, N. Inhibition of vacuolar adenosine triphosphatase antagonizes the effects of clostridial neurotoxins but not phospholipase A2 neurotoxins. *J. Pharmacol. Exp. Ther.* **1994**, *269*, 256–262. [PubMed]
38. Williamson, L.C.; Neale, E.A. Bafilomycin A1 inhibits the action of tetanus toxin in spinal cord neurons in cell culture. *J. Neurochem.* **1994**, *63*, 2342–2345. [CrossRef] [PubMed]
39. Sun, S.; Suresh, S.; Liu, H.; Tepp, W.H.; Johnson, E.A.; Edwardson, J.M.; Chapman, E.R. Receptor binding enables botulinum neurotoxin B to sense low pH for translocation channel assembly. *Cell Host Microbe* **2011**, *10*, 237–247. [CrossRef] [PubMed]
40. Fischer, A.; Montal, M. Crucial role of the disulfide bridge between botulinum neurotoxin light and heavy chains in protease translocation across membranes. *J. Biol. Chem.* **2007**, *282*, 29604–29611. [CrossRef] [PubMed]
41. Zanetti, G.; Azarnia Teheran, D.; Pirazzini, M.; Binz, T.; Shone, C.C.; Fillo, S.; Lista, F.; Rossetto, O.; Montecucco, C. Inhibition of botulinum neurotoxins interchain disulfide bond reduction prevents the peripheral neuroparalysis of botulism. *Biochem. Pharmacol.* **2015**, *98*, 522–530. [CrossRef] [PubMed]
42. Pirazzini, M.; Azarnia Teheran, D.; Zanetti, G.; Megighian, A.; Scorzeto, M.; Fillo, S.; Shone, C.C.; Binz, T.; Rossetto, O.; Lista, F.; et al. Thioredoxin and its reductase are present on synaptic vesicles, and their inhibition prevents the paralysis induced by botulinum neurotoxins. *Cell Rep.* **2014**, *8*, 1870–1878. [CrossRef] [PubMed]
43. Meyer, Y.; Buchanan, B.B.; Vignols, F.; Reichheld, J.P. Thioredoxins and glutaredoxins: Unifying elements in redox biology. *Annu. Rev. Genet.* **2009**, *43*, 335–367. [CrossRef] [PubMed]

44. Hanschmann, E.M.; Godoy, J.R.; Berndt, C.; Hudemann, C.; Lillig, C.H. Thioredoxins, glutaredoxins, and peroxiredoxins—Molecular mechanisms and health significance: From cofactors to antioxidants to redox signaling. *Antioxid. Redox Signal.* **2013**, *19*, 1539–1605. [CrossRef] [PubMed]
45. Berndt, C.; Lillig, C.H.; Holmgren, A. Thioredoxins and glutaredoxins as facilitators of protein folding. *Biochim. Biophys. Acta* **2008**, *1783*, 641–650. [CrossRef] [PubMed]
46. Montecucco, C.; Rasotto, M.B. On botulinum neurotoxin variability. *Mbio* **2015**, *6*, E02131-14. [CrossRef] [PubMed]
47. Pirazzini, M.; Leka, O.; Zanetti, G.; Rossetto, O.; Montecucco, C. On the translocation of botulinum and tetanus neurotoxins across the membrane of acidic intracellular compartments. *Biochim. Bioph. Acta Biomembr.* **2016**, *1858*, 467–474. [CrossRef] [PubMed]
48. Sim, W.S. Application of Botulinum Toxin in Pain Management. *Korean J. Pain* **2011**, *24*, 1–6. [CrossRef] [PubMed]
49. Rummel, A.; Eichner, T.; Weil, T.; Karnath, T.; Gutcaits, A.; Mahrhold, S.; Sandhoff, K.; Proia, R.L.; Acharya, K.R.; Bi galke, H.; et al. Identification of the receptor binding site of botulinum neurotoxins B and G proves the double-receptor concept. *Proc. Natl. Acad. Sci. USA* **2007**, *104*, 359–364. [CrossRef] [PubMed]
50. Nishiki, T.; Tokuyama, Y.; Kamata, Y.; Nemoto, Y.; Yoshida, A.; Sato, K.; Sekiguchi, M.; Takahashi, M.; Kozaki, S. The high-affinity binding of Clostridium botulinum type B neurotoxin to synaptotagmin II associated with gangliosides GT1b/GD1a. *FEBS Lett.* **1996**, *378*, 253–257. [CrossRef]
51. Dressler, D.; Saberi, F.A. Botulinum toxin: Mechanism of action. *Eur. Neurol.* **2005**, *53*, 3–9. [CrossRef] [PubMed]
52. Bahat, P.Y.; Çetin, B.A.; Turan, G. Vaginismus treatment with libido increase and practice. *Int. J. Reprod. Contracept. Obstet. Gynecol.* **2017**, *6*, 3167–3169. [CrossRef]
53. Lamont, J.A. Vaginismus. *Am. J. Obstet. Gynecol.* **1978**, *131*, 633–636. [CrossRef]
54. Ghazizadeh, S.; Nikzad, M. Botulinum Toxin in the Treatment of Refractory Vaginismus. *Obstet. Gynecol.* **2004**, *104*, 922–925. [CrossRef] [PubMed]
55. Shafik, A.; El-Sibai, O. Vaginismus: Results of treatment with botulin toxin. *J. Obstet. Gynaecol.* **2000**, *20*, 300–302. [CrossRef] [PubMed]
56. Bertolasi, L.; Frasson, E.; Cappelletti, J.Y.; Vicentini, S.; Bordignon, M.; Graziottin, A. Botulinum Neurotoxin Type A Injections for Vaginismus Secondary to Vulvar Vestibulitis Syndrome. *Obstet. Gynecol.* **2009**, *114*, 1008–1016. [CrossRef] [PubMed]
57. Pacik, P.T. Botox Treatment for Vaginismus. *Plast. Reconstr. Surg.* **2009**, *124*, 455e–456e. [CrossRef] [PubMed]
58. Pacik, P.T. Understanding and treating vaginismus: A multimodal approach. *Int. Urogynecol. J.* **2014**, *25*, 1613–1620. [CrossRef] [PubMed]
59. Pacik, P.T.; Geletta, S. Vaginismus Treatment: Clinical Trials Follow Up 241 Patients. *Sex. Med.* **2017**, *5*, e114–e123. [CrossRef] [PubMed]
60. Yoon, H.; Chung, W.S.; Shim, B.S. Botulinum toxin A for the management of vulvodynia. *Int. J. Impot. Res.* **2007**, *19*, 84–87. [CrossRef] [PubMed]
61. Dollery, C. *Therapeutic Drugs*, 2nd ed.; Churchill Livingstone: New York, NY, USA, 1999.
62. Goldstein, A.T.; Marinoff, S.C.; Haefner, H.K. Vulvodynia: Strategies for treatment. *Clin. Obstet. Gynecol.* **2005**, *48*, 769–785. [CrossRef] [PubMed]
63. Petersen, C.D.; Lundvall, L.; Kristensen, E.; Giraldi, A. Botulinum Toxin Type A- A Novel Treatment for Provoked Vestibulodynia? Results from a Randomized, Placebo Controlled, Double Blinded Study. *J. Sex. Med.* **2008**, *87*, 893–901. [CrossRef] [PubMed]
64. Zolnoun, D.; Hartmann, K.; Lamvu, G.; As-Sanie, S.; Maixner, W.; Steege, J. A conceptual model for the pathophysiology of vulvar vestibulitis syndrome. *Obstet. Gynecol. Surv.* **2006**, *61*, 395–401. [CrossRef] [PubMed]
65. Friedrich, E.G., Jr. Vulvar vestibulitis syndrome. *J. Reprod. Med.* **1987**, *32*, 110–114. [PubMed]
66. Pelletier., F.; Parratte, B.; Penz, S.; Moreno, J.P.; Aubin, F.; Humbert, P. Efficacy of high doses of botulinum toxin A for treating provoked vestibulodynia. *Br. J. Dermatol.* **2011**, *164*, 617–622. [CrossRef] [PubMed]
67. Jeon, Y.; Kim, Y.; Shim, B.; Yoon, H.; Park, Y.; Shim, B.; Jeong, W.; Lee, D. A retrospective study of the management of vulvodynia. *Korean J. Urol.* **2013**, *54*, 48–52. [CrossRef] [PubMed]

68. Moore, R.A.; Wiffen, P.J.; Derry, S.; McQuay, H.J. Gabapentin for chronic neuropathic pain and fibromyalgia in adults. *Cochrane Database Syst. Rev.* **2011**, *3*, CD007938.
69. Falsetta, M.L.; Foster, D.C.; Bonham, A.D.; Phipps, R.P. A review of the available clinical therapiers for vulvodynia management and new data implicating pro-inflammatory mediators in pain elicitation. *BJOG* **2017**, *124*, 210–218. [CrossRef] [PubMed]
70. Mathias, S.; Kupperman, M.; Liberman, R.F.; Lipschutz, R.C.; Steege, J.F. Chronic pelvic pain: Prevalence, health related quality and economic correlates. *Obstet. Gynecol.* **1996**, *87*, 321–327. [CrossRef]
71. Srinivasa, A.K.; Kaye, J.D.; Moldwin, R. Myofascial dysfunction associated with chronic pelvic floor pain: Management strategies. *Curr. Pain Headache Rep.* **2007**, *11*, 359–364. [CrossRef]
72. Qeramaa, E.; Fuglsang-Frederiksena, A.; Jensen, T.S. The role of botulinum toxin in management of pain: An evidencebased review. *Curr. Opin. Anaesthesiol.* **2010**, *23*, 602–610. [CrossRef] [PubMed]
73. Adelowo, A.; Hacker, M.R.; Shapiro, A.; Merport Modest, A.; Elkadry, E. Botulinum Toxin Type A (BOTOX) for Refractory Myofascial Pelvic Pain. *Female Pelvic. Med. Reconstr. Surg.* **2013**, *19*, 288–292. [CrossRef] [PubMed]
74. Abbott, J.A.; Jarvis, S.K.; Lyons, S.D.; Thomson, A.; Vancaille, T.G. Botulinum Toxin Type A for Chronic Pain and Pelvic Floor Spasm in Women. A Randomized Controlled Trial. *Obstet. Gynecol.* **2006**, *108*, 915–923. [CrossRef] [PubMed]
75. Klimek, L.; Bergmann, C.K.; Biedermann, T.; Bousquet, J.; Hellings, P.; Jung, K.; Merk, H.; Olze, H.; Schlenter, W.; Stock, P.; et al. Visual analogue scales (VAS): Measuring instruments for the documentation of symptoms and therapy monitoring in cases of allergic rhinitis in everyday health care. *Allergo. J. Int.* **2017**, *26*, 16–24. [CrossRef] [PubMed]
76. Gajraj, N.M. Botulinum Toxin a Injection of the Obturator Internus Muscle for Chronic Perineal Pain. *J. Pain.* **2005**, *6*, 333–337. [CrossRef] [PubMed]
77. Jarvis, S.K.; Abbott, J.A.; Lenart, M.B.; Steensma, A.; Vancaillie, T.G. Pilot study of botulinum toxin type A in the treatment of chronic pelvic pain associated with spasm of the levator ani muscles. *Aust. N. Z. J. Obstet. Gynaecol.* **2004**, *44*, 46–50. [CrossRef] [PubMed]
78. Morrissey, D.; El-Khawand, D.; Ginzburg, N.; Wehbe, S.; O'Hare, P.; Whitmore, K. Botulinum Toxin a Injections into Pelvic Floor Muscles under Electromyographic Guidance for Women with Refractory High-Tone Pelvic Floor Dysfunction: A 6-Month Prospective Pilot Study. *Female Pelvic. Med. Reconstr. Surg.* **2015**, *21*, 277–282. [CrossRef] [PubMed]
79. Charioni, G.; Nardo, A.; Vantini, I.; Romito, A.; Whitehead, W.E. Biofeedback Is Superior to Electrogalvanic Stimulation and Massage for Treatment of Levator Ani Syndrome. *Gastroenterol* **2010**, *138*, 1321–1329. [CrossRef] [PubMed]
80. Rao, S.C.C.; Paulson, J.; Mata, M.; Zimmerman, B. Clinical trial: Effects of botulinum toxin on levator ani syndrome—A double-blind, placebo-controlled study. *Aliment. Pharmacol. Ther.* **2009**, *29*, 985–991. [CrossRef] [PubMed]
81. Jhang, J.F.; Kuo, H.C. Novel treatment of chronic bladder pain syndrome and other pelvic pain disorders by onabotulinumtoxinA injection. *Toxins* **2015**, *7*, 2232–2250. [CrossRef] [PubMed]
82. Xiao, L.; Cheng, J.; Dai, J.; Zhang, D. Botulinum toxin decreases hyperalgesia and inhibits P2X3 receptor over-expression in sensory neurons induced by ventral root transection in rats. *Pain Med.* **2011**, *12*, 1385–1394. [CrossRef] [PubMed]
83. Montenegro, M.L.; Mateus-Vasconcelos, E.C.; Rosa e Silva, J.C.; Nogueira, A.A.; Dos Reis, F.J.; Poli Neto, O.B. Importance of pelvic muscle tenderness evaluation in women with chronic pelvic pain. *Pain* **2010**, *11*, 224–228. [CrossRef] [PubMed]
84. Tu, F.F.; As-Sanie, S.; Steege, J.F. Prevalence of pelvic musculoskeletal disorders in a female chronic pelvic pain clinic. *J. Reprod. Med.* **2006**, *51*, 185–189. [CrossRef] [PubMed]
85. Arezzo, J.C. Possible mechanisms for the effects of botulinum toxin on pain. *Clin. J. Pain.* **2002**, *18*, S125–S132. [CrossRef] [PubMed]
86. Hamilton, S.G.; McMahon, S.B. ATP as a peripheral mediator of pain. *J. Auton. Nerv. Syst.* **2000**, *81*, 187–194. [CrossRef]
87. Kaya, S.; Hermans, L.; Willems, T.; Roussel, N.; Meeus, M. Central sensitization in urogynecological chronic pelvic pain: A systematic literature review. *Pain Phys.* **2013**, *16*, 291–308.

88. Aoki, K.R. Evidence for antinociceptive activity of botulinum toxin type A in pain management. *Headache* **2003**, *43*, S9–S15. [CrossRef] [PubMed]
89. Foran, P.G.; Mohammed, N.; Lisk, G.O.; Nagwaney, S.; Lawrence, G.W.; Johnson, E.; Smith, L.; Aoki, K.R.; Dolly, J.O. Evaluation of the therapeutic usefulness of botulinum neurotoxin B, C1, E, and F compared with the long lasting type A. Basis for distinct durations of inhibition of exocytosis in central neurons. *J. Biol. Chem.* **2003**, *278*, 1363–1371. [CrossRef] [PubMed]
90. Deepali, S.; Arunkalaivanan, A.S. New developments Botulinum toxin type A: Applications in urogynaecology. *Obstet. Gynecol.* **2006**, *8*, 177–180. [CrossRef]
91. Apostolidis, A.; Dasgupta, P.; Denys, P.; Elneil, S.; Fowler, C.J.; Giannantoni, A.; Karsenty, G.; Schulte-Baukloh, H.; Schurch, B.; Wyndaele, J.J. Recommendations on the Use of Botulinum Toxin in the Treatment of Lower Urinary Tract Disorders and Pelvic Floor Dysfunctions: A European Consensus Report. *Eur. Urol.* **2009**, *55*, 100–120. [CrossRef] [PubMed]
92. Smith, C.P.; Radziszewski, P.; Borkowski, A.; Somogyi, G.T.; Boone, T.B.; Chancellor, M.B. Botulinum toxin a has antinociceptive effects in treating interstitial cystitis. *Urology* **2004**, *64*, 871–875. [CrossRef] [PubMed]
93. Pinto, R.A.; Silva, A.; Lopes, T.; Silva, J.F.; Silva, C.M.; Cruz, F.R.; O Dinis, P. Intratrigonal injection of botulinum toxin in patients with bladder pain syndrome- results at 9- months follow-up. *J. Urol.* **2009**, *181*, 20. [CrossRef]
94. Giannantoni, A.; Costantini, E.; Di Stasi, S.M.; Mearini, E.; Santaniello, F.; Vianello, A.; Porena, M. Intravesical passive delivery of botulinum a toxin in patients affected by painful bladder syndrome: A pilot study. *Eur. Urol. Suppl.* **2007**, *6*, 246. [CrossRef]
95. Giannantoni, A.; Porena, M.; Costantini, E.; Zucchi, A.; Mearini, L.; Mearini, E. Botulinum a Toxin Intravesical Injection in Patients with Painful Bladder Syndrome: 1-Year Followup. *J. Urol.* **2008**, *179*, 1031–1034. [CrossRef] [PubMed]
96. Kuo, H.C. Preliminary Results of Suburothelial Injection of Botulinum a Toxin in the Treatment of Chronic Interstitial Cystitis. *Urol. Int.* **2005**, *75*, 170–174. [CrossRef] [PubMed]
97. Carl, S.; Grosse, J.; Laschke, S. Treatment of Interstitial Cystitis with Botulinum toxin type A. *Eur. Urol. Suppl.* **2007**, *6*, 248. [CrossRef]
98. Ramsay, A.; Small, D.; Conn, G. Intravesical Botulinum Toxin type A in Interstitial Cystitis. *Eur. Urol. Suppl.* **2007**, *6*, 248. [CrossRef]
99. Pinto, R.; Lopes, T.; Silva, J.; Silva, C.; Dinis, P.; Cruz, F. Persistent Therapeutic Effect of Repeated Injections of Onabotulinum Toxin A in Refractory Bladder Pain Syndrome/Interstitial Cystitis. *J. Urol.* **2013**, *189*, 548–553. [CrossRef] [PubMed]
100. Apostolidis, A.; Dasgupta, P.; Fowler, C.J. Proposed mechanism for the efficacy of injected botulinum toxin in the treatment of human detrusor overactivity. *Eur. Urol.* **2006**, *49*, 644–650. [CrossRef] [PubMed]
101. Andersson, K.E.; Wein, A.J. Pharmacology of the lower urinary tract: Basis for current and future treatments of urinary incontinence. *Pharmacol. Rev.* **2004**, *56*, 581–631. [CrossRef] [PubMed]
102. Karsenty, G.; Denys, P.; Amarenco, G.; De Seze, M.; Gamé, X.; Haab, F.; Kerdraon, J.; Perrouin-Verbe, B.; Ruffion, A.; Saussine, C.; et al. Botulinum toxin A (Botox®) intradetrusor injections in adults with neurogenic detrusor overactivity/neurogenic overactive bladder: A systematic literature review. *Eur. Urol.* **2008**, *53*, 275–287. [CrossRef] [PubMed]
103. Hsieh, P.F.; Chiu, H.C.; Chen, K.C.; Chang, C.H.; Chou, E.C. Botulinum toxin A for the Treatment of Overactive Bladder. *Toxins* **2016**, *8*, 59. [CrossRef] [PubMed]
104. Atiemo, H.; Wynes, J.; Chuo, J.; Nipkow, L.; Sklar, G.N.; Chai, T.C. Effect of Botulinum toxin on detrusor overactivity induced by intravesical adenosine triphosphate and capsaicin in a rat model. *Urology* **2005**, *65*, 622–626. [CrossRef] [PubMed]
105. Brady, C.M.; Apostolidis, A.N.; Harper, M.; Yiangou, Y.; Beckett, A.; Jacques, T.S.; Freeman, A.; Scaravilli, F.; Fowler, C.J.; Anand, P. Parallel changes in bladder suburothelial vanilloid receptor TRPV1 (VR1) and pan-neuronal marker PGP9.5 immunoreactivity in patients with neurogenic detrusor overactivity (NDO) following intravesical resiniferatoxin treatment. *BJU Int.* **2004**, *93*, 770–776. [CrossRef] [PubMed]
106. Brady, C.; Apostolidis, A.; Yiangou, Y.; Baecker, P.A.; Ford, A.P.; Freeman, A.; Jacques, T.S.; Fowler, C.J.; Anand, P. P2X3-immunoreactive nerve fibres in neurogenic detrusor overactivity and the effect of intravesical resiniferatoxin (RTX). *Eur. Urol.* **2004**, *46*, 247–253. [CrossRef] [PubMed]

107. Apostolidis, A.; Popat, R.; Yiangou, Y.; Cockayne, D.; Ford, A.P.; Davis, J.B.; Dasgupta, P.; Fowler, C.J.; Anand, P. Decreased sensory receptors P2X3 and TRPV1 in suburothelial nerve fibers following intradetrusor injections of Botulinum toxin for human detrusor overactivity. *J. Urol.* **2005**, *174*, 977–983. [CrossRef] [PubMed]
108. Smet, P.J.; Moore, K.H.; Jonavicius, J. Distribution and colocalization of calcitonin gene-related peptide, tachykinins, and vasoactive intestinal peptide in normal and idiopathic unstable human urinary bladder. *Lab. Investig.* **1997**, *77*, 37–49. [CrossRef] [PubMed]
109. Chuang, Y.C.; Yoshimura, N.; Huang, C.C.; Chiang, P.H.; Chancellor, M.B. Intravesical Botulinum toxin A administration produces analgesia against acetic acid induced bladder pain responses in rats. *J. Urol.* **2004**, *172*, 1529–1532. [CrossRef] [PubMed]
110. Lavin, S.T.; Southwell, B.R.; Murphy, R.; Jenkinson, K.M.; Furness, J.B. Activation of neurokinin 1 receptors on interstitial cells of Cajal of the guinea-pig small intestine by substance P. Histochem. *Cell Biol.* **1998**, *110*, 263–271. [CrossRef]
111. Hannestad, Y.S.; Rortveit, G.; Sandvik, H.; Hunskaar, S. A community-based epidemiological survey of female urinary incontinence: The Norwegian EPINCONT study. Epidemiology of Incontinence in the County of NordTrondelag. *J. Clin. Epidemiol.* **2000**, *53*, 1150–1157. [CrossRef]
112. Cvach, K.; Dwyer, P. Overactive bladder in women: Achieving effective management. *Online Med. Today* **2015**, *16*, 41–51.
113. Le Normand, P.D.; Ghout, I.; Costa, P.; Chartier-Kastler, E.; Grise, P.; Hermieu, J.F.; Amarenco, G.; Karsenty, G.; Saussine, C.; Barbot, F. Efficacy and Safety of Low Doses of OnabotulinumtoxinA for the Treatment of Refractory Idiopathic Overactive Bladder: A Multicentre, Double-Blind, Randomised, Placebo-Controlled Dose-Ranging Study. *Eur. Urol.* **2012**, *61*, 520–529. [CrossRef]
114. Popat, R.; Apostolidis, A.; Kalsi, V.; Gonzales, G.; Fowler, C.J. A comparison between the response of patient with idiopathic detrusor overactivity and neurogenic detrusor overactivity to the first intradetrusor injection of botulinum- A toxin. *J. Urol.* **2005**, *174*, 984–989. [CrossRef] [PubMed]
115. Schmid, D.M.; Sauermann, P.; Werner, M.; Perucchini, D.; Sulser, T.; Schurch, B. Experiences including 5 year results of 180 cases treated with Botulinum-A Toxin Injections into the Detrusor muscle for Overactive Bladder refractory to Anticholinergics. *Eur. Urol. Suppl.* **2007**, *6*, 246. [CrossRef]
116. Brubaker, L.; Richter, H.E.; Visco, A.; Mahajan, S.; Nygaard, I.; Braun, T.M.; Barber, M.D.; Menefee, S.; Schaffer, J.; Weber, A.M.; et al. Refractory Idiopathic Urge Urinary Incontinence and Botulinum A Injection. *J. Urol.* **2008**, *180*, 217–222. [CrossRef] [PubMed]
117. Khanlow, S.; Kesslerlow, T.M.; Apostolidis, A.; Kalsi, V.; Panicker, J.; Roosen, A.; Gonzales, G.; Haslam, C.; Elneil, S. What a Patient with Refractory Idiopathic Detrusor Overactivity Should Know about Botulinum Neurotoxin Type A Injection. *J. Urol.* **2009**, *181*, 1773–1778. [CrossRef]
118. Dowson, C.; Watkins, J.; Khan, M.S.; Dasgupta, P.; Sahai, A. Repeated Botulinum Toxin Type A Injections for Refractory Overactive Bladder: Medium-Term Outcomes, Safety Profile, and Discontinuation Rates. *Eur. Urol.* **2011**, *61*, 834–839. [CrossRef] [PubMed]
119. Moga, M.A.; Banciu, S.; Dimienescu, O.; Bigiu, N.F.; Scarneciu, I. Botulinum-A Toxin's efficacy in the treatment of idiopathic overactive bladder. *J. Pak. Med. Assoc.* **2015**, *65*, 76–80. [PubMed]

toxins

MDPI

Review

Novel Applications of OnabotulinumtoxinA in Lower Urinary Tract Dysfunction

Jia-Fong Jhang and Hann-Chorng Kuo *

Department of Urology, Buddhist Tzu Chi General Hospital, and Tzu Chi University, Hualien 970, Taiwan; alur1984@hotmail.com

* Correspondence: hck@tzuchi.com.tw; Tel./Fax: +886-3865-1825 (ext. 2113)

Received: 25 April 2018; Accepted: 22 June 2018; Published: 26 June 2018

Abstract: OnabotulinumtoxinA (BoNT-A) was first used to treat neurogenic lower urinary tract dysfunction (LUTD) 30 years ago. Recently, application of BoNT-A in LUTD have become more common since the approval of intravesical BoNT-A injection for patients with both overactive bladders (OAB) and neurogenic detrusor overactivity (NDO) by regulatory agencies in many countries. Although unlicensed, BoNT-A has been recommended to treat patients with interstitial cystitis/bladder pain syndrome (IC/BPS) under different guidelines. BoNT-A delivery with liposome-encapsulation and gelation hydrogel intravesical instillation provided a potentially less invasive and more convenient form of application for patients with OAB or IC/BPS. BoNT-A injections into the urethral sphincter for spinal cord injury patients with detrusor-sphincter dyssynergia have been used for a long time. New evidence revealed that it could also be applied to patients with non-neurogenic dysfunctional voiding. Previous studies and meta-analyses suggest that BoNT-A injections for patients with benign prostate hyperplasia do not have a better therapeutic effect than placebo. However, new randomized and placebo-controlled trials revealed intraprostatic BoNT-A injection is superior to placebo in specific patients. A recent trial also showed intraprostatic BoNT-A injection could significantly reduce pain in patients with chronic prostatitis. Both careful selection of patients and prudent use of urodynamic evaluation results to confirm diagnoses are essential for successful outcomes of BoNT-A treatment for LUTD.

Keywords: botulinum toxin; clinical trial; human; urodynamics

Key Contribution: This article summarized recent novel applications of BoNT-A for LUTD, and suggested the possible further works to improve the therapeutic efficacy.

---

1. Introduction

Lower urinary tract dysfunction (LUTD) is a condition presented by patients suffering from LUTD linked to one or more structures and/or functions of the lower urinary tract [1]. LUTD is common in both men and women, and the incidence and prevalence increase as people age [2]. A recent large cross-sectional study in China revealed 61.1% of women and 61.2% of men reported LUTD [2]. In general, the pathophysiology of LUTD could be classified into bladder or bladder outlet dysfunction, and treatments of LUTD should focus on etiology. However, not all LUTDs could be treated effectively, even if the etiology is definite. Treatment of functional LUTD, such as interstitial cystitis/bladder pain syndrome (IC/BPS), overactive bladder (OAB), and dysfunctional voiding (DV), remains a challenge to the urologist.

Botulinum toxin (BoNT) is a potent poisonous neurotoxin, which is produced by the bacterium *Clostridium botulinum* and related species [3]. Ingestion of BoNT-poisoned food causes intoxication by inhibiting the release of the neurotransmitter acetylcholine from nerve fibers, thereby inhibiting muscle contractions, which was first described in the early 17th century [4]. BoNT was first isolated in 1895, and now could be classified antigenically and serologically into eight distinguishable exotoxins (A, B, C1, C2, D, E, F, and G) [5]. In 1981, Scott first used onabotulinumtoxinA (BoNT-A) by injecting it into human eye muscles to correct strabismus successfully [6]. Since then, BoNT-A has been widely used to treat many neuropathic pain syndromes and dystonic diseases. In LUTD, the first application of BoNT-A targeted the urethral sphincter. Dykstra used transperineal or cystoscopic injection of BoNT-A into the urethral sphincter in patients with spinal cord injury (SCI) and detrusor-sphincter dyssynergia (DSD) in 1988 [7]. Currently, BoNT-A has been widely used in different kinds of LUTDs, especially in diseases that could not be easily treated with oral medications. In the American Urology Association (AUA) guidelines, BoNT-A injection into the urinary bladder is now a standard treatment for patients with refractory OAB and IC/BPS [8,9]. Newly published clinical trials also revealed novel applications of BoNT-A in different LUTDs and exhibited promising results. The aim of the current article is to review important new applications of BoNT-A in LUTDs and the associated evidence supporting its use.

2. Mechanisms of BoNT-A in LUTDs

BoNT-A, a potent neurotoxic protein, is well known for its ability to inhibit the release of the neurotransmitter acetylcholine from presynaptic efferent nerves at neuromuscular junctions [5]. BoNT-A consists of a 50-kDa light chain and a 100-kDa heavy endocytosis [10]. Subsequently, the light chain and heavy chain separate in the endosomal vesicle [11,12]. The light chain is the biologically active moiety of BoNT-A. The light chain of BoNT-A cleaves synaptosome-associated protein 25 in the presynaptic nerve terminal, and inhibits the release of acetylcholine by disrupting the fusion of vesicles with the neuron's cell membrane, finally causing flaccid paralysis of muscles [13,14]. Traditionally, the effects of BoNT-A in treating LUTDs, such as OAB and DSD, were believed to be attributed to the inhibition of detrusor or urethral sphincter contractions. Recently, evidence also revealed BoNT-A injection into the bladder also could regulate sensory nerve function by blocking the release of various noxious neurotransmitters, including adenosine triphosphate, calcitonin gene-related peptide, calcitonin gene-related peptide, and substance P [15,16]. Modulation of sensory nerve function might be the mechanism of BoNT-A in some sensory problems predominantly LUTD, such as IC/BPS. In addition, studies showed an anti-inflammatory effect for BoNT-A. Immunohistochemical evidence revealed decreased tryptase expression in the bladder after BoNT-A injections, which suggests a reduction in active mast cells in bladders of IC/BPS patients [17].

3. Intravesical BoNT-A Injection in OAB and Neurogenic Detrusor Overactivity

OAB is a clinical syndrome, which is characterized by urinary urgency, usually accompanied by frequency and nocturia, with or without urgency, urinary incontinence, in the absence of urinary tract infection (UTI), or other obvious pathology [18]. According to a recent large cross-sectional study in Asia, the prevalence of OAB was 20.8% overall (men 19.5%, women 22.1%) and increased significantly with age [19]. Treatments of OAB are usually started with behavioral therapy and then oral medications such as antimuscarinics or beta-agonists [8]. Although oral medications might be effective, a large-scale study showed that 46.2% of OAB patients discontinued antimuscarinics and stated the reason for treatment discontinuation was "did not work as expected" [20]. In patients with neurogenic detrusor overactivity (NDO) due to SCI, oral antimuscarinics have been reported to increase bladder capacity and decrease intravesical pressure [21]. However, the effect of antimuscarinics is usually poor in NDO patients with severe urgency and incontinence symptoms. In a large series of NDO patients with urinary incontinence, only 32% of patients could become continent after using oxybutynin and trospium [22]. Thus, treatment for patients with OAB and NDO, who were refractory to oral medications, is a daily common challenging problem in the urology clinic.

Intravesical BoNT-A injection for treating patients with SCI and NDO have been reported since 2000 [23]. Schurch first injected 200 to 300 units (U) of BoNT-A into the detrusor muscle of NDO patients [23]. At six weeks of follow-up, complete continence was observed in 17 of 19 (89.4%) cases in which anticholinergic medication was markedly decreased or withdrawn. Evidence from basic and clinical researchers revealed BoNT-A injection could block acetylcholine release from efferent nerves ending by cleaving Synaptosomal-associated protein 25, thereby temporarily inhibiting detrusor muscle contraction and improve bladder storage symptoms [24]. Further investigation also revealed that BoNT-A injection could also inhibit both noradrenaline and adenosine triphosphate release, which have a powerful influence on bladder sensation [25,26]. After years of work by many researchers and clinicians, intravesical BoNT-A injection has provided evidence demonstrating its utility as standard therapy in patients with both OAB and NDO [8,27]. The application of BoNT-A in OAB and NDO has also been approved by regulatory agencies in most countries.

Patients with NDO and OAB who respond to BoNT-A usually need repeat injections every 6 to 12 months [28]. The long-term efficacy of repeat BoNT-A injections was doubtful before, but recent long-term follow-up studies (>5 years) revealed that BoNT-A could decrease urinary incontinence rate and improve quality of life in patients with both NDO and OAB [29,30]. However, treatment compliance might be not satisfactory. Rahnama'i reported that only 25% of patients continued treatment during the six years of follow-up [29]. Most of these patients could not tolerate voiding urinary tract symptoms, urine retention, or urethral catheterization [29].

4. Intravesical Liposome-Encapsulated BoNT-A Instillation in OAB

In our prospective pilot randomized controlled study, liposome-encapsulated BoNT-A (Lipotoxin) bladder installation was used to treat patients with OAB [31]. At one month after treatment, the change in urinary frequency and urgency significantly improved in the Lipotoxin group but not in the normal saline instillation group. More importantly, no adverse event such as post-voiding residual volume (PVR), urinary retention, or UTI significantly increased or was reported by patients during the follow-up period. Bladder instillation of Lipotoxin in patients with OAB seems to be an effective treatment without significant adverse effects, but the long-term efficacy still needs to be proved in the future. Although the use of Lipotoxin for treating OAB patients is promising, it has not been used in patients with NDO until now. The therapeutic effect of Lipotoxin in NDO might be not adequate in this case.

Management is usually difficult in some patients who are characterized by urinary urgency, incontinence with incomplete bladder emptying, and with a urodynamic diagnosis of detrusor hyperactivity with impaired contractile function (DHIC) [32]. Recently, we reported our experience with suburothelial injection of 100 U of BoNT-A in patients with DHIC [33]. At six months of follow-up, the subjective urgency symptom scores improved significantly, but urgency episodes did not significantly improve in 21 patients. Acute urinary retention developed in 7 (33.3%) and UTI was noted in eight patients with DHIC (38.1%). The incidence of adverse effects of BoNT-A injection in patients with DHIC was relatively higher than that in patients with OAB. We concluded that the efficacy of intravesical BoNT-A injection for DHIC patients was limited and short-term. Physicians should inform patients of both potential benefits and risks of BoNT-A injection for the treatment of DHIC. A comprehensive urodynamic study before decision-making is recommended to rule out the coexistence of LUTD such as bladder neck dysfunction.

5. Intravesical BoNT-A Injection in Interstitial Cystitis/Bladder Pain Syndrome

IC/BPS is a clinical syndrome and includes a large group of patients who are defined by the AUA as having "an unpleasant sensation (pain, pressure, discomfort) perceived to be related to the urinary bladder, associated with LUTD of more than six weeks duration, in the absence of infection or other identifiable causes" [9]. The estimated prevalence of IC/BPS among adult females in the US ranges from 2.7% to 6.53% [34]. Until now, the etiology of IC/BPS is still uncertain, and its management is both frustrating and difficult [35]. Smith et al. first treated female IC/BPS patients with intravesical 100 to 200 U BoNT-A injection plus cystoscopic hydrodistention at the same time [36]. We also conducted a prospective, randomized, double-blind clinical trial to investigate the clinical efficacy of

BoNT-A intravesical injection in patients with IC/BPS [37]. Our results showed a significantly greater reduction in pain and increase in cystometric bladder capacity in the BoNT-A group compared with the normal saline injection group at eight weeks of follow-up. Experimental studies conducted in both animals and humans provided laboratory evidence to support BoNT-A injections in the IC/BPS. BoNT-A injections into the bladder have been shown to block the release of noxious neurotransmitters including calcitonin, calcitonin gene-related peptide, glutamate, adenosine triphosphate, and substance P from neurons [38]. Now, intravesical BoNT-A injection is the fourth-line standard treatment in the AUA treatment guideline of IC/BPS [9].

A recent network meta-analysis compared BoNT-A injection with different intravesical therapy for IC/BPS, including bacillus Calmette-Guerin, resiniferatoxin, lidocaine, chondroitin sulfate, oxybutynin, and pentosan polysulfate [39]. The results indicate that in patients with IC/BPS BoNT-A injection has the highest probability of being the best therapy according to the global response assessment, and significantly improves bladder capacity. Recently, we conducted a double-blind, randomized trial to investigate the efficacy of intravesical Lipotoxin instillation in patients with IC/BPS [40]. Patients who received Lipotoxin therapy demonstrated a statistically significant decrease in O'Leary-Sant symptom scores and on the visual analog scale for pain. However, there was no significant difference in improvement between the Lipotoxin and normal saline instillation group. Nevertheless, no significant adverse effect developed in either group, the efficacy of Lipotxoin instillation in IC/BPS might be masked by the placebo effect, and further study is necessary to validate the actual effect. Rappaport et al. recently used TC-3 gel, a novel reverse-thermal gelation hydrogel to deliver BoNT-A into IC/BPS bladders [41]. A single intravesical instillation of 200 U of BoNT-A mixed with 40 mL TC-3 gel could significantly reduce both pain and O'Leary-Sant symptom scores at 12 weeks of follow-up. Preliminary results of instillation of a TC-3 gel-BoNT-A mixture are promising, but further prospective and randomized trials are necessary to prove its efficacy.

6. Urethral Sphincter BoNT-A Injection in Detrusor-Sphincter Dyssynergia

DSD is characterized by involuntary contractions of the external urethral sphincter during a detrusor contraction, which is caused by central nervous system injury between the pontine micturition center and the sacral spinal cord [42]. Patients with SCI and DSD usually suffer from incomplete bladder emptying and DO. Application of BoNT-A in DSD started as early as 1988 [7]. At that time, it was believed that the effect of BoNT-A could block acetylcholine release from presynaptic vesicles at the neuromuscular junction into the urethral sphincter [43]. However, clinical evidence to support its efficacy remains limited and randomized placebo-controlled trial data was limited until now. Our prospective study showed that 100 U of BoNT-A injection into the urethral sphincter could significantly decrease voiding detrusor pressure and increase maximum flow rate [44]. However, some patients might complain of an increase in incontinence grade and were dissatisfied with the BoNT-A injection. A recent prospective trial enrolled 59 SCI patients with both NDO and DSD. All these patients received both 200 U intravesical and 100 U urethral sphincter injections of BoNT-A at the same time [45]. Patients could experience a significant reduction of detrusor voiding pressure, urinary incontinence episode, and increased voiding volume at 12 weeks of follow-up. Twenty-five patients (42.4%) even reported complete dryness at follow-up. Patients with DSD may become incontinent after urethral sphincter BoNT-A injection, and it might adversely affect the quality of life in these patients. Simultaneously, BoNT-A injections in the detrusor and urethral sphincters are a reasonable treatment for SCI patients with both NDO and DSD. Using urodynamic study results to evaluate both urethral and bladder function in these patients and presenting a thorough explanation of all possible adverse effects as well as expectations is key to increase patient satisfaction.

7. Urethral Sphincter BoNT-A Injection in Dysfunctional Voiding

As urethral BoNT-A injection had been successfully used in the treatment of DSD in SCI patients, this treatment was further applied to adults with non-neurogenic voiding dysfunction due to bladder outlet obstruction and urethral sphincter overactivity. Fowler's syndrome consists of difficulty in passing urine or urinary retention due to failure to relax the urethral sphincter in patients without neurological or anatomical abnormality [46]. Treatment of Fowler's syndrome is complicated and patients usually need intermittent self-catheterization [46]. In 2016, an open-label, prospective study enrolled 10 women with difficult urination due to Fowler's syndrome and treated these patients with urethral injection of 100 U of BoNT-A [47]. At 10 weeks of follow-up, the maximal urinary flow rate was significantly increased and the residual volume was decreased. Even four of the five women, who initially had complete retention, could void spontaneously after the treatment. Recently, we also conducted a randomized, double-blind, and placebo-controlled study using BoNT-A injection into the urethral sphincter to treat patients with refractory DV (open bladder neck but a poorly relaxed urethral sphincter, and a normal-to-high voiding pressure with a low urinary flow) [48]. Our results revealed that patients who received BoNT-A injection had a significantly improved international prostate symptom score (IPSS), quality-of-life index, maximum flow rate, voided volume, and decreased detrusor voiding pressure at one month of follow-up. When compared with the normal saline injection group, however, only the total IPSS and voided volume improvement were significantly greater in the BoNT-A injection group. Improvement in other clinical parameters was not significantly different between the BoNT-A and normal saline injection groups. We concluded that urethral sphincter injection with either BoNT-A or placebo could safely and effectively ameliorate clinical symptoms and improve quality of life in patients with DV. Although the exact pathogenetic mechanism remains unknown, local injection itself might have a therapeutic effect on the relaxation of the urethral sphincter, regardless of pharmacologic effects of BoNT-A. Additional studies enrolling more patients with DV are necessary to elucidate the efficacy of BoNT-A urethral injection.

8. Intraprostatic BoNT-A Injection in Benign Prostate Hyperplasia

Benign prostate hyperplasia (BPH) resulting in bladder outlet obstruction is one of the most common conditions presented in the urology clinic. An epidemiological meta-analysis revealed the occurrence of BPH in age groups 40–49 years, 50–59 years, 60–69 years, 70–79 years, and 80 years and older was 2.9%, 29.0%, 44.7%, 58.1%, and 69.2%, respectively [49]. Mainstream treatment of BPH is usually started with oral medication including an α-adrenergic blocker and a 5-α-reductase inhibitor [50]. Surgical intervention such as transurethral prostate resection is indicated if BPH patients are refractory to treatment with oral medication [51]. The prostate is an organ composed of glandular tissue and fibromuscular stroma. The prostate may cause bladder outlet obstruction not only because of glandular hyperplasia, but also because it may be associated with the dysregulation of smooth muscle contractility in the stroma [52]. Relaxation of smooth muscle in the prostate stroma has been considered a potential target to treat patients with BPH in many pharmacological studies [52]. Given its inhibitory effect on neurotransmitter release from the neuromuscular junction, studies using 100 to 200 U intraprostatic injection of BoNT-A to treat patients with BPH started as early as 2003, and initial results showed promising therapeutic effects [53,54]. BPH patients who received intraprostatic BoNT-A injection experienced significant improvement in both symptom score and quality-of-life index at short-term follow-up (one month) [53,54]. In addition, evidence from both human and animal studies showed prostate apoptosis activity increased after BoNT-A injection [53,55]. However, two large, randomized, double-blind, placebo-controlled trials showed no significant difference between patients who received intraprostatic BoNT-A injection and placebo [56,57]. A meta-analysis including randomized, placebo-controlled trials also suggested that BoNT-A injection for patients with BPH does not have a significantly better therapeutic effect than does placebo [58]. On the other hand, a recent randomized placebo-controlled study, which enrolled only BPH patients with moderate to severe symptoms (IPSS $\geq$ 19) and pressure-flow study, indicated bladder outlet obstruction showed different results [59]. Patients received BoNT-A injection reported significantly greater improvement of IPSS, maximum flow rate, and PVR when compared with the placebo group at three months of follow-up. The follow-up urodynamic study in the BoNT-A injection group also showed a significant reduction in bladder outlet obstruction index (54%), which was not significantly changed in the placebo group. This study enrolled only BPH patients with evidence of bladder outlet obstruction and might be the reason why these results are different from previous studies. We suggested intraprostatic BoNT-A should be a reasonable treatment option for moderate to severe BPH patients who are refractory to oral medications and not willing to undergo surgical intervention. Careful selection of patients according to symptom severity and urodynamic study evaluation before treatment might be essential for successful outcome of this treatment.

9. Intraprostatic BoNT-A Injection in Chronic Prostatitis

Prostatitis is another common problem among many young and middle-aged male patients in the urology clinic. Male patients with chronic prostatitis usually present with pelvic pain/discomfort (perineal, testicular, penis, or pubic area) and voiding symptoms [60]. Treatments of chronic prostatitis should be treated first with oral antibiotics and an α-adrenergic blocker [61]. If there is no obvious symptomatic benefit, medications targeting neuropathic pain or neuromodulation procedures should be considered in these patients [61]. Giorgio et al. first used BoNT-A injection to treat voiding dysfunction in male patients with chronic prostatitis [62]. An animal study revealed the anti-inflammatory and analgesic effects of BoNT-A in prostatitis [63]. In rats with capsaicin-induced prostatitis, Chuang et al. showed that intraprostatic BoNT-A injection could both reduce pain and decrease infiltration of inflammatory cells in the prostate. Falahatkar et al. conducted a prospective, randomized, double-blind, placebo-controlled study to evaluate transurethral intraprostatic injection of 100 U of BoNT-A for patients with chronic prostatitis [64]. Significant improvement in pain score, National Institutes of Health chronic prostatitis symptom index, and quality of life were observed in the BoNT-A injection group at six months of follow-up. When compared with the placebo group, symptom improvements were significantly greater in the BoNT-A group. Another study compared the efficacy of transurethral and transrectal intraprostatic BoNT-A for chronic prostatitis [65]. Both groups demonstrated significant improvement in pain at six months of follow-up, but only patients in the transrectal injection group had significant improvement in the chronic prostatitis symptom index. Both anti-inflammatory and anti-nociceptive effects should be key factors for treating chronic prostatitis with BoNT-A. Although these pilot studies showed promising results of BoNT-A injection for treating chronic prostatitis, additional randomized placebo-controlled trials that enroll more patients are necessary to prove its efficacy.

In summary, both researchers and clinicians are determined to develop novel BoNT-A applications for treating LUTDs, improve the convenience of drug delivery, and decrease adverse effects. However, some patients continued to be dissatisfied with the outcome and opted to discontinue injections. For example, in a prospective study, only 68% of refractory OAB patients would like to continue to receive BoNT-A treatment after the first injection [66]. A study also detected neutralizing antibodies to BoNT-A in patients who had received bladder or urethral BoNT-A injections and suggested a possible cause of therapy failure [67]. Physicians should comprehensively evaluate voiding problems in patients and make diagnoses precisely before using BoNT-A to treat LUTDs. Further research that focuses on ways to improve BoNT-A with stronger effects and long-lasting formulations are necessary. Adjustment of BoNT-A dose according to urodynamics, study findings, or in combination with oral medications might improve the efficacy or prolong the duration of the therapeutic effect. A summary of novel applications of BoNT-A in LUTDs is provided in Table 1.

Table 1. Summary of novel applications of BoNT-A in Lower urinary tract dysfunctions (LUTDs).

LUTDs	Condition	BoNT-A Delivery Route	Study Design	Efficacy	Comment
LUTDs originated from bladder	IC/BPS	Intravesical injection	Randomized, placebo-controlled	Significantly greater reduction in pain and increase in bladder capacity in BoNT-A group compared with placebo group	First randomized, placebo-controlled trial for IC/BPS
		Instillation Lipotoxin	Randomized, placebo-controlled	No significant difference between Lipotoxin and placebo group	-
		Instillation gelation hydrogel	Prospective, non-controlled study	BoNT-A mixed with hydrogel significantly reduced the pain score at 12 weeks of follow up	-
	OAB	Instillation Lipotoxin	Randomized, placebo-controlled	Significantly improved frequency and urgency in Lipotoxin group but not in placebo group	-
	DHIC	Intravesical injection	Retrospective study	Subjective urgency symptom score significantly improved, but not incontinence episode	33% of patients experienced retention
LUTDs originated from bladder outlet	DV	Intrasphincter injection	Randomized, placebo-controlled	Significantly improved QoL, Qmax, IPSS, and VV in the study group. Only IPSS and VV improved greater than placebo group	-
	BPH	Intraprostatic injection	Randomized, placebo-controlled	Significantly greater improvement in IPSS, Qmax, and PVR compared with placebo group	Select patients with BPH urodynamic study
	Chronic prostatitis		Randomized, placebo-controlled	Significant improvement in pain score and QoL compared with placebo group	-

QoL: quality of life; Qmax: maximal urinary flow rate; IPSS: international prostate symptom score; VV: voided volume; PVR: post-voiding residual volume. IC/BPS: interstitial cystitis/bladder pain syndrome; OAB: overactive bladder; DHIC: detrusor hyperactivity with impaired contractile function; DV: dysfunctional voiding; BPH: benign prostate hyperplasia.

10. Conclusions

Since BoNT-A was first used to treat LUTD 30 years ago, applications have become increasingly prevalent and popular. Intravesical BoNT-A injection for patients with OAB or NDO has been widely used in daily urologic practice and proved by DHIC in the United States and many countries. For IC/BPS patients who have an inadequate response to initial treatment, intravesical BoNT-A injections also have been considered as standard treatment according to different clinical guidelines. BoNT-A delivery with liposome-encapsulation and gelation hydrogel intravesical installation provided a new class of less invasive and convenient application for patients with OAB or IC/BPS. Clinical trials revealed promising therapeutic results of novel BoNT-A applications, including DV, BPH, and chronic prostatitis. However, further randomized and placebo-controlled studies that enroll patients with accurate diagnoses are necessary to prove the efficacy of BoNT-A treatment. Both careful patient selection and prudent use of urodynamic study evaluation to confirm diagnoses are essential to achieve successful treatment outcomes.

Conflicts of Interest: The authors declare no conflicts of interest.

References

1. Yang, C.C.; Weinfurt, K.P.; Merion, R.M.; Kirkali, Z.; Group, L.S. Symptoms of lower urinary tract dysfunction research network. *J. Urol.* **2016**, *196*, 146–152. [CrossRef] [PubMed]
2. Wang, Y.; Hu, H.; Xu, K.; Wang, X.; Na, Y.; Kang, X. Prevalence, risk factors and the bother of lower urinary tract symptoms in China: A population-based survey. *Int. Urogynecol. J.* **2015**, *26*, 911–919. [CrossRef] [PubMed]
3. Montecucco, C.; Molgo, J. Botulinal neurotoxins: Revival of an old killer. *Curr. Opin. Pharmacol.* **2005**, *5*, 274–279. [CrossRef] [PubMed]
4. Erbguth, F.J.; Naumann, M. Historical aspects of botulinum toxin: Justinus Kerner (1786–1862) and the "sausage poison". *Neurology* **1999**, *53*, 1850–1853. [CrossRef] [PubMed]
5. Nigam, P.K.; Nigam, A. Botulinum toxin. *Indian J. Dermatol.* **2010**, *55*, 8–14. [CrossRef] [PubMed]
6. Scott, A.B. Botulinum toxin injection of eye muscles to correct strabismus. *Trans. Am. Ophthalmol. Soc.* **1981**, *79*, 734–770. [PubMed]
7. Dykstra, D.D.; Sidi, A.A.; Scott, A.B.; Pagel, J.M.; Goldish, G.D. Effects of botulinum A toxin on detrusor-sphincter dyssynergia in spinal cord injury patients. *J. Urol.* **1988**, *139*, 919–922. [CrossRef]
8. Gormley, E.A.; Lightner, D.J.; Faraday, M.; Vasavada, S.P.; American Urological Association; Society of Urodynamics, Female Pelvic Medicine. Diagnosis and treatment of overactive bladder (non-neurogenic) in adults: AUA/SUFU guideline amendment. *J. Urol.* **2015**, *193*, 1572–1580. [CrossRef] [PubMed]
9. Hanno, P.M.; Erickson, D.; Moldwin, R.; Faraday, M.M.; American Urological Association. Diagnosis and treatment of interstitial cystitis/bladder pain syndrome: AUA guideline amendment. *J. Urol.* **2015**, *193*, 1545–1553. [CrossRef] [PubMed]
10. Franciosa, G.; Floridi, F.; Maugliani, A.; Aureli, P. Differentiation of the gene clusters encoding botulinum neurotoxin type a complexes in clostridium botulinum type a, ab, and a(b) strains. *Appl. Environ. Microbiol.* **2004**, *70*, 7192–7199. [CrossRef] [PubMed]
11. Dolly, J.O.; O'Connell, M.A. Neurotherapeutics to inhibit exocytosis from sensory neurons for the control of chronic pain. *Curr. Opin. Pharmacol.* **2012**, *12*, 100–108. [CrossRef] [PubMed]
12. Rummel, A. The long journey of botulinum neurotoxins into the synapse. *Toxicon* **2015**, *107*, 9–24. [CrossRef] [PubMed]
13. Dong, M.; Yeh, F.; Tepp, W.H.; Dean, C.; Johnson, E.A.; Janz, R.; Chapman, E.R. SV2 is the protein receptor for botulinum neurotoxin A. *Science* **2006**, *312*, 592–596. [CrossRef] [PubMed]
14. Fdez, E.; Jowitt, T.A.; Wang, M.C.; Rajebhosale, M.; Foster, K.; Bella, J.; Baldock, C.; Woodman, P.G.; Hilfiker, S. A role for soluble N-ethylmaleimide-sensitive factor attachment protein receptor complex dimerization during neurosecretion. *Mol. Biol. Cell* **2008**, *19*, 3379–3389. [CrossRef] [PubMed]
15. Aoki, K.R. Evidence for antinociceptive activity of botulinum toxin type A in pain management. *Headache* **2003**, *43* (Suppl. S1), S9–S15. [CrossRef] [PubMed]

16. Kaya, S.; Hermans, L.; Willems, T.; Roussel, N.; Meeus, M. Central sensitization in urogynecological chronic pelvic pain: A systematic literature review. *Pain Phys.* **2013**, *16*, 291–308.
17. Shie, J.H.; Liu, H.T.; Wang, Y.S.; Kuo, H.C. Immunohistochemical evidence suggests repeated intravesical application of botulinum toxin A injections may improve treatment efficacy of interstitial cystitis/bladder pain syndrome. *BJU Int.* **2013**, *111*, 638–646. [CrossRef] [PubMed]
18. Haylen, B.T.; de Ridder, D.; Freeman, R.M.; Swift, S.E.; Berghmans, B.; Lee, J.; Monga, A.; Petri, E.; Rizk, D.E.; Sand, P.K.; et al. An International Urogynecological Association (IUGA)/International Continence Society (ICS) joint report on the terminology for female pelvic floor dysfunction. *Int. Urogynecol. J.* **2010**, *21*, 5–26. [CrossRef] [PubMed]
19. Chuang, Y.C.; Liu, S.P.; Lee, K.S.; Liao, L.; Wang, J.; Yoo, T.K.; Chu, R.; Sumarsono, B. Prevalence of overactive bladder in China, Taiwan and South Korea: Results from a cross-sectional, population-based study. *Low Urin. Tract Symptoms* **2017**. [CrossRef] [PubMed]
20. Benner, J.S.; Nichol, M.B.; Rovner, E.S.; Jumadilova, Z.; Alvir, J.; Hussein, M.; Fanning, K.; Trocio, J.N.; Brubaker, L. Patient-reported reasons for discontinuing overactive bladder medication. *BJU Int.* **2010**, *105*, 1276–1282. [CrossRef] [PubMed]
21. Madersbacher, H.; Murtz, G.; Stohrer, M. Neurogenic detrusor overactivity in adults: A review on efficacy, tolerability and safety of oral antimuscarinics. *Spinal Cord* **2013**, *51*, 432–441. [CrossRef] [PubMed]
22. Hadiji, N.; Previnaire, J.G.; Benbouzid, R.; Robain, G.; Leblond, C.; Mieusset, R.; Enjalbert, M.; Soler, J.M. Are oxybutynin and trospium efficacious in the treatment of detrusor overactivity in spinal cord injury patients? *Spinal Cord* **2014**, *52*, 701–705. [CrossRef] [PubMed]
23. Schurch, B.; Stohrer, M.; Kramer, G.; Schmid, D.M.; Gaul, G.; Hauri, D. Botulinum-A toxin for treating detrusor hyperreflexia in spinal cord injured patients: A new alternative to anticholinergic drugs? Preliminary results. *J. Urol.* **2000**, *164*, 692–697. [CrossRef]
24. Cruz, F. Targets for botulinum toxin in the lower urinary tract. *Neurourol. Urodyn.* **2014**, *33*, 31–38. [CrossRef] [PubMed]
25. Schulte-Baukloh, H.; Priefert, J.; Knispel, H.H.; Lawrence, G.W.; Miller, K.; Neuhaus, J. Botulinum toxin A detrusor injections reduce postsynaptic muscular M2, M3, P2X2, and P2X3 receptors in children and adolescents who have neurogenic detrusor overactivity: A single-blind study. *Urology* **2013**, *81*, 1052–1057. [CrossRef] [PubMed]
26. Andersson, K.E.; Arner, A. Urinary bladder contraction and relaxation: Physiology and pathophysiology. *Physiol. Rev.* **2004**, *84*, 935–986. [CrossRef] [PubMed]
27. Groen, J.; Pannek, J.; Castro Diaz, D.; Del Popolo, G.; Gross, T.; Hamid, R.; Karsenty, G.; Kessler, T.M.; Schneider, M.; t' Hoen, L.; et al. Summary of European Association of Urology (EAU) guidelines on neuro-urology. *Eur. Urol.* **2016**, *69*, 324–333. [CrossRef] [PubMed]
28. Tyagi, P.; Kashyap, M.; Yoshimura, N.; Chancellor, M.; Chermansky, C.J. Past, Present and future of chemodenervation with botulinum toxin in the treatment of overactive bladder. *J. Urol.* **2017**, *197*, 982–990. [CrossRef] [PubMed]
29. Rahnamai, M.S.; Marcelissen, T.A.T.; Brierley, B.; Schurch, B.; de Vries, P. Long-term compliance and results of intravesical botulinum toxin A injections in male patients. *Neurourol. Urodyn.* **2017**, *36*, 1855–1859. [CrossRef] [PubMed]
30. Ginsberg, D.A.; Drake, M.J.; Kaufmann, A.; Radomski, S.; Gousse, A.E.; Chermansky, C.J.; Magyar, A.; Nicandro, J.P.; Nitti, V.W.; 191622-096 Investigators. Long-Term treatment with onabotulinumtoxina results in consistent, durable improvements in health related quality of life in patients with overactive bladder. *J. Urol.* **2017**, *198*, 897–904. [CrossRef] [PubMed]
31. Kuo, H.C.; Liu, H.T.; Chuang, Y.C.; Birder, L.A.; Chancellor, M.B. Pilot study of liposome-encapsulated onabotulinumtoxina for patients with overactive bladder: A single-center study. *Eur. Urol.* **2014**, *65*, 1117–1124. [CrossRef] [PubMed]
32. Hoag, N.; Gani, J. Underactive bladder: Clinical features, urodynamic parameters, and treatment. *Int. Neurourol. J.* **2015**, *19*, 185–189. [CrossRef] [PubMed]
33. Wang, C.C.; Lee, C.L.; Kuo, H.C. Efficacy and safety of intravesical onabotulinumtoxina injection in patients with detrusor hyperactivity and impaired contractility. *Toxins* **2016**, *8*. [CrossRef] [PubMed]

34. Berry, S.H.; Elliott, M.N.; Suttorp, M.; Bogart, L.M.; Stoto, M.A.; Eggers, P.; Nyberg, L.; Clemens, J.Q. Prevalence of symptoms of bladder pain syndrome/interstitial cystitis among adult females in the United States. *J. Urol.* **2011**, *186*, 540–544. [CrossRef] [PubMed]
35. Bosch, P.C.; Bosch, D.C. Treating interstitial cystitis/bladder pain syndrome as a chronic disease. *Rev. Urol.* **2014**, *16*, 83–87. [PubMed]
36. Smith, C.P.; Radziszewski, P.; Borkowski, A.; Somogyi, G.T.; Boone, T.B.; Chancellor, M.B. Botulinum toxin a has antinociceptive effects in treating interstitial cystitis. *Urology* **2004**, *64*, 871–875. [CrossRef] [PubMed]
37. Kuo, H.C.; Jiang, Y.H.; Tsai, Y.C.; Kuo, Y.C. Intravesical botulinum toxin-A injections reduce bladder pain of interstitial cystitis/bladder pain syndrome refractory to conventional treatment—A prospective, multicenter, randomized, double-blind, placebo-controlled clinical trial. *Neurourol. Urodyn.* **2016**, *35*, 609–614. [CrossRef] [PubMed]
38. Jhang, J.F.; Kuo, H.C. Novel treatment of chronic bladder pain syndrome and other pelvic pain disorders by onabotulinumtoxina injection. *Toxins* **2015**, *7*, 2232–2250. [CrossRef] [PubMed]
39. Zhang, W.; Deng, X.; Liu, C.; Wang, X. Intravesical treatment for interstitial cystitis/painful bladder syndrome: A network meta-analysis. *Int. Urogynecol. J.* **2017**, *28*, 515–525. [CrossRef] [PubMed]
40. Chuang, Y.C.; Kuo, H.C. A prospective, multicenter, double-blind, randomized trial of bladder instillation of liposome formulation onabotulinumtoxina for interstitial cystitis/bladder pain syndrome. *J. Urol.* **2017**, *198*, 376–382. [CrossRef] [PubMed]
41. Rappaport, Y.H.; Zisman, A.; Jeshurun-Gutshtat, M.; Gerassi, T.; Hakim, G.; Vinshtok, Y.; Stav, K. Safety and feasibility of intravesical instillation of botulinum toxin-a in hydrogel-based slow-release delivery system in patients with interstitial cystitis-bladder pain syndrome: A pilot study. *Urology* **2018**, *114*, 60–65. [CrossRef] [PubMed]
42. Chancellor, M.B.; Kaplan, S.A.; Blaivas, J.G. Detrusor-external sphincter dyssynergia. *Ciba Found. Symp.* **1990**, *151*, 195–206. [PubMed]
43. Jhang, J.F.; Kuo, H.C. Botulinum toxin a and lower urinary tract dysfunction: Pathophysiology and mechanisms of action. *Toxins* **2016**, *8*, 120. [CrossRef] [PubMed]
44. Kuo, H.C. Satisfaction with urethral injection of botulinum toxin A for detrusor sphincter dyssynergia in patients with spinal cord lesion. *Neurourol. Urodyn.* **2008**, *27*, 793–796. [CrossRef] [PubMed]
45. Huang, M.; Chen, H.; Jiang, C.; Xie, K.; Tang, P.; Ou, R.; Zeng, J.; Liu, Q.; Li, Q.; Huang, J.; et al. Effects of botulinum toxin A injections in spinal cord injury patients with detrusor overactivity and detrusor sphincter dyssynergia. *J. Rehabil. Med.* **2016**, *48*, 683–687. [CrossRef] [PubMed]
46. Osman, N.I.; Chapple, C.R. Fowler's syndrome—A cause of unexplained urinary retention in young women? *Nat. Rev. Urol.* **2014**, *11*, 87–98. [CrossRef] [PubMed]
47. Panicker, J.N.; Seth, J.H.; Khan, S.; Gonzales, G.; Haslam, C.; Kessler, T.M.; Fowler, C.J. Open-label study evaluating outpatient urethral sphincter injections of onabotulinumtoxinA to treat women with urinary retention due to a primary disorder of sphincter relaxation (Fowler's syndrome). *BJU Int.* **2016**, *117*, 809–813. [CrossRef] [PubMed]
48. Jiang, Y.H.; Wang, C.C.; Kuo, H.C. OnabotulinumtoxinA urethral sphincter injection as treatment for non-neurogenic voiding dysfunction—A randomized, double-blind, placebo-controlled study. *Sci. Rep.* **2016**, *6*. [CrossRef] [PubMed]
49. Wang, W.; Guo, Y.; Zhang, D.; Tian, Y.; Zhang, X. The prevalence of benign prostatic hyperplasia in mainland China: Evidence from epidemiological surveys. *Sci. Rep.* **2015**, *5*. [CrossRef] [PubMed]
50. Nitti, V.W. Pressure flow urodynamic studies: The gold standard for diagnosing bladder outlet obstruction. *Rev. Urol.* **2005**, *7* (Suppl. S6), S14–S21. [PubMed]
51. McVary, K.T.; Roehrborn, C.G.; Avins, A.L.; Barry, M.J.; Bruskewitz, R.C.; Donnell, R.F.; Foster, H.E., Jr.; Gonzalez, C.M.; Kaplan, S.A.; Penson, D.F.; et al. Update on AUA guideline on the management of benign prostatic hyperplasia. *J. Urol.* **2011**, *185*, 1793–1803. [CrossRef] [PubMed]
52. Drescher, P.; Eckert, R.E.; Madsen, P.O. Smooth muscle contractility in prostatic hyperplasia: Role of cyclic adenosine monophosphate. *Prostate* **1994**, *25*, 76–80. [CrossRef] [PubMed]
53. Chuang, Y.C.; Chiang, P.H.; Huang, C.C.; Yoshimura, N.; Chancellor, M.B. Botulinum toxin type A improves benign prostatic hyperplasia symptoms in patients with small prostates. *Urology* **2005**, *66*, 775–779. [CrossRef] [PubMed]

54. Maria, G.; Brisinda, G.; Civello, I.M.; Bentivoglio, A.R.; Sganga, G.; Albanese, A. Relief by botulinum toxin of voiding dysfunction due to benign prostatic hyperplasia: Results of a randomized, placebo-controlled study. *Urology* **2003**, *62*, 259–264. [CrossRef]
55. Chuang, Y.C.; Huang, C.C.; Kang, H.Y.; Chiang, P.H.; Demiguel, F.; Yoshimura, N.; Chancellor, M.B. Novel action of botulinum toxin on the stromal and epithelial components of the prostate gland. *J. Urol.* **2006**, *175*, 1158–1163. [CrossRef]
56. McVary, K.T.; Roehrborn, C.G.; Chartier-Kastler, E.; Efros, M.; Bugarin, D.; Chen, R.; Patel, A.; Haag-Molkenteller, C. A multicenter, randomized, double-blind, placebo controlled study of onabotulinumtoxinA 200 U to treat lower urinary tract symptoms in men with benign prostatic hyperplasia. *J. Urol.* **2014**, *192*, 150–156. [CrossRef] [PubMed]
57. Marberger, M.; Chartier-Kastler, E.; Egerdie, B.; Lee, K.S.; Grosse, J.; Bugarin, D.; Zhou, J.; Patel, A.; Haag-Molkenteller, C. A randomized double-blind placebo-controlled phase 2 dose-ranging study of onabotulinumtoxinA in men with benign prostatic hyperplasia. *Eur. Urol.* **2013**, *63*, 496–503. [CrossRef] [PubMed]
58. Shim, S.R.; Cho, Y.J.; Shin, I.S.; Kim, J.H. Efficacy and safety of botulinum toxin injection for benign prostatic hyperplasia: A systematic review and meta-analysis. *Int. Urol. Nephrol.* **2016**, *48*, 19–30. [CrossRef] [PubMed]
59. Totaro, A.; Pinto, F.; Pugliese, D.; Vittori, M.; Racioppi, M.; Foschi, N.; Bassi, P.F.; Sacco, E. Intraprostatic botulinum toxin type "A" injection in patients with benign prostatic hyperplasia and unsatisfactory response to medical therapy: A randomized, double-blind, controlled trial using urodynamic evaluation. *Neurourol. Urodyn.* **2018**, *37*, 1031–1038. [CrossRef] [PubMed]
60. Wagenlehner, F.M.; van Till, J.W.; Magri, V.; Perletti, G.; Houbiers, J.G.; Weidner, W.; Nickel, J.C. National Institutes of Health Chronic Prostatitis Symptom Index (NIH-CPSI) symptom evaluation in multinational cohorts of patients with chronic prostatitis/chronic pelvic pain syndrome. *Eur. Urol.* **2013**, *63*, 953–959. [CrossRef] [PubMed]
61. Rees, J.; Abrahams, M.; Doble, A.; Cooper, A.; Prostatitis Expert Reference Group. Diagnosis and treatment of chronic bacterial prostatitis and chronic prostatitis/chronic pelvic pain syndrome: A consensus guideline. *BJU Int.* **2015**, *116*, 509–525. [CrossRef] [PubMed]
62. Maria, G.; Destito, A.; Lacquaniti, S.; Bentivoglio, A.R.; Brisinda, G.; Albanese, A. Relief by botulinum toxin of voiding dysfunction due to prostatitis. *Lancet* **1998**, *352*, 625. [CrossRef]
63. Chuang, Y.C.; Yoshimura, N.; Wu, M.; Huang, C.C.; Chiang, P.H.; Tyagi, P.; Chancellor, M.B. Intraprostatic capsaicin injection as a novel model for nonbacterial prostatitis and effects of botulinum toxin A. *Eur. Urol.* **2007**, *51*, 1119–1127. [CrossRef] [PubMed]
64. Falahatkar, S.; Shahab, E.; Gholamjani Moghaddam, K.; Kazemnezhad, E. Transurethral intraprostatic injection of botulinum neurotoxin type A for the treatment of chronic prostatitis/chronic pelvic pain syndrome: Results of a prospective pilot double-blind and randomized placebo-controlled study. *BJU Int.* **2015**, *116*, 641–649. [CrossRef] [PubMed]
65. El-Enen, M.A.; Abou-Farha, M.; El-Abd, A.; El-Tatawy, H.; Tawfik, A.; El-Abd, S.; Rashed, M.; El-Sharaby, M. Intraprostatic injection of botulinum toxin-A in patients with refractory chronic pelvic pain syndrome: The transurethral vs. transrectal approach. *Arab J. Urol.* **2015**, *13*, 94–99. [CrossRef] [PubMed]
66. Malde, S.; Dowson, C.; Fraser, O.; Watkins, J.; Khan, M.S.; Dasgupta, P.; Sahai, A. Patient experience and satisfaction with Onabotulinumtoxin A for refractory overactive bladder. *BJU Int.* **2015**, *116*, 443–449. [CrossRef] [PubMed]
67. Schulte-Baukloh, H.; Bigalke, H.; Miller, K.; Heine, G.; Pape, D.; Lehmann, J.; Knispel, H.H. Botulinum neurotoxin type A in urology: Antibodies as a cause of therapy failure. *Int. J. Urol.* **2008**, *15*, 407–415. [CrossRef] [PubMed]

toxins

MDPI

Review

Exploiting Botulinum Neurotoxins for the Study of Brain Physiology and Pathology

Matteo Caleo and Laura Restani *

CNR Neuroscience Institute, via G. Moruzzi 1, 56124 Pisa, Italy; caleo@in.cnr.it
* Correspondence: restani@in.cnr.it; Tel.: +39-050-315-3199

Received: 31 March 2018; Accepted: 23 April 2018; Published: 25 April 2018

Abstract: Botulinum neurotoxins are metalloproteases that specifically cleave *N*-ethylmaleimide-sensitive factor attachment protein receptor (SNARE) proteins in synaptic terminals, resulting in a potent inhibition of vesicle fusion and transmitter release. The family comprises different serotypes (BoNT/A to BoNT/G). The natural target of these toxins is represented by the neuromuscular junction, where BoNTs block acetylcholine release. In this review, we describe the actions of botulinum toxins after direct delivery to the central nervous system (CNS), where BoNTs block exocytosis of several transmitters, with near-complete silencing of neural networks. The use of clostridial neurotoxins in the CNS has allowed us to investigate specifically the role of synaptic activity in different physiological and pathological processes. The silencing properties of BoNTs can be exploited for therapeutic purposes, for example to counteract pathological hyperactivity and seizures in epileptogenic brain foci, or to investigate the role of activity in degenerative diseases like prion disease. Altogether, clostridial neurotoxins and their derivatives hold promise as powerful tools for both the basic understanding of brain function and the dissection and treatment of activity-dependent pathogenic pathways.

Keywords: synaptic transmission; SNAP-25; epilepsy; Parkinson's disease; neurotransmission blockade; electrical activity; prion disease

Key Contribution: This review describes the experimental use of botulinum neurotoxins as tools to block synaptic function in specific brain modules and dissect activity-dependent pathways in CNS pathologies.

1. Introduction

Botulinum neurotoxins (BoNTs) are the pathogenic agents responsible for the manifestation of botulism. The typical flaccid paralysis of botulism induced by BoNTs is due to blockade of cholinergic neurotransmission at the neuromuscular junction and autonomic terminals [1–3].

These toxins are produce by anaerobic bacteria of the genus Clostridium and are among the most potent naturally-occurring substances. The family of BoNTs comprises seven antigenically distinct botulinum neurotoxins (BoNT/A–BoNT/G). For serotypes A, B, E, and F, several subtypes have been described based on differences in amino-acid sequences. For BoNT/A, at least eight subtypes (named A1 to A8) are currently known with different enzymatic activity and toxicological properties [4–6].

BoNTs share a common molecular structure and are composed of a disulphide-linked, ~100-kDa heavy chain and ~50-kDa light chain. They are metalloproteases that bind to presynaptic terminals, enter the cytosol and block neurotransmitter release by specific cleavage of proteins of the soluble *N*-ethylmaleimide-sensitive factor attachment protein receptor (SNARE) complex. The SNARE complex is necessary for synaptic vesicles fusion, thus the net effect is blockade of neurotransmitter release [3,7,8]. The target protein differs according to BoNTs serotype. BoNT/A and E cleave synaptosomal associated protein of 25 kDa (SNAP-25); BoNT/C acts on both SNAP-25 and syntaxin; BoNT/B, D, F and G cleave vesicle-associated membrane proteins (VAMPs, also known as synaptobrevins).

Despite their toxicity, they produce a prolonged but reversible action at the synapses. Thus, it has been speculated, already decades ago, that small amount of BoNTs could be used therapeutically to treat disorders characterized by hyperexcitability. Historically, the first to make therapeutic use of BoNT/s was Alan B. Scott in the 1970s, for the treatment of strabismus [9]. Subsequently, the Food and Drug Administration has continuously increased the approved uses for botulinum neurotoxin A1 (BoNT/A1). BoNT/A1 is indeed the most used serotype in clinical practice, because the protease has a persistent activity and this allows long lasting duration of the therapeutic effects (months).

To date, approved indications include focal dystonias, spasticity, cosmetic treatments and migraine, and several other applications are emerging. In all of these cases, minute amounts of BoNT are administered in peripheral muscles to locally inhibit transmitter release.

However, BoNTs are also effective in blocking transmitter release at central synapses when directly delivered into the brain [10].

Here we will review literature data reporting BoNTs effects following direct injection into the central nervous system. Specifically, we will describe how these potent and selective synaptic blockers may be exploited to gain insight into mechanisms of brain physiology and dysfunction.

2. Action of BoNTs on Central Synaptic Terminals

BoNTs enter central neurons mainly via activity-dependent synaptic endocytosis, indeed depolarization increases toxins uptake [11–14]. At least for BoNT/A, neuronal entry also occurs via an alternative pathway independent of synaptic vesicle endocytosis [15,16], which may direct the toxin to the retroaxonal transport pathway [17,18].

Analyses on brain synaptosomes have demonstrated that BoNTs (mainly studies on BoNT/A) interfere with neurotransmitter release of acetylcholine, glutamate, noradrenaline, serotonin and dopamine from central synases ([10]). It is interesting to note that GABAergic terminals are more resistant to BoNT/A intoxication compared to excitatory (glutamatergic) terminals [19,20]. One reason could be that SNAP-25, the synaptic target of BoNT/A, is less expressed in inhibitory than in glutamatergic terminals [20,21]. For example, SNAP-25 is almost absent in perisomatic inhibitory terminals impinging onto principal neurons in the pyramidal layer of hippocampal CA1 [22]. However, recent electrophysiological recordings in embryonic stem cell-derived neurons (ESNs), showed that miniature Inhibitory Post Synaptic Currents (mIPSC) frequencies were already reduced more than 70% 30 min after BoNT/A intoxication, while decrease in miniature Excitatory Post Synaptic Currents (mEPSC) frequencies was detectable only after 70 min [23]. This finding supports the initial increase in frequency of mPSCs in the first hour after BoNT/A treatment, followed by basically a complete silencing of activity around 15 h [23].

Silencing of spontaneous and evoked excitatory postsynaptic potentials was already demonstrated in hippocampal neurons [24,25]. Accordingly, in vivo delivery of BoNT/A or BoNT/E in rodent hippocampus prevents neuronal spiking activity in hippocampal CA1 [26,27].

It is worth noting that BoNT/A produces an efficient blockade of neurotransmitter release by cleaving a small percentage (about 10%) of the SNAP-25. This seems to be due to the dominant negative effect of BoNT/A-truncated SNAP-25 [28]. However, it possible to rescue BoNT/A-induced blockade of neurotransmission by increasing extracellular calcium concentration. Although BoNT/A and BoNT/E share the same synaptic target (SNAP-25), this rescue with calcium is not possible with BoNT/E, probably because serotype E cleaves a larger fragment at the C-terminus of SNAP-25 [24,29].

At the ultrastructural level, our group investigated the morphological changes induced by local delivery of BoNT/A into the hippocampus [30,31]. Hippocampal samples were analyzed at different times following BoNT/A injection (2, 4, 8 weeks). Observation of electron microscope images, focused on the CA1 stratum radiatum, revealed that BoNT/A induced an accumulation of synaptic vesicles. This accumulation triggered an enlargement of presynaptic terminals which was maximal at 4 weeks [30]. It is noteworthy that these changes were detectable basically only in asymmetric, excitatory synapses, and not in symmetric, GABAergic synapses, confirming a preferential effect of BoNT/A on excitatory terminals [20–22,30]. Axonal enlargements were also observed within the striatum injected with BoNT/A. These enlargements result positive for choline acetyltransferase (ChAT) and tyrosine hydroxylase (TH) in rats, but positive only for ChAT in mice [32,33].

3. BoNTs for the Study of Brain Physiology

A typical feature of BoNTs is that their action is prolonged but reversible. These characteristics make BoNTs, in particular BoNT/E which produces a short-lived blockade, ideal tools to study brain physiology. BoNTs allow a transient "silencing" of specific brain regions after a single administration, which is experimentally more convenient compared to other drugs that need to be continuously infused (e.g., tetrodotoxin or muscimol) [34].

Luvisetto, Pavone and collaborators were among the first to test the impact of direct brain injections of BoNTs in mice. They performed intracerebroventricular (icv) injections of sub-lethal doses of BoNT/A or BoNT/B and assessed various behavioral responses [35], such as active avoidance and object recognition. They also analyzed BoNTs effects on pharmacologically induced locomotor activity. The results indicated no effect on active avoidance acquisition, while there were impairments in the novel object recognition task, and amplified effects of drugs which induce locomotor activity [35]. The same group also tested the effects of central administration of BoNT/A on pain mechanisms [36]. They used a mouse model of formalin-induced pain (injection of formalin into the hindpaw) and the licking response as an index of pain. The data showed that intracerebral BoNT/A affected the licking response in the second phase of formalin test, similar to the effects obtained with peripheral administration [36,37]. Anti-nociceptive effects of central administrations of BoNT/A were later confirmed by other groups in various models of pain [38,39].

Our group has exploited BoNT/E to obtain a sustained but reversible blockade of neurotransmission for about 2 weeks in specific brain regions [27,40]. In particular, to investigate the role of cortical activity in the maturation of visual function, we unilaterally injected BoNT/E into the visual cortex (V1) in rat pups, at the time of eye opening [40]. BoNT/E injection produced a unilateral silencing of V1 for about 2 weeks, completely abolishing visual responses during the so called "critical period" for development of cortical function [41]. We performed electrophysiological recordings 3 weeks following BoNT/E injection (when cleaved SNAP-25 was no longer detectable), in order to assess visual system development when electrical activity was recovered, i.e., at the completion of the normal critical period. We found that BoNT/E-induced silencing of cortical activity did not allow normal maturation of visual function, keeping visual acuity low and extending the duration of the critical period [40]. We also evaluated if these deficits were persistent, or if they reflected only a delay in visual function maturation. Thus we performed behavioral and electrophysiological analyses at a longer time point (more than 2 months following toxin injection), and we confirmed a persistent impairment in visual performance. In conclusion, exploiting BoNT/E delivery to induce a transient silencing of cortical activity during the critical period allowed us to demonstrate that intrinsic cortical activity is necessary for a correct development of visual function [40].

Long-lasting serotypes such as BoNT/A and BoNT/B could be useful to create animal models of pathologies (e.g., dementia, [42]) or to treat hyperexcitability [26] (see below). However, these models could also offer basic knowledge about the role of specific brain regions in behavioral performance. For example, BoNT/B injection into the entorhinal cortex in adult rats produce learning and memory impairments as assessed by maze tests [42].

Similarly, BoNT/E hippocampal injection in adult rats induces deficits in spatial learning during the Morris water maze task, but since BoNT/E action is short-lived, the impairments are completely reversible and confirm a key role of hippocampus in spatial learning [26].

Mapping of the spread of BoNT/E via immunostaining for intact and cleaved SNAP-25 [40,43] demonstrates that toxin action remains confined to the cortical areas close to the injection site, thus allowing regional specificity of the synaptic blockade. Toxin diffusion can be further limited via the use of convection-enhanced delivery (CED), which provides a more homogeneous distribution than conventional bolus injection and does not damage the surrounding tissue [44–47].

4. Exploiting BoNTs in Pathological Brain Conditions

We have already reported examples of how BoNTs could be exploited to study the role of electrical activity in physiological, developmental brain processes [40]. In addition, BoNTs delivery could be useful to address the impact of electrical activity in neurodegenerative pathologies. Indeed, while it is known that synaptic degeneration precedes cell loss (e.g., [48]), little is known about mechanisms that tag synapses for degeneration. In this context, our group hypothesized that in a hippocampal mouse model of prion disease (a neurodegenerative disease associated with aggregates of misfolded proteins), synaptic degeneration was activity-dependent. To verify this hypothesis, we injected BoNT/A into the hippocampus of mice with prion disease and we analyzed synaptic degeneration at the ultrastructural level by electron microscopy [30]. Contrary to our expectations, we failed to find differences in the density of degenerating synapses between BoNT/A- and vehicle-injected prion mice. The morphology of the degenerating synapses was also indistinguishable between the two groups. These experiments challenge the idea that dysfunctions in synaptic vesicle release trigger the elimination of synaptic boutons, at least in prion-induced neurodegeneration [30,31].

Recently, Spalletti et al. (2017) used BoNT/E to produce a transient silencing of the contralesional hemisphere in a mouse model of focal stroke in the motor cortex. One of the main hypothesis in the stroke field is the "inter-hemispheric competition model", which posits an enhanced transcallosal inhibition from the healthy to the lesioned side. To reduce this interhemispheric inhibition, the authors applied BoNT/E to block activity in the contralesional motor cortex immediately after the stroke. They found a significant recovery of motor function in the treated animals. Importantly, functional recovery was further enhanced when the silencing of the healthy side was coupled with physical rehabilitation of the affected arm [43].

Since BoNTs block neurotransmitter release, it is not unexpected that they have been exploited to treat, similarly to the peripheral nervous system, pathologies characterized by hyperexcitability. The most frequent category of central pathologies associated with hyperexcitability is epilepsy. About six millions of persons in Europe develop epilepsy, and around 30% of these are pharmaco-resistant [49]. This means that there are no drugs available to suppress or decrease their seizures. In the worst cases, the only clinical solution is a surgical intervention which physically removes the main epileptic focus. Consequently, efforts for discovering new therapeutic treatments are warranted. Our group and others have investigated whether central, local BoNTs delivery could suppress seizures in animal models of epilepsy [4,26,27,45,50]. The first serotype used was BoNT/E, tested in animal models of acute seizures, triggered by hippocampal administration of pro-convulsant agent kainic acid (KA) [26]. To measure BoNT/E effects, authors performed behavioral and electrographic analyses, demonstrating that BoNT/E delivery is effective in decreasing number and duration of seizures triggered by KA. BoNT/E effects were not limited to the electrophysiological level, but the toxin had an impact also on hippocampal histopathological changes, such as neuronal loss. This neuroprotection likely depends on blockade of excitoxicity phenomena occurring during prolonged electrical activity [26]. The neuroprotective action elicited by BoNT/E has been demonstrated also in a model of focal ischemia [51]. The potent vaso-constricting peptide endothelin-1 (ET-1) was delivered intrahippocampally in adult rats, followed 20 min later by BoNT/E injection in CA1. To evaluate BoNT/E action on excitoxicity, that is, on glutamate release, the authors performed in vivo microdialysis. Data showed that BoNT/E-injected rats had a decreased glutamate release. This synaptic effect was matched with a decrease in CA1 neuronal loss, as measured by immunohistochemistry [51]. Thus, the neuroprotective action by BoNT/E depends on the inhibition of the release of glutamate and occurs via downregulation of proapoptotic proteins, such as caspase-3 [52].

Based on these initial, encouraging data on acute seizures, BoNT/E was tested also in a mouse model of chronic seizures that resembles mesial temporal lobe epilepsy (MTLE), one of the most common pharmacoresistant forms of epilepsy in humans, obtained by intrahippocampal injection of KA [27,50]. The authors initially tested the impact of BoNT/E delivery on epileptogenesis (i.e., the development of spontaneous ictal events) following an episode of status epilepticus triggered by KA. The findings indicated that BoNT/E-mediated synaptic blockade during epileptogenesis was not effective in blocking the occurrence of spontaneous seizures. However, BoNT/E treatment was associated with histopatological protection; there was less neuronal loss in CA1 and the dispersion of granule cells in the dentate gyrus was potently prevented [27]. In a second work, the authors investigated if BoNT/E delivery was sufficient to reduce seizures during the chronic phase of epilepsy [50]. Mice injected with KA were implanted with bipolar electrodes, and after a period of baseline recording sessions, BoNT/E was infused directly into the epileptic hippocampus. Subsequent electrophysiological recordings clearly proved that BoNT/E delivery produces a reduction in total seizure duration and frequency [50].

One may argue that to be practically useful in the treatment of epilepsy, focal treatments require a long duration of action. Other serotypes of BoNTs with a prolonged proteolytic activity, like BoNT/A or BoNT/B, are ideal tools. Indeed, a couple of studies have used these serotypes to block seizures for longer periods in the amygdala kindling model, an experimental paradigm that allows to follow seizures for weeks to months. Gasior and colleagues (2013) directly infused BoNT/A or BoNT/B into the amygdala, via convection-enhanced delivery (CED) [45]. Therapeutic effects of both toxins were assessed by measuring after-discharge threshold and other parameters of the amygdala-kindled seizures at different times (3, 7, 10, 15, 21, 35, 50, and 64 days) after the administration. Results pointed to the anti-convulsant effects of both toxins, as assessed with EEG measures (i.e., elevation in after-discharge threshold of stimulation and seizures duration). The anti-convulsant action persisted until day 50. It interesting to note that, whilst BoNT/B was also effective in reduction of behavioral seizures, BoNT/A did not reach significance values in this parameter [45].

Another manuscript exploited infusion of BoNT/A (specifically serotype A2) to reduce seizures in kindled mice [53]. In half of the animals, BoNT/A2 was able to completely block the appearance of seizures. In addition, the toxin decreases the level of seizures, at least until 18 days following injection.

Taken together, these results suggest that BoNTs are quite effective in amelioration of epileptic activity, and they could be potentially used as focal antiepileptic treatments.

One might envision another possible "diagnostic" use of BoNTs in epilepsy, especially for BoNT/E, which has the shorter duration of action. In patients eligible for resection surgery, it is fundamental to precisely map brain epileptic foci, to remove all the hyperexcitable areas and render the patient seizure-free after surgery. The mapping is usually performed by non-invasive imaging techniques (such as magnetoencephalography (MEG) and functional MRI (fMRI)), or by EEG with chronically implanted electrodes [54], however the results are not always satisfactory, and patient could suffer of residual seizures also after surgery. In this context, local delivery of botulinum toxins could represent a strategy to functionally map the epileptogenic areas, and check whether the silencing of the presumptive focus is effective in abolishing seizures.

Another promising application of local delivery of BoNT/A is the therapeutic treatment of movement disorders and neurotransmission dysfunction typical of Parkinson's disease (PD). PD is characterized by an imbalanced cholinergic hyperactivity in the striatum, due to the loss of dopaminergic neurons of the substantia nigra. Since BoNT/A blocks neurotransmitter release, including acetylcholine (ACh), the toxin was injected directly into the striatum, in animal models of PD [32,33,55–57]. In particular, the rodent model of 6-hydroxydopamine (6-OHDA) produces a hemi-parkinsonism. Wree and colleagues (2011) tested effects of BoNT/A injected 6 weeks following lesion with 6-OHDA. BoNT/A action was evaluated using the apomorphine-induced contralateral rotation test. Apomorphine is a dopamine (DA) receptor agonist and stimulates the supersensitive dopamine receptor D2 (DRD2) in the lesioned hemisphere, causing a net rotation away from the side of the lesion, that is, anti-clockwise [58]. Infusion of BoNT/A into the ipsilateral, lesioned striatum is able to reverse this rotation movement until 3 months [32]. Authors observed also enlarged axonal varicosities in BoNT/A (BiVs) injected-animals (possibly due to synaptic vesicles accumulation as seen in hippocampus by Caleo and co-authors [30]). Immunohistochemical analysis revealed that these axonal varicosities were cholinergic, but some of the BiVs were found to be positive for tyrosine hydroxylase (TH) [32,55]. In a subsequent work, these cholinergic varicosities induced by BoNT/A were investigated in detail [55]. They evaluated the number of ChAT-positive interneurons as well as the density and the volumetric size of the BiVs. In the ipsilateral side of BoNT/A-injected rats, with 6-OHDA lesion, the numeric density of BiVs reached a maximum 3 months after BoNT/A, while their volume increased during the whole time course of the experiment. However, no differences were detectable in the number of ChAT-positive neurons, up to 1 year following BoNT/A injection. This last result is important because it speaks in favor of a lack of cytotoxic effects of BoNT/A [55].

A similar study has been performed in mice, to extend possible therapeutic BoNT/A applications to genetics mouse models of PD [33]. Authors injected increasing doses of BoNT/A, finding no differences in the number of ChAT-positive interneurons. Increasing BoNT/A doses (from 25 pg to 200 pg), led to an increased BiV volume, and a decreased number of small BiVs. It is noteworthy that, in contrast to rats, TH-immunoreactive BiVs were not found in BoNT/A-infused mice [33].

Intrastriatally injected BoNT/A appears also to induce changes in receptor expression, likely due to activity silencing. For example, BoNT/A reduced density of dopamine receptor D2/D3, whereas other key receptors (such as dopamine 1 (D1), noradrenergic (a1 and a2) and serotonergic (5HT2A) receptors) remained basically unaltered in rats [57]. Since authors found few weeks after unilateral 6-hydroxydopamine (6-OHDA) lesion a significant increase of D2/D3 receptor ratio, the therapeutic effects of BoNT/A probably resides in reducing the interhemispheric imbalance in D2/D3 receptor density in lesioned rats.

Altogether, these results indicate how intracerebrally injected BoNTs could induce synaptic silencing and long-lasting changes in neurotransmitter-related proteins, that ultimately produce therapeutic benefits (see Table 1 for a summary).

Table 1. Exploiting botulinum neurotoxins (BoNTs) in pathological brain conditions. The table summarizes the main studies that have exploited central delivery of botulinum neurotoxins to treat pathological brain conditions.

Disease	Animal Model	Species	BoNT Serotype	Reported Effects	Reference
Epilepsy	intrahippocampal KA	rat	BoNT/E	decreased number and duration of seizures triggered by KA; decreased neuronal loss	Costantin et al, 2005 [26]
	intrahippocampal KA	rat	BoNT/E	downregulation of caspase 3	Manno et al, 2007 [52]
	intrahippocampal KA	mouse	BoNT/E	decreased neuronal loss and dispersion of granule cells (BoNT/E tested during epileptogenesis)	Antonucci et al, 2008 [27]
	intrahippocampal KA	mouse	BoNT/E	reduction of total seizure duration and frequency (BoNT/E tested during chronic phase)	Antonucci et al, 2009 [50]
	amygdala kindling model	rat	BoNT/A BoNT/B	anti-convulsant effects of both toxins (BoNT/B also at behavioral level)	Gasior et al, 2013 [45]
	amygdala kindling model	mouse	BoNT/A2	decreased seizures (in 50% of animals)	Kato et al, 2013 [53]

Table 1. *Cont.*

Disease	Animal Model	Species	BoNT Serotype	Reported Effects	Reference
Ischemia	endothelin 1	rat	BoNT/E	neuroprotective effect (decrease of glutamate release)	Antonucci et al, 2010 [48]
	phototrombotic stroke	mouse	BoNT/E	synaptic silencing of contralateral hemisphere improved motor recovery	Spalletti et al, 2017 [43]
Parkinson's disease	6-OHDA model	rat	BoNT/A	abolished pathologic rotational behavior; induced ChAT and TH axonal varicosities	Wree et al, 2011 [32]
	6-OHDA model	rat	BoNT/A	induced ChAT and TH axonal varicosities; no changes in ChAT-positive neurons	Mehlan et al, 2016 [55]
	6-OHDA model	mouse	BoNT/A	induced ChAT axonal varicosities;	Hawlitschka et al, 2017 [33]
	6-OHDA model	rat	BoNT/A	changes in receptor expression (rebalance of D2/D3 receptor density)	Mann et al, 2018 [57]
Prion disease	ME7 prion disease	mouse	BoNT/A	electrical activity does not impact on synaptic degeneration	Caleo et al, 2012 [30]
Pain	formalin-induced pain	mouse	BoNT/A	decreased licking response in the second phase of formalin test	Luvisetto et al, 2006 [36]

5. Intracerebral BoNTs: Future Directions

BoNT clinical indications are continuously increasing, thanks to advantages such as very long duration, high potency, and complete reversibility of action [3].

There is currently considerable interest in developing novel forms of BoNTs with optimized therapeutic properties and neuronal selectivity (i.e., neuromuscular junction vs. sensory endings), which could offer new treatment opportunities. On one hand, the natural repertoire of BoNTs offers a wide variety of molecules with specific actions in neuronal cells and in vivo mouse models [59]. Second, an engineering approach has been taken to modify the pharmacological properties of native toxins by specific mutations. For example, a mutated BoNT/A1 has been created with faster onset and a shorter duration of action than BoNT/A1 wild type [60], opening the way to design BoNT variants with novel and useful properties.

The group of Bazbek Davletov has quite recently developed a new technology, named "protein-stapling", by which it is possible to re-assemble chimeric clostridial neurotoxins starting from two separate modules, that is, the light chain/translocation domain and the receptor-binding domain [61,62]. This technology is not only useful to safely produce active toxins, but also allows engineering of toxins. The first engineered toxin was an analogue of the botulinum neurotoxin type A, called BiTox. The structural evaluation of BiTox suggests that the re-assembled BoNT/A could be substantially longer than the native molecule. However, BiTox demonstrated similar efficiency to that of native BoNT/A in proteolytic cleavage of SNAP-25 in vitro and in vivo, and thus in neurotransmitter silencing [61]. Interestingly, and clinically relevant, potency of BiTox at the neuromuscular junction is reduced, probably because of the bigger size of the molecule. Thus, systemic toxicity is reduced in BiTox injected subjects, and this represents a considerable advantage for clinical applications [61].

Engineered neurotoxins could also be exploited to enhance the selectivity for selected neuronal populations, combining the receptor-binding domain with different catalytic chains. For example, the same group has combined BoNT/A protease with the TeNT binding domain, allowing intoxication of different neuron populations compared to the native BoNT/A [62]. This chimera has a nociceptive action at central level, but has no action on motoneurons (as it caused neither flaccid nor spastic paralysis), resulting safer and potentially relevant for medical applications. On the other side, engineered toxins are interesting also for basic neuroscience research. Indeed, this chimera, following direct delivery into the rat visual cortex, was able to modulate sensory function [62].

Author Contributions: M.C. and L.R. wrote and discussed the manuscript.

Acknowledgments: We acknowledge financial support from AIRC (Italian Association for Cancer Research) grant #IG18925, Regione Toscana (RONDA Project, "Programma Attuativo Regionale" financed by FAS—now FSC), CNR InterOmics project, and CNR NanoMax project.

Conflicts of Interest: The authors declare no conflict of interest. The founding sponsors had no role in the design of the study; in the collection, analyses, or interpretation of data; in the writing of the manuscript, and in the decision to publish the results.

References

1. Van der Kloot, W.; Molgó, J. Quantal acetylcholine release at the vertebrate neuromuscular junction. *Physiol. Rev.* **1994**, *74*, 899–991. [CrossRef] [PubMed]
2. Rossetto, O.; Pirazzini, M.; Montecucco, C. Botulinum neurotoxins: Genetic, structural and mechanistic insights. *Nat. Rev. Microbiol.* **2014**, *12*, 535–549. [CrossRef] [PubMed]
3. Pirazzini, M.; Rossetto, O.; Eleopra, R.; Montecucco, C. Botulinum Neurotoxins: Biology, Pharmacology, and Toxicology. *Pharmacol. Rev.* **2017**, *69*, 200–235. [CrossRef] [PubMed]
4. Akaike, N.; Shin, M.-C.; Wakita, M.; Torii, Y.; Harakawa, T.; Ginnaga, A.; Kato, K.; Kaji, R.; Kozaki, S. Transsynaptic inhibition of spinal transmission by A2 botulinum toxin. *J. Physiol.* **2013**, *591*, 1031–1043. [CrossRef] [PubMed]
5. Whitemarsh, R.C.M.; Tepp, W.H.; Bradshaw, M.; Lin, G.; Pier, C.L.; Scherf, J.M.; Johnson, E.A.; Pellett, S. Characterization of botulinum neurotoxin A subtypes 1 through 5 by investigation of activities in mice, in neuronal cell cultures, and in vitro. *Infect. Immun.* **2013**, *81*, 3894–3902. [CrossRef] [PubMed]
6. Peck, M.W.; Smith, T.J.; Anniballi, F.; Austin, J.W.; Bano, L.; Bradshaw, M.; Cuervo, P.; Cheng, L.W.; Derman, Y.; Dorner, B.G.; et al. Historical Perspectives and Guidelines for Botulinum Neurotoxin Subtype Nomenclature. *Toxins* **2017**, *9*. [CrossRef] [PubMed]
7. Schiavo, G.; Matteoli, M.; Montecucco, C. Neurotoxins affecting neuroexocytosis. *Physiol. Rev.* **2000**, *80*, 717–766. [CrossRef] [PubMed]
8. Montal, M. Botulinum neurotoxin: A marvel of protein design. *Annu. Rev. Biochem.* **2010**, *79*, 591–617. [CrossRef] [PubMed]
9. Scott, A.B.; Rosenbaum, A.; Collins, C.C. Pharmacologic weakening of extraocular muscles. *Investig. Ophthalmol.* **1973**, *12*, 924–927.
10. Bozzi, Y.; Costantin, L.; Antonucci, F.; Caleo, M. Action of botulinum neurotoxins in the central nervous system: Antiepileptic effects. *Neurotox. Res.* **2006**, *9*, 197–203. [CrossRef] [PubMed]
11. Dong, M.; Yeh, F.; Tepp, W.H.; Dean, C.; Johnson, E.A.; Janz, R.; Chapman, E.R. SV2 is the protein receptor for botulinum neurotoxin A. *Science* **2006**, *312*, 592–596. [CrossRef] [PubMed]
12. Verderio, C.; Rossetto, O.; Grumelli, C.; Frassoni, C.; Montecucco, C.; Matteoli, M. Entering neurons: Botulinum toxins and synaptic vesicle recycling. *EMBO Rep.* **2006**, *7*, 995–999. [CrossRef] [PubMed]
13. Harper, C.B.; Papadopulos, A.; Martin, S.; Matthews, D.R.; Morgan, G.P.; Nguyen, T.H.; Wang, T.; Nair, D.; Choquet, D.; Meunier, F.A. Botulinum neurotoxin type-A enters a non-recycling pool of synaptic vesicles. *Sci. Rep.* **2016**, *6*, 19654. [CrossRef] [PubMed]
14. Kroken, A.R.; Blum, F.C.; Zuverink, M.; Barbieri, J.T. Entry of Botulinum Neurotoxin Subtypes A1 and A2 into Neurons. *Infect. Immun.* **2017**, *85*. [CrossRef] [PubMed]
15. Restani, L.; Giribaldi, F.; Manich, M.; Bercsenyi, K.; Menendez, G.; Rossetto, O.; Caleo, M.; Schiavo, G. Botulinum Neurotoxins A and E Undergo Retrograde Axonal Transport in Primary Motor Neurons. *PLoS Pathog.* **2012**, *12*. [CrossRef] [PubMed]
16. Bomba-Warczak, E.; Vevea, J.D.; Brittain, J.M.; Figueroa-Bernier, A.; Tepp, W.H.; Johnson, E.A.; Yeh, F.L.; Chapman, E.R. Interneuronal Transfer and Distal Action of Tetanus Toxin and Botulinum Neurotoxins A and D in Central Neurons. *Cell Rep.* **2016**, *16*, 1974–1987. [CrossRef] [PubMed]
17. Antonucci, F.; Rossi, C.; Gianfranceschi, L.; Rossetto, O.; Caleo, M. Long-distance retrograde effects of botulinum neurotoxin A. *J. Neurosci.* **2008**, *28*, 3689–3696. [CrossRef] [PubMed]

18. Restani, L.; Novelli, E.; Bottari, D.; Leone, P.; Barone, I.; Galli-Resta, L.; Strettoi, E.; Caleo, M. Botulinum neurotoxin A impairs neurotransmission following retrograde transynaptic transport. *Traffic* **2012**, *13*, 1083–1089. [CrossRef] [PubMed]
19. Ashton, A.C.; Dolly, J.O. Characterization of the inhibitory action of botulinum neurotoxin type A on the release of several transmitters from rat cerebrocortical synaptosomes. *J. Neurochem.* **1988**, *50*, 1808–1816. [CrossRef] [PubMed]
20. Verderio, C.; Grumelli, C.; Raiteri, L.; Coco, S.; Paluzzi, S.; Caccin, P.; Rossetto, O.; Bonanno, G.; Montecucco, C.; Matteoli, M. Traffic of botulinum toxins A and E in excitatory and inhibitory neurons. *Traffic* **2007**, *8*, 142–153. [CrossRef] [PubMed]
21. Garbelli, R.; Inverardi, F.; Medici, V.; Amadeo, A.; Verderio, C.; Matteoli, M.; Frassoni, C. Heterogeneous expression of SNAP-25 in rat and human brain. *J. Comp. Neurol.* **2008**, *506*, 373–386. [CrossRef] [PubMed]
22. Verderio, C.; Pozzi, D.; Pravettoni, E.; Inverardi, F.; Schenk, U.; Coco, S.; Proux-Gillardeaux, V.; Galli, T.; Rossetto, O.; Frassoni, C.; et al. SNAP-25 Modulation of Calcium Dynamics Underlies Differences in GABAergic and Glutamatergic Responsiveness to Depolarization. *Neuron* **2004**, *41*, 599–610. [CrossRef]
23. Beske, P.H.; Scheeler, S.M.; Adler, M.; McNutt, P.M. Accelerated intoxication of GABAergic synapses by botulinum neurotoxin A disinhibits stem cell-derived neuron networks prior to network silencing. *Front. Cell. Neurosci.* **2015**, *9*, 159. [CrossRef] [PubMed]
24. Capogna, M.; McKinney, R.A.; O'Connor, V.; Gähwiler, B.H.; Thompson, S.M. Ca^{2+} or Sr^{2+} partially rescues synaptic transmission in hippocampal cultures treated with botulinum toxin A and C, but not tetanus toxin. *J. Neurosci.* **1997**, *17*, 7190–7202. [CrossRef] [PubMed]
25. Sutton, M.A.; Wall, N.R.; Aakalu, G.N.; Schuman, E.M. Regulation of dendritic protein synthesis by miniature synaptic events. *Science* **2004**, *304*, 1979–1983. [CrossRef] [PubMed]
26. Costantin, L.; Bozzi, Y.; Richichi, C.; Viegi, A.; Antonucci, F.; Funicello, M.; Gobbi, M.; Mennini, T.; Rossetto, O.; Montecucco, C.; et al. Antiepileptic effects of botulinum neurotoxin E. *J. Neurosci.* **2005**, *25*, 1943–1951. [CrossRef] [PubMed]
27. Antonucci, F.; Di Garbo, A.; Novelli, E.; Manno, I.; Sartucci, F.; Bozzi, Y.; Caleo, M. Botulinum neurotoxin E (BoNT/E) reduces CA1 neuron loss and granule cell dispersion, with no effects on chronic seizures, in a mouse model of temporal lobe epilepsy. *Exp. Neurol.* **2008**, *210*, 388–401. [CrossRef] [PubMed]
28. Montecucco, C.; Schiavo, G.; Pantano, S. SNARE complexes and neuroexocytosis: How many, how close? *Trends Biochem. Sci.* **2005**, *30*, 367–372. [CrossRef] [PubMed]
29. Keller, J.E.; Neale, E.A. The role of the synaptic protein snap-25 in the potency of botulinum neurotoxin type A. *J. Biol. Chem.* **2001**, *276*, 13476–13482. [CrossRef] [PubMed]
30. Caleo, M.; Restani, L.; Vannini, E.; Siskova, Z.; Al-Malki, H.; Morgan, R.; O'Connor, V.; Perry, V.H. The role of activity in Synaptic degeneration in a protein misfolding disease, prion disease. *PLoS ONE* **2012**, *7*. [CrossRef] [PubMed]
31. Caleo, M.; Restani, L.; Perry, V.H. Silencing synapses: A route to understanding synapse degeneration in chronic neurodegenerative disease. *Prion* **2013**, *7*, 147–150. [CrossRef] [PubMed]
32. Wree, A.; Mix, E.; Hawlitschka, A.; Antipova, V.; Witt, M.; Schmitt, O.; Benecke, R. Intrastriatal botulinum toxin abolishes pathologic rotational behaviour and induces axonal varicosities in the 6-OHDA rat model of Parkinson's disease. *Neurobiol. Dis.* **2011**, *41*, 291–298. [CrossRef] [PubMed]
33. Hawlitschka, A.; Holzmann, C.; Witt, S.; Spiewok, J.; Neumann, A.-M.; Schmitt, O.; Wree, A.; Antipova, V. Intrastriatally injected botulinum neurotoxin-A differently effects cholinergic and dopaminergic fibers in C57BL/6 mice. *Brain Res.* **2017**, *1676*, 46–56. [CrossRef] [PubMed]
34. Davletov, B.; Bajohrs, M.; Binz, T. Beyond BOTOX: Advantages and limitations of individual botulinum neurotoxins. *Trends Neurosci.* **2005**, *28*, 446–452. [CrossRef] [PubMed]
35. Luvisetto, S.; Marinelli, S.; Rossetto, O.; Montecucco, C.; Pavone, F. Central injection of botulinum neurotoxins: Behavioural effects in mice. *Behav. Pharmacol.* **2004**, *15*, 233–240. [CrossRef] [PubMed]
36. Luvisetto, S.; Marinelli, S.; Lucchetti, F.; Marchi, F.; Cobianchi, S.; Rossetto, O.; Montecucco, C.; Pavone, F. Botulinum neurotoxins and formalin-induced pain: Central vs. peripheral effects in mice. *Brain Res.* **2006**, *1082*, 124–131. [CrossRef] [PubMed]
37. Cui, M.; Khanijou, S.; Rubino, J.; Aoki, K.R. Subcutaneous administration of botulinum toxin A reduces formalin-induced pain. *Pain* **2004**, *107*, 125–133. [CrossRef] [PubMed]

38. Bach-Rojecky, L.; Lacković, Z. Central origin of the antinociceptive action of botulinum toxin type A. *Pharmacol. Biochem. Behav.* **2009**, *94*, 234–238. [CrossRef] [PubMed]
39. Matak, I.; Lacković, Z. Botulinum toxin A, brain and pain. *Prog. Neurobiol.* **2014**, *119–120*, 39–59. [CrossRef] [PubMed]
40. Caleo, M.; Restani, L.; Gianfranceschi, L.; Costantin, L.; Rossi, C.; Rossetto, O.; Montecucco, C.; Maffei, L. Transient synaptic silencing of developing striate cortex has persistent effects on visual function and plasticity. *J. Neurosci.* **2007**, *27*, 4530–4540. [CrossRef] [PubMed]
41. Takesian, A.E.; Hensch, T.K. Balancing plasticity/stability across brain development. *Prog. Brain Res.* **2013**, *207*, 3–34. [PubMed]
42. Ando, S.; Kobayashi, S.; Waki, H.; Kon, K.; Fukui, F.; Tadenuma, T.; Iwamoto, M.; Takeda, Y.; Izumiyama, N.; Watanabe, K.; et al. Animal model of dementia induced by entorhinal synaptic damage and partial restoration of cognitive deficits by BDNF and carnitine. *J. Neurosci. Res.* **2002**, *70*, 519–527. [CrossRef] [PubMed]
43. Spalletti, C.; Alia, C.; Lai, S.; Panarese, A.; Conti, S.; Micera, S.; Caleo, M. Combining robotic training and inactivation of the healthy hemisphere restores pre-stroke motor patterns in mice. *Elife* **2017**, *6*. [CrossRef] [PubMed]
44. Rogawski, M.A. Convection-enhanced delivery in the treatment of epilepsy. *Neurotherapeutics* **2009**, *6*, 344–351. [CrossRef] [PubMed]
45. Gasior, M.; Tang, R.; Rogawski, M.A. Long-lasting attenuation of amygdala-kindled seizures after convection-enhanced delivery of botulinum neurotoxins A and B into the amygdala in rats. *J. Pharmacol. Exp. Ther.* **2013**, *346*, 528–534. [CrossRef] [PubMed]
46. Zhang, C.; Mastorakos, P.; Sobral, M.; Berry, S.; Song, E.; Nance, E.; Eberhart, C.G.; Hanes, J.; Suk, J.S. Strategies to enhance the distribution of nanotherapeutics in the brain. *J. Control. Release* **2017**, *267*, 232–239. [CrossRef] [PubMed]
47. Barua, N.U.; Gill, S.S.; Love, S. Convection-enhanced drug delivery to the brain: Therapeutic potential and neuropathological considerations. *Brain Pathol.* **2014**, *24*, 117–127. [CrossRef] [PubMed]
48. Cunningham, C.; Deacon, R.; Wells, H.; Boche, D.; Waters, S.; Diniz, C.P.; Scott, H.; Rawlins, J.N.P.; Perry, V.H. Synaptic changes characterize early behavioural signs in the ME7 model of murine prion disease. *Eur. J. Neurosci.* **2003**, *17*, 2147–2155. [CrossRef] [PubMed]
49. Van Vliet, E.A.; Aronica, E.; Gorter, J.A. Role of blood-brain barrier in temporal lobe epilepsy and pharmacoresistance. *Neuroscience* **2014**, *277*, 455–473. [CrossRef] [PubMed]
50. Antonucci, F.; Bozzi, Y.; Caleo, M. Intrahippocampal infusion of botulinum neurotoxin E (BoNT/E) reduces spontaneous recurrent seizures in a mouse model of mesial temporal lobe epilepsy. *Epilepsia* **2009**, *50*, 963–966. [CrossRef] [PubMed]
51. Antonucci, F.; Cerri, C.; Maya Vetencourt, J.F.; Caleo, M. Acute neuroprotection by the synaptic blocker botulinum neurotoxin E in a rat model of focal cerebral ischaemia. *Neuroscience* **2010**, *169*, 395–401. [CrossRef] [PubMed]
52. Manno, I.; Antonucci, F.; Caleo, M.; Bozzi, Y. BoNT/E prevents seizure-induced activation of caspase 3 in the rat hippocampus. *Neuroreport* **2007**, *18*, 373–376. [CrossRef] [PubMed]
53. Kato, K.; Akaike, N.; Kohda, T.; Torii, Y.; Goto, Y.; Harakawa, T.; Ginnaga, A.; Kaji, R.; Kozaki, S. Botulinum neurotoxin A2 reduces incidence of seizures in mouse models of temporal lobe epilepsy. *Toxicon* **2013**, *74*, 109–115. [CrossRef] [PubMed]
54. Dorfer, C.; Widjaja, E.; Ochi, A.; Carter Snead, O., III; Rutka, J.T. Epilepsy surgery: Recent advances in brain mapping, neuroimaging and surgical procedures. *J. Neurosurg. Sci.* **2015**, *59*, 141–155. [PubMed]
55. Mehlan, J.; Brosig, H.; Schmitt, O.; Mix, E.; Wree, A.; Hawlitschka, A. Intrastriatal injection of botulinum neurotoxin-A is not cytotoxic in rat brain—A histological and stereological analysis. *Brain Res.* **2016**, *1630*, 18–24. [CrossRef] [PubMed]
56. Wedekind, F.; Oskamp, A.; Lang, M.; Hawlitschka, A.; Zilles, K.; Wree, A.; Bauer, A. Intrastriatal administration of botulinum neurotoxin A normalizes striatal D2R binding and reduces striatal D1R binding in male hemiparkinsonian rats. *J. Neurosci. Res.* **2018**, *96*, 75–86. [CrossRef] [PubMed]
57. Mann, T.; Zilles, K.; Dikow, H.; Hellfritsch, A.; Cremer, M.; Piel, M.; Rösch, F.; Hawlitschka, A.; Schmitt, O.; Wree, A. Dopamine, Noradrenaline and Serotonin Receptor Densities in the Striatum of Hemiparkinsonian Rats following Botulinum Neurotoxin-A Injection. *Neuroscience* **2018**, *374*, 187–204. [CrossRef] [PubMed]

58. Ungerstedt, U.; Butcher, L.L.; Butcher, S.G.; Andén, N.E.; Fuxe, K. Direct chemical stimulation of dopaminergic mechanisms in the neostriatum of the rat. *Brain Res.* **1969**, *14*, 461–471. [CrossRef]
59. Pellett, S.; Bradshaw, M.; Tepp, W.H.; Pier, C.L.; Whitemarsh, R.C.M.; Chen, C.; Barbieri, J.T.; Johnson, E.A. The Light Chain Defines the Duration of Action of Botulinum Toxin Serotype A Subtypes. *MBio* **2018**, *9*. [CrossRef] [PubMed]
60. Scheps, D.; López de la Paz, M.; Jurk, M.; Hofmann, F.; Frevert, J. Design of modified botulinum neurotoxin A1 variants with a shorter persistence of paralysis and duration of action. *Toxicon* **2017**, *139*, 101–108. [CrossRef] [PubMed]
61. Ferrari, E.; Maywood, E.S.; Restani, L.; Caleo, M.; Pirazzini, M.; Rossetto, O.; Hastings, M.H.; Niranjan, D.; Schiavo, G.; Davletov, B. Re-assembled botulinum neurotoxin inhibits CNS functions without systemic toxicity. *Toxins* **2011**, *3*, 345–355. [CrossRef] [PubMed]
62. Ferrari, E.; Gu, C.; Niranjan, D.; Restani, L.; Rasetti-Escargueil, C.; Obara, I.; Geranton, S.M.; Arsenault, J.; Goetze, T.A.; Harper, C.B.; et al. Synthetic self-assembling clostridial chimera for modulation of sensory functions. *Bioconjug. Chem.* **2013**, *24*, 1750–1759. [CrossRef] [PubMed]

toxins

MDPI

Article

Unilateral Botulinum Neurotoxin-A Injection into the Striatum of C57BL/6 Mice Leads to a Different Motor Behavior Compared with Rats

Veronica Antipova [1,2], Andreas Wree [1,*], Carsten Holzmann [3], Teresa Mann [1], Nicola Palomero-Gallagher [4,5], Karl Zilles [4,5,6], Oliver Schmitt [1] and Alexander Hawlitschka [1]

1 Institute of Anatomy, Rostock University Medical Center, Gertrudenstrasse 9, D-18057 Rostock, Germany; veronica.antipova@medunigraz.at (V.A.); Teresa.Mann@med.uni-rostock.de (T.M.); oliver.schmitt@med.uni-rostock.de (O.S.); alexander.hawlitschka@med.uni-rostock.de (A.H.)

2 Gottfried Schatz Research Center for Cell Signaling, Metabolism and Aging, Macroscopic and Clinical Anatomy, Medical University of Graz, Harrachgasse 21/1, A-8010 Graz, Austria

3 Institute of Medical Genetics, Rostock University Medical Center, Ernst-Heydemann-Strasse 8, D-18057 Rostock, Germany; carsten.holzmann@med.uni-rostock.de

4 Institute of Neuroscience and Medicine INM-1, Research Center Jülich, D-52425 Jülich, Germany; n.palomero-gallagher@fz-juelich.de (N.P.-G.); k.zilles@fz-juelich.de (K.Z.)

5 Department of Psychiatry, Psychotherapy and Psychosomatics, Medical Faculty, RWTH Aachen, D-52062 Aachen, Germany

6 JARA—Translational Brain Medicine, D-52062 Aachen, Germany

* Correspondence: andreas.wree@med.uni-rostock.de; Tel.: +49-381-4948400; Fax: +49-381-4948402

Received: 5 July 2018; Accepted: 15 July 2018; Published: 17 July 2018

Abstract: Different morphological changes in the caudate-putamen (CPu) of naïve rats and mice were observed after intrastriatal botulinum neurotoxin-A (BoNT-A) injection. For this purpose we here studied various motor behaviors in mice (n = 46) longitudinally up to 9 months after intrastriatal BoNT-A administration as previously reported for rats, and compared both outcomes. Apomorphine- and amphetamine-induced rotational behavior, spontaneous motor behavior, as well as lateralized neglect were studied in mice after the injection of single doses of BoNT-A into the right CPu, comparing them with sham-injected animals. Unilateral intrastriatal injection of BoNT-A in mice induced significantly increased contralateral apomorphine-induced rotations for 1 to 3 months, as well as significantly increased contralateral amphetamine-induced rotations 1 to 9 months after injection. In rats (n = 28), unilateral BoNT-A injection also induced significantly increased contralateral apomorphine-induced rotations 3 months after injection, but did not provoke amphetamine-induced rotations at all. Lateralized sensorimotor integration, forelimb preference, and forelimb stepping were significantly impaired on the left side. The differences in motor behaviors between rats and mice may be caused by different BoNT-A effects on cholinergic and catecholaminergic fibers in rat and mouse striata, interspecies differences in striatal receptor densities, and different connectomes of the basal ganglia.

Keywords: botulinum neurotoxin-A; basal ganglia; interspecies differences in motor behavior; mouse; rat; interneurons

Key Contribution: We investigated the effect of intrastriatal BoNT-A application on motor behavior in naïve mice for the first time. To interpret the differences of the BoNT-A effect in mice and rats, multi-receptor fingerprints of Wistar rats and C57Bl/6 mice as well as their basal ganglia connectomes were compared.

1. Introduction

Parkinson's disease (PD) is a common chronic progressive age-related neurodegenerative movement disorder characterized by the loss of dopaminergic neurons in the substantia nigra pars compacta and, subsequently, of dopamine in the caudate-putamen (CPu) [1–3]. Dopamine deficit causes a profound impairment of neuronal circuits in the basal ganglia [4–7], and particularly an increased release of acetylcholine by tonically active striatal interneurons [8–12]. Anticholinergic drugs are used to antagonize striatal hypercholinism in PD, but this treatment often elicits adverse side effects [13–15]. In order to circumvent general anticholinergic drug effects, we tested a local intrastriatal injection of botulinum neurotoxin-A (BoNT-A) [16–20].

Indeed, in the experimental 6-OHDA-induced hemiparkinsonian (hemi-PD) rat model, intrastriatal application of BoNT-A abolished apomorphine-induced rotational behavior—most probably by blocking acetylcholine, the release of cholinergic terminals, and/or inducing changes in receptor densities [16–23]. Moreover, the unilateral intrastriatal BoNT-A injection induced rotational behavior in naïve rats without 6-OHDA-induced hemi-PD. Following the injection of 1 ng BoNT-A into the right CPu, rats showed 2–4 apomorphine-induced rotations per min in the direction of the injection site for two months, and rotated tentatively to the contralateral side thereafter [19].

To date, behavioral effects of intrastriatal BoNT-A injections were studied in rats, but not in mice. This would be interesting, as comparative morphological studies of the striata of BoNT-A-injected rats and mice striata showed obvious differences in the structural changes of choline acetyltransferase-immunoreactive (ChAT-ir) and tyrosine hydroxylase-immunoreactive (TH-ir) fibers [19,20,24], in addition to similarities concerning unchanged CPu volume and the number of cholinergic interneurons. Rats and mice differed in the induction of BoNT-A-induced varicosities: both kinds of these varicosities were found in rats [16,17,19–21], whereas only ChAT-ir BoNT-A-induced varicosities were observed in mice [24].

As naïve mice and rats reacted morphologically in a different manner following intrastriatal BoNT-A injection, we sought to determine whether these species differences would also hold true for motor behavior. Thus, mouse motor behavior was scored after unilateral BoNT-A injection into the right CPu using apomorphine- and amphetamine-induced rotations. Spontaneous behavior was tested using the cylinder and stepping tests, lateralized sensorimotor activity by the corridor task, and cerebellar ataxia by hindlimb clasping. To evaluate temporally restricted effects, mice were tested up to 9 months after BoNT-A injection. A potential dose-dependency was evaluated by using dosages of 25 and 50 pg BoNT-A.

It is known that mice are very sensitive to botulinum toxins and also differ in many respects from rats [25–33]. However, there are currently no studies evaluating the behavioral outcome of intrastriatally applied BoNT-A in naïve mice. Moreover, the effect of BoNT-A in naïve mice must be understood prior to evaluation of intrastriatal BoNT-A application in mice models of hemi-PD and genetic PD. The BoNT-A dosage used for intrastriatal injection for the treatment of experimental hemi-PD in rats was based on the LD50 and recent intracerebral BoNT-A injections [34–38]. In Wistar rats we found a well-tolerated and effective dosage at 1 ng BoNT-A per CPu, whereas 5 ng were mortal [19]. In the C57BL/6 mice, dosages of 25–50 pg BoNT-A per striatum were found to be appropriate [24].

Studying the behavioral effect of unilateral intrastriatal BoNT-A application in naïve mice also seemed to be important, since the effect of therapeutic BoNT-A applications is explored in increasingly studied genetic Parkinsonian mouse models [39–45].

2. Results

2.1. Body Weight

Changes in body weight were evaluated as an index of general adverse effects of BoNT-A application. The mice weighed 18–24 g at the time of BoNT-A or vehicle injection. Thereafter, body weight increased in all experimental groups (Figure 1). Increase in body weight over time was significantly ($F_{2,50} = 15.5999$, $p < 0.001$) lower in mice injected with BoNT-A than in those receiving vehicle substance. However, 9 months after BoNT-A injection, the 25 pg BoNT-A mice weighed 31.85 ± 0.37 g (mean ± SEM), the 50 pg BoNT-A mice 33.72 ± 0.40 g, and thus did not differ from the sham group, which weighed 34.66 ± 0.35 g (Figure 1).

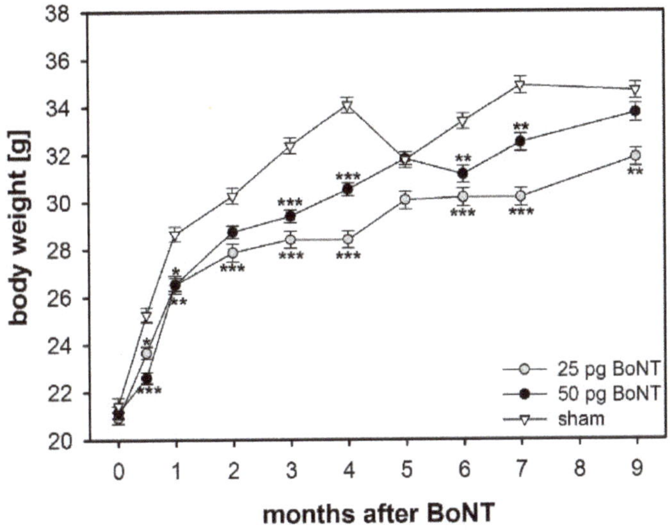

Figure 1. Body weight over time. Asterisks indicate significant differences (25 pg, $n = 15$; 50 pg, $n = 20$) compared to the sham group ($n = 11$) (* $p < 0.05$, ** $p < 0.01$, *** $p < 0.001$). Data are means ± SEM.

2.2. Apomorphine-Induced Rotations

2.2.1. Mice

In order to test the effect of a unilateral intrastriatal BoNT-A injection on drug-induced motor behavior we used apomorphine- and amphetamine-induced rotation tests. Half a month after injection of 25 or 50 pg BoNT-A or vehicle into the right CPu mice showed no apomorphine-induced rotation behavior (Figure 2A). Vehicle application did not induce rotational behavior in the subsequent 9 months. However, both applications of 25 and 50 pg BoNT-A resulted in significant ($F_{2,50} = 6.150$, $p = 0.004$) anti-clockwise, i.e., contralateral, apomorphine-induced rotations with net rotations of about 2 per minute after a post-injection survival of 1 and 3 months (Figure 2A). Six and 9 months after BoNT-A, rotational behavior decreased to values similar to those observed in the vehicle-treated group.

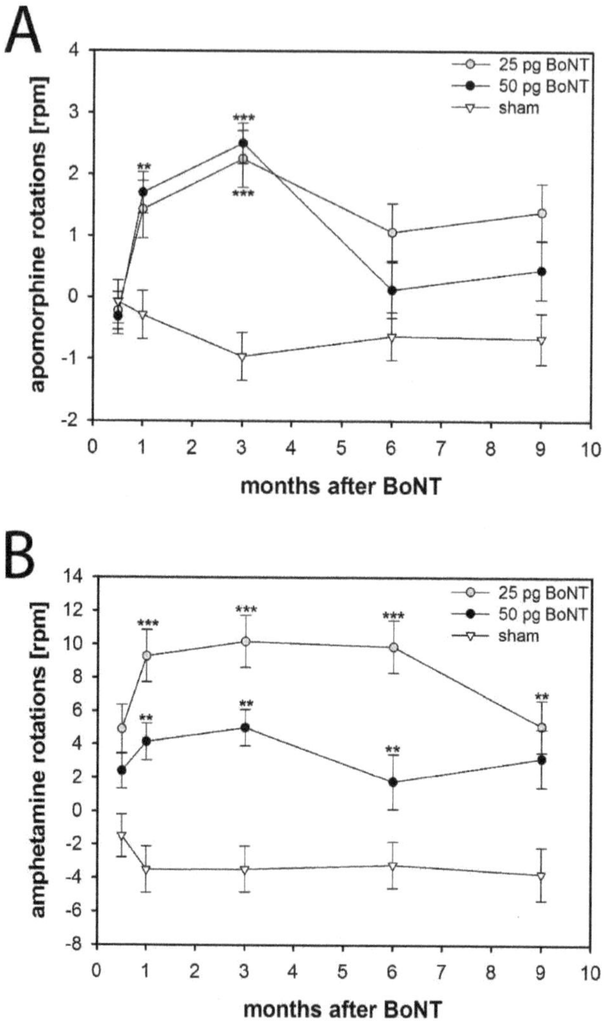

Figure 2. (**A**) Apomorphine- and (**B**) amphetamine-induced rotations in mice treated with intrastriatal BoNT-A (25 pg, $n = 15$; 50 pg, $n = 20$) or vehicle ($n = 11$). (**A**) BoNT-A in either dosage caused a significant increase of the apomorphine-induced turning rate 1 and 3 months after injection. (**B**) BoNT-A in both dosages resulted in significantly increased amphetamine-induced rotations 1–9 months after injection, while sham injections did not change rotational behavior. Asterisks indicate significant differences compared with the sham group (** $p < 0.01$, *** $p < 0.001$). Data are means ± SEM.

2.2.2. Rats

Following apomorphine injection rats significantly rotated contralaterally to the intrastriatal BoNT-A application with rotations of approximately 1.5 to 2 per minute 3 months after 1 ng BoNT-A (Figure 3A).

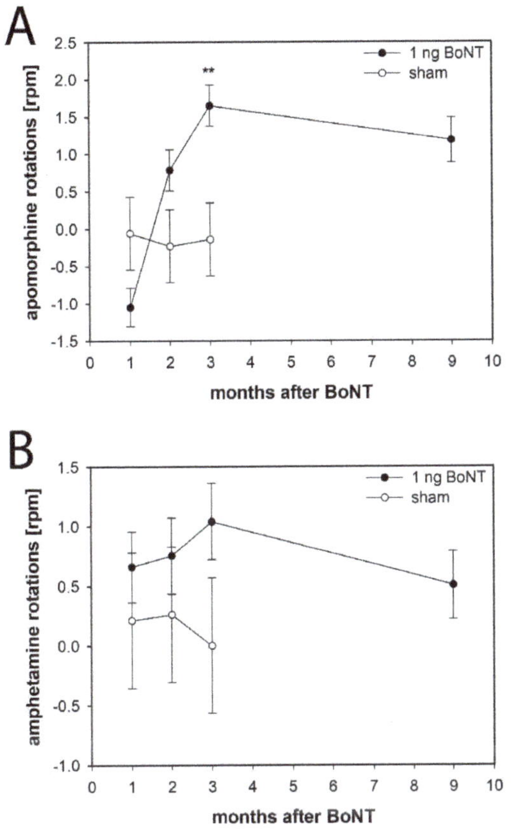

Figure 3. (**A**) Apomorphine- and (**B**) amphetamine-induced rotations in rats intrastriatally injected with BoNT-A (n = 22) or vehicle (n = 6). (**A**) 1 ng BoNT-A caused a significant anti-clockwise apomorphine-induced turning 3 months after injection, (**B**) but did not influence amphetamine-induced rotation behavior significantly 1–9 months after BoNT-A as compared to the sham group. Asterisks indicate significant differences compared with the sham group (** $p < 0.01$). Data are means ± SEM.

2.3. *Amphetamine-Induced Rotations*

2.3.1. Mice

After intrastriatal injection of 25 or 50 pg BoNT-A, the mice showed significantly increased ($F_{2,48} = 15.360$, $p < 0.001$) amphetamine-induced rotations compared to the vehicle group from 1 to 9 months post injection (Figure 2B). Whereas application of BoNT-A was associated with strong amphetamine-induced anti-clockwise net rotations of approximately 4–10 per min, vehicle injection resulted in clockwise rotations of approximately 3 per min (Figure 2B).

2.3.2. Rats

In rats, amphetamine application revealed no significant effect of unilateral intrastriatal BoNT-A as compared with vehicle injection (Figure 3B).

2.4. *Cylinder Test*

The cylinder test evaluates asymmetries in spontaneous forelimb use during exploratory activity in a novel environment. Sham injection did not induce any laterality of forepaw usage during the whole testing period up to 9 months; left and right forepaws were used equally often in the sham group (Figure 4A). In contrast, BoNT-A-injected mice, irrespective of the dosage and survival time, exhibited a significantly reduced ($F_{2, 52} = 31.971$, $p < 0.001$) use of the left forepaw of about 40% (Figure 4A).

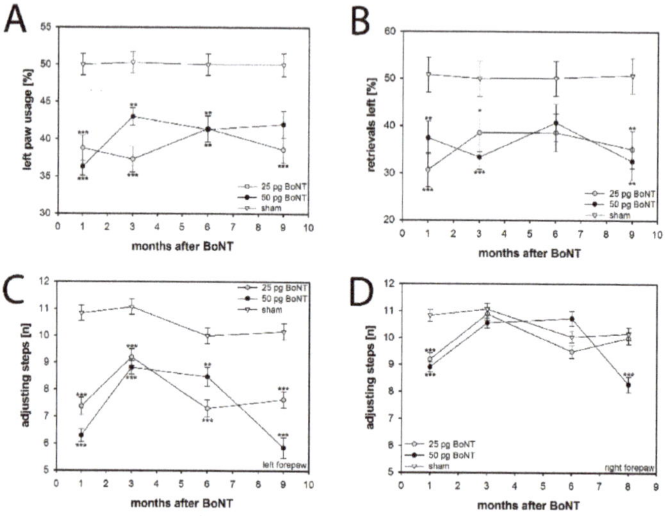

Figure 4. (**A**) The cylinder test of BoNT-A-injected mice (25 pg, n = 15; 50 pg, n = 20) of both dosages revealed a significantly lower use of the left forepaw at all time points compared with sham-injected mice (n = 11). (**B**) In the corridor task, BoNT-A-injected mice of both dosages (25 pg, n = 11; 50 pg, n = 12) retrieved pellets significantly less often from the left side compared to the sham group (n = 10). (**C**,**D**) The stepping test revealed constant adjusting steps of sham-treated mice (n = 10). (**C**) Right side BoNT-A-injected mice of both dosages (25 pg, n = 11; 50 pg, n = 10) displayed significantly decreased left forepaw adjusting steps 1–9 months after surgery, whereas (**D**) the number of adjusting steps of the right forepaw only differed significantly from the sham group one month after BoNT-A injection. However, the 50 pg BoNT-A group also showed significantly fewer right forepaw adjusting steps 9 months after injection. Asterisks indicate significant differences compared with the sham group (* $p < 0.05$, ** $p < 0.01$, *** $p < 0.001$). Data are means ± SEM.

2.5. *Corridor Task*

Lateralized sensorimotor integration was assessed using the corridor test, which depends on the rodent's ability to retrieve food from either side of its body. Animals of the vehicle group made an equivalent number of retrievals (about 50% of total retrievals from both the left and right sides of the corridor) over the whole testing period (Figure 4B). However, mice of both BoNT-A groups showed a significant neglect ($F_{2, 40} = 11.506$, $p < 0.001$) of the corridor side contralateral to the BoNT-A injection side. These mice retrieved only about 35% of the sugar pellets from the left corridor side during the whole observation period (Figure 4B).

2.6. *Stepping Test*

The motor activity of the forelimbs was estimated using a mouse-friendly version of the stepping test. Adjusting forepaw steps were measured on the injected (right) and noninjected (left) sides. Mice of the sham group made approximately 10–11 steps with either forepaw during the whole testing time

(Figure 4C,D). Mice of both BoNT-A groups exhibited significantly fewer adjusting steps ($F_{2, 42} = 99.773$, $p < 0.001$) with their left forepaws up to 9 months after BoNT-A (Figure 4C). A reduction in adjusting steps with the right forepaw was seen in BoNT-A-injected mice of both dosages 1 month after BoNT-A (Figure 4D).

2.7. Hindlimb Clasping

We evaluated neurological abnormalities using the hindlimb clasping test. Mice of the two BoNT-A groups and the sham group did not show any pathological hindlimb clasping during the whole testing period from 1 to 9 months; the hindlimbs of all mice were consistently splayed outward and away from the abdomen resulting in an assigned score of 0.

3. Discussion

Previous studies of unilateral injections of BoNT-A into the CPu of male C57BL/6 mice showed that the number of ChAT-ir interneurons was unaltered in the CPu, and ChAT-ir BoNT-A-induced varicosities were visible. Both results are comparable with findings in the rat [16–20]. However, in contrast to rats, there were no TH-ir BoNT-A-induced varicosities in BoNT-A-injected mouse. As BoNT-A application seemed to have a different influence on cholinergic and dopaminergic axons in the mouse striatum [24], the CPu-associated motor behavior was studied. Moreover, a possible temporally occurring BoNT-A effect as seen in previous studies in rats [16–21] was evaluated by testing mice up to 9 months after BoNT-A injection. Dose dependency was studied by using dosages of 25 and 50 pg BoNT-A. As a significant dose dependency within the evaluated parameters was not obvious, the results of mice receiving dosages of 25 and 50 pg BoNT-A will be discussed together.

We found that unilateral intrastriatal BoNT-A injection in naïve mice led to significant contralateral amphetamine- and apomorphine-induced rotations as well as to significant impairments of the left (i.e., contralateral) side with respect to lateralized sensorimotor integration, forelimb usage, and forelimb stepping.

3.1. Basal Ganglia Circuitry after BoNT-A Injection

Locally injected BoNT-A is thought to act in two main ways in the striatum, where it blocks the acetylcholine release of the tonically active cholinergic interneurons [46–48], counteracts the D_2 receptor upregulation found in hemi-PD rats, and reduces D_2 receptor concentrations in naïve rats [22,23]. The assumed BoNT-A-induced reduction of acetylcholine concentration in the injected CPu reduces the firing activity of medium spiny neurons projecting to (i) the external globus pallidus, i.e., those which are part of the indirect basal ganglia loop, and (ii) to the internal globus pallidus, i.e., those which are part of the direct basal ganglia loop [49–53].

The effects of BoNT-A on the reduction of cholinergic transmission and of D_2 receptor concentrations seemingly underlie movement initiation deficits, akinesia and reduced spontaneous use of the contralateral forelimbs [54–57].

3.2. Body Weight

Body weight increased in all three experimental groups from two weeks up to 9 months after intrastriatal BoNT-A or vehicle injection. However, mice injected with either of the BoNT-A dosages weighed less compared to the sham group two weeks after injection onwards, although the differences diminished after 9 months. These differences might point at a mild temporal toxicity of BoNT-A after the stereotactic injection.

3.3. Spontaneous Motor Tests

3.3.1. Spontaneous Forelimb Use

The cylinder test evaluates locomotor asymmetry and forelimb use in rodent models of central nervous system disorders by assessing the innate drive to explore a novel environment by rearing and leaning their forepaw against the wall of the glass cylinder [58]. Unilaterally sham-injected mice used the left and right paws symmetrically, i.e., about 50% each. Right side intrastriatal application of BoNT-A significantly reduced the use of the left paw.

Seemingly, the impairment of motor initiation deficit for voluntary movements of the contralateral forelimb is a specific result of BoNT-A injection into the CPu since it decreases firing of GABAergic medium spiny neurons to the internal globus pallidus in the direct loop, and therefore inhibits the ventrolateral thalamic nucleus. On the other hand D_2 receptor-bearing medium spiny neurons increase inhibition of the external globus pallidus in the indirect loop, and resulted in a more actively firing internal globus pallidus via reduced inhibition of the spontaneously active subthalamic nucleus. Therefore, the inhibited neurons of the ventrolateral thalamic nucleus are not able to sufficiently activate the premotor cortex via both loops.

3.3.2. Sensorimotor Integration

The corridor task, originally designed to study unilateral sensorimotor integration impairments in rats [59,60], was adapted for experiments in mice [61]. Mice injected with 25 or 50 pg BoNT-A into the right striatum retrieved pellets significantly less often from the left side during the testing period up to 9 months after BoNT-A, whereas sham-injected mice behaved symmetrically. As is the case for the forepaw preference studied in the cylinder test, the motor initiation deficit for voluntary movements of the contralateral forelimb is probably a specific result of the BoNT-A injection into the CPu. Both the reduction of striatal cholinergic transmission and the reduction of D_2 receptor density causes changes in the basal ganglia circuitry resulting in a reduced initiation of movements of the contralateral body via crossed motor efferents [57,62,63].

3.3.3. Forelimb Adjusting Steps

In our study, we used the mouse-friendly version of the stepping test described by Blume et al. [64] and modified by Heuer et al. [65]. Right sided intrastriatal application of 25 and 50 pg BoNT-A clearly reduced the stepping frequency of the left forepaw up to 9 months after injection compared to sham group. A reduced initiation of movements of the paw contralateral to the BoNT-A application via crossed motor efferents is reasonable for the outcome of this behavioral test [66–68]. Interestingly, the intrastriatal BoNT-A injection into the right CPu also results in a short-term reduction of right paw adjusting steps. One month after vehicle injection mice made 10.8 ± 0.2 steps; at the same time the 25 pg BoNT-A group made 9.2 ± 0.2, and the 50 pg BoNT-A group 8.9 ± 0.2 steps. This phenomenon is not fully understood, as the right forepaw steps should be unaltered. The mouse-friendly design of the stepping test has also been applied in the mouse MTPT model [64] resulting in bilateral impairment, and also following different right side models of dopaminergic lesioning to induce unilateral parkinsonian-like symptoms [65,69,70]. Unilateral dopaminergic depletion, however, led to contradicting results in the same test. Heuer et al. [65] stated that the number of steps is reduced in both paws to about 80% compared to sham-injected mice irrespective of the experimental approach inducing unilateral or bilateral striatal dopamine reduction. In contrast, Glajch et al. [69] reported a ratio of contralateral-to-ipsilateral steps of about 0.2 after unilateral 6-OHDA lesion of the medial forebrain bundle. Boix et al. [70] reported a ratio of approximately 6 to 27%, depending on the 6-OHDA dosage used. Thus, both groups show a clear unilateral effect. However, neither Glajch et al. [69] nor Boix et al. [70] mention the absolute number of steps made by the ipsilateral paw, which would be important for comparison with our results.

3.3.4. Hindlimb Clasping

Hindlimb clasping has been shown to occur in various neurodegenerative mouse models [71,72] including PD models [73,74]. All our mice, irrespective of BoNT-A or vehicle injection, never showed pathological hindlimb clasping during the whole testing period from 1 to 9 months. We interpret the absence of this pathological behavior in our model as indirect evidence that the BoNT-A dosages used are not generally toxic in the striatum.

3.4. Drug-Induced Rotation Tests

3.4.1. Apomorphine-Induced Rotations

There is an apomorphine-induced rotational behavior of BoNT-A-treated mice and rats. Mice with 25 and 50 pg BoNT-A injected intrastriatally showed significant contralateral apomorphine-induced rotations after a survival of 1 and 3 months with rotations of about 2 per minute. Thereafter, rotational behavior decreased to values not significantly different from those of the vehicle group. These measurements corroborate data obtained in rats (Figure 3A), which also showed a significantly altered behavior with rotations of approximately 1.5 to 2 per minute 3 months after intrastriatal injection of 1 ng BoNT-A.

Apomorphine-induced rotations are mainly due to binding of the drug to D_2 receptors that are distributed unequally in both striata. Following apomorphine application, hemi-PD rats and hemi-PD mice rotate to the body side contralateral to the dopamine-depleted hemisphere, which has a higher D_2 receptor concentration than the contralateral one [65,70,75]. Acetylcholine is reduced in BoNT-A-injected striata, and thus, the activation of all medium spiny neurons is reduced. Moreover, striatal receptor concentration measurements investigated in BoNT-A-treated hemi-PD rats speak in favor of a BoNT-A-induced reduction of D_2 receptors in the respective CPu [22,23].

Considering that the majority of striatal D_2 receptors are located on the D_2 receptor bearing medium spiny neuron, an unaltered dopamine concentration in the CPu would result in a movement deficit of the contralateral body side via the indirect basal ganglia loop in BoNT-A-treated striata. However, if the majority of striatal D_2 receptors are located on the presynaptic terminals of the dopamine afferents from the substantia nigra pars compacta, then dopamine release should be increased due to reduced inhibition by D_2 autoreceptors on dopamine terminals [76]. The hypothetically increased striatal dopamine concentration in the BoNT-A-injected CPu would result in an increased movement of the contralateral body side via the indirect basal ganglia loop as suggested by Da Cunha et al. [77]. As all tests for spontaneous motor behavior after striatal BoNT-A revealed an initiation deficit in the contralateral forelimb, the functional significance of D_2 autoreceptors for these non-drug-induced behaviors seemed limited.

Since apomorphine is mainly a D_2 receptor agonist, its application possibly reverses the alterations in basal ganglia circuitry induced by BoNT-A by shifting the dopamine-mediated functional significance from D_2 receptor-bearing medium spiny neuron to D_2 autoreceptor-bearing dopamine terminals, thus resulting in a stronger movement initiation in the contralateral body musculature. If dopamine release by the disinhibited dopamine terminals exceeds the apomorphine-induced disinhibition of the D_2 receptor-bearing medium spiny neuron, then we can assume the occurrence of a mildly increased contralateral forelimb activity via deactivation of the medium spiny neuron of the indirect basal ganglia loop, which would result in the contralateral rotation behavior [66,67].

3.4.2. Amphetamine-Induced Rotations

Mice with intrastriatal injection of 25 or 50 pg BoNT-A show clear anti-clockwise rotations of about 4–10 per min following the application of amphetamine (Figure 2B). In contrast, comparable experiments in rats revealed no significant effect of BoNT-A injections as compared with vehicle injection (Figure 3B). The obvious difference in BoNT-A-inducible amphetamine rotations between mice and rats is not fully understood.

Amphetamine mainly increases the extracellular dopamine concentration by different mechanisms: it competitively inhibits dopamine uptake via dopamine transporter, facilitates the movement of dopamine from the vesicle into the cytoplasm, and promotes DAT-mediated reverse transport of dopamine into the synaptic cleft independent of action potential-induced vesicular release [78]. Additionally, microdialysis studies in rats revealed amphetamine-induced increased extracellular concentrations of glutamate, aspartate, GABA, taurine, glycine, serotonin, acetylcholine, and of different peptides [79–86].

There is a notable species difference regarding amphetamine-induced contralateral rotation behavior in unilaterally BoNT-A-injected animals, since it is present in mice, but not in rats. Three aspects will be discussed: (1) different effects on axon terminals after intrastriatal BoNT-A injections in mice and rats, (2) the concentrations of the most frequent transmitter receptors in the CPu of naïve mice and rats, and (3) the connectome of the basal ganglia of mice and rats.

Hawlitschka et al. [24] showed that striata from mice and rats react differently after BoNT-A injection with respect to the appearance of TH-ir BoNT-A -induced varicosities [24], since they are consistently found in rats, but were never seen in mice [19,24]. BoNT-A-induced varicosities can be interpreted as a sign of structural alterations induced by BoNT-A. The difference in the occurrence of BoNT-A-induced varicosities between mice and rats might be based on the synaptic vesicle glycoprotein C (SV2C) receptor responsible for the internalization of BoNT-A into the neuron [87,88]. Unfortunately, no data exist concerning differences of SV2C affinity or susceptibility between the CPu of rats and mice [87–95]. It cannot be ruled out that the dopaminergic fibers are differently influenced by BoNT-A and thus the balance or interaction of various transmitter systems on the functional outcome underlying the amphetamine-induced rotation behavior of intrastriatally applied BoNT-A may differ [79,96–101]. In contrast to the interspecies differences in BoNT-A-induced varicosities, ChAT-ir BoNT-A-induced varicosities were consistently found in CPu of both rats and mice following intrastriatal BoNT-A.

3.4.3. Receptors and Connectomics of the CPu

To analyze possible interspecies differences of transmitter systems in the CPu of control rats and mice, we compared the multireceptor fingerprints (Figure S1) of Wistar rats ($n = 6$, data from [23,102, 103]) and of C57Bl/6 mice ($n = 6$; data from [40]). Additionally, the connectome of the mouse basal ganglia generated in a high throughput tract tracing study published as Alan Atlas connectome [104] is compared with rat data (Figure S2). Details to multireceptor fingerprints and connectomes are provided in the Supplement.

4. Conclusions and Future Perspectives

BoNT-A unilaterally injected into the CPu in naïve mice differentially affected various motor behaviors. Lateralized sensorimotor integration, forelimb preference, and forelimb stepping were significantly impaired contralateral to the injected side. Unilateral intrastriatal BoNT-A induced significant contralateral amphetamine-induced rotations from 1 to 9 months post injection, which is completely opposite to the reaction found in rats. The differences in motor behavior induced by unilateral intrastriatal BoNT-A injections between rats and mice is possibly caused by different effects of BoNT-A on TH-ir fibers in rat and mouse striata, interspecies differences in striatal receptor densities, and different connectomes of the basal ganglia between mice and rats.

Local injection of BoNT-A into the striatum of hemi-PD rats is thought to decrease the local release of acetylcholine therein. Hypercholinism of the striatum caused by acetylcholine released from disinhibited tonically active cholinergic interneurons is held responsible for a disturbed basal ganglia circuitry and, consequently, for motor and behavioral dysfunctions [9,46,48,105]. One possible approach to treat PD is the reduction of the hypercholinism using oral anticholinergic drugs [106,107]. Due to the systemic drug application, adverse side effects such as anticholinergic syndrome and dyskinesia are common [13–15,108]. In the experimental hemi-PD rats, BoNT-A injected locally into the CPu is beneficial for 3 to 6 months with respect to apomorphine-induced rotational behavior [16–21]. Future experiments will cover two topics: First, repeated intrastriatal BoNT-A injections in hemi-PD rats every 6 months should test whether motor behavior could be improved for a longer time period, which would be a prerequisite for the clinical application of BoNT-A [109–112]. Second, extending our studies of intrastriatal BoNT-A injections to naïve mice, BoNT-A will be injected into mice of various parkinsonian models including those with alterations of relevant PD-associated genes to obtain further insights into PD-related etiology [39,40,113–115].

In conclusion, locally applied BoNT-A, or other botulinum neurotoxins, could be useful in treating brain dysfunctions requiring a deactivation of local brain activity [116]. Advantageously, the effect of local BoNT-A is time-limited and reversible. It can be speculated that following prospective experiments in primates botulinum neurotoxins might be applied as an effective and individually-tailored "chemical neurosurgical approach" [116,117].

5. Materials and Methods

5.1. Animals

A total of 46 young adult male C57BL/6 mice (Charles River Wiga, Sulzfeld, Germany) weighing 18–24 g and 28 Wistar rats (strain Crl: WI BR, Charles River Wiga, Sulzfeld, Germany) with a body weight of 280–320 g were used in this study. Animals were housed in standard cages in a temperature-controlled room (22 ± 2 °C) under 12 h light/12 h dark conditions with free access to food and water. All procedures were approved by the State Animal Research Committee of Mecklenburg-Western Pomerania (LALLF M-V/TSD/7221.3-1.1-053/08, LALLF M-V/TSD/7221.3-1.1-003/13 from 26 April 2013 and 13 April 2016).

5.2. BoNT-A application

In the mice, surgery was conducted under aseptic conditions and animals were deeply anesthetized with ketamine (75 mg/kg, bela-pharm Vechta, Germany)/xylazine (5.8 mg/kg, Rompun®, Bayer, Germany), mounted in a mouse adapter (Stoelting, Wood Dale, IL, USA), and fixed in a rat stereotactic apparatus (Kopf, Tujunga, CA, USA). The skull was opened with a dental drill and the mice received an injection of 1 µL BoNT-A solution (Lot No. 13028A1A; List, Campbell, CA, USA, purchased via Quadratech Diagnostics, Surrey, UK) containing a total of 25 pg or 50 pg BoNT-A dissolved in PBS + 0.1% BSA into the right CPu delivered over 4 min using a 26-gauge 5 µL Hamilton syringe, at a rate of 0.25 µL per minute (Figure 5). The sham group received 1 µL BoNT-A vehicle solution. The injection coordinates with reference to bregma were: anterior-posterior = +0.65 mm, lateral = −1.6 mm, and vertical = −3.0 mm from dura, respectively [118] (Figure 5).

Rats were injected either with 1 ng BoNT-A (n = 22) or the vehicle solution (sham, n = 6) into the right striatum under ketamine (50 mg/kg)/xylazine (4 mg/kg) anesthesia. The BoNT-A solution was injected at two sites, each injection consisting of 0.5 ng BoNT-A solved in 1 µL PBS + 0.1% BSA. Sham-injected rats received the vehicle solution. The coordinates according to bregma were: anterior-posterior = +1.3 mm/−0.4 mm, lateral = −2.6 mm/−3.6 mm and ventral = −5.5 mm/−5.5 mm, respectively [119].

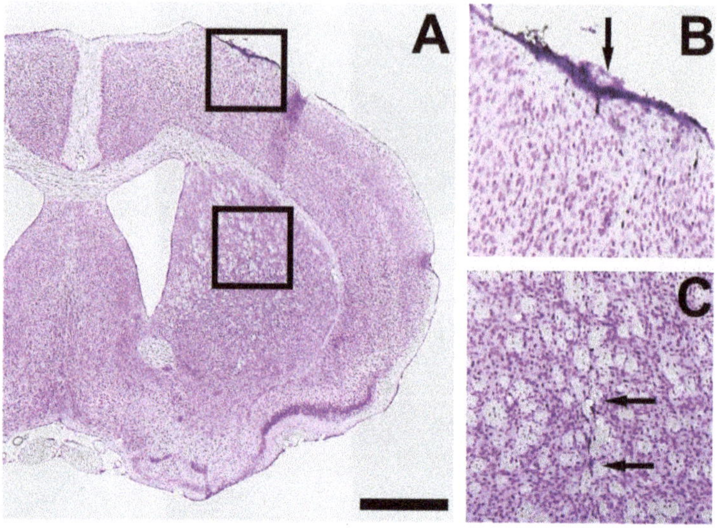

Figure 5. (**A**) A coronal Nissl-stained brain section 30 μm thick of a mouse treated intrastriatally with 25 pg BoNT-A 6 months before sacrifice. (**B**,**C**) Higher magnifications of the boxes in (**A**). In (**B**) the needle tract through the cortex is marked by an arrow, in (**C**) the injection channel in the striatum is indicated by two arrows. Scale bar applies to (**A**): 1 mm.

We founded our experiments on the weight values of BoNT-A, i.e., 25 to 50 pg per mouse CPu and 1 ng per rat CPu. In mice the LD_{50} value after intraperitoneal injection is about 0.25–1.15 ng/kg BoNT-A [120]. Thus, in our experiments a dosage of 50 pg BoNT-A per mouse, injected intrastriatally, is below the classical LD_{50}, and well tolerated. In clinical use the normal amount of BoNT-A (Xeomin, Dysport, Botox and others) is about 200 to 300 units at maximum per patient per session depending on the clinical symptoms and site of application. Remarkably, the clinical efficacy of a "unit" is reported differently by the various manufactures (Botox: 5 ng correspond to 100 units; Dysport: 4.35 ng correspond to 500 units; Xeomin: 0.6 ng correspond to 100 units) [121]. These uncertainties relay on the nonstandardized LD_{50} bioassays required to achieve the median lethal dose = LD_{50} (depending on mouse strain, sex, age, volume and route of injection) [122].

5.3. Body Weight

Body weights were measured before stereotactic surgery and 0.5, 1, 2, 3, 4, 5, 6, 7, and 9 months after injection of BoNT-A or vehicle.

5.4. Behavioral Testing

Three experimental mouse groups were behaviorally tested: (1) animals receiving 25 pg BoNT-A (25 pg BoNT-A group, n = 15), (2) animals receiving 50 pg BoNT-A (50 pg BoNT-A group, n = 20), and (3) animals receiving vehicle (sham group, n = 11). During the experimental period 5 mice died. Smaller groups were evaluated for the stepping test and the corridor task (25 pg, n = 11; 50 pg, n = 12; sham, n = 10). All mice were adapted to the examination room for 1 h before testing. All tests were performed at 4 time points (1, 3, 6, and 9 months) after the injection of BoNT-A or vehicle, and drug-induced rotations were additionally scored 0.5 months after BoNT-A or vehicle, always according to an identical time schedule (Figure 6). In rats drug-induced rotation tests were carried out 1, 2, 3, and 9 months after BoNT (n = 22) or vehicle (n = 6) injection.

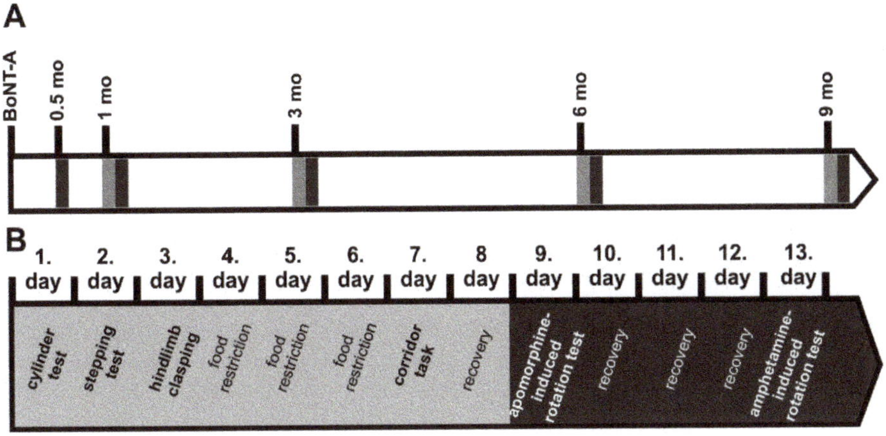

Figure 6. (**A**) Time schedule of the stereotactic application of BoNT-A in mice and behavioral tests. Light grey rectangles symbolize batteries of non-drug-induced behavior tests, dark grey rectangles the subsequently performed apomorphine- and amphetamine-induced rotation tests. (**B**) Detailed visualization of single behavior test batteries. Non-drug-induced tests were performed on the days presented in the light grey part of the time line, drug-induced tests on the days of the dark grey part. The non-drug-induced tests were performed as follows: On the first day the mice underwent the cylinder test until 30 consecutive touches of the glass wall with the forepaws were done. On the second day the stepping test and on the third day the hindlimb clasping were carried out three times per mouse, respectively. On the following 3 days mice underwent food restriction and on the seventh day the corridor task was performed. Following recovery the drug-induced rotation tests were conducted.

5.4.1. Drug-Induced Rotation Tests (Apomorphine, Amphetamine)

Mice rotations were assessed using an automated rotometer system (Rotometer UGO BASILE 43000; Ugo Basile Sri, Gemonio, Varese, Italy). Apomorphine was injected subcutaneously at a dosage of 0.5 mg/kg [123–125] (Teclapharm, Lüneburg, Germany) dissolved in 0.9% sterile saline. Three days later, D-amphetamine sulphate (Sigma Aldrich, München, Germany) was injected intraperitoneally at a dosage of 2.5 mg/kg [124,126,127] (Figure 6). Recording of apomorphine- and amphetamine-induced rotations began 5 min after drug injection and lasted 40 min. Rotations were defined as complete 360° turns and registered as net difference between the two directions per minute [128]. Anti-clockwise rotations were expressed by positive values, rotations in clockwise direction by negative values. Respective rotations in rats were induced by either 0.25 mg/kg apomorphine applied subcutaneously (Teclapharm, Germany) or 2.5 mg d-amphetamine sulfate (intraperitoneal; Sigma Aldrich, München, Germany), both solved in saline. Rotations were measured over 40 min after apomorphine and over 60 min after amphetamine in a self-constructed rotometer according to Ungerstedt and Arbuthnott [128].

5.4.2. Spontaneous Motor Tests

Mice were tested in the cylinder test, stepping test, hindlimb clasping, and corridor task at 1, 3, 6, and 9 months after injection of BoNT-A or vehicle following a constant time table (Figure 6).

Cylinder Test

Forelimb preference was evaluated with the cylinder test as previously described [58,129]. Mice were placed in a glass cylinder (diameter 19 cm, height 20 cm) with mirrors placed behind to allow for a 360° view of every contact with the side of the cylinder. Sessions were taped with a video camera system (JVC, GZ-MG255E, Yokohama, Japan), and scored later. For each animal thirty consecutive forepaw contacts with the glass cylinder were evaluated by counting the initial contacts of the right or left paw. Then the ratio of left and right forepaw use was calculated. Evaluation of the videotapes was performed by an observer blinded to the animals' identities.

Corridor Task

Lateralized sensorimotor integration and neglect were examined using the corridor task [61]. For our study we used a custom-made 60 cm long, 4 cm wide, and 15 cm high alleyway equipped with 10 pairs of adjacent pots with a diameter of 1 cm, placed at 5 cm intervals and containing 5 sugar pellets (Ain-76A Rodent Tablet 20 mg TestDiet, Richmond, IN, USA). Prior to testing, the mice were food-restricted for three days and maintained at 90% of free-feeding bodyweight during habituation and testing [130]. Animals were adapted to the apparatus for 10 min each on two consecutive days with some scattered sugar pellets along the floor of the corridor and started from different ends of the corridor each day. On the test day, mice were at first positioned in an identical, but empty corridor for 5 min for adaptation and then placed at the end of the testing corridor with bowls containing the pellet. Animals were allowed to move freely along the apparatus for 5 min to retrieve pellets placed on either side of their body. The number of ipsilateral (right side) and contralateral (left side) retrievals made by each mouse was calculated and the data were expressed as a percentage of left and right retrievals of the total number of retrievals. A "retrieval" was defined as a nose poke into a bowl, whether or not pellets were taken, and a new retrieval was counted by investigating a new pot [59,61].

Stepping Test

Forelimb akinesia was assessed according to Blume et al. [64] and modified by Heuer et al. [65] using an open table (1.5 m in length). Mice were tested three times in one day during the day light cycle. Each trial was recorded on video. As a first step for habituation to the test, mice were allowed to settle at one end of the table for 1–2 s, with all limbs on the table. Secondly, the experimenter gently lifted up the hindlimbs by pulling up on the tail leaving only the forepaws touching the table surface. Then, at a steady pace of 1 m in 3–4 s the experimenter pulled the animal the total test distance of 1 m backwards by the tail. Finally, the numbers of adjusting steps made with the left and right forepaws were counted offline in the videos.

Hindlimb Clasping

Hindlimb clasping is a marker of disease progression in a number of mouse models of neurodegeneration, including certain cerebellar ataxias [131] and parkinsonian mouse models [73,74], and was performed as previously described [72,73]. Outside the cage, each mouse was slowly lifted by the tail for 10 s and then lowered back to the surface. The hindlimbs were observed and the position of the hindlimbs was scored for each trial [72]. A score of 0 indicated that the hindlimbs were consistently splayed outwards and away from the abdomen. A score of 1 indicated that one hindlimb was retracted inwards towards the abdomen more than 50% of the trial period, a score of 2 indicated that both hindlimbs were partially retracted inwards towards the abdomen for at least 50% of the observation period. Mice were tested three times on one day and each trial was recorded on video.

5.5. Receptor Autoradiography and Histology

The autoradiographic procedure was performed according to standard protocols already published [132–136]. Cryosections of the respective brains were stained with cresyl-violet acetate (SIGMA C1791-5G) to verify the injection sites.

5.6. Statistical Analysis

Data of all behavioral tests were subjected to two-way ANOVA with repeated measurements. The Holm–Sidak test was used for post-hoc comparisons. The level of significance was set at $p \leq 0.05$ for all statistical analyses. All statistical tests were done using SigmaPlot 11 Software (Systat Software, Inc., San Jose, CA 95110, USA).

Supplementary Materials: The following are available online at http://www.mdpi.com/2072-6651/10/7/295/s1, Figure S1: Multi-receptor fingerprints of the caudate-putamen of mouse (blue) and rat (red), Figure S2: (A) Differential adjacency matrix of the rat and mouse basal ganglia. (B) Differential reciprocity matrix of rat and mouse basal ganglia.

Author Contributions: Conceptualization and Supervision, V.A., A.H., O.S. and A.W.; Investigation, A.H., V.A. and A.W.; Visualization, C.H., O.S. and A.H.; Methodology, K.Z., N.P.-G. and T.M.; Writing-Original Draft Preparation , V.A., C.H., O.S., A.W., A.H., N.P.-G. and K.Z.; Writing-Review & Editing, V.A., C.H., A.W., N.P.-G. and K.Z.; Funding Acquisition, A.H., K.Z.

Funding: Rostock University Medical Center internal funding FORUN 889005 and 889014, European Union's Horizon 2020 Framework Programme for Research and Innovation under Grant Agreement No 720270 (Human Brain Project SGA1) (K.Z.), and Portfolio Theme "Supercomputing and Modeling for the Human Brain" of the Helmholtz Association.

Acknowledgments: We gratefully acknowledge S. Lehmann, F. Winzer, M. Cremer, S. Wilms, S. Buller, J. Bausch, S. Krause and A. Börner for their excellent technical assistance.

Conflicts of Interest: The authors declare no conflicts of interest.

Abbreviations

6-OHDA	6-hydroxydopamine
BoNT-A	botulinum neurotoxin-A
ChAT	choline acetyltransferase
CPu	caudate-putamen
D_1	dopamine D_1 receptor
D_2	dopamine D_2 receptor
GABA	α-amino butyric acid
hemi-PD	hemiparkinsonian
ir	immunoreactive
nic	acetylcholine nicotinic $\alpha_4\beta_2$ receptor
PD	Parkinson's disease
SV2C	synaptic vesicle glycoprotein C
TH	tyrosine hydroxylase

References

1. Siderowf, A.; Stern, M. Update on Parkinson Disease. *Ann. Intern. Med.* **2003**, *138*, 651–658. [CrossRef] [PubMed]
2. Moore, D.J.; West, A.B.; Dawson, V.L.; Dawson, T.M. Molecular Pathophysiology of Parkinson's Disease. *Annu. Rev. Neurosci.* **2005**, *28*, 57–87. [CrossRef] [PubMed]
3. Morin, N.; Jourdain, V.A.; Di Paolo, T. Modeling dyskinesia in animal models of Parkinson disease. *Exp. Neurol.* **2014**, *256*, 105–116. [CrossRef] [PubMed]
4. Albin, R.L.; Young, A.B.; Penney, J.B. The functional anatomy of basal ganglia disorders. *Trends Neurosci.* **1989**, *12*, 366–375. [CrossRef]
5. DeLong, M.R.; Wichmann, T. Circuits and circuit disorders of the basal ganglia. *Arch. Neurol.* **2007**, *64*, 20–24. [CrossRef] [PubMed]
6. Marsden, C.D. The mysterious motor function of the basal ganglia: The Robert Wartenberg Lecture. *Neurology* **1982**, *32*, 514–539. [CrossRef] [PubMed]
7. Obeso, J.A.; Rodriguez-Oroz, M.C.; Rodriguez, M.; DeLong, M.R.; Olanow, C.W. Pathophysiology of levodopa-induced dyskinesias in Parkinson's disease: Problems with the current model. *Ann. Neurol.* **2000**, *47*, S22–S32. [PubMed]

8. Coffield, J.A.; Yan, X. Neuritogenic actions of botulinum neurotoxin A on cultured motor neurons. *J. Pharmacol. Exp. Ther.* **2009**, *330*, 352–358. [CrossRef] [PubMed]
9. Pisani, A.; Bernardi, G.; Ding, J.; Surmeier, D.J. Re-emergence of striatal cholinergic interneurons in movement disorders. *Trends Neurosci.* **2007**, *30*, 545–553. [CrossRef] [PubMed]
10. Ding, J.; Guzman, J.N.; Tkatch, T.; Chen, S.; Goldberg, J.A.; Ebert, P.J.; Levitt, P.; Wilson, C.J.; Hamm, H.E.; Surmeier, D.J. RGS4-dependent attenuation of M4 autoreceptor function in striatal cholinergic interneurons following dopamine depletion. *Nat. Neurosci.* **2006**, *9*, 832–842. [CrossRef] [PubMed]
11. Oldenburg, I.A.; Ding, J.B. Cholinergic modulation of synaptic integration and dendritic excitability in the striatum. *Curr. Opin. Neurobiol.* **2011**, *21*, 425–432. [CrossRef] [PubMed]
12. Ztaou, S.; Maurice, N.; Camon, J.; Guiraudie-Capraz, G.; Kerkerian-Le Goff, L.; Beurrier, C.; Liberge, M.; Amalric, M. Involvement of Striatal Cholinergic Interneurons and M1 and M4 Muscarinic Receptors in Motor Symptoms of Parkinson's Disease. *J. Neurosci.* **2016**, *36*, 9161–9172. [CrossRef] [PubMed]
13. Clarke, C.E. Medical Management of Parkinson's Disease. *J. Neurol. Neurosurg. Psychiatry* **2002**, *72*, i22–i27. [CrossRef] [PubMed]
14. Fernandez, H.H. Updates in the medical management of Parkinson disease. *Clevel. Clin. J. Med.* **2012**, *79*, 28–35. [CrossRef] [PubMed]
15. Connolly, B.S.; Lang, A.E. Pharmacological treatment of Parkinson disease: A review. *JAMA* **2014**, *311*, 1670–1683. [CrossRef] [PubMed]
16. Antipova, V.; Hawlitschka, A.; Mix, E.; Schmitt, O.; Dräger, D.; Benecke, R.; Wree, A. Behavioral and structural effects of unilateral intrastriatal injections of botulinum neurotoxin a in the rat model of Parkinson's disease. *J. Neurosci. Res.* **2013**, *91*, 838–847. [CrossRef] [PubMed]
17. Hawlitschka, A.; Antipova, V.; Schmitt, O.; Witt, M.; Benecke, R.; Mix, E.; Wree, A. Intracerebrally applied botulinum neurotoxin in experimental neuroscience. *Curr. Pharm. Biotechnol.* **2013**, *14*, 124–130. [CrossRef] [PubMed]
18. Holzmann, C.; Dräger, D.; Mix, E.; Hawlitschka, A.; Antipova, V.; Benecke, R.; Wree, A. Effects of intrastriatal botulinum neurotoxin A on the behavior of Wistar rats. *Behav. Brain Res.* **2012**, *234*, 107–116. [CrossRef] [PubMed]
19. Wree, A.; Mix, E.; Hawlitschka, A.; Antipova, V.; Witt, M.; Schmitt, O.; Benecke, R. Intrastriatal botulinum toxin abolishes pathologic rotational behaviour and induces axonal varicosities in the 6-OHDA rat model of Parkinson's disease. *Neurobiol. Dis.* **2011**, *41*, 291–298. [CrossRef] [PubMed]
20. Mehlan, J.; Brosig, H.; Schmitt, O.; Mix, E.; Wree, A.; Hawlitschka, A. Intrastriatal injection of botulinum neurotoxin-A is not cytotoxic in rat brain—A histological and stereological analysis. *Brain Res.* **2016**, *1630*, 18–24. [CrossRef] [PubMed]
21. Antipova, V.A.; Holzmann, C.; Schmitt, O.; Wree, A.; Hawlitschka, A. Botulinum Neurotoxin A Injected Ipsilaterally or Contralaterally into the Striatum in the Rat 6-OHDA Model of Unilateral Parkinson's Disease Differently Affects Behavior. *Front. Behav. Neurosci.* **2017**, *11*, 119. [CrossRef] [PubMed]
22. Wedekind, F.; Oskamp, A.; Lang, M.; Hawlitschka, A.; Zilles, K.; Wree, A.; Bauer, A. Intrastriatal administration of botulinum neurotoxin A normalizes striatal D_2R binding and reduces striatal D_1R binding in male hemiparkinsonian rats. *J. Neurosci. Res.* **2018**, *96*, 75–86. [CrossRef] [PubMed]
23. Mann, T.; Zilles, K.; Dikow, H.; Hellfritsch, A.; Cremer, M.; Piel, M.; Rösch, F.; Hawlitschka, A.; Schmitt, O.; Wree, A. Dopamine, Noradrenaline and Serotonin Receptor Densities in the Striatum of Hemiparkinsonian Rats following Botulinum Neurotoxin-A Injection. *Neuroscience* **2018**, *374*, 187–204. [CrossRef] [PubMed]
24. Hawlitschka, A.; Holzmann, C.; Witt, S.; Spiewok, J.; Neumann, A.M.; Schmitt, O.; Wree, A.; Antipova, V. Intrastriatally injected botulinum neurotoxin-A differently effects cholinergic and dopaminergic fibers in C57BL/6 mice. *Brain Res.* **2017**, *1676*, 46–56. [CrossRef] [PubMed]
25. Corchs, F.; Nutt, D.J.; Hince, D.A.; Davies, S.J.; Bernik, M.; Hood, S.D. Evidence for serotonin function as a neurochemical difference between fear and anxiety disorders in humans? *J. Psychopharmacol.* **2015**, *29*, 1061–1069. [CrossRef] [PubMed]
26. Ellenbroek, B.; Youn, J. Rodent models in neuroscience research: Is it a rat race? *Dis. Model. Mech.* **2016**, *9*, 1079–1087. [CrossRef] [PubMed]
27. Jaramillo, S.; Zador, A.M. Mice and rats achieve similar levels of performance in an adaptive decision-making task. *Front. Syst. Neurosci.* **2014**, *8*, 173. [CrossRef] [PubMed]

28. Klein, C.; Westenberger, A.; Hollingworth, P.; Harold, D.; Jones, L.; Owen, M.J.; Williams, J.; Marques, S.C.F.; Oliveira, C.R.; Pereira, C.M.F.; et al. Genetics of Parkinson's Disease. *Int. J. Geriatr. Psychiatry* **2012**, *26*, a008888. [CrossRef] [PubMed]
29. Lazarov, O.; Hollands, C. Hippocampal neurogenesis: Learning to remember. *Prog. Neurobiol.* **2016**, *138–140*, 1–18. [CrossRef] [PubMed]
30. Lindström, M.; Korkeala, H. Laboratory diagnostics of botulism. *Clin. Microbiol. Rev.* **2006**, *19*, 298–314. [CrossRef] [PubMed]
31. Overgaard, A.; Tena-Sempere, M.; Franceschini, I.; Desroziers, E.; Simonneaux, V.; Mikkelsen, J.D. Comparative analysis of kisspeptin-immunoreactivity reveals genuine differences in the hypothalamic Kiss1 systems between rats and mice. *Peptides* **2013**, *45*, 85–90. [CrossRef] [PubMed]
32. Sesardic, D.; Das, R.G. Alternatives to the LD50 assay for botulinum toxin potency testing: Strategies and progress towards refinement, reduction and replacement. *AATEX* **2008**, *14*, 581–585.
33. Wheeler, C.; Inami, G.; Mohle-Boetani, J.; Vugia, D. Sensitivity of mouse bioassay in clinical wound botulism. *Clin. Infect. Dis.* **2009**, *48*, 1669–1673. [CrossRef] [PubMed]
34. Antonucci, F.; Rossi, C.; Gianfranceschi, L.; Rossetto, O.; Caleo, M. Long-distance retrograde effects of botulinum neurotoxin A. *J. Neurosci.* **2008**, *28*, 3689–3696. [CrossRef] [PubMed]
35. De Leonibus, E.; Costantini, V.J.A.; Massaro, A.; Mandolesi, G.; Vanni, V.; Luvisetto, S.; Pavone, F.; Oliverio, A.; Mele, A. Cognitive and neural determinants of response strategy in the dual-solution plus-maze task. *Learn. Mem.* **2011**, *18*, 241–244. [CrossRef] [PubMed]
36. Caleo, M.; Restani, L.; Gianfranceschi, L.; Costantin, L.; Rossi, C.; Rossetto, O.; Montecucco, C.; Maffei, L. Transient Synaptic Silencing of Developing Striate Cortex Has Persistent Effects on Visual Function and Plasticity. *J. Neurosci.* **2007**, *27*, 4530–4540. [CrossRef] [PubMed]
37. Schiavo, G.; Montecucco, C. Tetanus and Botulism Neurotoxins: Isolation and Assay. *Methods Enzymol.* **1995**, *248*, 643–652. [CrossRef] [PubMed]
38. Montecucco, C.; Schiavo, G. Structure and Function of Tetanus and Botulinum Neurotoxins. *Q. Rev. Biophys.* **1995**, *28*, 423–472. [CrossRef] [PubMed]
39. Cremer, J.N.N.; Amunts, K.; Schleicher, A.; Palomero-Gallagher, N.; Piel, M.; Rösch, F.; Zilles, K. Changes in the expression of neurotransmitter receptors in Parkin and DJ-1 knockout mice—A quantitative multireceptor study. *Neuroscience* **2015**, *311*, 539–551. [CrossRef] [PubMed]
40. Cremer, J.N.; Amunts, K.; Graw, J.; Piel, M.; Rösch, F.; Zilles, K. Neurotransmitter receptor density changes in Pitx3ak mice—A model relevant to parkinson's disease. *Neuroscience* **2015**, *285*, 11–23. [CrossRef] [PubMed]
41. Orth, M.; Tabrizi, S.J. Models of Parkinson's disease. *Mov. Disord.* **2003**, *18*, 729–737. [CrossRef] [PubMed]
42. Le, W.; Jankovic, J. Animal models of Parkinson's disease. *Park. Dis. Diagn. Mot. Symptoms Non-Mot. Features* **2013**, *115*, 115–135. [CrossRef]
43. Wong, P.C.; Cai, H.; Borchelt, D.R.; Price, D.L. Genetically engineered mouse models of neurodegenerative diseases. *Nat. Neurosci.* **2002**, *5*, 633–639. [CrossRef] [PubMed]
44. Magen, I.; Chesselet, M.-F. Genetic mouse models of Parkinson's disease. *Recent Adv. Park. Dis. Clin. Res.* **2010**, *184*, 53–87. [CrossRef]
45. Blandini, F.; Armentero, M.-T. Animal models of Parkinson's disease. *FEBS J.* **2012**, *279*, 1156–1166. [CrossRef] [PubMed]
46. Day, M.; Wang, Z.; Ding, J.; An, X.; Ingham, C.A.; Shering, A.F.; Wokosin, D.; Ilijic, E.; Sun, Z.; Sampson, A.R.; et al. Selective elimination of glutamatergic synapses on striatopallidal neurons in Parkinson disease models. *Nat. Neurosci.* **2006**, *9*, 251–259. [CrossRef] [PubMed]
47. Obeso, J.Á.; Marin, C.; Rodriguez-Oroz, C.; Blesa, J.; Benitez-Temiño, B.; Mena-Segovia, J.; Rodríguez, M.; Olanow, C.W. The basal ganglia in Parkinson's disease: Current concepts and unexplained observations. *Ann. Neurol.* **2008**, *64*, S30–S46. [CrossRef] [PubMed]
48. Obeso, J.Á.; Rodríguez-Oroz, M.C.; Benitez-Temino, B.; Blesa, F.J.; Guridi, J.; Marin, C.; Rodriguez, M. Functional organization of the basal ganglia: Therapeutic implications for Parkinson's disease. *Mov. Disord.* **2008**, *23*, S548–S559. [CrossRef] [PubMed]
49. Bordia, T.; Zhang, D.; Perez, X.A.; Quik, M. Striatal cholinergic interneurons and D_2 receptor-expressing GABAergic medium spiny neurons regulate tardive dyskinesia. *Exp. Neurol.* **2016**, *286*, 32–39. [CrossRef] [PubMed]

50. Hurley, M.J.; Jenner, P. What has been learnt from study of dopamine receptors in Parkinson's disease? *Pharmacol. Ther.* **2006**, *111*, 715–728. [CrossRef] [PubMed]
51. Mamaligas, A.A.; Cai, Y.; Ford, C.P. Nicotinic and opioid receptor regulation of striatal dopamine D_2-receptor mediated transmission. *Sci. Rep.* **2016**, *6*, 37834. [CrossRef] [PubMed]
52. Perreault, M.L.; Hasbi, A.; O'Dowd, B.F.; George, S.R. The dopamine D_1–D_2 receptor heteromer in striatal medium spiny neurons: Evidence for a third distinct neuronal pathway in basal ganglia. *Front. Neuroanat.* **2011**, *5*, 31. [CrossRef] [PubMed]
53. Rico, A.J.; Dopeso-Reyes, I.G.; Martínez-Pinilla, E.; Sucunza, D.; Pignataro, D.; Roda, E.; Marín-Ramos, D.; Labandeira-García, J.L.; George, S.R.; Franco, R.; et al. Neurochemical evidence supporting dopamine D_1–D_2 receptor heteromers in the striatum of the long-tailed macaque: Changes following dopaminergic manipulation. *Brain Struct. Funct.* **2017**, *222*, 1767–1784. [CrossRef] [PubMed]
54. Ariano, M.A.; Stromski, C.J.; Smyk-Randall, E.M.; Sibley, D.R. D_2 dopamine receptor localization on striatonigral neurons. *Neurosci. Lett.* **1992**, *144*, 215–220. [CrossRef]
55. Brock, J.W.; Farooqui, S.; Ross, K.; Prasad, C. Localization of dopamine D_2 receptor protein in rat brain using polyclonal antibody. *Brain Res.* **1992**, *578*, 244–250. [CrossRef]
56. Yung, K.K.L.; Bolam, J.P.; Smith, A.D.; Hersch, S.M.; Ciliax, B.J.; Levey, A.I. Immunocytochemical localization of D_1 and D_2 dopamine receptors in the basal ganglia of the rat: Light and electron microscopy. *Neuroscience* **1995**, *65*, 709–730. [CrossRef]
57. Li, N.; Chen, T.-W.; Guo, Z.V.; Gerfen, C.R.; Svoboda, K. A motor cortex circuit for motor planning and movement. *Nature* **2015**, *519*, 51–56. [CrossRef] [PubMed]
58. Kirik, D.; Rosenblad, C.; Bjorklund, A. Preservation of a functional nigrostriatal dopamine pathway by GDNF in the intrastriatal 6-OHDA lesion model depends on the site of administration of the trophic factor. *Eur. J. Neurosci.* **2000**, *12*, 3871–3882. [CrossRef] [PubMed]
59. Dowd, E.; Monville, C.; Torres, E.M.; Dunnett, S.B. The Corridor Task: A simple test of lateralised response selection sensitive to unilateral dopamine deafferentation and graft-derived dopamine replacement in the striatum. *Brain Res. Bull.* **2005**, *68*, 24–30. [CrossRef] [PubMed]
60. Fitzsimmons, D.F.; Moloney, T.C.; Dowd, E. Further validation of the corridor task for assessing deficit and recovery in the hemi-Parkinsonian rat: Restoration of bilateral food retrieval by dopamine receptor agonism. *Behav. Brain Res.* **2006**, *169*, 352–355. [CrossRef] [PubMed]
61. Grealish, S.; Mattsson, B.; Draxler, P.; Björklund, A. Characterisation of behavioural and neurodegenerative changes induced by intranigral 6-hydroxydopamine lesions in a mouse model of Parkinson's disease. *Eur. J. Neurosci.* **2010**, *31*, 2266–2278. [CrossRef] [PubMed]
62. Starkey, M.L.; Barritt, A.W.; Yip, P.K.; Davies, M.; Hamers, F.P.T.; McMahon, S.B.; Bradbury, E.J. Assessing behavioural function following a pyramidotomy lesion of the corticospinal tract in adult mice. *Exp. Neurol.* **2005**, *195*, 524–539. [CrossRef] [PubMed]
63. Welniarz, Q.; Dusart, I.; Gallea, C.; Roze, E. One hand clapping: Lateralization of motor control. *Front. Neuroanat.* **2015**, *9*, 75. [CrossRef] [PubMed]
64. Blume, S.R.; Cass, D.K.; Tseng, K.Y. Stepping test in mice: A reliable approach in determining forelimb akinesia in MPTP-induced Parkinsonism. *Exp. Neurol.* **2009**, *219*, 208–211. [CrossRef] [PubMed]
65. Heuer, A.; Smith, G.A.; Lelos, M.J.; Lane, E.L.; Dunnett, S.B. Unilateral nigrostriatal 6-hydroxydopamine lesions in mice I: Motor impairments identify extent of dopamine depletion at three different lesion sites. *Behav. Brain Res.* **2012**, *228*, 30–43. [CrossRef] [PubMed]
66. Baskin, Y.K.; Dietrich, W.D.; Green, E.J. Two effective behavioral tasks for evaluating sensorimotor dysfunction following traumatic brain injury in mice. *J. Neurosci. Methods* **2003**, *129*, 87–93. [CrossRef]
67. Cohen, N.R.; Taylor, J.S.; Scott, L.B.; Guillery, R.W.; Soriano, P.; Furley, A.J. Errors in corticospinal axon guidance in mice lacking the neural cell adhesion molecule L1. *Curr. Biol.* **1998**, *8*, 26–33. [CrossRef]
68. Steward, O.; Zheng, B.; Ho, C.; Anderson, K.; Tessier-Lavigne, M. The Dorsolateral Corticospinal Tract in Mice: An Alternative Route for Corticospinal Input to Caudal Segments following Dorsal Column Lesions. *J. Comp. Neurol.* **2004**, *472*, 463–477. [CrossRef] [PubMed]
69. Glajch, K.E.; Fleming, S.M.; Surmeier, D.J.; Osten, P. Sensorimotor assessment of the unilateral 6-hydroxydopamine mouse model of Parkinson's disease. *Behav. Brain Res.* **2012**, *230*, 309–316. [CrossRef] [PubMed]

70. Boix, J.; Padel, T.; Paul, G. A partial lesion model of Parkinson's disease in mice—Characterization of a 6-OHDA-induced medial forebrain bundle lesion. *Behav. Brain Res.* **2015**, *284*, 196–206. [CrossRef] [PubMed]
71. Fernagut, P.O.; Diguet, E.; Bioulac, B.; Tison, F. MPTP potentiates 3-nitropropionic acid-induced striatal damage in mice: Reference to striatonigral degeneration. *Exp. Neurol.* **2004**, *185*, 47–62. [CrossRef] [PubMed]
72. Guyenet, S.J.; Furrer, S.A.; Damian, V.M.; Baughan, T.D.; La Spada, A.R.; Garden, G.A. A simple composite phenotype scoring system for evaluating mouse models of cerebellar ataxia. *J. Vis. Exp.* **2010**, 2–4. [CrossRef] [PubMed]
73. Morris, M.; Koyama, A.; Masliah, E.; Mucke, L. Tau reduction does not prevent motor deficits in two mouse models of Parkinson's disease. *PLoS ONE* **2011**, *6*, e29257. [CrossRef] [PubMed]
74. Lieu, C.A.; Chinta, S.J.; Rane, A.; Andersen, J.K. Age-Related Behavioral Phenotype of an Astrocytic Monoamine Oxidase-B Transgenic Mouse Model of Parkinson's Disease. *PLoS ONE* **2013**, *8*, e54200. [CrossRef] [PubMed]
75. Winkler, J.D.; Weiss, B. Reversal of supersensitive apomorphine-induced rotational behavior in mice by continuous exposure to apomorphine. *J. Pharmacol. Exp. Ther.* **1986**, *238*, 242–247. [PubMed]
76. Ford, C.P. The role of D_2-autoreceptors in regulating dopamine neuron activity and transmission. *Neuroscience* **2014**, *282*, 13–22. [CrossRef] [PubMed]
77. Da Cunha, C.; Wietzikoski, E.C.; Ferro, M.M.; Martinez, G.R.; Vital, M.A.B.F.; Hipólide, D.; Tufik, S.; Canteras, N.S. Hemiparkinsonian rats rotate toward the side with the weaker dopaminergic neurotransmission. *Behav. Brain Res.* **2008**, *189*, 364–372. [CrossRef] [PubMed]
78. Fleckenstein, A.E.; Volz, T.J.; Riddle, E.L.; Gibb, J.W.; Hanson, G.R. New insights into the mechanism of action of amphetamines. *Annu. Rev. Pharmacol. Toxicol.* **2007**, *47*, 681–698. [CrossRef] [PubMed]
79. Del Arco, A.; González-Mora, J.L.; Armas, V.R.; Mora, F. Amphetamine increases the extracellular concentration of glutamate in striatum of the awake rat: Involvement of high affinity transporter mechanisms. *Neuropharmacology* **1999**, *38*, 943–954. [CrossRef]
80. Del Arco, A.; Castañeda, T.R.; Mora, F. Amphetamine releases GABA in striatum of the freely moving rat: Involvement of calcium and high affinity transporter mechanisms. *Neuropharmacology* **1998**, *37*, 199–205. [CrossRef]
81. Hernandez, L.; Lee, F.; Hoebel, B.G. Simultaneous microdialysis and amphetamine infusion in the nucleus accumbens and striatum of freely moving rats: Increase in extracellular dopamine and serotonin. *Brain Res. Bull.* **1987**, *19*, 623–628. [CrossRef]
82. Mandel, R.J.; Leanza, G.; Nilsson, O.G.; Rosengren, E. Amphetamine induces excess release of striatal acetylcholine in vivo that is independent of nigrostriatal dopamine. *Brain Res.* **1994**, *653*, 57–65. [CrossRef]
83. Mora, F.; Porras, A. Effects of amphetamine on the release of excitatory amino acid neurotransmitters in the basal ganglia of the conscious rat. *Can. J. Physiol. Pharmacol.* **1993**, *71*, 348–351. [CrossRef] [PubMed]
84. Miele, M.; Mura, M.A.; Enrico, P.; Esposito, G.; Serra, P.A.; Migheli, R.; Zangani, D.; Miele, E.; Desole, M.S. On the mechanism of d-amphetamine-induced changes in glutamate, ascorbic acid and uric acid release in the striatum of freely moving rats. *Br. J. Pharmacol.* **2000**, *129*, 582–588. [CrossRef] [PubMed]
85. Sulzer, D.; Sonders, M.S.; Poulsen, N.W.; Galli, A. Mechanisms of neurotransmitter release by amphetamines: A review. *Prog. Neurobiol.* **2005**, *75*, 406–433. [CrossRef] [PubMed]
86. Butcher, S.P.; Fairbrother, I.S.; Kelly, J.S.; Arbuthnott, G.W. Amphetamine-Induced Dopamine Release in the Rat Striatum: An In Vivo Microdialysis Study. *J. Neurochem.* **1988**, *50*, 346–355. [CrossRef] [PubMed]
87. Kroken, A.R.; Blum, F.C.; Zuverink, M.; Barbieri, J.T. Entry of Botulinum neurotoxin subtypes A1 and A2 into neurons. *Infect. Immun.* **2016**, *85*, IAI.00795-16. [CrossRef] [PubMed]
88. Dong, M.; Yeh, F.; Tepp, W.H.; Dean, C.; Johnson, E.A.; Janz, R.; Chapman, E.R. SV2 Is the Protein Receptor for Botulinum Neurotoxin A. *Science* **2006**, *312*, 592–596. [CrossRef] [PubMed]
89. Dardou, D.; Dassesse, D.; Cuvelier, L.; Deprez, T.; De Ryck, M.; Schiffmann, S.N. Distribution of SV2C mRNA and protein expression in the mouse brain with a particular emphasis on the basal ganglia system. *Brain Res.* **2011**, *1367*, 130–145. [CrossRef] [PubMed]
90. Dardou, D.; Monlezun, S.; Foerch, P.; Courade, J.P.; Cuvelier, L.; De Ryck, M.; Schiffmann, S.N. A role for SV2C in basal ganglia functions. *Brain Res.* **2013**, *1507*, 61–73. [CrossRef] [PubMed]
91. Janz, R.; Südhof, T.C. SV2C is a synaptic vesicle protein with an unusually restricted localization: Anatomy of a synaptic vesicle protein family. *Neuroscience* **1999**, *94*, 1279–1290. [CrossRef]

92. Bajjalieh, S.M.; Peterson, K.; Linial, M.; Scheller, R.H. Brain contains two forms of synaptic vesicle protein 2. *Proc. Natl. Acad. Sci. USA* **1993**, *90*, 2150–2154. [CrossRef] [PubMed]
93. Miyauchi, N.; Saito, A.; Karasawa, T.; Harita, Y.; Suzuki, K.; Koike, H.; Han, G.D.; Shimizu, F.; Kawachi, H. Synaptic vesicle protein 2B is expressed in podocyte, and its expression is altered in proteinuric glomeruli. *J. Am. Soc. Nephrol.* **2006**, *17*, 2748–2759. [CrossRef] [PubMed]
94. Wang, M.M.; Janz, R.; Belizaire, R.; Frishman, L.J.; Sherry, D.M. Differential distribution and developmental expression of synaptic vesicle protein 2 isoforms in the mouse retina. *J. Comp. Neurol.* **2003**, *460*, 106–122. [CrossRef] [PubMed]
95. Hayashi, M.; Yamamoto, A.; Yatsushiro, S.; Yamada, H.; Futai, M.; Yamaguchi, A.; Moriyama, Y. Synaptic vesicle protein SV2B, but not SV2A, is predominantly expressed and associated with microvesicles in rat pinealocytes. *J. Neurochem.* **1998**, *71*, 356–365. [CrossRef] [PubMed]
96. Ashton, A.C.; Dolly, J.O. Characterization of the Inhibitory Action of Botulinum Neurotoxin Type A on the Release of Several Transmitters from Rat Cerebrocortical Synaptosomes. *J. Neurochem.* **1988**, *50*, 1808–1816. [CrossRef] [PubMed]
97. Bigalke, H.; Heller, I.; Bizzini, B.; Habermann, E. Tetanus toxin and botulinum A toxin inhibit release and uptake of various transmitters, as studied with particulate preparations from rat brain and spinal cord. *Naunyn. Schmiedebergs. Arch. Pharmacol.* **1981**, *316*, 244–251. [CrossRef] [PubMed]
98. Bozzi, Y.; Costantin, L.; Antonucci, F.; Caleo, M. Action of botulinum neurotoxins in the central nervous system: Antiepileptic effects. *Neurotox. Res.* **2006**, *9*, 197–203. [CrossRef] [PubMed]
99. Dunn, A.R.; Stout, K.A.; Ozawa, M.; Lohr, K.M.; Hoffman, C.A.; Bernstein, A.I.; Li, Y.; Wang, M.; Sgobio, C.; Sastry, N.; et al. Synaptic vesicle glycoprotein 2C (SV2C) modulates dopamine release and is disrupted in Parkinson disease. *Proc. Natl. Acad. Sci. USA* **2017**, *114*, E2253–E2262. [CrossRef] [PubMed]
100. Mahrhold, S.; Rummel, A.; Bigalke, H.; Davletov, B.; Binz, T. The synaptic vesicle protein 2C mediates the uptake of botulinum neurotoxin A into phrenic nerves. *FEBS Lett.* **2006**, *580*, 2011–2014. [CrossRef] [PubMed]
101. Pearce, L.B.; First, E.R.; MacCallum, R.D.; Gupta, A. Pharmacologic characterization of botulinum toxin for basic science and medicine. *Toxicon* **1997**, *35*, 1373–1412. [CrossRef]
102. Mann, T.; Zilles, K.; Klawitter, F.; Cremer, M.; Hawlitschka, A.; Palomero-Gallagher, N.; Schmitt, O.; Wree, A. Acetylcholine neurotransmitter receptor densities in the striatum of hemiparkinsonian rats following Botulinum neurotoxin-A injection. *Front. Neuroanat.* **2018**, in press.
103. Mann, T.; Zilles, K.; Frederike, V.; Höhmann, K.; Hellfritsch, A.; Van Bonn, S.; Cremer, M.; Schmitt, O.; Hawlitschka, A.; Wree, A. Glutamate, GABA and adenosine neurotransmitter receptor densities in the striatum of hemiparkinsonian rats following Botulinum neurotoxin-A injection. 2018; in press.
104. Oh, S.W.; Harris, J.A.; Ng, L.; Winslow, B.; Cain, N.; Mihalas, S.; Wang, Q.; Lau, C.; Kuan, L.; Henry, A.M.; et al. A mesoscale connectome of the mouse brain. *Nature* **2014**, *508*, 207–214. [CrossRef] [PubMed]
105. Gerfen, C.R. Basal Ganglia. In *The Rat Nervous System*; Toga, A.W., Ed.; Elsevier Academic: Amsterdam, The Netherlands, 1994; pp. 217–227. ISBN 9780123970251.
106. Klockgether, T. Medikamentöse behandlung der idiopathischen Parkinson-krankheit. *Nervenarzt* **2003**, *74*, S12–S21. [CrossRef] [PubMed]
107. Horstink, M.; Tolosa, E.; Bonuccelli, U.; Deuschl, G.; Friedman, A.; Kanovsky, P.; Larsen, J.P.; Lees, A.; Oertel, W.; Poewe, W.; et al. Review of the therapeutic management of Parkinson's disease. Report of a joint task force of the European Federation of Neurological Societies and the Movement Disorder Society-European Section. Part I: Early (uncomplicated) Parkinson's disease. *Eur. J. Neurol.* **2006**, *13*, 1170–1185. [CrossRef] [PubMed]
108. Whitney, C.M. Medications for Parkinson's disease. *Neurologist* **2007**, *13*, 387–388. [CrossRef] [PubMed]
109. Orsini, M.; Leite, M.A.A.; Chung, T.M.; Bocca, W.; de Souza, J.A.; de Souza, O.G.; Moreira, R.P.; Bastos, V.H.; Teixeira, S.; Oliveira, A.B.; et al. Botulinum neurotoxin type A in neurology: Update. *Neurol. Int.* **2015**, *7*, 79–84. [CrossRef] [PubMed]
110. Chen, S. Clinical uses of botulinum neurotoxins: Current indications, limitations and future developments. *Toxins* **2012**, *4*, 913–939. [CrossRef] [PubMed]
111. Jankovic, J. An update on new and unique uses of botulinum toxin in movement disorders. *Toxicon* **2017**, *147*, 84–88. [CrossRef] [PubMed]
112. Jankovic, J. Botulinum toxin: State of the art. *Mov. Disord.* **2017**, *32*, 1131–1138. [CrossRef] [PubMed]

113. Bezard, E.; Yue, Z.; Kirik, D.; Spillantini, M.G. Animal models of Parkinson's disease: Limits and relevance to neuroprotection studies. *Mov. Disord.* **2013**, *28*, 61–70. [CrossRef] [PubMed]
114. Deng, H.; Yuan, L. Genetic variants and animal models in SNCA and Parkinson disease. *Ageing Res. Rev.* **2014**, *15*, 161–176. [CrossRef] [PubMed]
115. Pickrell, A.M.; Pinto, M.; Moraes, C.T. Mouse models of Parkinson's disease associated with mitochondrial dysfunction. *Mol. Cell. Neurosci.* **2013**, *55*, 87–94. [CrossRef] [PubMed]
116. Gasior, M.; Tang, R.; Rogawski, M.A. Long-lasting attenuation of amygdala-kindled seizures after convection-enhanced delivery of botulinum neurotoxins a and B into the amygdala in rats. *J. Pharmacol. Exp. Ther.* **2013**, *346*, 528–534. [CrossRef] [PubMed]
117. Antonucci, F.; Bozzi, Y.; Caleo, M. Intrahippocampal infusion of botulinum neurotoxin E (BoNT/E) reduces spontaneous recurrent seizures in a mouse model of mesial temporal lobe epilepsy. *Epilepsia* **2009**, *50*, 963–966. [CrossRef] [PubMed]
118. Paxinos, G.; Franklin, K.B.J. *The Mouse Brain in Stereotaxic Coordinates*; Academic Press: Amsterdam, The Netherlands, 2001; ISBN 0125476361.
119. Paxinos, G.; Watson, C. *The Rat Brain in Stereotaxic Coordinates*, 5th ed.; Elsevier Academic Press: Amsterdam, The Netherlands; London, UK, 2005; ISBN 0120885727.
120. Pirazzini, M.; Rossetto, O.; Eleopra, R.; Montecucco, C. Botulinum Neurotoxins: Biology, Pharmacology, and Toxicology. *Pharmacol. Rev.* **2017**, *69*, 200–235. [CrossRef] [PubMed]
121. Frevert, J. Content of botulinum neurotoxin in botox®vistabel®, dysport®azzalure®, and xeomin®bocouture. *Drugs R D* **2010**, *10*, 67–73. [CrossRef] [PubMed]
122. Scaglione, F. Conversion ratio between botox®, dysport®, and xeomin® in clinical practice. *Toxins* **2016**, *8*, 65. [CrossRef] [PubMed]
123. Bensadoun, J.C.; Deglon, N.; Tseng, J.L.; Ridet, J.L.; Zurn, A.D.; Aebischer, P. Lentiviral vectors as a gene delivery system in the mouse midbrain: Cellular and behavioral improvements in a 6-OHDA model of Parkinson's disease using GDNF. *Exp. Neurol.* **2000**, *164*, 15–24. [CrossRef] [PubMed]
124. Iancu, R.; Mohapel, P.; Brundin, P.; Paul, G. Behavioral characterization of a unilateral 6-OHDA-lesion model of Parkinson's disease in mice. *Behav. Brain Res.* **2005**, *162*, 1–10. [CrossRef] [PubMed]
125. Da Conceição, F.S.L.; Ngo-Abdalla, S.; Houzel, J.-C.; Rehen, S.K. Murine model for Parkinson's disease: From 6-OH dopamine lesion to behavioral test. *J. Vis. Exp.* **2010**, *35*, 9–11. [CrossRef] [PubMed]
126. Brundin, P.; Isacson, O.; Gage, F.H.; Prochiantz, A.; Björklund, A. The rotating 6-hydroxydopamine-lesioned mouse as a model for assessing functional effects of neuronal grafting. *Brain Res.* **1986**, *366*, 346–349. [CrossRef]
127. Fu, A.; Zhou, Q.H.; Hui, E.K.W.; Lu, J.Z.; Boado, R.J.; Pardridge, W.M. Intravenous treatment of experimental Parkinson's disease in the mouse with an IgG-GDNF fusion protein that penetrates the blood-brain barrier. *Brain Res.* **2010**, *1352*, 208–213. [CrossRef] [PubMed]
128. Ungerstedt, U.; Arbuthnott, G.W. Quantitative recording of rotational behavior in rats after 6-hydroxy-dopamine lesions of the nigrostriatal dopamine system. *Brain Res.* **1970**, *24*, 485–493. [CrossRef]
129. Schallert, T.; Tillerson, J.L. Intervention Strategies for Degeneration of Dopamine Neurons in Parkinsonism: Optimizing Behavioral Assessment of Outcome. In *Central Nervous System Diseases*; Emerich, D.F., Dean, R.L., Sanberg, P.R., Eds.; Humana Press: Totowa, NJ, USA, 2000; pp. 131–151, ISBN 978-1-59259-691-1.
130. Schackel, S.; Pauly, M.-C.; Piroth, T.; Nikkhah, G.; Döbrössy, M.D. Donor age dependent graft development and recovery in a rat model of Huntington's disease: Histological and behavioral analysis. *Behav. Brain Res.* **2013**, *256*, 56–63. [CrossRef] [PubMed]
131. Chou, A.H.; Chen, C.Y.; Chen, S.Y.; Chen, W.J.; Chen, Y.L.; Weng, Y.S.; Wang, H.L. Polyglutamine-expanded ataxin-7 causes cerebellar dysfunction by inducing transcriptional dysregulation. *Neurochem. Int.* **2010**, *56*, 329–339. [CrossRef] [PubMed]
132. Zilles, K.; Qü, M.S.; Schröder, H.; Schleicher, A. Neurotransmitter receptors and cortical architecture. *J. Hirnforsch.* **1991**, *32*, 343–356. [PubMed]
133. Zilles, K.; Werner, L.; Qü, M.; Schleicher, A.; Gross, G. Quantitative auto radiography of 11 different transmitter binding sites in the basal forebrain region of the rat-evidence of heterogeneity in distribution patterns. *Neuroscience* **1991**, *42*, 473–481. [CrossRef]

134. Zilles, K.; Gross, G.; Schleicher, A.; Schildgen, S.; Bauer, A.; Bahro, M.; Schwendemann, G.; Zech, K.; Kolassa, N. Regional and laminar distributions of alpha 1-adrenoceptors and their subtypes in human and rat hippocampus. *Neuroscience* **1991**, *40*, 307–320. [CrossRef]
135. Zilles, K.; Palomero-Gallagher, N.; Grefkes, C.; Scheperjans, F.; Boy, C.; Amunts, K.; Schleicher, A. Architectonics of the human cerebral cortex and transmitter receptor fingerprints: Reconciling functional neuroanatomy and neurochemistry. *Eur. Neuropsychopharmacol.* **2002**, *12*, 587–599. [CrossRef]
136. Zilles, K.; Schleicher, A.; Palomero-Gallagher, N.; Amunts, K. Quantitative Analysis of Cyto- and Receptor Architecture of the Human Brain. In *Brain Mapping: The Methods*; Toga, A.W., Mazziotta, J.C., Eds.; Elsevier Academic Press: London, UK, 2002; Volume 58, pp. 573–602, ISBN 9780126930191. 0385-5600 (Print) 0385-5600 (Linking).

toxins MDPI

Communication

Detection of *Clostridium tetani* Neurotoxins Inhibited In Vivo by Botulinum Antitoxin B: Potential for Misleading Mouse Test Results in Food Controls

Luca Bano [1,*], Elena Tonon [1], Ilenia Drigo [1], Marco Pirazzini [2], Angela Guolo [1], Giovanni Farina [1], Fabrizio Agnoletti [1] and Cesare Montecucco [2]

1 Istituto Zooprofilattico Sperimentale delle Venezie, 35020 Legnaro, Italy; etonon@izsvenezie.it (E.T.); idrigo@izsvenezie.it (I.D.); aguolo@izsvenezie.it (A.G.); gfarina@izsvenezie.it (G.F.); fagnoletti@izsvenezie.it (F.A.)

2 Department of Biomedical Sciences, University of Padova, 35131 Padua, Italy; marco.pirazzini@unipd.it (M.P.); cesare.montecucco@unipd.it (C.M.)

* Correspondence: lbano@izsvenezie.it; Tel.: +39-0422-302-302

Received: 14 May 2018; Accepted: 13 June 2018; Published: 19 June 2018

Abstract: The presence of botulinum neurotoxin-producing Clostridia (BPC) in food sources is a public health concern. In favorable environmental conditions, BPC can produce botulinum neurotoxins (BoNTs) outside or inside the vertebrate host, leading to intoxications or toxico-infectious forms of botulism, respectively. BPC in food are almost invariably detected either by PCR protocols targeted at the known neurotoxin-encoding genes, or by the mouse test to assay for the presence of BoNTs in the supernatants of enrichment broths inoculated with the tested food sample. The sample is considered positive for BPC when the supernatant contains toxic substances that are lethal to mice, heat-labile and neutralized in vivo by appropriate polyclonal antibodies raised against purified BoNTs of different serotypes. Here, we report the detection in a food sample of a *Clostridium tetani* strain that produces tetanus neurotoxins (TeNTs) with the above-mentioned characteristics: lethal for mice, heat-labile and neutralized by botulinum antitoxin type B. Notably, neutralization occurred with two different commercially available type B antitoxins, but not with type A, C, D, E and F antitoxins. Although TeNT and BoNT fold very similarly, evidence that antitoxin B antiserum can neutralize the neurotoxic effect of TeNT in vivo has not been documented before. The presence of *C. tetani* strains in food can produce misleading results in BPC detection using the mouse test.

Keywords: mouse test; *Clostridium tetani*; botulinum antitoxin; food safety

Key Contribution: *Clostridium tetani* may contaminate foodstuffs and it can interfere with the detection of botulinum neurotoxin-producing Clostridia by the mouse bioassay, considered the gold standard for detecting botulinum neurotoxins in culture supernatants.

1. Introduction

Botulism is a neuroparalytic illness caused by the action of heat-labile botulinum neurotoxins (BoNT) produced by Gram-positive, spore-forming, anaerobe microorganisms belonging to the genus *Clostridium*. Seven confirmed BoNT serotypes (types A–G) have been recognized, characterized by the continuous isolation of intratypic variants known as subtypes and indicated with an Arabic number (BoNT/A1, BoNT/A2, BoNT/B1, BoNT/B2, etc.) [1,2]. A potential eighth type ("type H") was reported in 2013 and a new toxin, displaying the lowest degree of similarities among BoNTs, dubbed BoNT/X, has been recently described [3,4].

Botulism is characterized by the flaccid paralysis of cranial and skeletal muscles, possibly leading to death by respiratory failure [5]. The disease may occur following the intake of BoNTs preformed outside (intoxication) or produced inside the host (toxico-infection). The most frequent form of BoNT intoxication in humans is food-borne botulism due to consumption of food where BoNT-producing Clostridia (BPC) have found adequate conditions for spore germination and neurotoxin production [6]. This requires rigorous testing in food preparations considered at risk of botulism, to search for preformed BoNTs or BPC. BPC in food can be conveniently detected by PCR, with protocols targeted at BoNT-encoding genes, or through the mouse test, which can detect BoNTs in the supernatant of suitable enrichment media inoculated with the tested food sample [7]. A food sample is considered positive for BPC through the mouse test when the supernatant contains toxic substances that are lethal to mice, is heat-labile and neutralized in vivo by appropriate polyclonal antibodies raised against purified BoNTs of different serotypes [8]. When clinical signs consistent with botulism are displayed despite the use of specific antitoxins, the sample requires further investigation as botulism could be due to unknown BoNT serotypes.

A strict relative of BoNTs is tetanus neurotoxin (TeNT), produced by *Clostridium tetani*. TeNT is responsible for tetanus which is characterized by a spastic paralysis [9]. TeNT and BoNTs are very similar protein toxins, both in terms of structure and cellular mechanism of action [10,11], yet they display little homology in terms of amino acid composition. Such variability accounts for their different antigenicity.

Here we report the relevant observation that a TeNT produced by a *C. tetani* strain present in a food sample is neutralized by antisera raised against BoNT/B. The implications of this finding in the detection of BPC from food samples are discussed.

2. Results

The mouse test revealed the presence of a heat-labile neurotoxin neutralized by the trivalent A, B, E antitoxin and by two type-B monovalent antitoxins. Mice died between 10 and 24 h and the clinical signs were not observed; however, see below.

The PCR tests to detect BoNT genes (A to F) were negative.

Bacteriological examination revealed the presence of lipase-positive and lipase-negative anaerobic colonies in EYA (Figure 1) and uniform, weakly haemolytic, rhizoid and swarming colonies in BAB2. Both lipase-positive and lipase-negative colonies were lecithinase-negative. These two types of colonies were sub-cultured on EYA and, 24 h later, the two subcultures appeared to be morphologically identical and lipase-negative. Forty-eight hours later, lipase-positive colonies appeared in both subcultures. One week later, all the colonies that appeared were lipase-positive (Figure 1).

All the isolates were identified as *Clostridium tetani* by MALDI TOF MS with scores equal or higher than 2.489. The first best match of the strain was with the spectrum of the *C. tetani* reference strain DSM 11745 included in the default-database (Figure 2). This *C. tetani* strain was dubbed TV1277. We concluded that, for unknown reasons, there was an initial difference (dimorphism) in the appearance of the colonies cultured in EYA due to the lipase-reaction.

The mouse test was subsequently repeated with the supernatant obtained from TPGY containing a 4-day-old pure culture of the TV1277 strain. The results were the same as the ones described for the TPGY inoculated with the polenta sample but sternal recumbency, general paralysis and dyspnea were observed at 12 h post inoculation. No specific clinical signs referable to tetanus were noted. Postmortem examination revealed pulmonary lesions compatible with respiratory failure.

The neurotoxic effect of the tetanus neurotoxin (TeNT) produced by the pure culture of the *C. tetani* strain TV1277 was neutralized by 100 and 1000 UI/mL antitoxin type B (NIBSC), but not by 10 UI/mL. All the experiments in animals are summarized in Table 1.

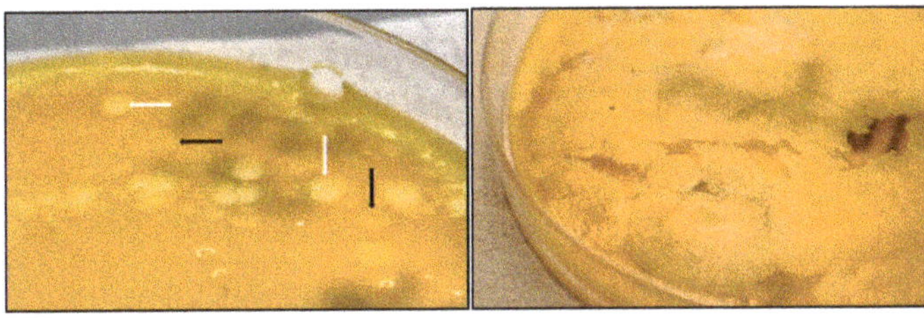

(**a**) (**b**)

Figure 1. Macroscopic aspect of *Clostridium tetani* strain TV1277. (**a**) Lipase-positive (white arrows) and lipase-negative (black arrows) colonies in a 48 h-old pure culture (dimorphism). (**b**) After one week of incubation all colonies appear lipase-positive.

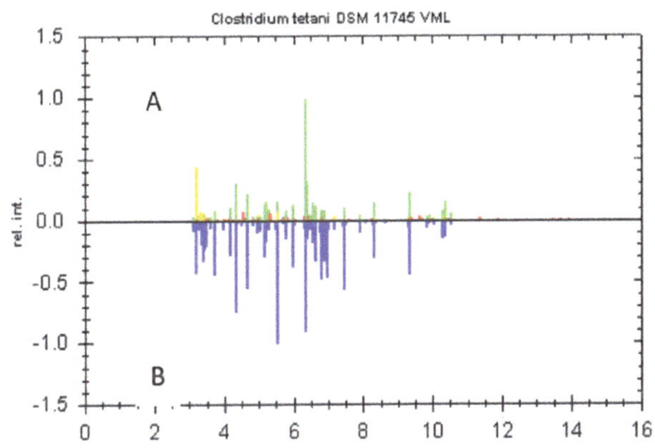

Figure 2. The peak list of the strain TV1277 spectrum is displayed in the upper half of the graphic. The color of the peaks reflects the degree of matching with the reference MSP (green = full match, yellow = partial match, red = no match). The lower half of the graphic displays the peak list of the reference MSP (*C. tetani* DSM 11745) in blue using an inverted intensity scale.

Table 1. Experiments in animals with filtrated supernatant of a 4-day-old culture of *C. tetani* TV1277. For each experiment, two mice were injected intraperitoneally.

Antitoxin	Producer	Antitoxin Titre	Number of Dead Mice at 24, 48 and 72 h Post Inoculation		
			24 h	**48 h**	**72 h**
Botulinum trivalent antitoxin A, B, E	CDC	>10 UI/mL	0	0	0
Botulinum antitoxin A	CDC	>10 UI/mL	2	-	-
Botulinum antitoxin B	CDC	>10 UI/mL	0	0	0
Botulinum antitoxin C	CDC	>10 UI/mL	2	-	-
Botulinum antitoxin D	CDC	>10 UI/mL	2	-	-
Botulinum antitoxin E	CDC	≥10 UI/mL	2	-	-
Botulinum antitoxin F	CDC	≥10 UI/mL	2	-	-
Botulinum antitoxin B	NIBSC	10 UI/mL	1	1	-
Botulinum antitoxin B	NIBSC	100 UI/mL	0	0	0
Botulinum antitoxin B	NIBSC	1000 UI/mL	0	0	0
Tetanus antitoxin	NIBSC	10 UI/mL	0	0	0
Further samples tested					
Untreated supernatant	-	-	2	-	-
Heat treated supernatant	-	-	0	0	0

The ELISA showed that both trivalent (A, B, E) and monovalent (B) antitoxins reacted with TeNTs produced by the *C. tetani* reference strain (ATCC 10779) (Figure 3). Notably, trivalent antitoxin cross-reacts with TeNT to a similar extent with respect to BoNT/A1 and BoNT/B1. Monovalent antitoxin displays higher affinity for BoNT/B and sizeable cross activity with TeNT, that is practically equal with high toxin amount. A minimal cross reactivity with BoNT/A is also present.

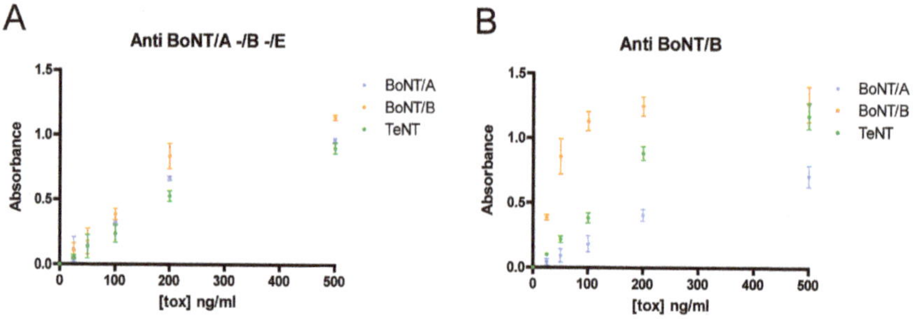

Figure 3. Cross reactivity of trivalent (**A**) and monovalent (**B**) BoNT-antitoxin with TeNT. Indicated concentrations of BoNT/A1 (cyan), BoNT/B1 (orange) and TeNT (green) were immobilized onto 96-well. Trivalent botulinum antitoxin (types A, B, E) from CDC (**A**) or monovalent antitoxin type B from the National Institute for Biological Standards and Control (NIBSC code: 60/001) (**B**) were used to assay immunoreactivity by indirect ELISA. Values reported were normalized subtracting background absorbance and are expressed as mean values of triplicates.

3. Discussion

The present report describes the isolation of a *C. tetani* strain (TV1277) producing a neurotoxin that is neutralized by two different commercially available type B botulinum antitoxins in the mouse test.

Although *C. tetani* is not considered a food-borne pathogen, it can be present in foodstuff and interfere with the detection of BPC by the mouse test, considered the gold standard for BoNT detection from culture supernatants, giving rise to misleading results.

The protocols for performing the mouse test specify that death without clinical signs is not adequate evidence that botulinum toxin was present in the injected material [12]. The mice should be observed for 4 days but death preceded by neurological signs can occur in the absence of animal facility personnel, as initially happened to us. Furthermore, clinical signs of tetanus and botulism can be indistinguishable in mice when a large amount of TeNT has been injected [13,14]. It is therefore advisable to perform the mouse assay with progressive dilutions of the sample until a concentration where the progression of the symptoms is obvious, but this may raise ethical issues.

We do not know if CDC antitoxins are produced in animals that are regularly vaccinated against tetanus neurotoxin (TeNT). However, NIBSC antitoxin B is produced in horses reported to be unvaccinated for tetanus [15]. Moreover, any interference from tetanus vaccine antibodies should be observed with all types of antitoxin tested, not just antitoxin type B.

One explanation for this "off-target" neutralization of the TeNT effect with botulinum type B antitoxin might be the existence of common epitopes between these two neurotoxins. This possibility is reinforced by some findings reporting that TeNT shares common antigenic sites with BoNTs types B, C, D and E, recognized by specific monoclonal antibodies [16]. However, in the present study, only monovalent type B antitoxin showed an in vivo neutralizing capability towards the TeNT produced by strain TV1277. Furthermore, BoNTs and TeNT exhibit a very similar folding of the three domains composing their structure, making it very likely that some sequential and conformational epitopes of BoNT/B may be present in TeNT [2]. This conclusion is further supported by the close overlapping of the alpha-carbon chain folding of BoNT/B (in red) and that of TeNT (in blue) showed in Figure 4 [11]. Panel 2A shows the similar three-domain structure of the two toxins with the different spatial position of their binding domains HC with respect to domains L and HN. Panel 2B shows that when the single HC and L-HN domains of TeNT (blue trace) and BoNT/B (red trace) are overlapped a substantial similarity is found. Clearly, as antigenic sites are determined also by the lateral amino acid chains, this superimposition should be analyzed further. However, the overall similar folding speaks in favor of the possibility that common antigenic determinants, playing a major role in the neuronal paralysis induced by these potent neurotoxins, do exist.

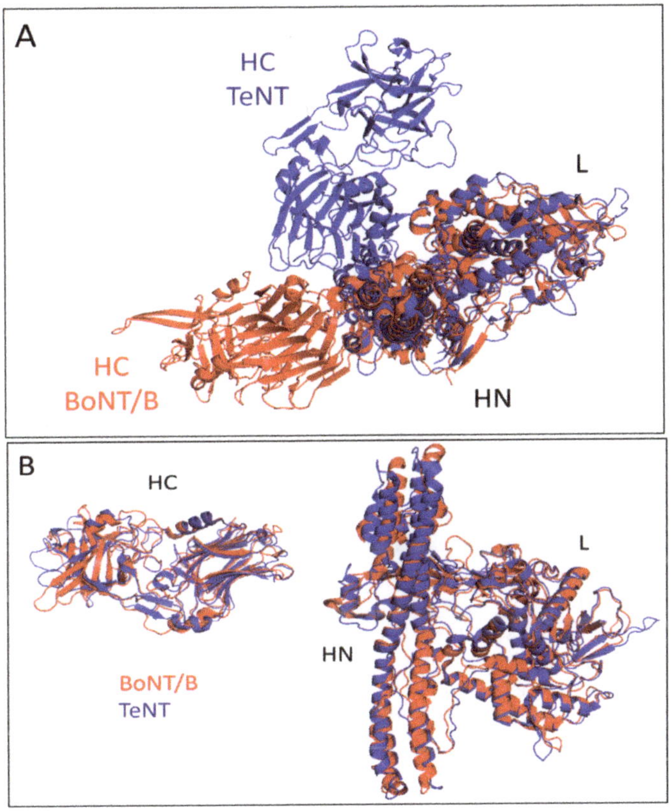

Figure 4. Spatial folding of tetanus (blue) and botulinum B (red) neurotoxins. (**A**) Notice the different position of the HC domain with respect to the other two domains (HN and L) in the two neurotoxins. (**B**) Overlapping of the two HC domain (**left**) and of the L-HN domains (**right**) of the two neurotoxins. The almost complete overlapping of the folding of the alpha-carbon chains of the two toxins supports the possibility of the existence of common antigenic determinants in the two toxins.

Despite the above common characteristics, a cross-neutralization effect of TeNT in vivo due to botulinum antitoxin type B has never, to the best of our knowledge, been reported before.

In future studies we will investigate whether this "in vivo" neutralizing effect of botulinum antitoxin B is observed only for the TeNT produced by strain TV1277 or if it is a common characteristic of TeNTs produced by different strains. The results of the ELISA test obtained with the TeNT produced by the Harvard E88 strain support the second hypothesis. In addition, the amino acid sequence of TV1277 TeNT revealed only 17 mutations out of 1315 amino acids of the reference TeNT produced by the Harvard E88 strain (data not shown).

Curiously, the lipase-positive reaction of strain TV1277 contrasts with the published biochemical properties of *C. tetani* [17], but is characteristic of *C. botulinum* groups I, II and III [18]. We subsequently repeated isolation of lipase-different colonies three times and, after one week, all the subcultures showed a uniform, lipase-positive reaction.

PCR proved to be a reliable tool that should replace the mouse test for BPC detection, partly for ethical considerations. However, this method is instead inadequate for detecting unknown BoNT-encoding genes.

The presence of TeNTs that react with botulinum antitoxin might also interfere with immune-enzymatic methods for detecting BoNTs in culture supernatants. Accordingly, these kits should additionally be validated for specificity towards such TeNTs.

Humans are not usually vaccinated against BoNT type B but citizens in many countries are regularly vaccinated for tetanus. It might be interesting to investigate whether the human vaccine for type B botulism also protects from certain isoforms of TeNTs. It is possible that people vaccinated for type B botulism could be simultaneously protected against tetanus.

In conclusion, our results demonstrate that *C. tetani* may present in foodstuffs and can interfere with the detection of BPC by the mouse bioassay, considered the gold standard for detecting BoNT in culture supernatants.

4. Materials and Methods

4.1. Detection of Botulinum Neurotoxin-Producing Clostridia by the Mouse Bioassay

In December 2016, a food producer located in the province of Trento prepared a batch of vacuum-packed polenta, a maize porridge preparation typical of the North of Italy. The polenta was vacuum-packed in glass jars and one aliquot of the stock was sent to the laboratory for the routine microbiology testing that precedes consumption of the product.

The sample was screened for the presence of BPC through the mouse bioassay (or mouse test) as previously described [8,12]. Briefly, 25 g of the sample were introduced into 225 mL of trypticase peptone-glucose yeast extract (TPGY), heated to 80 °C for 10 min and incubated at 30 °C for 4 days [19]. The supernatant was collected, centrifuged at 8000× *g* and filtered with a 0.45 µm filter (Millipore, Tullagreen, Ireland). Two mice were intraperitoneally injected with 0.4 mL of the untreated supernatant and two with 0.5 mL of the supernatant previously heated to 100 °C for 10 min. Next, 0.25 mL of the trivalent botulinum antitoxin (types A, B, E) supplied by the Center for Disease Control (CDC) was mixed with 1 mL of supernatant and, after 45 min, 0.5 mL were intraperitoneally injected into two mice. This step was then repeated with monovalent CDC antitoxins types A, B, C, D, E, F and titrated monovalent antitoxin type B supplied by the National Institute for Biological Standards and Control (NIBSC, code: 60/001). Mice were injected at 9.00 a.m. and observed at 4, 6, 8, 10 and 24 h post inoculation. The surviving mice were monitored for a further 48 h.

The mouse test was then repeated with the supernatant obtained from TPGY containing a 4-day-old pure neurotoxic culture isolated as reported in paragraph 2.3. The NIBSC antitoxin was used in this supernatant at 10, 100 and 1000 UI/mL to determine the neutralization titer after inoculation of two mice for each dilution. A volume of 0.25 mL of tetanus antitoxin (NIBSC, 60/113) containing 10 UI/mL, was mixed with 1 mL of the filtered supernatant of a 4-day-old neurotoxic culture. Forty-five minutes later, 0.5 mL were inoculated intraperitoneally in two mice.

Dead mice underwent postmortem examination.

4.2. PCR Protocols for Detecting and Characterizing BoNT-Encoding Genes

After 48 h of incubation, 175 µL of the inoculated TPGY broth were collected from the bottom of the tube and DNA was automatically extracted (Microlab Starlet, Hamilton, Bonaduz, Switzerland) using the MagMax Total Nucleic Acid Isolation kit (Ambion/Life Technologies, Carsland, CA, USA).

Real-time PCR and PCR methods for *C. botulinum* neurotoxin genes types A to F were applied in accordance with previously published protocols [20,21].

4.3. Bacteriological Examination

Fifty microliters of TPGY were plated on egg yolk agar (EYA) produced as previously described [22] and incubated for 48 h at 37 °C in an anaerobic cabinet (Shel Lab, Cornelius, OR, USA) with an atmosphere composed of 5% hydrogen, 5% carbon dioxide and 90% nitrogen. Single colonies with different macroscopic morphology and/or different lipase/lecithinase reactions, were collected and streaked on 2 different plates of Blood Agar Base No.2 (BAB2) (Oxoid, Hampshire, UK) and 2 plates of EYA. One plate for each medium was incubated in aerobic and one in anaerobic conditions at 37 °C for 48 h. Colonies growing only in anaerobic conditions were then identified by MALDI TOF MS (Biotyper Microflex LT, Bruker Daltonics, Bremen, Germany), using the MALDI Biotyper software package (version 3.0, Bruker Daltonics, Bremen, Germany) and an "in house" database created with *C. botulinum* reference and field strains [23]. As specified by the manufacturer, a score value of <1.7 indicated that identification was unreliable; scores between 1.7 and 2.0 that identification was reliable at the genus level; scores between 2.0 and 2.3 that it was reliable at the genus level and probable at the species level; scores higher than 2.3 indicated highly probable species identification.

4.4. ELISA Assay

Ninety six-well polystyrene plates (Sarstedt, Nümbrecht, Germany) were coated with 100 µL of BoNT/A1, BoNT/B1 or TeNT (E88 strain) solutions at the concentrations: 25, 50, 100, 150 and 500 ng/mL diluted with PBS and incubated overnight at 4 °C [24]. Toxins were purified as described previously [23]. Thereafter, wells were treated with 2% BSA for 1 h, washed with PBS 0.05% Tween 20 (PBST) and incubated for 2 h at room temperature with indicated antitoxins (CDC) diluted 1:200 in PBST supplemented with 0.1% BSA (Sigma Aldrich, St. Louis, MI, USA). Samples were then extensively washed with PBST and incubated 1 h with HRP-conjugated secondary antibody. After washing, 100 µL of 2,2′-Azino-bis(3-ethylbenzothiazoline-6-sulfonic acid) (ABTS) was added and absorbance read at 405 nm with a microplate reader. Values reported were normalized for the absorbance of the wells coated without toxins.

4.5. Experiments on Animals

The mouse test was conducted in accordance with Italian and European legislation on ethical standards (European Communities Council Directive [2010/63/EU] on the protection of animals used for scientific purposes).

The mouse test was approved by the Ethics Committee of the Istituto Zooprofilattico Sperimentale delle Venezie (opinion No. 24/2014) and officially authorized by the Italian Ministry of Health (authorization No. 239/2015-PR) on 9 April 2015.

Author Contributions: L.B. and C.M. conceived and designed the experiments and wrote the manuscript; E.T., I.D. and A.G. performed the mouse test and the biomolecular tests; M.P. performed the ELISA and analyzed the superimposition of the neurotoxins; G.F. contributed the diagnostic samples and the case history; F.A. analyzed the data and supervised the experiments in animals.

Funding: This research received no external funding.

Acknowledgments: This research did not receive any specific grant from funding agencies in the public, commercial, or not-for-profit sectors.

Conflicts of Interest: The authors declare no conflict of interest.

References

1. Peck, M.W.; Smith, T.J.; Anniballi, F.; Austin, J.W.; Bano, L.; Bradshaw, M.; Cuervo, P.; Cheng, L.W.; Derman, Y.; Dorner, B.G.; et al. Historical Perspectives and Guidelines for Botulinum Neurotoxin Subtype Nomenclature. *Toxins* **2017**, *9*, 38. [CrossRef] [PubMed]
2. Rossetto, O.; Pirazzini, M.; Montecucco, C. Botulinum Neurotoxins: Genetic, Structural and Mechanistic Insights. *Nat. Rev. Microbiol.* **2014**, *12*, 535–549. [CrossRef] [PubMed]
3. Barash, J.R.; Arnon, S.S. A Novel Strain of *Clostridium Botulinum* that Produces Type B and Type H Botulinum Toxins. *J. Infect. Dis.* **2013**, *209*, 183–191. [CrossRef] [PubMed]
4. Zhang, S.; Masuyer, G.; Zhang, J.; Shen, Y.; Lundin, D.; Henriksson, L.; Miyashita, S.; Martínez-Carranza, M.; Dong, M.; Stenmark, P. Identification and Characterization of a Novel Botulinum Neurotoxin. *Nat. Commun.* **2017**, *8*, 14130. [CrossRef] [PubMed]
5. Johnson, E.A.; Montecucco, C. Botulism. In *Handbook of Clinical Neurology*; Goudin, D.S., Ed.; Elsevier: New York, NY, USA, 2008; pp. 333–368.
6. Peck, M.W. Biology and Genomic Analysis of Clostridium Botulinum. *Adv. Microb. Physiol.* **2009**, *55*, 183–320. [PubMed]
7. Lindstrom, M.; Korkeala, H. Laboratory Diagnostics of Botulism. *Clin. Microbiol. Rev.* **2006**, *19*, 298–314. [CrossRef] [PubMed]
8. AOAC International. AOAC International. AOAC Official Method 977.26 (sec 17.7.01) *Clostridium botulinum* and its toxins in food. In *Official Methods of Analysis*, 17th ed.; AOAC International: Gaithersburg, MD, USA, 2001.
9. Montecucco, C.; Schiavo, G. Structure and Function of Tetanus and Botulinum Neurotoxins. *Q. Rev. Biophys.* **1995**, *28*, 423–472. [CrossRef] [PubMed]
10. Eisel, U.; Jarausch, W.; Goretzki, K.; Henschen, A.; Engels, J.; Weller, U.; Hudel, M.; Habermann, E.; Niemann, H. Tetanus Toxin: Primary Structure, Expression in *E. Coli*, and Homology with Botulinum Toxins. *EMBO J.* **1986**, *5*, 2495–2502. [PubMed]
11. Masuyer, G.; Conrad, J.; Stenmark, P. The Structure of the Tetanus Toxin Reveals pH-Mediated Domain Dynamics. *EMBO Rep.* **2017**, *18*, 1306–1317. [CrossRef] [PubMed]
12. Centers for Disease Control and Prevention. Botulism in the United States, 1899–1996. Handbook for Epidemiolosts, Clinicians and Laboratory Workers. 1998. Available online: http://www.cdc.gov/ncidod/dbmd/diseaseinfo/files/botulism.pdf (accessed on 2 February 2018).
13. Matsuda, M.; Sugimoto, N.; Ozutsumi, K.; Hirai, T. Acute Botulinum-Like Intoxication by Tetanus Neurotoxin in Mice. *Biochem. Biophys. Res. Commun.* **1982**, *104*, 799–805. [CrossRef]
14. Konig, K.; Ringe, H.; Dorner, B.G.; Diers, A.; Uhlenberg, B.; Muller, D.; Varnholt, V.; Gaedicke, G. Atypical Tetanus in a Completely Immunized 14-Year-Old Boy. *Pediatrics* **2007**, *120*, e1355-8. [CrossRef] [PubMed]
15. Sesardic, T.; (National Institute for Biological Standards and Control, Hertfordshire, UK). Personal communication, 2017.
16. Tsuzuki, K.; Yokosawa, N.; Syuto, B.; Ohishi, I.; Fujii, N.; Kimura, K.; Oguma, K. Establishment of a Monoclonal Antibody Recognizing an Antigenic Site Common to Clostridium Botulinum Type B, C1, D, and E Toxins and Tetanus Toxin. *Infect. Immun.* **1988**, *56*, 898–902. [PubMed]
17. Jousimies-Somer, R.H.; Summanen, P.; Citron, D.M.; Baron, E.J.; Waxler, H.M.; Finegold, S.M. Advanced identification methods. In *Wadsworth-KTL Anaerobic Bacteriology Manual*, 6th ed.; Hoffman, S., Ed.; Star Publ.: Seoul, Korea, 2002; pp. 81–132, ISBN 978-0898632095.
18. Hatheway, C.L. Toxigenic Clostridia. *Clin. Microbiol. Rev.* **1990**, *3*, 66–98. [CrossRef] [PubMed]
19. Lilly, T., Jr.; Harmon, S.; Kautter, D.; Solomon, H.; Lynt, R., Jr. An Improved Medium for Detection of *Clostridium Botulinum* Type E. *J. Milk Food Technol.* **1971**, *34*, 492–497. [CrossRef]
20. De Medici, D.; Anniballi, F.; Wyatt, G.M.; Lindström, M.; Messelhäußer, U.; Aldus, C.F.; Delibato, E.; Korkeala, H.; Peck, M.W.; Fenicia, L. Multiplex PCR for Detection of Botulinum Neurotoxin-Producing Clostridia in Clinical, Food, and Environmental Samples. *Appl. Environ. Microbiol.* **2009**, *75*, 6457–6461. [CrossRef] [PubMed]
21. Woudstra, C.; Skarin, H.; Anniballi, F.; Fenicia, L.; Bano, L.; Drigo, I.; Koene, M.; Bäyon-Auboyer, M.; Buffereau, J.; De Medici, D. Neurotoxin Gene Profiling of *Clostridium Botulinum* Types C and D Native to Different Countries within Europe. *Appl. Environ. Microbiol.* **2012**, *78*, 3120–3127. [CrossRef] [PubMed]

22. Bano, L.; Drigo, I.; Tonon, E.; Berto, G.; Tavella, A.; Woudstra, C.; Capello, K.; Agnoletti, F. Evidence for a Natural Humoral Response in Dairy Cattle Affected by Persistent Botulism Sustained by Non-Chimeric Type C Strains. *Anaerobe* **2015**, *36*, 25–29. [CrossRef] [PubMed]
23. Bano, L.; Drigo, I.; Tonon, E.; Pascoletti, S.; Puiatti, C.; Anniballi, F.; Auricchio, B.; Lista, F.; Montecucco, C.; Agnoletti, F. Identification and Characterization of *Clostridium Botulinum* Group III Field Strains by Matrix-Assisted Laser Desorption-Ionization Time-of-Flight Mass Spectrometry (MALDI-TOF MS). *Anaerobe* **2017**, *48*, 126–134. [CrossRef] [PubMed]
24. Shone, C.; Tranter, H. Growth of clostridia and preparation of their neurotoxins. In *Clostridial Neurotoxins*; Springer: Berlin, Germany, 1995; pp. 143–160.

MDPI
St. Alban-Anlage 66
4052 Basel
Switzerland
Tel. +41 61 683 77 34
Fax +41 61 302 89 18
www.mdpi.com

Toxins Editorial Office
E-mail: toxins@mdpi.com
www.mdpi.com/journal/toxins

www.ingramcontent.com/pod-product-compliance
Lightning Source LLC
LaVergne TN
LVHW070236100526
838202LV00015B/2135
* 9 7 8 3 0 3 9 4 3 4 5 6 5 *